WONG'S SEVENTH EDITION

Clinical Manual of PEDIATRIC NURSING

David Wilson, MS, RNC
Staff, Children's Hospital Urgent Care Center
Saint Francis Hospital;
Faculty, Langston University School of Nursing
Tulsa, Oklahoma

Marilyn J. Hockenberry, PhD, RN-CS, PNP, FAAN
Director, Center for Research and Evidence-Based Practice
Nurse Scientist, Texas Children's Hospital;
Director of Nurse Practitioners, Texas Children's Cancer Center;
Professor, Department of Pediatrics, Baylor College of Medicine
Houston, Texas

With 280 illustrations

MOSBY

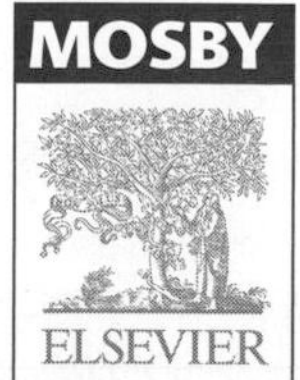

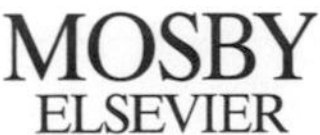

ELSEVIER

11830 Westline Industrial Drive
St. Louis, Missouri 63146

WONG'S CLINICAL MANUAL OF PEDIATRIC NURSING,
SEVENTH EDITION ISBN: 978-0-323-04713-5

Notice

Knowledge and best practice in this field are constantly changing. As new research and experience broaden our knowledge, changes in practice, treatment, and drug therapy may become necessary or appropriate. Readers are advised to check the most current information provided (i) on procedures featured or (ii) by the manufacturer of each product to be administered, to verify the recommended dose or formula, the method and duration of administration, and contraindications. It is the responsibility of the practitioner, relying on his or her own experience and knowledge of the patient, to make diagnoses, to determine dosages and the best treatment for each individual patient, and to take all appropriate safety precautions. To the fullest extent of the law, neither the Publisher nor the Authors assume any liability for any injury and/or damage to persons or property arising out of or related to any use of the material contained in this book.

The Publisher

Library of Congress Control Number: 2007934627

Acquisitions Editor: Catherine Jackson
Managing Editor: Michele D. Hayden
Developmental Editor: Amanda Sunderman Politte
Publishing Services Manager: Deborah L. Vogel
Senior Project Manager: Deon Lee
Book Designer: Maggie Reid

Printed in the United States of America

Last digit is the print number: 9 8 7 6 5 4 3 2 1

Contributors and Reviewers

CONTRIBUTING EDITORS

Patrick Barrera, BS
Assistant Director
Center for Research and Evidence-Based Practice
Texas Children's Hospital
Houston, Texas

Terri L. Brown, MSN, RN, CPN
Faculty, Evidence-Based Practice Specialist
Center for Research and Evidence Based Practice
Texas Children's Hospital
Houston, Texas

CONTRIBUTORS

Rosalind Bryant, MN, APRN, BC, PNP
Pediatric Nurse Practitioner
Texas Children's Cancer Center
Texas Children's Hospital;
Clinic Instructor, Department of Pediatrics
Baylor College of Medicine
Houston, Texas

Kathleen E. Carberry, RN, BSN
Research Nurse
Congenital Heart Surgery Service
Texas Children's Hospital
Houston, Texas

Janet DeJean, RN, CPON
Cancer Center and Hematology Service
Texas Children's Hospital
Houston, Texas

Joy Hesselgrave, RN, MSN, CPON
Clinical Specialist
Cancer Center and Hematology Service
Texas Children's Hospital
Houston, Texas

Brandi Horvath, BSN, RN, CPON
Cancer Center and Hematology Service
Texas Children's Hospital
Houston, Texas

Jessica A. Kouba, RN, BSN
Department of Pediatric Orthopaedics & Scoliosis
Texas Children's Hospital
Houston, Texas

Shannon Stone McCord, RN, MS, CPNP, CNS, WOCN, CCRN
Pediatric Nurse Practitioner
Wound, Ostomy, & Continence
Texas Children's Hospital
Houston, Texas

Kathleen M. McLane, MSN, RN, CPNP, CWCN, COCN
Pediatric Nurse Practitioner
Wound, Ostomy, & Continence
Texas Children's Hospital
Houston, Texas

Barbara A. Montagnino, MS, RN, CNS
Clinical Nurse Specialist—Progressive Care Unit
Texas Children's Hospital
Houston, Texas

Angela C. Morgan, MS, RN, CCRN
Clinical Nurse Specialist
Texas Children's Hospital
Houston, Texas

Shelly Nalbone, RN, MS, CPNP
Assistant Director
Texas Children's Hospital
Houston, Texas

Rebecca Owens, RN
Nurse Manager
Neurology/Neurosurgery
Texas Children's Hospital
Houston, Texas

Kerri L. Phelps, BSN, RN
Education Coordinator
Surgical/Orthopedic Unit
Texas Children's Hospital
Houston, Texas

Ivy Razmus, RN, MS
Nurse Manager, Newborn Nursery
Saint Francis Hospital
Tulsa, Oklahoma

Jennifer L. Sanders, RN, BSN
Nurse Manager, General Medicine/Transplant Unit
Texas Children's Hospital
Houston, Texas

Kelly D. Wallin, RN, MS
Assistant Director, Congenital Heart Surgery
Texas Children's Hospital
Houston, Texas

Carmen Watrin, RN, MSN
Clinical Specialist, Congenital Heart Surgery
Texas Children's Hospital
Houston, Texas

REVIEWERS

Melissa Parker, BS, CCLS
Child Life Coordinator
Saint John Medical Center
Tulsa, Oklahoma

Kerstin West-Wilson, RNC, MS, IBCLC
Lactation Consultant and Discharge Coordinator
Eastern Oklahoma Perinatal Center
Saint Francis Children's Hospital, Saint Francis Hospital
Tulsa, Oklahoma

Barbara Wheeler, RN, MN, IBCLC
Neonatal Clinical Nurse Specialist
Certified Lactation Consultant
St. Boniface General Hospital
Winnipeg, Manitoba
Canada

Preface

The seventh edition of ***Wong's Clinical Manual of Pediatric Nursing,*** like its previous editions, serves a unique function in the study and practice of pediatric nursing. This work benefits from the addition of several contributors whose expertise in pediatric nursing is reflected in this new edition. The manual is a practical guide for practicing nurses and students engaged in the care of children and their families—a compendious collection of clinical information, resources, and data packaged for convenient use and easy access. For the practicing nurse, the book is a ready resource of material that is otherwise available only in a wide array of journal articles, texts, federal publications, professional association recommendations, and brochures. Examples of current "cutting edge" information are recommendations from the American Academy of Pediatrics, Agency for Healthcare Research and Quality, American Pain Society, National Center for Health Statistics, and Centers for Disease Control and Prevention. For the student, it is an indispensable guide to the care of children and their families.

As an adjunct to clinical practice, the ***Manual*** assumes the thorough preparation and basic theoretical knowledge only a textbook can provide. Although it is not designed to accompany any particular textbook, it serves as a valuable addition to ***Wong's Nursing Care of Infants and Children*** and ***Wong's Essentials of Pediatric Nursing.*** The ***Manual*** contains twice as many care plans as these texts, and the outlined information and the Patient and Family Education guidelines provide easy methods of self-learning for students.

The ***Manual*** is authoritative and up to date. An **evidence-based practice** approach is used to present existing knowledge relevant to nursing care. Its content reflects the latest research and current clinical practice. The nursing care plans have been completely revised and include the current North American Nursing Diagnosis Association (NANDA), Nursing Interventions Classification (NIC), and Nursing Outcomes Classification (NOC) nomenclature. The Patient and Family Education guidelines reflect increasing family participation in the care of the child in the home setting; many of these have been translated into Spanish and are available on the Evolve website. Users will appreciate access to the latest information on childhood immunizations; end-of-life care interventions; asthma management; central line care; arterial blood gas interpretation; management of the patient requiring mechanical ventilation; neonatal and child pain assessment and management; new blood pressure guidelines based on age, height, and gender; and a comprehensive resource of standard laboratory values. This edition provides Evidence-Based Practice boxes, which provide the latest research information on issues such as appropriate needle length for intramuscular injections and reduction of minor procedural pain in infants. The Evidence-Based Practice features serve to further enhance the practicing nurse's role in the provision of quality pediatric patient care.

The ***Manual*** is designed to ensure that specific information can be located quickly and easily when it is needed. Color tabs printed on the cover facilitate quick access to each of the six units, which have coordinating black thumbtabs. In addition to a detailed table of contents in the front of the book, a unit outline with page references is included at the beginning of each unit. A list of related topics found elsewhere in the book is included in most units. Vital reference data appear inside the front and back covers, where they can be located at a moment's notice.

As in past editions, material designed to be distributed to families is clearly identified. Permission is given to photocopy this material and provide it to caregivers to ensure that they have access to accurate, current information; to improve the quality of care; and to facilitate the nurse's teaching responsibilities.

Greater attention is given to **critical thinking** by emphasizing essential nursing observations and interventions in **Safety Alert** boxes. These call the reader's attention to considerations which, if ignored, could lead to a deteriorating or emergency situation. Key assessment data, risk factors, and danger signs are among the kinds of information in this feature. The concept of **atraumatic care**—the provision of therapeutic care in settings by personnel and through the use of interventions that eliminate or minimize the psychologic and physical distress experienced by children and their families in the health care system—is incorporated throughout the text and highlighted as boxed material.

Unit 1 focuses on the **assessment of the child and family.** It includes history taking; assessment of present and past physical health; and a summary of developmental achievements, both general and age specific. New information to this unit includes the addition of a cultural assessment tool, a revised discussion of temperature measurement, and history taking regarding alternative therapies. The new CDC growth charts are included in this section, and the body mass index formula is provided.

Unit 2 emphasizes **health promotion** in the areas of preventive care, nutrition, immunization, safety and injury prevention, parental guidance, and play. The material on childhood immunizations and on current car restraint guidelines is completely revised to reflect current recommendations. Some of the material on nutrition, childhood injury prevention, and play may be photocopied and given to families.

Unit 3 outlines **basic nursing procedures** adapted for the child. This section has been revised and provides **Evidence-Based Practice** summaries on numerous nursing interventions. Unit 3 includes an extensive collection of skills and procedures including preparation for procedures, collection of specimens, administration of medicine, venous access devices, invasive and noninvasive oxygen monitoring, and cardiopulmonary resuscitation. New sections have been added on end-of-life care interventions, mechanical ventilation, arterial blood gas interpretation, blood product administration, and chest tube management.

Unit 4 is devoted to **health problems,** primarily those requiring hospitalization. More than 40 care plans are included.

Each nursing care plan consists of assessment guidelines specific to the condition, relevant nursing diagnoses, patient/family goals, interventions, and expected patient/family outcomes. The nursing diagnoses conform to the most recent nomenclature accepted by NANDA, and they are prioritized within the care plans. The nursing diagnoses include Defining Characteristics and Subjective and Objective Data, which assist the student in the validation of assumptions that lead to selected relevant nursing diagnoses. In addition, NOC and NIC nomenclature has been added to further standardize and validate nursing care. The revised nursing care plans have been written to provide the student with a general guideline for critical thinking to encourage further problem solving and meet the patient's individualized care needs. The student may use the care plans as a springboard for developing outcomes and interventions that are applicable to the individual pediatric patient. The Nursing Care Plan on pain can be used to meet The Joint Commission's current pain standards. The health problems were selected to avoid repetition while including a variety of pediatric disorders.

Unit 5 consists of a collection of instructions for those who provide care for a child in the ambulatory setting, outpatient clinic, and home setting. These detailed Patient and Family Education guidelines are designed to be copied and distributed to the parent or other care provider. The instructions are written in simple and clear language to accommodate users with a low reading level. They can be used for client teaching, for facilitating discharge planning, or for promoting continuity of care in the home or community. The Patient and Family Education guides may be further individualized to meet the patient's and family's needs. New additions include administering nebulized medications, drawing up and administering insulin, monitoring blood glucose levels, caring for the child in a cast, treating newborn jaundice, and preventing accidental poisoning. The latest American Heart Association recommendations for performing cardiopulmonary resuscitation on an infant or child and for caring for a choking infant or child are included.

Unit 6 includes basic resource information for interpretation of **laboratory data,** including values in International Units. The extensive list of **abbreviations** and **acronyms** used in health care settings has been expanded and updated.

Although the information in the ***Manual*** is carefully researched, references are included only when citations are required to appropriately credit the work. The reader is directed to the current editions of ***Wong's Nursing Care of Infants and Children*** and ***Wong's Essentials of Pediatric Nursing*** for additional references and discussion of material, especially for growth and development, interviewing, and health problems.

Every effort has been made to ensure that the information is accurate and up to date at the time of publication. However, as new research and experience broaden our practice, standards of care change accordingly. Therefore, the reader may find some differences in local and regional practices.

A number of people have contributed time and expertise to this edition. We are grateful to Patrick Barrera and Terri Brown, whose contributions to the Wong nursing textbooks greatly benefit the ***Clinical Manual.*** Numerous reviewers and contributors have provided invaluable expertise for updating the material in this ***Manual.*** These outstanding experts have helped us achieve our goal of presenting data that are both current and accurate. And finally, we are so fortunate to have an outstanding Elsevier team—Shelly Hayden, Deon Lee, and Amanda Politte—who make the book a reality.

A special debt of gratitude is expressed to Donna Wong, whose knowledge and expertise of pediatric nursing have made us all better nurses.

David Wilson
Marilyn J. Hockenberry

Contents

UNIT 1

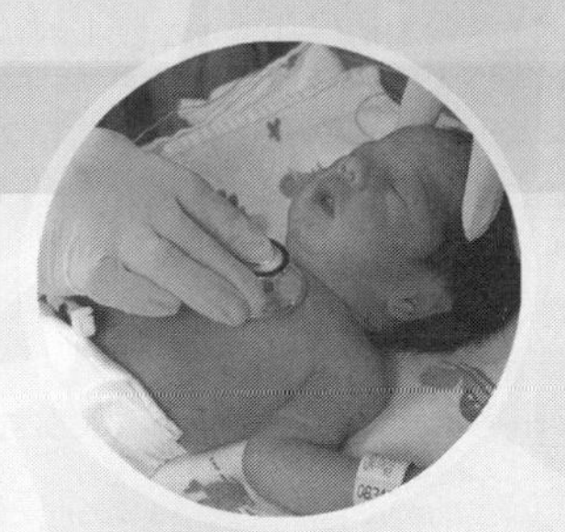

Assessment

RELATED TOPICS

Symbol ▶ indicates material that may be photocopied and distributed to families.

Health History

One of the most significant aspects of a health assessment is the health history. To take a thorough history, the nurse must be well versed in communication and interviewing principles. An overview of the process is presented in terms of general guidelines for communication and interviewing, with additional specific guidelines for children. Because of the frequent need for interpreters with non–English-speaking families, guidelines for using interpreters are included.

The history furnishes information about the child's physical health since birth, details the events of the present problem, and includes social and family history facts that are essential for providing comprehensive care. The objective of each assessment area is the identification of nursing diagnoses.

The summary is primarily intended for the recording of data, not the acquisition of information from the informant. Therefore it is not meant to be used as a questionnaire. The column entitled "Comments" is intended to enhance and detail sections of the history, as well as to emphasize areas of possible intervention. For a more comprehensive discussion of approaches to taking a history, see *Wong's Nursing Care of Infants and Children* or *Wong's Essentials of Pediatric Nursing.**

General Guidelines for Communication and Interviewing

Assess ability to speak and understand English.

Conduct the interview in a private, quiet area.

Begin the interview with appropriate introductions.

- Address each person by name.

Clarify the purpose of the interview.

Inform the interviewees of the confidential limits of the interview.

Demonstrate interest in the interview by sitting at eye level and close to interviewees (not across a desk), leaning slightly forward, and speaking in a calm, steady voice.

Begin with general conversation to put the interviewees at ease.

- Use comments such as, "How have things been since we talked last?" or (to the child) "What do you think is going to happen today?" to let the family express the main concern.

Include all parties in the interview.

- Direct age-appropriate questions to children (e.g., "What grade are you in at school?" or "What do you like to eat?").
- Be sensitive to instances in which family members, such as adolescents, may wish to be interviewed separately.
- Recognize and respect cultural patterns of communication, e.g., avoiding direct eye contact (American Indian) or nodding for courtesy rather than to express actual agreement or understanding (many Asian cultures).
- Use open-ended questions or statements that begin with "What," "How," "Tell me about," or "You were saying," and reflect back key words or phrases to encourage discussion.
- Encourage continued discussion with nodding and eye contact, saying "Uh-huh," "I see," or "Yes."
- Use focused questions (questions that ask for a specific response, e.g., "What did you try next?") and closed-ended questions (questions that ask for a single answer, e.g., "Did you call the doctor?") to direct the focus of the interview.
- Ensure mutual understanding by frequently clarifying and summarizing information.
- Use active listening to attend to the verbal and nonverbal aspects of the communication.
- Verbal cues to important issues include these techniques:
  - Frequent reference to a topic
  - Repetition of key words
  - Special reference to an event or person
- Nonverbal cues to important issues include the following:
  - Changes in body position (e.g., looking away or leaning forward)
  - Changes in pitch, rate, intonation, and volume of speech (e.g., speaking rapidly, frequent pauses, whispering, or shouting)
- Use silence to allow persons to do the following:
  - Sort out thoughts and feelings.
  - Search for responses to questions.
  - Share feelings expressed by another.
- Break silence constructively with statements such as, "Is there anything else you wish to say?", "I see you find it difficult to continue; how may I help?", or "I don't know what this silence means. Perhaps there is something you would like to put into words but find difficult to say."
- Convey empathy by attending to the verbal and nonverbal language of the interviewee and reflecting back the feeling of the communication (e.g., "I can see how upsetting that must have been for you").

*Hockenberry M, Wilson D: *Wong's nursing care of infants and children,* ed 8, St Louis, 2007, Mosby; Hockenberry M, Wilson D, Winkelstein M: *Wong's essentials of pediatric nursing,* ed 7, St Louis, 2005, Mosby.

- Provide reassurance to acknowledge concerns and any positive efforts used to deal with problems.
- Avoid blocks to communication:
  - Socializing
  - Giving unrestricted and sometimes unasked-for advice
  - Offering premature or inappropriate reassurance
  - Giving overready encouragement
  - Defending a situation or opinion
  - Using stereotyped comments or clichés
  - Limiting expression of emotion by asking directed, close-ended questions
  - Interrupting and finishing the person's sentence
  - Talking more than the interviewee
  - Forming prejudged conclusions
  - Deliberately changing the focus
- Watch for signs of information overload:
  - Long periods of silence
  - Wide eyes and fixed facial expression
  - Constant fidgeting or attempting to move away
  - Nervous habits (e.g., tapping, playing with hair)
  - Sudden disruptions (e.g., asking to go to the bathroom)
  - Looking around
  - Yawning, eyes drooping
  - Frequently looking at a watch or clock
  - Attempting to change topic of discussion

Close the interview with an opportunity for others to bring up overlooked or sensitive concerns with a statement such as, "Have we covered everything?"

Summarize the interview, especially if problems were identified or interventions were planned.

Discuss the need for follow-up, and schedule a time.

Express appreciation for each person's participation.

Specific Guidelines for Communicating with Children

Allow children time to feel comfortable.

Avoid sudden or rapid advances, broad smiles, extended eye contact, or other gestures that may be seen as threatening.

Talk to the parent if the child is initially shy.

Communicate through transition objects such as dolls, puppets, or stuffed animals before questioning a young child directly.

Give older children the opportunity to talk without the parents present.

Assume a position that is at eye level with the child.

Speak in a quiet, unhurried, and confident voice.

Speak clearly, be specific, use simple words and short sentences.

State directions and suggestions *positively.*

Offer a choice only when one exists.

Be honest with children.

Allow children to express their concerns and fears.

Use a variety of communication techniques.

Creative Communication Techniques with Children

VERBAL TECHNIQUES

"I" Messages

Relate a feeling about a behavior in terms of "I."

Describe the effect the behavior had on the person.

Avoid use of "you."

- "You" messages are judgmental and provoke defensiveness.
  - **Example:** "You" message—"You are being very uncooperative about doing your treatments."
  - **Example:** "I" message—"I am concerned about how the treatments are going because I want to see you get better."

Third-Person Technique

Involves expressing a feeling in terms of a third person ("he," "she," "they")

Is less threatening than directly asking children how they feel, because it gives them an opportunity to agree or disagree without being defensive

- **Example:** "Sometimes when a person is sick a lot, he feels angry and sad because he cannot do what others can." Either wait silently for a response or encourage a reply with a statement such as, "Did you ever feel that way?"

Approach allows children three choices: (1) to agree and, hopefully, express how they feel; (2) to disagree; or (3) to remain silent, in which case they probably have such feelings but are unable to express them at this time.

Facilitative Responding

Involves careful listening and reflecting back to patients the feelings and content of their statements.

Responses are empathic and nonjudgmental and legitimize the person's feelings.

Formula for facilitative responses: "You feel ________ because ________."

- **Example:** If child states, "I hate coming to the hospital and getting needles," a facilitative response is, "You feel unhappy because of all the things that are done to you."

Storytelling

Uses the language of children to probe into areas of their thinking while bypassing conscious inhibitions or fears.

Simplest technique is asking children to relate a story about an event, such as being in the hospital.

Other approaches:

- Show children a picture of a particular event, such as a child in a hospital with other people in the room, and ask them to describe the scene.
- Cut out comic strips, remove words, and have child add statements for scenes.

Mutual Storytelling

Reveals child's thinking and attempts to change child's perceptions or fears by retelling a somewhat different story (more therapeutic approach than storytelling)

Begins by asking child to tell a story about something, followed by another story told by the nurse that is similar to child's tale but with differences that help child in problem areas

- **Example:** Child's story is about going to the hospital and never seeing his or her parents again. Nurse's story is also about a child (using different names but similar circumstances) in a hospital whose parents visit every day, but in the evening after work, until the child is better and goes home with them.

Bibliotherapy

Uses books in a therapeutic and supportive process (Box 1-1)

Provides children with an opportunity to explore an event that is similar to their own but sufficiently different to allow them to distance themselves from it and remain in control

General guidelines for using bibliotherapy are:

- Assess child's emotional and cognitive development in terms of readiness to understand the book's message.
- Be familiar with the book's content (intended message or purpose) and the age for which it is written.
- Read the book to the child if child is unable to read.
- Explore the meaning of the book with the child by having child:
  - Retell the story.
  - Read a special section with the nurse or parent.
  - Draw a picture related to the story and discuss the drawing.
  - Talk about the characters.
  - Summarize the moral or meaning of the story.

Dreams

Often reveal unconscious and repressed thoughts and feelings

- Ask child to talk about a dream or nightmare.
- Explore with child what meaning the dream could have.

"What If" Questions

Encourage child to explore potential situations and to consider different problem-solving options.

- **Example:** "What if you got sick and had to go to the hospital?" Children's responses reveal what they know already and what they are curious about and provide an opportunity for helping children learn coping skills, especially in potentially dangerous situations.

Three Wishes

Involves asking, "If you could have any three things in the world, what would they be?"

If child answers, "That all my wishes come true," ask child for specific wishes.

Rating Game

Uses some type of rating scale (numbers, sad to happy faces) to rate an event or feeling

- **Example:** Instead of asking youngsters how they feel, ask how their day has been "on a scale of 1 to 10, with 10 being the best."

BOX 1-1 | Sources of Books for Bibliotherapy

Doll B, Doll CA: *Bibliotherapy with young people: librarians and mental health professionals working together,* Westport, Conn, 1997, Teacher Ideas Press. (800) 225-5800. *http://www.lu.com.*

Grindler MC, and others: *The right book, the right time: helping children cope,* Boston, 1997, Allyn & Bacon. (617) 848-6000.

Jones EH: *Bibliotherapy for bereaved children: healing reading,* London, 2001, Jessica Kingsley Publishing. +44 (020) 7833-2307. *http://www.jkp.com.*

Kaywell JF: *Using literature to help troubled teenagers cope with family issues (using literature to help troubled teenagers),* Westport, Conn, 1998, Greenwood Publishing Group. (800) 225-5800 or (203) 226-3571. *http://www.greenwood.com.*

Pardeck JT, Pardek JA: *Children in foster care and adoption: a guide to bibliotherapy,* Westport, Conn, 1998, Greenwood Publishing Group. (800) 225-5800 or (203) 226-3571. *http://www.greenwod.com.*

Pearl P: *Helping children through books, a selected booklist,* Portland, Ore, 2001, Church & Synagogue Library Association. (503) 244-6919 or (800) 542-2752. *http://www.worldaccessnet.com/~clsa.*

Philpot JG: *Bibliotherapy for classroom use,* Nashville, Tenn, 1997, Incentive Publications. (800) 421-2830.

Silvey A: *100 best books for children,* New York, 2004, Houghton Mifflin. *http://www.houghtonmifflinbooks.com.*

Word Association Game

Involves stating key words and asking children to say the first word they think of when they hear each word

- Start with neutral words, then introduce more anxiety-producing words, such as "illness," "needles," "hospitals," and "operation."
- Select key words that relate to some relevant event in child's life.

Sentence Completion

Involves presenting a partial statement and having child complete it

Some sample statements are:

- The thing I like best (least) about school is ______________________.
- The best (worst) age to be is ______________________.
- The most (least) fun thing I ever did was ______________________.
- The thing I like most (least) about my parents is ______________________.
- The one thing I would change about my family is ______________________.
- If I could be anything I wanted, I would be ______________________.
- The thing I like most (least) about myself is ______________________.

Pros and Cons

Involves selecting a topic, such as being in the hospital, and having child list five good things and five bad things about it

Is an exceptionally valuable technique when applied to relationships, such as things family members like and dislike about each other

NONVERBAL TECHNIQUES

Writing

Is an alternative communication approach for older children and adults

Specific suggestions include:

- Keep a journal or diary.
- Write down feelings or thoughts that are difficult to express.
- Write letters that are never mailed (a variation is making up a pen pal to write to).
- Keep an account of child's progress from both a physical and an emotional viewpoint.

Drawing

One of the most valuable forms of communication, it provides both nonverbal (from looking at the drawing) and verbal (from child's story of the picture) information.

Children's drawings tell a great deal about them because they are projections of their inner selves.

Spontaneous drawing involves giving child a variety of art supplies and providing the opportunity to draw.

Directed drawing involves a more specific direction, such as "draw a person" or the "three themes" approach (state three things about child and ask child to choose one and draw a picture).

Guidelines for Evaluating Drawings

Use spontaneous drawings, and evaluate more than one drawing whenever possible.

Interpret drawings in light of other available information about child and family.

Interpret drawings as a whole rather than concentrating on specific details of the drawing.

Consider individual elements of the drawing that may be significant:

Gender of figure drawn first—Usually relates to child's perception of own gender role

Size of individual figures—Expresses importance, power, or authority

Order in which figures are drawn—Expresses priority in terms of importance

Child's position in relation to other family members—Expresses feelings of status or alliance

Exclusion of a member—May denote feeling of not belonging or desire to eliminate

Accentuated parts—Usually express concern for areas of special importance (e.g., large hands may be a sign of aggression)

Absence of or rudimentary arms and hands—Suggests timidity, passivity, or intellectual immaturity; tiny, unstable feet may be an expression of insecurity, and hidden hands may mean guilt feelings

Placement of drawing on the page and type of stroke—Free use of paper and firm, continuous strokes express security, whereas drawings restricted to a small area and lightly drawn in broken or wavering lines may be a sign of insecurity

Erasures, shading, or cross-hatching—Expresses ambivalence, concern, or anxiety with a particular area

Magic

Uses simple magic tricks to help establish rapport with child, encourage compliance with health interventions, and provide effective distraction during painful procedures

Although "magician" talks, no verbal response from child is required.

Play

Is universal language and "work" of children

Tells a great deal about children because they project their inner selves through the activity

Spontaneous play involves giving child a variety of play materials and providing the opportunity to play.

Directed play involves a more specific direction, such as providing medical equipment, a doll, or a dollhouse for focused reasons, such as exploring child's fear of injections or exploring family relationships.

Guidelines for Using an Interpreter

Explain to interpreter the reason for the interview and the type of questions that will be asked.

Clarify whether a detailed or brief answer is required and whether the translated response can be general or literal.

Introduce interpreter to family, and allow some time before the actual interview so that they can become acquainted.

Give reassurance that interpreter will maintain confidentiality.

Communicate directly with family members when asking questions to reinforce interest in them and to observe nonverbal expressions, but do not ignore interpreter.

Pose questions to elicit only one answer at a time, such as "Do you have pain?" rather than "Do you have any pain, tiredness, or loss of appetite?"

Refrain from interrupting family members and interpreter while they are conversing.

Avoid commenting to interpreter about family members, since they may understand some English.

Be aware that some medical words, such as "allergy," may have no similar word in another language; avoid medical jargon whenever possible.

Respect cultural differences; it is often best to pose questions about sex, marriage, or pregnancy indirectly—ask about "child's father" rather than "mother's husband."

Allow time after the interview for interpreter to share something that he or she felt could not be said earlier; ask about interpreter's impression of nonverbal clues to communication and family members' reliability or ease in revealing information.

Arrange for family to speak with same interpreter on subsequent visits whenever possible.

Outline of a Health History

A. Identifying information
1. Name
2. Address
3. Telephone number
4. Age and birth date
5. Birth place
6. Race or ethnic group
7. Gender
8. Religion
9. Nationality
10. Date of interview
11. Informant

B. Chief complaint

C. Present illness
1. Onset
2. Characteristics
3. Course since onset

D. Past history
1. Pregnancy (maternal)
2. Labor and delivery
3. Perinatal period
4. Previous illnesses, operations, or injuries
5. Allergies
6. Current medications
7. Cultural remedies
8. Pain
9. Immunizations
10. Growth and development
11. Habits

E. Review of systems
1. General
2. Integument
3. Head
4. Eyes
5. Nose
6. Ears
7. Mouth
8. Throat
9. Neck
10. Chest
11. Respiratory
12. Cardiovascular
13. Gastrointestinal
14. Genitourinary
15. Gynecologic
16. Musculoskeletal
17. Neurologic
18. Endocrine
19. Lymphatic

F. Nutrition history*
1. Patterns of eating
2. Dietary intake

G. Family medical history
1. Family pedigree
2. Familial diseases
3. Family members with congenital anomalies
4. Family habits
5. Geographic location

H. Alternative therapies

I. Family personal and social history*
1. Family structure
2. Family function
3. Daycare

*Because of the importance of the nutrition history and family personal and social history, separate sections devoted to assessment of these two topics are on pp. 129 and 126, respectively.

J. **Sexual history**
   1. Sexual concerns and activity of youngster
   2. Sexual concerns and activity of adults if warranted

K. **Patient profile (summary)**
   1. Health status
   2. Psychologic status
   3. Socioeconomic status

Summary of a Health History

Information | **Comments**

Identifying Information

Information

1. Name
2. Address
3. Telephone number
4. Age
5. Birth date
6. Race or ethnic group
7. Gender
8. Religion or spiritual beliefs
9. Nationality
10. Date of interview
11. Informant

Comments

Additional information appropriate to older adolescent may include occupation, marital status, and temporary and permanent addresses.

Under "informant" include subjective impression of reliability, general attitude, willingness to communicate, overall accuracy of data, and any special circumstances, such as use of an interpreter.

Informants should include parent and child, as well as others who may be primary caregivers, such as grandparent.

Chief Complaint (CC)

Information

To establish the major specific reason for the individual's seeking professional health attention

Comments

Record in patient's own words; include duration of symptoms.

If informant has difficulty isolating *one* problem, ask which problem or symptom led person to seek help *now*.

In case of routine physical examination, state *CC* as reason for visit.

Present Illness (PI)

Information

To obtain all details related to the chief complaint

1. Onset
   a. Date of onset
   d. Manner of onset (gradual or sudden)
   c. Precipitating and predisposing factors related to onset (emotional disturbance, physical exertion, fatigue, bodily function, pregnancy, environment, injury, infection, toxins and allergens, therapeutic agents)
2. Characteristics
   a. Character (quality, quantity, consistency, or other)
   b. Location and radiation (e.g., pain)
   c. Intensity or severity
   d. Timing (continuous or intermittent, duration of each, temporal relationship to other events)
   e. Aggravating and relieving factors
   f. Associated symptoms
3. Course since onset
   a. Incidence
      (1) Single acute attack
      (2) Recurrent acute attacks
      (3) Daily occurrences
      (4) Periodic occurrences
      (5) Continuous chronic episode

Comments

In its broadest sense, *illness* denotes any problem of a physical, emotional, or psychosocial nature.

Present information in chronologic order; may be referenced according to one point in time, such as *prior to admission* (PTA).

Concentrate on reason for seeking help now, especially if problem has existed for some time.

Summary of a Health History–cont'd

Information	Comments
Present Illness (PI)—cont'd	
b. Progress (better, worse, unchanged) c. Effect of therapy	
Past History (PH)	
To elicit a profile of the individual's previous illnesses, injuries, or operations 1. Pregnancy (maternal) a. Number (gravida) (1) Dates of delivery b. Outcome (parity) (1) Gestation (full-term, premature, postmature) (2) Stillbirths, abortions c. Health during pregnancy d. Medications taken	Importance of perinatal history depends on child's age; the younger the child, the more important the perinatal history. Explain relevance of obstetric history in revealing important factors relating to the child's health. Assess parents' emotional attitudes toward the pregnancy and birth.
2. Labor and delivery a. Duration of labor b. Type of delivery c. Place of delivery d. Medications	Assess parents' feelings regarding delivery; investigate factors that may affect bonding, such as separation from infant.
3. Perinatal period a. Weight and length at birth b. Time of regaining birth weight c. Condition of health immediately after birth d. Apgar score e. Presence of problems including congenital anomalies f. Date of discharge from nursery	If birth problems are reported, inquire about treatment, such as use of oxygen, phototherapy, and surgery, and parents' emotional response to the event.
4. Previous illnesses, operations, or injuries a. Onset, symptoms, course, termination b. Occurrence of complications c. Incidence of disease in other family members or in community d. Emotional response to previous hospitalization e. Circumstances and nature of injuries	Ask about diphtheria, scarlet fever, measles, rubella, chickenpox, mumps, tonsillitis, strep throat, pertussis, allergies, and common illnesses such as colds and earaches. Elicit a description of disease to verify the diagnosis. Be alert to areas of injury prevention.
5. Allergies a. Hay fever, asthma, or eczema b. Unusual reactions to foods, drugs, animals, plants, latex products, or household products	Have parent describe the type of allergic reaction and its severity.
6. Current medications a. Name, dose, schedule, duration, and reason for administration	Assess parents' knowledge of correct dosage of common drugs, such as acetaminophen; note underuse or overuse.
7. Cultural remedies* a. Herbs, natural products, special foods, drinks	Ask about names of the products used, frequency given, and dosages.
8. Pain a. Previous experiences b. Reactions c. Effective management d. Cultural Influences	When age-appropriate, elicit information from the child as well as parent. Does the child tend to be stoic or expressive with pain? What is the family's attitude about taking pain medications?

*From American Academy of Pediatrics, Committee on Children with Disabilities: Counseling families who choose complementary and alternative medicine for their child with chronic illness or disability, *Pediatrics* 107(3):598-601, 2001.

Continued

Summary of a Health History–cont'd

Information	Comments
Past History (PH)—cont'd	
9. Immunizations a. Name, number of doses, age when given b. Occurrence of reaction c. Administration of horse or other foreign serum, gamma-globulin, or blood transfusion	Parents may refer to immunizations as "baby shots." Whenever possible, confirm information by checking medical or school records. **SAFETY ALERT** Inquire about previous administration of any horse or other foreign serum, recent administration of gamma globulin or blood transfusion, and anaphylactic reactions to neomycin or chicken eggs.
10. Growth and development a. Weight at birth, 6 months, 1 year, and present b. Dentition (1) Age of eruption/shedding (2) Number (3) Problems with teething c. Age of head control, sitting unsupported, walking, first words	Compare parents' responses with own observations of child's achievement and results from objective tests, such as Denver II or DASE (see pp. 160 and 167).
d. Present grade in school, scholastic achievement e. Interaction with peers and adults f. Participation in organized activities, such as Scouting, sports	School and social history can be more thoroughly explored under Family Assessment.
11. Habits a. Behavior patterns (1) Nail biting (2) Thumb sucking	Assess parents' attitudes toward habits and any remedies used to curtail them, such as punishment for bed-wetting.
(3) Pica	Pica, the habitual ingestion of nonfood items, may be risk factor for lead poisoning.
(4) Rituals, such as use of security blanket (5) Unusual movements (head banging, rocking) (6) Temper tantrums b. Activities of daily living (1) Hour of sleep and arising (2) Duration of nighttime sleep or naps (3) Age of toilet training	
(4) Pattern of stools and urination; occurrence of enuresis or encopresis (5) Type of exercise	Record child's usual terms for defecation and urination.
c. Use or abuse of drugs, alcohol, coffee (caffeine), tobacco, vitamins and supplements, or alternative therapies. d. Usual disposition; response to frustration	With adolescents, ask about quantity and frequency of chemicals used.
Review of Systems (ROS)	
To elicit information concerning any potential health problem (Box 1-2)	Explain relevance of questioning to parents (similar to pregnancy section) in composing total health history of child. Make positive statements about each system (e.g., "Mother denies headaches, bumping into objects, squinting, or excessive rubbing of eyes"). Use terms parents are likely to understand, such as "bruises" for ecchymoses.

Summary of a Health History–cont'd

Information	Comments
Nutrition History	
To elicit information about adequacy of child's dietary intake and eating patterns (see p. 129)	
Family Medical History	
To identify the presence of genetic traits or diseases that have familial tendencies; to assess family habits and exposure to a communicable disease that may affect family members	Choose terms wisely when asking about child's parentage: for example, inquire about paternal history by referring to the child's "father" rather than mother's husband; use term "partner" rather than spouse.
1. Family pedigree (Figure 1-1) and guidelines for construction (Guidelines box)	A pedigree is a pictorial representation or diagram of a family tree to visualize patterns of disease transmission.

Continued

BOX 1-2 | Review of Systems

General—Overall state of health, fatigue, recent and/or unexplained weight gain or loss (period of time for either), contributing factors (change of diet, illness, altered appetite), exercise tolerance, fevers (time of day), chills, night sweats (unrelated to climatic conditions), frequent infections, general ability to carry out activities of daily living

Integument—Pruritus, pigment or other color changes, acne, moles, discoloration, eruptions, rashes (location), tendency toward bruising, petechiae, excessive dryness, general texture, disorders or deformities of nails, hair growth or loss, hair color change (for adolescent, use of hair dyes or other potentially toxic substances such as hair straighteners)

Head—Headaches, dizziness, injury (specific details)

Eyes—Visual problems (ask about behaviors indicative of blurred vision, such as bumping into objects, clumsiness, sitting very close to the television, holding a book close to the face, writing with head near desk, squinting, rubbing the eyes, bending the head in an awkward position), cross-eye (strabismus), eye infections, edema of lids, excessive tearing, use of glasses or contact lenses, date of last optic examination

Nose—Nosebleeds (epistaxis), constant or frequent running or stuffy nose, nasal obstruction (difficulty breathing), alteration or loss of sense of smell

Ears—Earaches, discharge, evidence of hearing loss (ask about behaviors such as need to repeat requests, loud speech, inattentive behavior), results of any previous auditory testing, pulling or rubbing ear

Mouth—Mouth breathing, gum bleeding, toothaches, toothbrushing, use of fluoride, difficulty with teething (symptoms), last visit to dentist (especially if temporary dentition is complete), response to dentist

Throat—Sore throats, difficulty in swallowing, choking (especially when chewing food—may be from poor chewing habits), hoarseness or other voice irregularities

Neck—Pain, limitation of movement, stiffness, difficulty in holding head straight (torticollis), thyroid enlargement, enlarged nodes or other masses

Chest—Breast enlargement, discharge, masses, enlarged axillary nodes (for adolescent female, ask about breast self-examination)

Respiratory—Chronic cough, frequent colds (number per year), wheezing, shortness of breath at rest or on exertion, difficulty in breathing, sputum production, infections (pneumonia, tuberculosis), date of last chest x-ray examination, and skin reaction from tuberculin testing

Cardiovascular—Cyanosis or fatigue on exertion, history of heart murmur or rheumatic fever, anemia, date of last blood count, blood type, recent transfusion

Gastrointestinal—Nausea, vomiting (not associated with eating, may be indicative of brain tumor or increased intracranial pressure), jaundice or yellowing skin or sclera, belching, flatulence, recent change in bowel habits (blood in stools, change in color, diarrhea, and constipation)

Genitourinary—Pain on urination, frequency, hesitancy, urgency, hematuria, nocturia, polyuria, unpleasant odor to urine, force of stream, discharge, change in size of scrotum, date of last urinalysis (for adolescent, sexually transmitted disease, type of treatment; for male adolescent, ask about testicular self-examination)

Gynecologic—Menarche, date of last menstrual period, regularity or problems with menstruation, vaginal discharge, pruritus, date and result of last Pap smear (include obstetric history as discussed under birth history when applicable); if sexually active, type of contraception

Musculoskeletal—Weakness, clumsiness, lack of coordination, unusual movements, back or joint stiffness, muscle pains or cramps, abnormal gait, deformity, fractures, serious sprains, activity level, redness, swelling, tenderness

Neurologic—Seizures, tremors, dizziness, loss of memory, general affect, fears, nightmares, speech problems, any unusual habit

Endocrine—Intolerance to weather changes, excessive thirst and urination, excessive sweating, salty taste to skin, signs of early puberty

Lymphatic—History of frequent infections, enlarged lymph nodes in any region, swelling, tenderness, red streaks

Summary of a Health History—cont'd

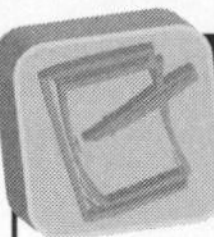

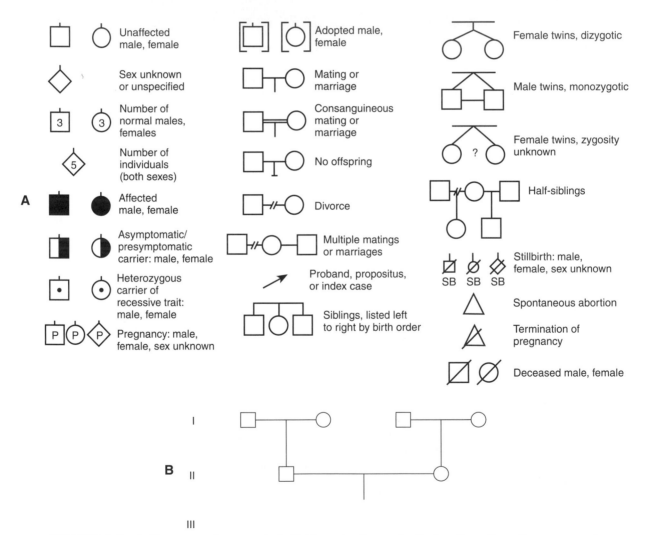

GUIDELINES

Pedigree Construction

1. Begin diagram in the middle of a large sheet of paper.
2. Represent males by placing a square to the left and females by placing a circle to the right (Figure 1-1, *A*).
3. Represent the proband (index case, original patient) with an arrow (if the counselee or patient is different, place a *C* under that person's symbol).
4. Use a horizontal line between a square and a circle for a mating or marriage.
5. Suspend offspring vertically from the mating line and place in order of birth with oldest to the left (regardless of gender).
6. Symbolize generations by Roman numerals with the earliest generation at the top.
7. Include three generations: (1) grandparents, (2) parents, and (3) offspring; may include aunts, uncles, and first cousins of proband (Figure 1-1, *B*).
8. Include name of each person (maiden names for married women), the person's date of birth, health problems, and date and cause of death.
9. Date the pedigree.

A

Unaffected male, female

Sex unknown or unspecified

3 3 Number of normal males, females

5 Number of individuals (both sexes)

Affected male, female

Asymptomatic/presymptomatic carrier: male, female

Heterozygous carrier of recessive trait: male, female

P P P Pregnancy: male, female, sex unknown

Adopted male, female

Mating or marriage

Consanguineous mating or marriage

No offspring

Divorce

Multiple matings or marriages

Proband, propositus, or index case

Siblings, listed left to right by birth order

Female twins, dizygotic

Male twins, monozygotic

? Female twins, zygosity unknown

Half-siblings

SB SB SB Stillbirth: male, female, sex unknown

Spontaneous abortion

Termination of pregnancy

Deceased male, female

B

I

II

III

FIGURE **1-1** **A,** Common pedigree symbols. **B,** Example of a standardized pedigree form. Roman numerals indicate generations: I—grandparents; II—parents; and III—offspring.

Summary of a Health History–cont'd

Information	Comments
Family Medical History—cont'd	
2. ***Familial diseases*** such as heart disease, hypertension, cancer, diabetes mellitus, obesity, congenital anomalies, allergy, asthma, tuberculosis, seizures, sickle cell disease, depression, mental retardation, mental illness or other emotional problems, syphilis, or rheumatic fever; indicate symptoms, treatment, and sequelae	
3. ***Family members*** with congenital anomalies	
4. ***Family habits,*** such as smoking or chemical use	Important for identification of endemic disease
5. ***Geographic location,*** including birth place, present location, and travel or contact with foreign visitors	
Alternative Therapies*	
The American Academy of Pediatrics (2001) has the following recommendations when discussing alternative, complementary, and unproven therapies: 1. ***Obtain*** information for yourself, and be prepared to share it with families. 2. ***Evaluate*** the scientific merits of specific therapeutic approaches. 3. ***Identify*** risks or potential harmful effects. 4. ***Provide*** families with information on treatment options. 5. ***Educate*** families to evaluate information and treatment options. 6. ***Avoid*** dismissal of complementary and alternative therapies (CAM) in ways that indicate a lack of sensitivity or concern. 7. ***Recognize*** feeling threatened, and guard against becoming defensive. 8. ***If the CAM approach is endorsed, offer*** to provide monitoring and evaluate the response. 9. ***Actively listen*** to the family and child with chronic illness or disability.	These recommendations should be used by nurses when discussing CAM with families. Remember, introducing the subject of CAM requires tactful communication skills. An approach such as, "I am very interested in how nontraditional or alternative therapies can be used to help children. What things have you tried?" is a positive and nonthreatening entrée to a discussion with the family. When families are using an unfamiliar intervention, ask for their sources of information and review them before giving advice. In general, if a therapy produces no adverse effect, including significant financial burden, do not discourage its use. Maintaining a trusting, supportive relationship with the family generally outweighs any benefit from trying to disprove the value of nonconventional therapy.
Family Personal and Social History	
To gain an understanding of the family's structure and function (see p. 126)	
Sexual History	
To elicit information concerning young person's concerns and/or activities and any pertinent data regarding adult's sexual activity that influence child 1. Sexual concerns and activity of youngster 2. Sexual concerns and activity of adults if warranted	Sexual history is an essential component of preadolescents' and adolescents' health assessments. Degree of investigation into parents' sexual history depends on its relevance to the child's health. It may be limited to family planning concerns, or it may be more detailed if overt sexual activity or abuse is suspected. Investigate toward end of history when rapport is greatest. Respect sensitive and complex nature of questioning. Give parents and youngster option of discussing sexual matters alone with nurse. Ensure confidentiality. Clarify terms such as "sexually active" or "having sex."

*From American Academy of Pediatrics, Committee on Children with Disabilities: Counseling families who choose complementary and alternative medicine for their child with chronic illness or disability, *Pediatrics* 107(3):598-601, 2001.

Continued

Summary of a Health History–cont'd

Information	Comments
Sexual History—cont'd	
	Refer to sexual contacts as "partners" not "girlfriends" or "boyfriends" to avoid biasing discussion of homosexual activity. Discussion may flow easily after review of genitourinary tract, such as asking female about menstruation or male about urinary problems. Suggestions for beginning discussion include the following: "Tell me about your social life." "Who are your closest friends?" "Is there one very special friend?" "Some teenagers have decided to have sex. What do you think about that?" Take detailed history of all contacts if sexually transmitted disease is suspected or diagnosed.
Patient Profile (Summary)	
To summarize the interviewer's overall impression of the child's and family's physical, psychologic, and socioeconomic background 1. Health status 2. Psychologic status 3. Socioeconomic status	A comprehensive summary often identifies nursing diagnoses based on subjective and objective findings.

HABITS TO ASSESS DURING A HEALTH INTERVIEW*

Behavior patterns such as nail biting, thumb sucking, pica (habitual ingestion of nonfood substances), rituals ("security" blanket or toy), and unusual movements (head banging, rocking, overt masturbation, and walking on toes)

Activities of daily living, such as hour of sleep and arising, duration of nighttime sleep and naps, type and duration of exercise, regularity of stools and urination, age of toilet training, and occurrences of daytime or nighttime bed-wetting

Unusual disposition, as well as response to frustration

Use or abuse of alcohol, drugs, coffee, or tobacco

TAKING AN ALLERGY HISTORY*

Has your child ever taken any drugs or tablets that have disagreed with him or her or caused an allergic reaction (Guidelines box)? If yes, can you remember the name(s) of these drugs?

Can you describe the reaction?

Was the drug taken by mouth (as a tablet or medicine), or was it an injection?

How soon after starting the drug did the reaction happen?

How long ago did this happen?

Did anyone tell you it was an allergic reaction, or did you decide for yourself?

Has your child ever taken this drug, or a similar one, again? If yes, did your child experience the same problems?

Have you told the doctors or nurses about your child's reaction or allergy?

GUIDELINES

Identifying Allergy

Does the child have any symptoms (e.g., sneezing, coughing, rashes, wheezing) when handling rubber products (balloons, tennis or Koosh balls, adhesive bandage strips) or when in contact with rubber hospital products, such as gloves and catheters?

Has your child ever had an allergic reaction during surgery?

Does the child have a history of rashes, asthma, or allergic reactions to medication or foods, especially milk, kiwi fruit, bananas, or chestnuts?

How would you identify or recognize an allergic reaction in your child?

What would you do if an allergic reaction occurred?

Has anyone ever discussed latex or rubber allergy or sensitivity with you?

Has the child had any allergy testing?

When did the child last come in contact with any type of rubber product? Were you present?

*Modified from Cantrill JA, Cottrell WN: Accuracy of drug allergy documentation, *Am J Health Syst Pharm* 54:1627-1629, 1997.

Cultural Assessment

Cultural assessment helps identify the family's understanding of the health-related problem in relation to how their culture may affect the plan of care. The cultural assessment identifies the family beliefs, values, and practices that may facilitate or interfere with health care. Careful assessment can assist the nurse in better understanding the patient and family.

Strategies for Gathering Cultural Information

Listen to the patient and family's understanding of the health problem.
Use cultural resources to promote understanding of different ethnic and religious cultures.
Assess cultural influences throughout the comprehensive nursing assessment.

CULTURALLY SENSITIVE INTERACTIONS

Nonverbal Strategies

Invite family members to choose where they would like to sit or stand, allowing them to select a comfortable distance.
Observe interactions with others to determine which body gestures (e.g., shaking hands) are acceptable and appropriate. Ask when in doubt. Know when physical contact is prohibited.
Avoid appearing rushed.
Be an active listener.
Observe for cues regarding appropriate eye contact.
Avoiding eye contact may be a sign of respect.
Learn appropriate use of pauses or interruptions for different cultures.
Ask for clarification if nonverbal meaning is unclear.
Learn if smiling indicates friendliness.

Verbal Strategies

Learn proper terms of address.
Use a positive tone of voice to convey interest.
Speak slowly and carefully, not loudly, when families have poor language comprehension.
Encourage questions.
Learn basic words and sentences of family's language, if possible.
Avoid professional terms.
When asking questions, tell family why the questions are being asked, the way in which the information they provide will be used, and how it might benefit their child.
Repeat important information more than once.
Always give the reason or purpose for a treatment or prescription.
Use information written in the family's language.
Arrange for the services of an interpreter when necessary.
Learn from families and representatives of their culture methods of communicating information without creating discomfort.
Address intergenerational needs (e.g., family's need to consult with others).
Be sincere, open, and honest and, when appropriate, share personal experiences, beliefs, and practices to establish rapport and trust.

Cultural Assessment Outline

COMMUNICATION

What language is spoken at home?
How does the family demonstrate respect or disrespect?
How well does the family understand English (spoken and written)?
Is an interpreter needed?

HEALTH BELIEFS

How are health and illness defined by the family?
How are feelings expressed regarding illness or death?
What are the attitudes toward sickness?
Who makes the decisions regarding health practices in the family?
Are there cultural practices that would restrict the type of care needed?
Is a health professional of the same gender or ethnic background an issue for the family?

RELIGIOUS PRACTICES AND RITUALS

What is the family's religious preference?
Who does the family turn to for support and counseling?
Are there special practices or rituals that may affect care?
Are there special rituals or ceremonies when a patient is ill or dying?
Are special rituals or ceremonies attached to birth, baptism, puberty, or death?

DIETARY PRACTICES

Are some foods restricted by the family's culture?
Are there cultural practices in observance of certain occasions or events?
How is food prepared?
Who is responsible for food preparation?
Do certain foods have special meaning to the family or child?
Are special foods believed to cause or cure an illness or disease?
Are there times of required food fasting?
How are the periods of fasting defined, and who fasts in the family?

FAMILY CHARACTERISTICS

Who makes the decisions in the family?
How many generations are considered to be a single family?
Which relatives comprise the family unit?
When are children disciplined or punished?
How is affection demonstrated in the family?
How are emotions exhibited in the family?
What is the attitude toward children?

SOURCES OF SUPPORT

To what ethnic or cultural organizations does the family belong?
How do the organizations influence the family's approach to health care?
Who is most responsible for influencing the family's health beliefs?
Is there a specific cultural group with which the family identifies?
Is the specific cultural group identified by where the child was born and has lived?

RESOURCES FOR CULTURAL INFORMATION

Giger & Davidhizar. (2004). Transcultural Nursing: Assessment and Intervention.
Leininger & McFarland. (2002). Transcultural Nursing: Concepts, Theories and Practice.
Lipson, & Dibble. (2005). Culture & Clinical Care.
Purnell & Paulanka. (2003). Transcultural Health Care: A Culturally Competent Approach
Spector. (2003). Cultural Diversity in Health and Illness.
http://ethnomed.org
http://www.ggalanti.com/cultural_profiles
http://www.tcns.org

Cultural Characteristics Related to Health Care of Children and Families

Health Beliefs	Health Practices	Family Relationships	Communication
African-American			
Illness classified as: Natural—affected by forces of nature without adequate protection (e.g., cold air, pollution, food, and water) Unnatural—God's punishment for improper behavior May see illness as "will of God"	Self-care and folk medicine prevalent Folk therapies usually religious in origin Folk therapies often not shared with medical provider Prayer is common means for prevention and treatment	Strong kinship bonds in extended family, with members coming to aid of others in crisis Less likely to view illness as a burden Place strong emphasis on work and ambition Older adults cared for and respected	Alert to any evidence of discrimination Place importance on nonverbal behavior Affection shown by touching and hugging Silence may indicate lack of trust Eye contact important to establish trust Best to use direct, but caring approach
Chinese			
View healthy body as gift from parents and ancestors that must be cared for Health one result of balance between the forces of *yin* (cold) and *yang* (hot)—energy forces that rule world Illness caused by imbalance	Goal of therapy: to restore balance of yin and yang *Acupuncture:* needles applied to appropriate meridians identified in terms of yin and yang *Acupressure* and *t'ai chi* replacing acupuncture in some areas	Extended family pattern common Strong concept of loyalty of young to old Respect for elders taught at early age—acceptance without questioning or talking back Children's behavior a reflection on family	Open expression of emotions unacceptable Often smile when they do not comprehend

Data from Lipson JG, Dibble SL, Minarik PA: *Culture and nursing care: a pocket guide*, San Francisco, 1998, UCSF Nursing Press; Spector RE: *Cultural diversity in health and illness*, Upper Saddle River, NJ, 2000, Prentice Hall.

Cultural Characteristics Related to Health Care of Children and Families–cont'd

Health Beliefs	Health Practices	Family Relationships	Communication
Chinese—cont'd			
Believe blood is source of life and is not regenerated *Chi* is innate energy	*Moxibustion:* application of heat to skin over specific meridians Wide use of medicinal herbs procured and applied in prescribed ways Meals sometimes planned to balance "hot" and "cold"	Family and individual honor and "face" important Self-reliance and self-esteem highly valued; self-expression repressed	
Filipino			
Health a result of balance Illness a result of imbalance To be healthy again is to correct an evil deed	May not respond to illness until it is advanced May use herbal medicine Eating appropriate amounts, not necessarily eating right, promotes good health Physical ailment possibly caused by the supernatural	Family highly valued, with strong family ties Multigenerational family structure common, often including collateral members Avoid behavior that would bring shame on family	Immigrants and older persons may not be able to speak or understand English Sensitive to tone and manner of speaker Limited direct eye contact
Haitian			
Illness a punishment Natural cause (*maladi bone die*—disease of the Lord) caused by environmental factors, movement of blood within body, changes between "hot" and "cold," and bone displacement Supernatural (*loa*—spirits' anger) Good health: maintenance of equilibrium Prayer and good spiritual habits important	Health seen as personal responsibility Foods have properties of "hot"/"cold" and "light"/"heavy" and must be in harmony with one's life cycle and bodily states Natural illnesses treated by home and folk remedies first May use religious medallions, rosary beads, or figure of saint to pray with	Maintenance of family reputation paramount Lineal authority supreme; children in subordinate position in family hierarchy Children valued for parental social security in old age and expected to contribute to family welfare at early age	Recent immigrants and older persons may speak only Haitian Creole Often smile and nod in agreement when do not understand Quiet and gentle communication style and lack of assertiveness, leading health care providers to falsely believe they comprehend health teaching and are compliant May not ask questions if health care provider is busy or rushed
Japanese			
Shinto religious influence Humans inherently good Evil caused by outside spirits Illness caused by contact with polluting agents (e.g., blood, corpses, skin diseases) Health achieved through harmony and balance between self and society	Energy restored by means of acupuncture, acupressure, massage, and moxibustion along affected meridians *Kampõ* medicine—use of natural herbs Believe in removal of diseased parts Trend to use both Western and Asian healing methods	Close intergenerational relationships Generational categories: *Issei*—first generation to live in United States *Nisei*—second generation *Sansei*—third generation *Yonsei*—fourth generation Family tendency to keep problems to self	*Issei*—born in Japan; usually speak Japanese only *Nisei, Sansei,* and *Yonsei* have few language difficulties Make significant use of nonverbal communication with subtle gestures and facial expression Tend to suppress emotions Will often wait silently

Continued

Cultural Characteristics Related to Health Care of Children and Families–cont'd

Health Beliefs	Health Practices	Family Relationships	Communication
Japanese—cont'd			
Disease caused by disharmony with society and not caring for body	Care for disabled viewed as family's responsibility Take pride in child's good health Seek preventive care, medical care for illness	Value self-control and self-sufficiency Concept of *haji* (shame) imposes strong control; unacceptable behavior of children reflects on family	
Mexican-American			
Health controlled by environment, fate, and will of God Certain illnesses considered "hot" and "cold" states and are treated with food that complements those states Disease based on imbalance between individual and environment	Seek help from *curandero* or *curandera,* especially in rural areas *Curandero(a)* receives position by birth, apprenticeship, or "calling" via dream or vision Treatments with herbs, rituals, and religious artifacts For severe illness, make promises, visit shrines, offer medals and candles, offer prayers Adhere to "hot" and "cold" food prescriptions and prohibitions for prevention and treatment of illness	Strong kinship ties; extended families include *compadres* (godparents) established by ritual kinship Children valued highly and desired, taken everywhere with family Elderly treated with respect	Spanish speaking or bilingual May have strong preference for native language and revert to it in times of stress May shake hands or engage in introductory embrace Interpret prolonged eye contact as disrespectful Relaxed concept of time—may be late to appointments
Native Americans			
Believe health is state of harmony with nature and universe Respect of bodies through proper management Depends on individual belief in traditional culture Traditional health beliefs holistic and wellness oriented	Distinction made between indigenous health problem requiring native healer or practice and Western disease requiring other medical care Promote health by participating in religious ceremonies and prayer	Cultures vary in kinship structure Extended family structure—usually includes relative from both sides of family Older members assume leadership roles	Most continue to speak their Indian language as well as English Nonverbal communication Individuals usually speak for themselves
Puerto Rican			
Subscribe to "hot-cold" theory of causation of illness Believe some illness caused by evil forces Destiny (*Si Dios quiere*—if God wants) in control of health	Infrequent use of health care system Seek folk healers (*espiritistas*)—use of herbs, rituals Treatment classified as "hot" or "cold" Many varieties of herbal teas used to treat illness and promote healing	Family usually large and home centered—core of existence Father has authority in family Great respect for elders Children valued—seen as gift from God Children taught to obey and respect parents	Spanish speaking or bilingual Strong sense of family privacy—may view questions regarding family as impudent

Cultural Characteristics Related to Health Care of Children and Families—cont'd

Health Beliefs	Health Practices	Family Relationships	Communication
Vietnamese			
Good health considered balance between yin and yang Concept of health based on harmony and balance Many use rituals to prevent illness	Family uses all means possible before using outside agencies for health care Regard health as family responsibility; outside aid sought when resources run out Use herbal medicine, spiritual practices, and acupuncture May use cupping, coin rubbing, or pinching skin May inhale aromatic oils, drink herbal teas, or wear strings tied on body	Family revered institution and chief social network Multigenerational families Children highly valued Individual needs and interests subordinate to those of family group Father main decision maker Women taught submission to men Parents expect respect and obedience from children	Many immigrants not proficient in speaking and understanding English May hesitate to ask questions Questioning authority seen as a sign of disrespect; asking questions considered impolite May avoid eye contact with health professionals as sign of respect

Physical Assessment

Physical assessment is a continuous process that begins during the interview, primarily by using inspection or observation. During the more formal examination, the tools of percussion, palpation, and auscultation are added to enhance and refine the assessment of body systems. Like the health history, the objective of the physical assessment is to formulate nursing diagnoses and evaluate the effectiveness of therapeutic interventions.

Because of important differences in physical assessment of the child and newborn, separate guidelines and summaries for conducting the physical examination of each age-group are presented.

The summary of the physical assessment of the newborn is also presented according to the area to be assessed, usual findings, common variations and minor abnormalities, and potential signs of distress or major abnormalities. Common variations and minor abnormalities should be recorded but generally do not require further evaluation. Potential signs of distress or major abnormalities are recorded and need to be reported for further evaluation. The procedures for assessment are not presented here but in the summary of physical assessment of the child. In addition to the newborn summary, assessment of clinical gestational age is also described.

The summary of the physical assessment of the child is presented according to the area to be assessed, the procedure for assessment, usual findings, and comments. The comments column includes findings that deviate from the normal and should be reported, special significance of certain findings, and areas for nursing intervention. This section includes detailed instructions for various assessment procedures.

For a more comprehensive discussion of performing a physical assessment, see *Wong's Nursing Care of Infants and Children* or *Wong's Essentials of Pediatric Nursing.**

General Guidelines for Physical Examination of the Newborn

Provide a comfortably warm and nonstimulating examination area.

- To prevent heat loss, undress only the body area to be examined unless the newborn is already under a heat source, such as a radiant warmer.

Proceed in an orderly sequence (usually head to toe) with the following exceptions:

- Perform first all procedures that require quiet observation (position, attitude, skin color); then proceed with quiet procedures, such as auscultating the lungs, heart, and abdomen.

*Hockenberry M, Wilson D: *Wong's nursing care of infants and children*, ed 8, St Louis, 2007, Mosby; Hockenberry M, Wilson D, Winkelstein M: *Wong's essentials of pediatric nursing*, ed 7, St Louis, 2005, Mosby.

- Perform disturbing procedures, such as testing reflexes, last.
- Measure head and length at same time to compare results.

Proceed quickly to avoid stressing the infant.

- Check that equipment and supplies are working properly and are accessible.

Comfort the infant during and after the examination if upset.

- Talk softly.
- Hold infant's hands against his or her chest.
- Swaddle and hold.
- Provide nonnutritive sucking.

Summary of Physical Assessment of the Newborn

Usual Findings	Common Variations and Minor Abnormalities	Potential Signs of Distress or Major Abnormalities
General Measurements		
Head circumference—33-35 cm (13-14 inches); about 2-3 cm (1 inch) larger than chest circumference	Molding after birth may decrease head circumference. Head and chest circumference may be equal for first 1-2 days after birth.	Head circumference <10th or >90th percentile
Chest circumference—30.5-33 cm (12-13 inches).		
Crown-to-rump length—31-35 cm (12.5-14 inches); approximately equal to head circumference		
Head-to-heel length—48-53 cm (19-21 inches)		
Birth weight—2700-4000 g (6-9 pounds)	Loss of 10% of birth weight in first week; regained in 10-14 days	Birth weight <10th or >90th percentile
Vital Signs		
Temperature (axillary)—36.5°-37° C (97.9°-98° F)	Crying may increase body temperature slightly. Radiant warmer may falsely increase axillary temperature.	Hypothermia Hyperthermia
Heart rate (apical)—120-140 beats/min	Crying will increase heart rate; sleep will decrease heart rate. During first period of reactivity (6-8 hours), rate can reach 180 beats/min.	Bradycardia—Resting rate below 80-100 beats/min Tachycardia—Rate above 180 beats/min Irregular rhythm
Respirations—30-60 breaths/min	Crying will increase respiratory rate; sleep will decrease respiratory rate. During first period of reactivity (6-8 hours), rate can reach 80 breaths/min.	Irregular rhythm Apnea >15 seconds
Blood pressure (BP) (oscillometric)—65/41 mm Hg in arm and calf	Crying and activity will increase BP. Placing cuff on thigh may agitate infant; thigh BP may be higher than arm or calf BP by 4-8 mm Hg and is least preferred method. See Guidelines Box.	Oscillometric systolic pressure in calf 6-9 mm Hg less than in upper extremity (possible sign of coarctation of aorta—correlate extremity pulses and pulse oximeter readings as well). Recommend taking BP in same limb each time for consistent comparisons. BP in preterm infants may vary according to age and illness factors.
General Appearance		
Posture—Flexion of head and extremities, which rest on chest and abdomen	***Frank breech***—Extended legs, abducted and fully rotated thighs, flattened occiput, extended neck	Limp posture, extension of extremities

Summary of Physical Assessment of the Newborn—cont'd

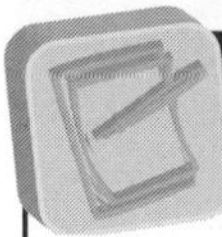

GUIDELINES

Using the Blood Pressure Tables

1. Use the standard height charts to determine the height percentile.
2. Measure and record the child's systolic blood pressure (SBP) and diastolic blood pressure (DBP).
3. Use the correct gender table for SBP and DBP.
4. Find the child's age on the left side of the table. Follow the age row horizontally across the table to the intersection of the line for the height percentile (vertical column).
5. There, find the 50th, 90th, 95th, and 99th percentiles for SBP in the left columns and for DBP in the right columns.
   - BP <90th percentile is normal.
   - BP between the 90th and 95th percentile is prehypertension. In adolescents, BP ≥120/80 mm Hg is prehypertension, even if this figure is <90th percentile.
   - BP >95th percentile may be hypertension.
6. If the BP is >90th percentile, the BP should be repeated twice at the same office visit, and an average SBP and DBP should be used.
7. If the BP is >95th percentile, BP should be staged. If stage 1 (95th percentile to 99th percentile plus 5 mm Hg), BP measurements should be repeated on two more occasions. If hypertension is confirmed, evaluation should proceed. If BP is stage 2 (>99th percentile plus 5 mm Hg), prompt referral should be made for evaluation and therapy. If the patient is symptomatic, immediate referral and treatment are indicated.

From National High Blood Pressure Education Program Working Group on High Blood Pressure in Children and Adolescents: The fourth report on the diagnosis, evaluation, and treatment of high blood pressure in children and adolescents, *Pediatrics* 114:555-576, 2004.

Usual Findings	Common Variations and Minor Abnormalities	Potential Signs of Distress or Major Abnormalities
Skin		
At birth, bright red, puffy, smooth Second to third day, pink, flaky, dry Vernix caseosa Lanugo Edema around eyes, face, legs, dorsa of hands, feet, and scrotum or labia *Acrocyanosis*—Cyanosis of hands and feet *Cutis marmorata*—Transient mottling when infant is exposed to stress, decreased temperature, or overstimulation	Neonatal jaundice after first 24 hours Ecchymoses or petechiae caused by birth trauma *Milia*—Distended sebaceous glands that appear as tiny white papules on cheeks, chin, and nose *Miliaria* or *sudamina*—Distended sweat (eccrine) glands that appear as minute vesicles, especially on face *Erythema toxicum*—Pink papular rash with vesicles superimposed on thorax, back, buttocks, and abdomen; may appear in 24-48 hours and resolve after several days *Harlequin color change*—Clearly outlined color change as infant lies on side; lower half of body becomes pink or red, and upper half is pale *Mongolian spots*—Irregular areas of deep blue pigmentation, usually in sacral and gluteal regions; seen predominantly in newborns of African, Native American, Asian, or Hispanic descent *Telangiectatic nevi ("stork bites")*—Flat, deep pink, localized areas usually seen on back of neck	Progressive jaundice, especially in first 24 hours Cracked or peeling skin Generalized cyanosis Cyanosis of one extremity that persists Pallor Mottling Grayness Plethora Hemorrhage, ecchymoses, or petechiae that persist *Sclerema*—Hard and stiff skin Poor skin turgor Rashes, pustules, or blisters *Café-au-lait spots*—Light brown spots *Nevus flammeus*—Port-wine marks Lacerations or abrasions

Continued

Summary of Physical Assessment of the Newborn—cont'd

Usual Findings	Common Variations and Minor Abnormalities	Potential Signs of Distress or Major Abnormalities
Head		
Anterior fontanel—Diamond shaped, 2.5-4 cm (1-1.75 inches) (Figure 1-2)	Molding following vaginal delivery Third sagittal (parietal) fontanel Bulging fontanel because of crying	Fused sutures Bulging or depressed fontanels when quiet Widened sutures and fontanels. Occipital or generalized scalp edema associated with vacuum delivery
Posterior fontanel—Triangular, 0.5-1 cm (0.2-0.4 inch) Fontanels should be flat, and firm. Widest part of fontanel measured from bone to bone, not suture to suture	***Caput succedaneum***—Edema of soft scalp tissue ***Cephalhematoma*** (uncomplicated)—Hematoma between periosteum and skull bone	***Craniotabes***—Snapping sensation along lambdoidal suture that resembles indentation of Ping-Pong ball
Eyes		
Lids usually edematous Iris color—Slate gray, dark blue, brown Absence of tears Presence of red reflex Corneal reflex in response to touch Pupillary reflex in response to light Blink reflex in response to light or touch Rudimentary fixation on objects and ability to follow to midline	Epicanthal folds in Asian infants Searching nystagmus or strabismus ***Subconjunctival (scleral) hemorrhages***—Ruptured capillaries, usually at limbus	Pink color of iris Purulent discharge Upward slant in non-Asians Hypertelorism (3 cm or greater) Hypotelorism Congenital cataracts—unilateral or bilateral Constricted or dilated fixed pupil Absence of red reflex Absence of pupillary or corneal reflex Inability to follow object or bright light to midline Blue sclera Yellow sclera
Ears		
Position—Top of pinna on horizontal line with outer canthus of eye Startle reflex elicited by a loud, sudden noise Pinna flexible, cartilage present	Inability to visualize tympanic membrane because of filled aural canals Pinna flat against head Irregular shape or size Pits or skin tags	Low placement of ears Absence of startle reflex in response to loud, sudden noise Minor abnormalities may be signs of various syndromes, especially renal

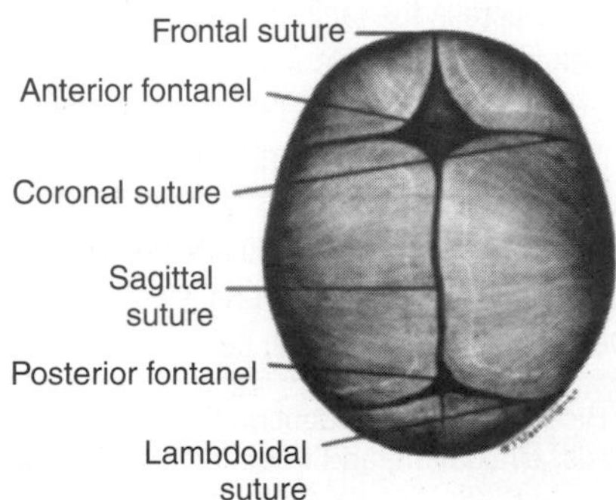

FIGURE **1-2** Locations of sutures and fontanels.

Summary of Physical Assessment of the Newborn—cont'd

Usual Findings	Common Variations and Minor Abnormalities	Potential Signs of Distress or Major Abnormalities
Nose		
Nasal patency	Flattened and bruised	Nonpatent canals—Inability to pass nasogastric tube Transient cyanosis and apnea with nonpatent canal may be sign of co-anal atresia
Nasal discharge—Thin, white mucus Sneezing Milia		Thick, bloody nasal discharge Flaring of nares (alae nasi) Copious nasal secretions or stuffiness (may be minor)
Mouth and Throat		
Intact, high arched palate Uvula in midline Frenulum of tongue Frenulum of upper lip Sucking reflex—Strong and coordinated Rooting reflex Gag reflex Extrusion reflex Absent or minimal salivation Vigorous cry	***Natal teeth***—Teeth present at birth; benign but may be associated with congenital defects ***Epstein pearls***—Small, white epithelial cysts along midline of hard palate Lingual frenulum extends to tip of tongue limiting tongue movement	Cleft lip Cleft palate Large, protruding tongue or posterior displacement of tongue Profuse salivation or drooling ***Candidiasis (thrush)***—White, adherent patches on tongue, palate, and buccal surfaces Inability to pass orogastric tube Hoarse, high-pitched, weak, absent, or other abnormal cry
Neck		
Short, thick, usually surrounded by skinfolds Tonic neck reflex	***Torticollis*** (wry neck)—Head held to one side with chin pointing to opposite side Fractured clavicle	Excessive skinfolds Resistance to flexion Absence of tonic neck reflex
Chest		
Anteroposterior and lateral diameters equal Slight sternal retractions evident during inspiration Xiphoid process evident Breast enlargement	Funnel chest (pectus excavatum) Pigeon chest (pectus carinatum) Supernumerary nipples Secretion of milky substance from breasts ("witch's milk")	Depressed sternum Marked retractions of chest and intercostal spaces during respiration Asymmetric chest expansion Redness and firmness around nipples Wide-spaced nipples
Lungs		
Respirations chiefly abdominal Cough reflex absent at birth, present by 1-2 days Bilateral, equal bronchial breath sounds	Rate and depth of respirations may be irregular; periodic breathing. Crackles shortly after birth	Inspiratory stridor Expiratory grunt Retractions Persistent irregular breathing Periodic breathing with repeated apneic spells (>15 seconds) Seesaw respirations (paradoxic) Unequal breath sounds Persistent fine crackles Wheezing Diminished breath sounds Peristaltic sounds on one side with diminished breath sounds on same side

Continued

Summary of Physical Assessment of the Newborn–cont'd

Usual Findings	Common Variations and Minor Abnormalities	Potential Signs of Distress or Major Abnormalities
Heart		
Apex—Fourth to fifth intercostal space, lateral to left sternal border S_2 slightly sharper and higher in pitch than S_1	***Sinus arrhythmia***—Heart rate increases with inspiration and decreases with expiration. Transient cyanosis on crying or straining	***Dextrocardia***—Heart on right side Displacement of apex, muffled Cardiomegaly Abdominal bruit Murmurs Thrills Persistent cyanosis Hyperactive precordium Unequal peripheral pulses
Abdomen		
Cylindric shape Bowel sounds present in all four quadrants ***Liver***—Palpable 2-3 cm below right costal margin ***Spleen***—Tip palpable at end of first week of age ***Kidneys***—Palpable 1-2 cm above umbilicus ***Umbilical cord***—Bluish white at birth with two arteries and one vein ***Femoral pulses***—Equal bilaterally	Umbilical hernia ***Diastasis recti***—Midline gap between recti muscles ***Wharton's jelly***—Unusually thick umbilical cord	Abdominal distention Localized bulging Distended veins Absent bowel sounds Enlarged liver and spleen Ascites Visible peristaltic waves Scaphoid or concave abdomen Green umbilical cord Presence of only one artery in cord Urine or stool leaking from cord Palpable bladder distention following scanty voiding Absent femoral pulses Cord bleeding, hematoma, or mass contained within cord (possible omphalocele) ***Bladder exstrophy***—externalization of bladder (possibly with epispadias) with widely separated symphysis pubis
Female Genitalia		
Labia and clitoris usually edematous Urethral meatus behind clitoris Vernix caseosa between labia Urination within 24 hours	***Pseudomenstruation***—Blood-tinged or mucoid discharge Hymenal tag Edema, petechiae, bruising from breech presentation (or delivery)	Enlarged clitoris with urethral meatus at tip Fused labia Absence of vaginal opening Meconium from vaginal opening, urethral opening, or perineum No urination within 24 hours Masses in labia Ambiguous genitalia
Male Genitalia		
Urethral opening at tip of glans penis Testes palpable in each scrotum Scrotum usually large, edematous, pendulous, and covered with rugae; usually deeply pigmented in dark-skinned ethnic groups	Urethral opening covered by prepuce Inability to retract foreskin ***Epithelial pearls***—Small, firm, white lesions at tip of prepuce Erection or priapism Testes palpable in inguinal canal	***Hypospadias***—Urethral opening on ventral surface of penis ***Epispadias***—Urethral opening on dorsal surface of penis ***Chordee***—Ventral curvature of penis

Summary of Physical Assessment of the Newborn–cont'd

Usual Findings	Common Variations and Minor Abnormalities	Potential Signs of Distress or Major Abnormalities
Male Genitalia—cont'd		
Smegma Urination within 24 hours	Scrotum small Edema, ecchymoses, bruising with breech presentation (or delivery)	Testes not palpable in scrotum or inguinal canal Micropenis (two standard deviations below the mean of length and width for age) No urination within 24 hours Inguinal hernia Hypoplastic or absent scrotum ***Hydrocele***—Fluid in scrotum Masses in scrotum Meconium from scrotum, raphe, or perineum Discoloration of testes—(bluish-red) possible testicular torsion Ambiguous genitalia
Back and Rectum		
Spine intact; no openings, masses, or prominent curves Trunk incurvation reflex Anal reflex Patent anal opening Passage of meconium within 48 hours	Green liquid stools in infant under phototherapy Delayed passage of meconium in very low–birth-weight or sick neonates	Anal fissures or fistulas Imperforate anus Absence of anal reflex No meconium within 36 hours Pilonidal cyst or sinus Tuft of hair along spine Spina bifida (any degree)
Extremities		
Ten fingers and 10 toes Full range of motion Nail beds pink, with transient cyanosis immediately after birth Creases on anterior two thirds of sole Sole usually flat Symmetry of extremities Equal muscle tone bilaterally, especially resistance to opposing flexion Equal bilateral brachial and femoral pulses	Partial syndactyly between second and third toes Second toe overlapping into third toe Wide gap between first (hallux) and second toes Deep crease on plantar surface of foot between first and second toes Asymmetric length of toes Dorsiflexion and shortness of hallux	***Polydactyly***—Extra digits ***Syndactyly***—Fused or webbed digits ***Phocomelia***—Hands or feet attached close to trunk ***Hemimelia***—Absence of distal part of extremity Hyperflexibility of joints Persistent cyanosis of nail beds Yellowing of nail beds Transverse palmar (simian) crease Fractures, abrasions, bruises Decreased or absent range of motion (ROM) Dislocated or subluxated hip Limitation in hip abduction Unequal gluteal or leg folds (Figure 1-3) Unequal knee height (Allis or Galeazzi sign) Audible clunk on abduction (Ortolani sign) Asymmetry of extremities Unequal muscle tone or ROM

Continued

Summary of Physical Assessment of the Newborn–cont'd

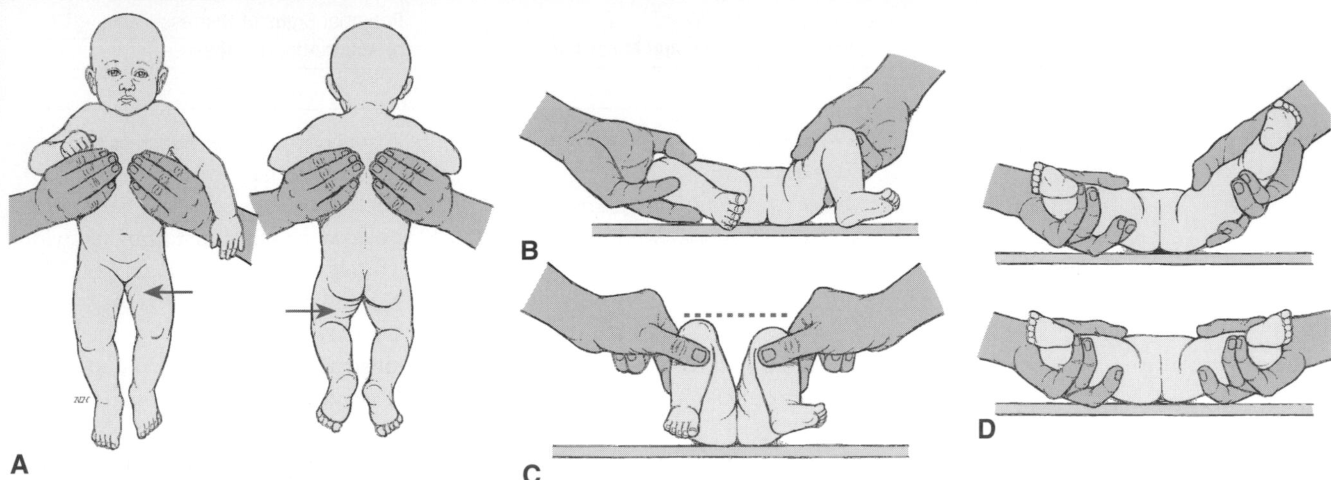

FIGURE **1-3** Signs of developmental dysplasia of the hip. **A**, Asymmetry of gluteal and thigh folds. **B**, Limited hip abduction, as seen in flexion. **C**, Apparent shortening of the femur, as indicated by the level of the knees in flexion. **D**, Ortolani clunk, heard when affected leg is abducted in infant under 4 weeks of age. NOTE: It is recommended that only the experienced clinician perform this maneuver to prevent further subluxation.

Usual Findings	Common Variations and Minor Abnormalities	Potential Signs of Distress or Major Abnormalities
Neuromuscular System		
Extremities usually maintain some degree of flexion. Extension of an extremity followed by previous position of flexion Head lag while sitting, but momentary ability to hold head erect Able to turn head from side to side when prone Able to hold head in horizontal line with back when held prone	Quivering or momentary tremors	***Hypotonia***—Floppy, poor head control, extremities limp ***Hypertonia***—Jittery, arms and hands tightly flexed, legs stiffly extended, startles easily Asymmetric posturing (except tonic neck reflex) Opisthotonic posturing—Arched back Signs of paralysis Tremors, twitches, and myoclonic jerks Marked head lag in all positions

COMMUNITY FOCUS

Newborn Home Care Following Early Discharge*

Wet diapers—Six to 10 per day

Breast-feeding—Successful latch-on and milk transfer at breast and feeding every 1½ to 3 hours daily

Formula feeding—Successfully, voiding as above, taking 3 to 4 ounces every 3 to 4 hours

Circumcision—Wash with warm water only; yellow exudate forming, nonbleeding; Plastibell intact 48 hours

Stools—At least one every 48 hours (bottle-feeding), or two to three per day (breast-feeding)

Color—Pink to ruddy when crying; pink centrally when at rest or asleep

Activity—Has four or five wakeful periods per day and is alert to environmental sounds and voices

Jaundice—Physiologic jaundice (not appearing in first 24 hours), feeding, voiding, and stooling as noted above; perform risk assessment using hour-specific nomogram (see Figure 1-5)

Cord—Kept above diaper line; nonodorous; drying process evident; no signs or symptoms of infection

Vital signs—Heart rate 120 to 140 beats/min at rest; respiratory rate 30 to 60 breaths/min at rest without evidence of sternal retractions, grunting, or nasal flaring; temperature 36.5° to 37° C (97.9° to 98° F) axillary

Position of sleep—Back

*Any deviation from this list and/or suspicion of poor newborn adaptation should be reported to the practitioner at once.

Assessment of Reflexes

Reflexes	Expected Behavioral Responses
Localized	
Eyes	
Blinking or corneal reflex	Infant blinks at sudden appearance of a bright light or at approach of an object toward cornea; persists throughout life.
Pupillary	Pupil constricts when a bright light shines toward it; persists throughout life.
Doll's eye	As head is moved slowly to right or left, eyes lag behind and do not immediately adjust to new position of head; disappears as fixation develops; if persists, indicates neurologic damage.
Nose	
Sneeze	Spontaneous response of nasal passages to irritation or obstruction; persists throughout life.
Glabellar	Tapping briskly on glabella (bridge of nose) causes eyes to close tightly.
Mouth and Throat	
Sucking	Infant begins strong sucking movements of circumoral area in response to stimulation; persists throughout infancy, even without stimulation, such as during sleep.
Gag	Stimulation of posterior pharynx by food, suction, or passage of a tube causes infant to gag; persists throughout life.
Rooting	Touching or stroking the cheek along side of mouth causes infant to turn head toward that side and begin to suck; should disappear at about age 3-4 months but may persist for up to 12 months.
Extrusion	When tongue is touched or depressed, infant responds by forcing it outward; disappears by age 4 months.
Yawn	Spontaneous response to decreased oxygen by increasing amount of inspired air; persists throughout life.
Cough	Irritation of mucous membranes of larynx or tracheobronchial tree causes coughing; persists throughout life; usually present 1 day after birth.
Extremities	
Grasp	Touching palms of hands or soles of feet near base of digits causes flexion of hands and toes; palmar grasp lessens after age 3 months, to be replaced by voluntary movement; plantar grasp lessens by 8 months of age.
Babinski	Stroking outer sole of foot upward from heel and across ball of foot causes toes to hyperextend and hallux to dorsiflex; disappears after age 1 year.
Ankle clonus	Briskly dorsiflexing foot while supporting knee in partially flexed position results in one or two oscillating movements ("beats"); eventually no beats should be felt.
Mass (Body)	
Moro*	Sudden jarring or change in equilibrium causes sudden extension and abduction of extremities and fanning of fingers, with index finger and thumb forming a C shape, followed by flexion and adduction of extremities; legs may weakly flex; infant may cry; disappears after age 3-4 months, usually strongest during first 2 months.
Startle*	A sudden loud noise causes abduction of the arms with flexion of elbows; hands remain clenched; disappears by age 4 months.
Perez	While infant is prone on a firm surface, thumb is pressed along spine from sacrum to neck; infant responds by crying, flexing extremities, and elevating pelvis and head; lordosis of the spine, as well as defecation and urination, may occur; disappears by age 4-6 months.
Asymmetric tonic neck	When infant's head is turned to one side, arm and leg extend on that side, and opposite arm and leg flex; disappears by age 3-4 months, to be replaced by symmetric positioning of both sides of body.

*Some authorities consider Moro and startle reflexes to be the same response.

Continued

Assessment of Reflexes–cont'd

Reflexes	Expected Behavioral Responses
Mass (Body)—cont'd	
Trunk incurvation (Galant)	Stroking infant's back alongside spine causes hips to move toward stimulated side; reflex disappears by age 4 weeks.
Dance or step	If infant is held so that sole of foot touches a hard surface, there is a reciprocal flexion and extension of the leg, simulating walking; disappears after age 3-4 weeks, to be replaced by deliberate movement.
Crawl	When placed on abdomen, infant makes crawling movements with arms and legs; disappears at about age 6 weeks.
Placing	When infant is held upright under arms and dorsal side of foot is briskly placed against hard object, such as table, leg lifts as if foot is stepping on table; age of disappearance varies.

Assessment of Gestational Age

Assessment of gestational age is an important criterion because perinatal morbidity and mortality are related to gestational age and birth weight. One of the most frequently used methods of determining gestational age is based on physical and neurologic findings. The scale in Figure 1-4, *A*, assesses six external physical and six neuromuscular signs. Each sign has a number score, and the cumulative score correlates with a maturity rating from 20 to 44 weeks (see maturity rating box on scale).

The new Ballard Scale, a revision of the original scale, can be used with newborns as young as 20 weeks of gestation. The tool has the same physical and neuromuscular sections but includes −1 and −2 scores that reflect signs of extremely premature infants, such as fused eyelids; imperceptible breast tissue; sticky, friable, transparent skin; no lanugo; and square-window (flexion of wrist) angle of greater than 90 degrees. The examination of infants with a gestational age of 20 weeks or less should be performed at a postnatal age of less than 12 hours. For infants with a gestational age of at least 26 weeks, the examination can be performed up to 96 hours after birth, although shortly after birth, preferably within 2 to 8 hours, is suggested. The scale overestimates gestational age by 2 to 4 days in infants less than 37 weeks' gestation, especially between 32 and 37 weeks' gestation. Neurologic maturity may require retesting once the infant's condition has stabilized. The new Ballard gestational age scale has greater validity when performed before 96 hours of age in preterm infants. It is also important to note that the infant's state and period of reactivity will affect the neuromuscular rating. An infant in the second stage of the first period of reactivity may not have an accurate neuromuscular score. (After the initial stage of alertness and activity [may last the first 6 to 8 hours of life], the infant enters the second stage of the first reactive period, which generally lasts 2 to 4 hours. Heart and respiratory rates decrease, temperature continues to fall, mucus production decreases, and urine or stool is usually not passed. The infant is in a state of sleep and relative calm. Any attempt at stimulation usually elicits a minimal response.)

Classification of infants at birth by both weight and gestational age provides a more satisfactory method for predicting mortality risks and providing guidelines for management of the neonate. The infant's birth weight, length, and head circumference are plotted on standardized graphs that identify normal values for gestational age. The infant whose weight is appropriate for gestational age (AGA) (between the 10th and 90th percentiles) can be presumed to have grown at a normal rate regardless of the length of gestation—preterm, term, or postterm. The infant who is large for gestational age (LGA) (above the 90th percentile) can be presumed to have grown at an accelerated rate during fetal life; the small-for-gestational-age (SGA) infant (below the 10th percentile) can be presumed to have grown at a restricted rate during intrauterine life. When gestational age is determined according to the Ballard scale, the newborn will fall into one of the following nine possible categories for birth weight and gestational age: AGA—term, preterm, postterm; SGA—term, preterm, postterm; or LGA—term, preterm, postterm. Figure 1-4, *B*, is a classification of newborns based on intrauterine growth.

To facilitate the use of Figure 1-4, *A*, the following tests and observations are described:

Test	Assessment or Description
Posture	With the infant quiet and in a supine position, observe the degree of flexion in the arms and legs. Muscle tone and degree of flexion increase with maturity. Full flexion of the arms and legs = 4.
Square window	With the thumb supporting the back of the arm below the wrist, apply gentle pressure with index and third fingers on dorsum of hand without rotating the infant's wrist. Measure the angle between the base of the thumb and forearm. Full flexion (hand lies flat on ventral surface of forearm) = 4.
Arm recoil	With the infant supine, fully flex both forearms on upper arms, hold for 5 seconds; pull down on hands to fully extend and rapidly release arms. Observe the rapidity and intensity of recoil to a state of flexion. A brisk return to full flexion = 4.
Popliteal angle	With the infant supine and the pelvis flat on a firm surface, flex lower leg on thigh, then flex thigh on abdomen. While holding knee with thumb and index finger, extend lower leg with index finger of other hand. Measure the degree of the angle behind the knee (popliteal angle). An angle <90 degrees = 5.
Scarf sign	With the infant supine, support the head in the midline with one hand; use other hand to pull infant's arm across the shoulder so that infant's hand touches the opposite shoulder. Determine location of elbow in relation to midline. Elbow does not reach midline = 4.
Heel to ear	With the infant supine and the pelvis flat on a firm surface, pull the foot as far as possible up toward the ear on the same side. Measure the distance of the foot from the ear and degree of knee flexion (same as popliteal angle). Knees flexed with a popliteal angle <90 degrees = 4.

ESTIMATION OF GESTATIONAL AGE BY MATURITY RATING

NEUROMUSCULAR MATURITY

	−1	0	1	2	3	4	5
Posture							
Square Window (wrist)	> 90°	90°	60°	45°	30°	0°	
Arm Recoil		180°	140° - 180°	110° 140°	90° - 110°	< 90°	
Popliteal Angle	180°	160°	140°	120°	100°	90°	< 90°
Scarf Sign							
Heel to Ear							

PHYSICAL MATURITY

Skin	sticky friable transparent	gelatinous red, translucent	smooth pink, visible veins	superficial peeling &/or rash, few veins	cracking pale areas rare veins	parchment deep cracking no vessels	leathery cracked wrinkled
Lanugo	none	sparse	abundant	thinning	bald areas	mostly bald	
Plantar Surface	heel-toe 40-50 mm: -1 <40 mm: -2	>50 mm no crease	faint red marks	anterior transverse crease only	creases ant. 2/3	creases over entire sole	
Breast	imperceptible	barely perceptible	flat areola no bud	stippled areola 1-2 mm bud	raised areola 3-4 mm bud	full areola 5-10 mm bud	
Eye/Ear	lids fused loosely: -1 tightly: -2	lids open pinna flat stays folded	sl. curved pinna; soft; slow recoil	well-curved pinna; soft but ready recoil	formed & firm instant recoil	thick cartilage ear stiff	
Genitals (male)	scrotum flat, smooth	scrotum empty faint rugae	testes in upper canal rare rugae	testes descending few rugae	testes down good rugae	testes pendulous deep rugae	
Genitals (female)	clitoris prominent labia flat	prominent clitoris small labia minora	prominent clitoris enlarging minora	majora & minora equally prominent	majora large minora small	majora cover clitoris & minora	

MATURITY RATING

score	weeks
-10	20
-5	22
0	24
5	26
10	28
15	30
20	32
25	34
30	36
35	38
40	40
45	42
50	44

A

FIGURE **1-4** **A**, New Ballard Scale for newborn maturity rating. Expanded scale includes extremely premature infants and has been refined to improve accuracy in more mature infants.

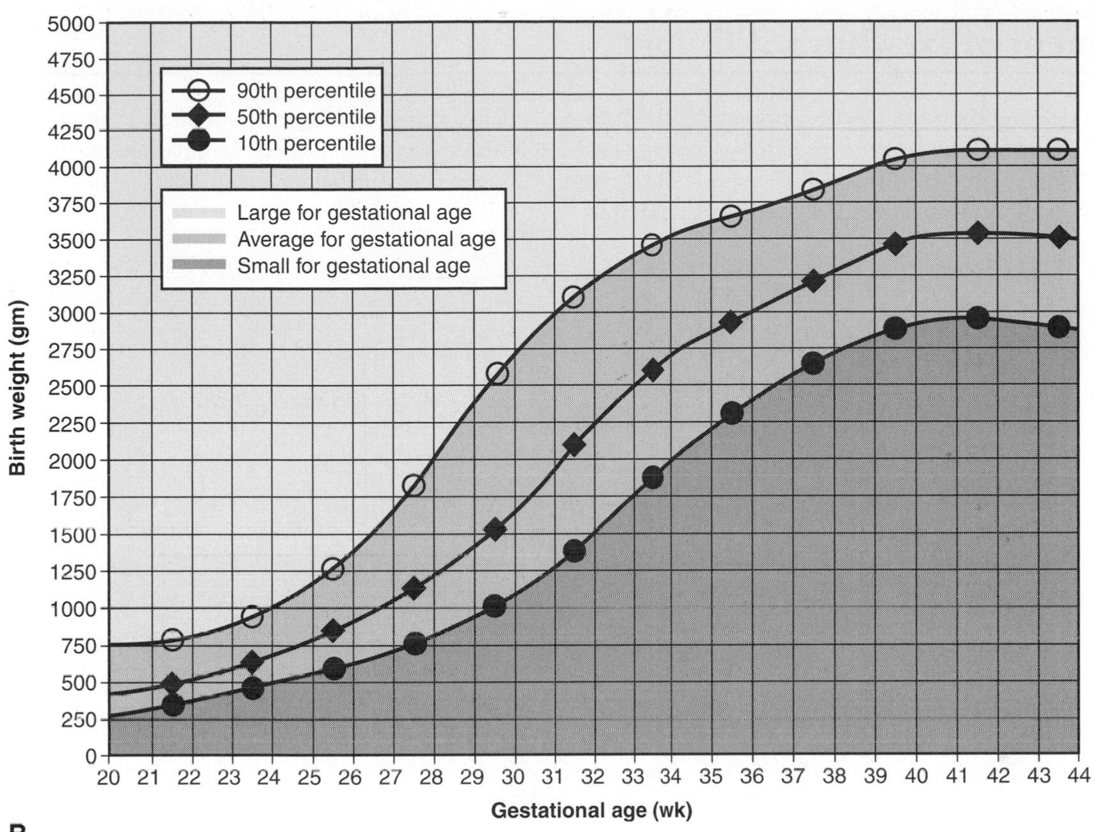

FIGURE **1-4, cont'd** B, Intrauterine growth: birth weight percentiles based on live single births at gestational ages 20 to 44 weeks. (Data from Alexander GR and others: A United States national reference for fetal growth, *Obstet Gynecol* 87(2):163-168, 1996.)

Assessment of Newborn Bilirubin

Hour-specific serum bilirubin levels to predict newborns at risk for rapidly rising levels may be used as a screening tool before discharge from the hospital. Using a nomogram (Figure 1-5) with three designated risk levels (high, intermediate, and low risk) for hour-specific total serum bilirubin values assists in the determination of which newborns might need further evaluation before and after discharge.

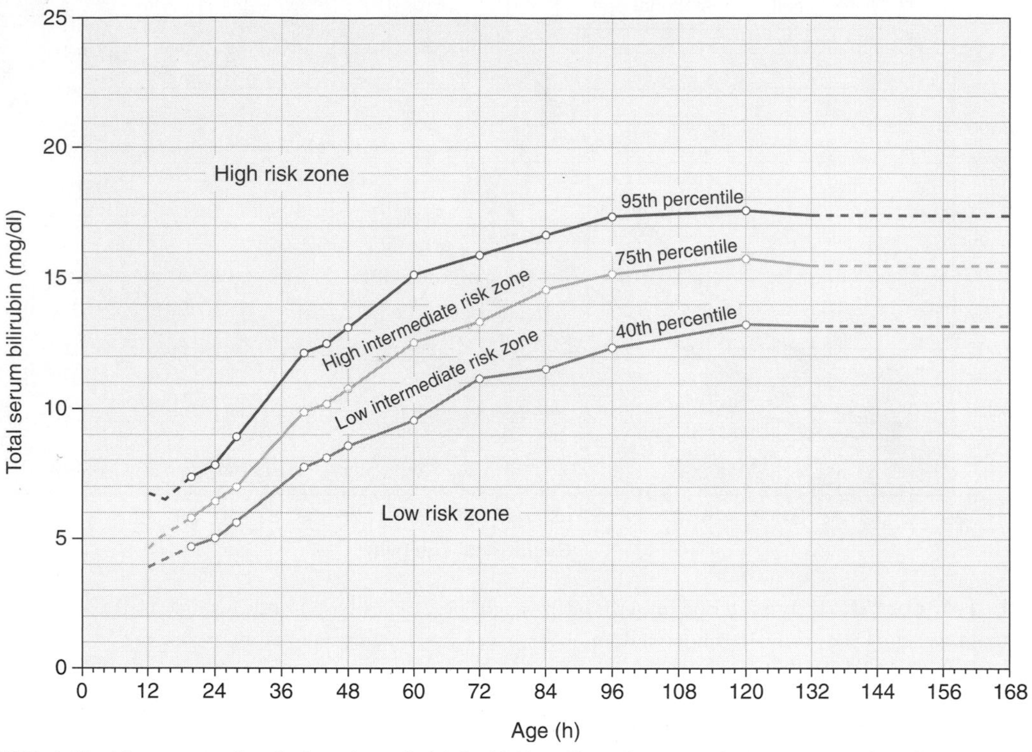

FIGURE **1-5** Nomogram for designation of risk in 2840 well newborns at 36 or more weeks of gestational age with birth weight of 2000 g (4.4 pounds) or more, or 35 or more weeks of gestational age and birth weight of 2500 g (5.5 pounds) or more, based on the hour-specific serum bilirubin values. (This nomogram should not be used to represent the natural history of neonatal hyperbilirubinemia.) (From Bhutani VK, Johnson L, Sivieri EM: Predictive ability of a predischarge hour-specific serum bilirubin for subsequent significant hyperbilirubinemia in healthy term and near-term newborns, *Pediatrics* 103[1]:6-14, 1999.)

General Guidelines for Physical Examination During Childhood

Perform examination in pleasant, nonthreatening area.
- Have room well lit and decorated.
- Have room temperature comfortably warm.
- Place all strange and potentially frightening equipment out of sight.
- Have some toys, dolls, stuffed animals, and games available for the child.
- If possible, have rooms decorated and equipped for different-age children.
- Provide privacy, especially for school-age children and adolescents.
- Check that equipment and supplies are working properly and are accessible to avoid disruption.

Provide time for play and becoming acquainted:
- Talking to the nurse
- Making eye contact
- Accepting the offered equipment
- Allowing physical touching
- Choosing to sit on examining table rather than parent's lap

If signs of readiness are not observed, use the following techniques:
- Talk to the parent while essentially "ignoring" the child; gradually focus on the child or a favorite object, such as a doll.
- Make complimentary remarks about the child, for instance, about his or her appearance, dress, or a favorite object.
- Tell a funny story or perform a simple magic trick.
- Have a nonthreatening "friend," such as a hand or finger puppet, available to "talk" to the child for the nurse.

If the child refuses to cooperate, use the following techniques:
- Assess reason for uncooperative behavior; consider that a child who is unduly afraid of a male examiner may have had a previous traumatic experience, including sexual abuse.
- Try to involve child and parent in process or, if appropriate, ask parent to leave.
- Avoid prolonged explanations about examining procedure.
- Use a firm, direct approach regarding expected behavior.
- Perform examination as quickly as possible.
- Have attendant gently restrain child.
- Minimize any disruptions or stimulation:
  - Limit number of people in room.
  - Use isolated room.
  - Use quiet, calm, confident voice.

Begin the examination in a nonthreatening manner for young children or children who are fearful (Atraumatic Care box).
- Use those activities that can be presented as games, such as tests for cranial nerves (see p. 77) or parts of developmental testing (see p. 160).
- Use approaches such as "Simon says" to encourage child to make a face, squeeze a hand, stand on one foot, and so on.
- Use the paper-doll technique:
  - Lay the child supine on an examining table or floor that is covered with a large sheet of paper.
  - Trace outline around the child's body.
  - Use the body outline to demonstrate what will be examined, such as drawing a heart and listening with the stethoscope before performing the activity on the child.

If several children in the family will be examined, begin with the most cooperative child.

Involve child in the examination process:
- Provide choices, such as sitting either on the table or on the parent's lap.
- Allow child to handle or hold equipment.
- Encourage child to use equipment on a doll, family member, or examiner.
- Explain each step of the procedure in simple language.

Examine child in a comfortable and secure position:
- Sitting in parent's lap
- Sitting upright if in respiratory distress

Proceed to examine the body in an organized sequence (usually head to toe) with following exceptions:
- Alter sequence to accommodate needs of different-age children (see p. 34).
- Examine painful areas last.
- In emergency situation, examine vital functions (airway, breathing, circulation) and injured area first.

Reassure child throughout examination, especially about bodily concerns that arise during puberty.

Discuss the findings with the family at the end of the examination.

Praise child for cooperation during examination; give reward such as an inexpensive toy or paper sticker.

ATRAUMATIC CARE

Reducing Young Children's Fears

Young children, especially preschoolers, fear intrusive procedures because of their poorly defined body boundaries. Therefore avoid invasive procedures, such as measuring rectal temperature, whenever possible. Also, avoid using the word *take* when measuring vital signs, because young children interpret words literally and may think that their temperature or other function will be taken away. Instead, say, "I want to know how warm you are."

Age-Specific Approaches to Physical Examination During Childhood

Position	Sequence	Preparation
Infant		
Before sits alone: supine or prone, preferably in parent's lap; before 4-6 months: can place on examining table After sits alone: sit in parent's lap whenever possible If on table, place with parent in full view	If quiet, auscultate heart, lungs, abdomen. Record heart and respiratory rates. Palpate and percuss same areas. Proceed in usual head-to-toe direction. Perform traumatic procedures last (eyes, ears, mouth [while infant is crying]). Elicit reflexes as body part examined. Elicit Moro reflex last.	Completely undress infant if room temperature permits. Leave diaper on male. Gain cooperation with distraction, bright objects, rattles, talking. Have older infants hold a small block in each hand; until voluntary release develops toward end of the first year, infants will be unable to grasp other objects (e.g., stethoscope, otoscope). Smile at infant; use soft, gentle voice. Pacify with bottle of sugar water or feeding. Enlist parent's aid in restraining to examine ears, mouth. Avoid abrupt, jerky movements.
Toddler		
Sitting or standing on or by parent Prone or supine in parent's lap	Inspect body area through play: count fingers, tickle toes. Use minimal physical contact initially. Introduce equipment slowly. Auscultate, percuss, palpate whenever quiet. Perform traumatic procedures last (same as for infant).	Have parent remove child's outer clothing. Remove underwear as body part is examined. Allow child to inspect equipment; demonstrating use of equipment is usually ineffective. If uncooperative, perform procedures quickly. Use restraint when appropriate; request parent's assistance. Talk about examination if cooperative; use short phrases. Praise for cooperative behavior.
Preschool Child		
Prefers standing or sitting Usually cooperative prone or supine Prefers parent's closeness	If cooperative, proceed in head-to-toe direction. If uncooperative, proceed as with toddler.	Request self-undressing. Allow to wear underpants. Offer equipment for inspection; briefly demonstrate use. Make up story about procedure: "I'm seeing how strong your muscles are" (blood pressure). Use paper-doll technique. Give choices when possible. Expect cooperation; use positive statements: "Open your mouth."
School-Age Child		
Prefers sitting Cooperative in most positions Younger child prefers parent's presence Older child may prefer privacy	Proceed in head-to-toe direction. May examine genitalia last in older child. Respect need for privacy.	Request self-undressing. Allow to wear underpants. Give gown to wear. Explain purpose of equipment and significance of procedure, such as otoscope to see eardrum, which is necessary for hearing. Teach about body functioning and care.

Age-Specific Approaches to Physical Examination During Childhood–cont'd

Position	Sequence	Preparation
Adolescent		
Same as for school-age child Offer option of parent's presence	Same as for older school-age child	Allow to undress in private. Give gown. Expose only area to be examined. Respect need for privacy. Explain findings during examination: "Your muscles are firm and strong." Matter-of-factly comment about sexual development: "Your breasts are developing as they should be." Emphasize normalcy of development. Examine genitalia as any other body part; may leave for end.

Outline of a Physical Assessment

- **A. Growth measurements**
  1. Length and height
  2. Crown-to-rump length or sitting height
  3. Weight
  4. Head circumference
  5. Chest circumference
  6. Skinfold thickness and arm circumference
- **B. Physiologic measurements**
  1. Temperature
  2. Pulse
  3. Respiration
  4. Blood pressure
- **C. General appearance**
- **D. Skin**
- **E. Accessory structures**
- **F. Lymph nodes**
- **G. Head**
- **H. Neck**
- **I. Eyes**
- **J. Ears**
- **K. Nose**
- **L. Mouth and throat**
- **M. Chest**
- **N. Lungs**
- **O. Heart**
- **P. Abdomen**
- **Q. Genitalia**
  1. Male
  2. Female
- **R. Anus**
- **S. Back and extremities**
- **T. Neurologic assessment**
  1. Mental status
  2. Motor functioning
  3. Sensory functioning
  4. Reflexes (deep tendons)
  5. Cranial nerves

Summary of Physical Assessment of the Child

Assessment	Procedure
Growth Measurements	
See Figure 1-6, *A* and *B*.	Plot length, weight, and head circumference on standard percentile charts (see pp. 147-158). Charts for 0-36 months and 2 to 20 years both include children ages 24-36 months; record only recumbent length on 0- to 36-month chart and only stature on 2- to 20-year chart. The prepubescent charts are appropriate only for plotting values for prepubescent boys and girls, regardless of chronologic age, and not for any child showing signs of pubescence, such as breast budding, testicular enlargement, or growth of axillary or pubic hair.

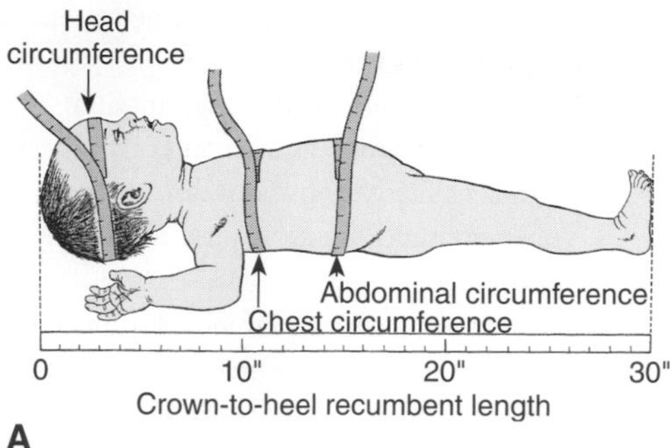

FIGURE **1-6** **A**, Measurement of head, chest, and abdominal circumference and crown-to-heel (recumbent) length.

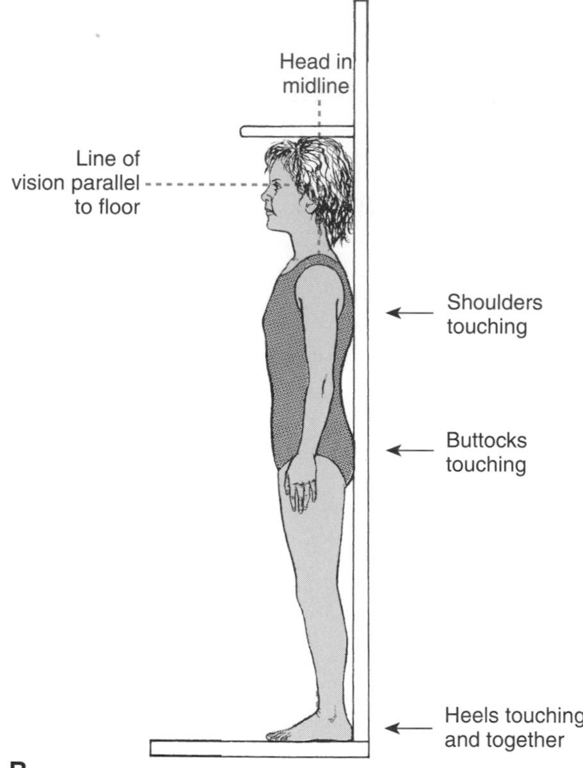

FIGURE **1-6, cont'd** **B**, Measurement of height (stature). (Redrawn from *Human growth and growth disorders: an update*, South San Francisco, 1989, Genentech.)

Usual Findings	Comments
Measurements of length, weight, and head circumference between the 25th and 75th percentiles are likely to represent normal growth (Safety Alert). Measurements between the 10th and 25th and between the 75th and 90th percentiles may or may not be normal, depending on previous and subsequent measurements and on genetic and environmental factors. Growth curve remains generally within same percentile, except during rapid growth periods.	Questionable results may include the following: 1. Children whose height and weight percentiles are widely disparate, for example, height in the 10th percentile and weight in the 90th percentile, especially with above-average skinfold thickness 2. Children who fail to show the expected gain in height and weight, especially during the rapid growth periods of infancy and adolescence 3. Children who show a sudden increase, except during puberty, or decrease in a previously steady growth pattern Compare findings with growth patterns of other family members: consider genetic influence on growth determination (see Chinese growth chart, p. 159). Compare children's growth trends (height and weight) with midparental height (MPH). Most children with normal birth weights and heights and normal childhood growth will achieve an adult height within ±2 inches of MPH. Special charts are available for parent-specific adjustments for evaluation of the child's height. To calculate MPH, use the following formulas: For girls: $\frac{\text{Father's height} - 13\text{ cm or 5 inches} + \text{Mother's height}}{2}$ For boys: $\frac{\text{Father's height} + 13\text{ cm or 5 inches} + \text{Mother's height}}{2}$

SAFETY ALERT

The 50th percentile represents the median growth (or midpoint of all the growth measurements for each age). The 5th percentile represents the lowest 5%, and the 95th percentile represents the highest 5% of growth measurements for each age.

Continued

Summary of Physical Assessment of the Child–cont'd

Assessment	Procedure
Length and Height	Recumbent length in children below 24-36 months: Place supine with head in midline. Grasp knees and push gently toward table to *fully* extend legs. Measure from vertex (top) of head to heels of feet (toes pointing upward). Standing height (stature) in children over 24-36 months: Remove socks and shoes. Have child stand as tall as possible, back straight, head in midline, and eyes looking straight ahead (see Figure 1-6, *B.*) Check for flexion of knees, slumping shoulders, raising of heels. Measure from top of head to standing surface. Measure to the nearest cm or ⅛ inch.
Weight	Weigh infants and young children nude on platform-type scale; protect infant by placing hand above body to prevent falling off scale. Weigh older children in underwear (and gown if privacy is a concern; no shoes) on standing-type upright scale. Check that scale is balanced before weighing. Cover scale with clean sheet of paper for each child. Measure to the nearest 10 g or ½ ounce for infants and 100 g or ¼ pound for children.
Head Circumference (HC)	Measure with paper or steel tape at greatest circumference, from top of the eyebrows and pinna of the ear to occipital prominence of skull.
Chest Circumference	Measure around chest at nipple line. Ideally, take measurements during inhalation and expiration; record the average of the two values.
Pulse	Take apical pulse in children younger than 2-3 years. Point of maximum intensity located lateral to nipple at fourth to fifth interspace at or near midclavicular line. Take radial pulse in children older than 2-3 years. Count pulse for 1 full minute, especially if any irregularity is present. For repeated measurement, count pulse for 15 or 30 seconds and multiply by 4 or 2, respectively.

Usual Findings	Comments
Plot on growth chart (pp. 150-158). Compare value with percentile for weight. Rule of thumb guide*: At 1 year = 1.5 × birth length 2-12 years = Age (years) 2.5 + 30 = length (inches)	For accurate measurements, use infant-measuring device for recumbent length and stadiometer for standing height. Normally height is less if measured in the afternoon than in the morning. To minimize this variation, apply modest upward pressure under the jaw or the mastoid processes.

Expected Growth Rates at Various Ages*

Age	Expected Growth Rate (cm/year)
1-6 months	18-22
6-12 months	14-18
Second year	11
Third year	8
Fourth year	7
Fifth to tenth years	5-6

*From *Human growth and disorders: an update,* South San Francisco, 1989, Genentech.

Usual Findings	Comments
Plot on growth chart (see pp. 150-158). Compare value with percentile for length. Rule of thumb guides*: At 1 year = 3 × birth weight 1-9 years: age (years) × 5 + 17 = weight (pounds) 9-12 years: age (years) × 9 − 20 = weight (pounds)	Compare weight with appearance, for example, excessive fat, well-developed musculature, flabby, loose skin, bony prominences (for skinfold measurement, see below). Assess nutritional status; compare with weight.
Plot on growth chart (see p. 147). Compare percentile with those of height and weight. Compare with chest circumference: At birth, HC exceeds chest circumference by 2-3 cm (1 inch). At 1-2 years, HC equals chest circumference. During childhood, chest circumference exceeds HC by about 5-7 cm (2-3 inches).	Usually taken in children under 36 months of age Taken in any child whose head size appears abnormal
Compare with head circumference (see earlier).	May be measured during examination of chest
(For average pulse rates at rest, see inside front cover.)	Pulse rate normally may increase with inspiration and decrease with expiration (sinus arrhythmia) (See also Box 1-6.) May grade pulses: **Grade 0** Not palpable **Grade +1** Difficult to palpate, thready, weak, easily obliterated with pressure **Grade +2** Difficult to palpate, may be obliterated with pressure **Grade +3** Easy to palpate, not easily obliterated with pressure (normal) **Grade +4** Strong, bounding, not obliterated with pressure

*Based on NCHS growth charts for boys, 50th percentile (see pp. 150-153) For explanation of percentiles, see Safety Alert, p. 37.

Continued

Summary of Physical Assessment of the Child–cont'd

Assessment	Procedure
Respiration	Observe rate of breathing for 1 full minute. In infants and young children, observe abdominal movement. In older children, observe thoracic movement.
Blood Pressure	*Selection of Cuff*

No matter what type of noninvasive technique is used, the most important factor in accurately measuring BP is the use of an appropriately sized cuff (cuff size refers only to the inner inflatable bladder, not the cloth covering) (Table 1-1). A technique to establish an appropriate cuff size is to choose a cuff having a bladder width that is approximately 40% of the arm circumference midway between the olecranon and the acromion. This will usually be a cuff bladder that covers 80% to 100% of the circumference of the arm (Figure 1-7). Researchers have found that selection of a cuff with a bladder width equal to 40% of the upper arm circumference most accurately reflects directly measured radial arterial pressure.

Cuffs that are either too narrow or too wide affect the accuracy of BP measurements. If the cuff size is too small, the reading on the device is falsely high. If the cuff size is too large, the reading is falsely low.

When another site is used, BP measurements using noninvasive techniques may differ. Generally, systolic pressure in the lower extremities (thigh or calf) is greater than pressure in the upper extremities, and systolic BP in the calf is higher than that in the thigh (see Figure 1-7). These differences are listed in Table 1-2 and apply to oscillometric measurements taken on the right extremities with the child supine and the cuff size based on the circumference method.

TABLE 1-1 Recommended Dimensions for Blood Pressure Cuff Bladders

Age Range	Width (cm)	Length (cm)	Maximum Arm Circumference (cm)*
Newborn	4	8	10
Infant	6	12	15
Child	9	18	22
Small adult	10	24	26
Adult	13	30	34
Large adult	16	38	44
Thigh	20	42	52

From National High Blood Pressure Education Program Working Group on High Blood Pressure in Children and Adolescents: The fourth report on the diagnosis, evaluation, and treatment of high blood pressure in children and adolescents, *Pediatrics* 114:555-576, 2004.

*Calculated so that the largest arm would still allow the bladder to encircle arm by at least 80%.

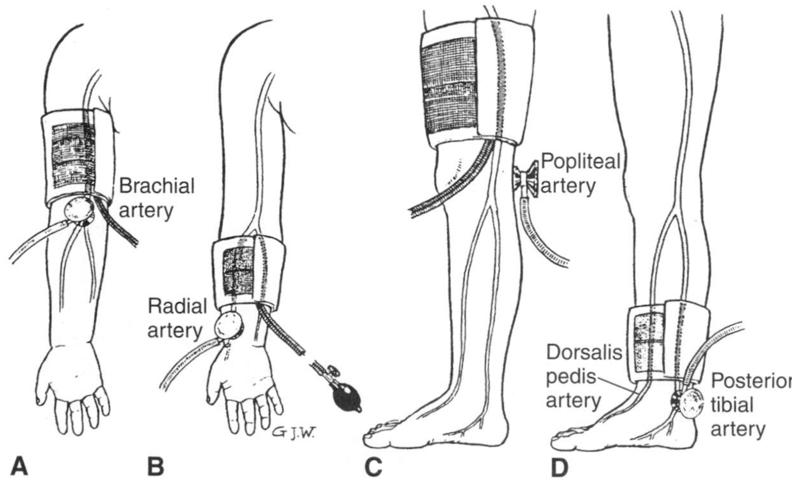

FIGURE **1-7** Sites for measuring blood pressure. **A,** Upper arm. **B,** Lower arm or forearm. **C,** Thigh. **D,** Calf or ankle.

Usual Findings	Comments
(For average respiratory rates at rest, see inside front cover.)	

SAFETY ALERT

Published norms for BP, such as those on the inside front cover, are valid only if the same method of measurement (auscultation and cuff size determination) is used in clinical practice.

SAFETY ALERT

When taking blood pressure, use an appropriately sized cuff. When the correct size is not available, use an oversized cuff rather than an undersized one or use another site that more appropriately fits the cuff size. Do not choose a cuff based on the name of the cuff (e.g., an "infant" cuff may be too small for some infants).

Repeat measurements above 95th percentile later during initial visit when child is least anxious; if a high reading persists, repeat measurements at least three times during subsequent visits to detect hypertension

Significant hypertension: Blood pressure persistently between 95th and 99th percentile for age, gender, and height

Severe hypertension: Blood pressure persistently at or above 99th percentile for age, gender, and height

Refer children with consistently high blood pressure readings or significant differences in pressure between upper and lower extremities for further evaluation (e.g., in newborns a calf pressure less than 6-9 mm Hg compared with upper arm pressure).*

Blood pressure readings using oscillometry are generally higher than those using auscultation but correlate better with direct radial artery blood pressure than auscultation readings (Table 1-3).†

TABLE 1-2 Differences in Oscillometric Systolic BP Between Arm and Lower Extremity Sites in Normal Children

	Systolic BP × (Mean ± SD)	
Age-Group (years)	Arm-Thigh	Arm-Calf
4-8	−7.1 ± 6.8	−9.3 ± 7.4
9-16	−2.4 ± 7.7	−5 ± 26.9

From Park M, Lee D, Johnson GA: Oscillometric blood pressures in the arm, thigh, and calf in healthy children and those with aortic coarctation, *Pediatrics* 91(4):761-765, 1993.

TABLE 1-3 Normative Dinamap (Oscillometry) Blood Pressure Values (Systolic/Diastolic, Mean in Parentheses)

Age-Group	Mean	90th Percentile	95th Percentile
Newborn (1-3 days)	65/41(50)	75/49(59)	78/52(62)
1-24 months	95/58(72)	106/68(83)	110/71(86)
2-5 years	101/57(74)	112/66(82)	115/68(85)

Data from Park M, Menard S: Normative oscillometric blood pressure values in the first five years in an office setting, *Am J Dis Child* 143(7):860-864, 1989.

*Park M, Lee D: Normative arm and calf blood pressure values in the newborn, *Pediatrics* 83(2):240-243, 1989.

†Park M, Menard S: Accuracy of blood pressure measurement by the Dinamap monitor in infants and children, *Pediatrics* 79(6):907-914, 1987.

Continued

Summary of Physical Assessment of the Child–cont'd

Assessment	Procedure
General Appearance	
	Observe the following: Facies Posture Body movement Hygiene Nutrition Behavior Development State of awareness
Skin	
	Observe skin in natural daylight or neutral artificial light.
	Color—Most reliably assessed in sclera, conjunctiva, nail beds, tongue, buccal mucosa, palms, and soles
	Texture—Note moisture, smoothness, roughness, integrity of skin, and temperature. *Temperature*—Compare each part of body for even temperature.

Usual Findings	Comments
Evaluated in terms of a comprehensive assessment; often gives clues to underlying problems such as poor hygiene and nutrition from parental neglect or poverty	Record actual observations that lead to a conclusion, such as signs of poor hygiene; give examples of present development milestones. Follow up on clues that may indicate problems, for example, investigate feeding practices of family if child appears undernourished.
	Reveals significant clues to problems such as poor hygiene, child abuse, inadequate nutrition, and serious physical disorders.
Genetically determined: Light-skinned—From milky white to rosy colored Dark-skinned—Various shades of brown, red, yellow, olive, and bluish tones	Observe for abnormalities such as pallor, cyanosis, erythema, ecchymosis, petechiae, and jaundice (Table 1-4). Factors affecting color include natural skin tone, melanin production, edema, hygiene, hemoglobin levels of blood, amount of lighting, color of room, atmospheric temperature, and use of cosmetics.
Smooth, slightly dry to touch, with even temperature	Note obvious changes, such as clammy skin, oily skin, obvious lesions, and excessive dryness (Boxes 1-3 and 1-4).
Usually same all over body, although exposed parts, such as hands, may be cooler	Note obvious differences, such as warm upper extremities and cold lower extremities.

TABLE 1-4 Differences in Color Changes of Racial Groups

Color Change	Appearance in Light Skin	Appearance in Dark Skin
Cyanosis	Bluish tinge, especially in palpebral conjunctiva (lower eyelid), nail beds, earlobes, lips, oral membranes, soles, and palms	Ashen gray lips and tongue
Pallor	Loss of rosy glow in skin, especially face	Ashen gray appearance in black skin More yellowish brown color in brown skin
Erythema	Redness easily seen anywhere on body	Much more difficult to assess; palpate for warmth or edema
Ecchymoses	Purplish to yellow-green areas; may be seen anywhere on skin	Very difficult to see unless in mouth or conjunctiva
Petechiae	Purplish pinpoints most easily seen on buttocks, abdomen, and inner surfaces of the arms or legs	Usually invisible except in oral mucosa, conjunctiva of eyelids, and conjunctiva covering eyeball
Jaundice	Yellow staining seen in sclera of eyes, skin, fingernails, soles, palms, and oral mucosa	Most reliably assessed in sclera, hard palate, palms, and soles

Continued

Summary of Physical Assessment of the Child–cont'd

Assessment	Procedure
Skin—cont'd	
	Turgor—Grasp skin on abdomen between thumb and index finger, pull taut, and release quickly. Indent skin with finger.

BOX 1-3 | PRIMARY SKIN LESIONS

Macule

Flat, circumscribed area of color change (red, brown, purple, white, tan); less than 1 cm in diameter; nonpalpable
Example: Freckle, flat mole, rubella, rubeola

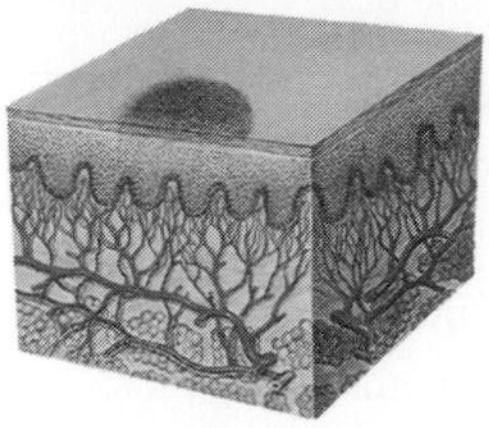

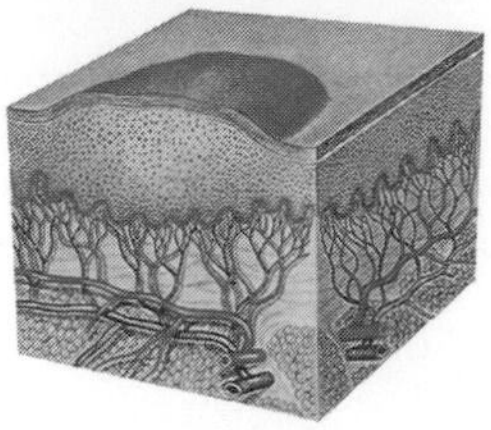

Wheal

Elevated, irregularly shaped area of cutaneous edema; solid, transient, changing; variable diameter; pale pink with lighter center
Example: Insect bites, urticaria

Papule

Small, circumscribed, firm, elevated, palpable discoloration (red, pink, tan, brown, bluish); less than 1 cm in diameter; the more superficial it is, the more distinct are the borders
Example: Wart, drug-related eruptions, pigmented nevi

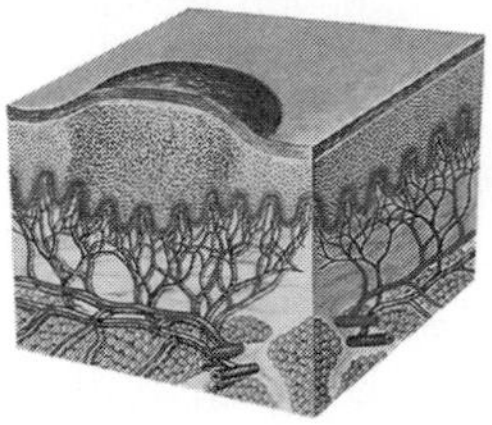

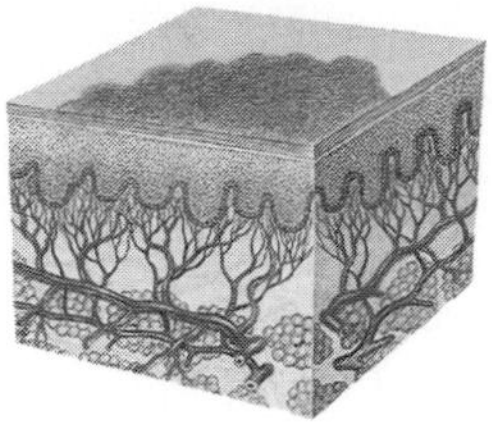

Patch

Flat, circumscribed, irregularly shaped, discoloration; nonpalpable; greater than 1 cm in diameter
Example: Vitiligo, port-wine marks

Nodule

Circumscribed, firm elevation; palpable: round or ellipsoid; located deeper in dermis than papules; 1-2 cm in diameter
Example: Erythema nodosum, lipoma

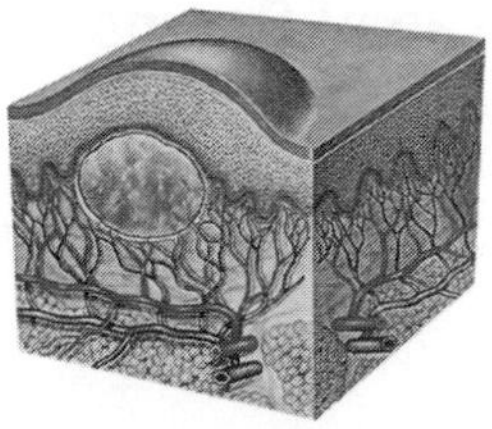

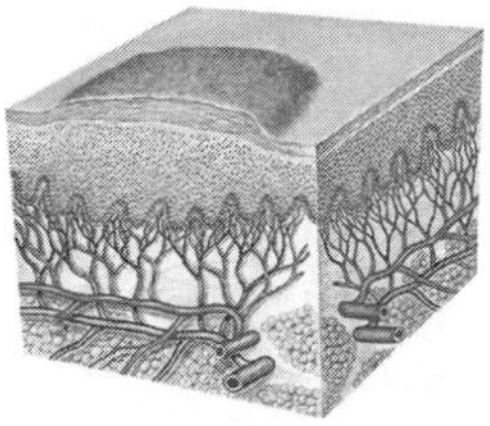

Plaque

Elevated; flat topped; firm; rough; superficial papule; greater than 1 cm in diameter
Example: Psoriasis, seborrheic and actinic keratoses

Cyst

Elevated, circumscribed, palpable, encapsulated, filled with liquid or semisolid material
Example: Sebaceous cyst

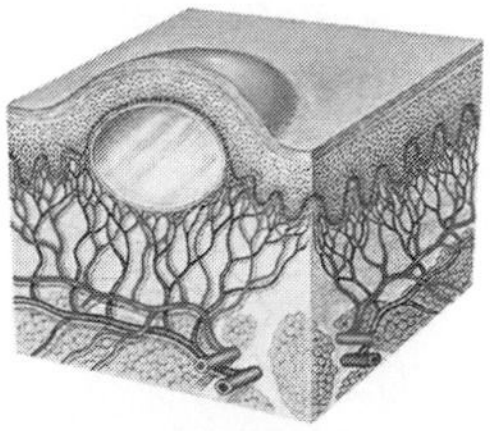

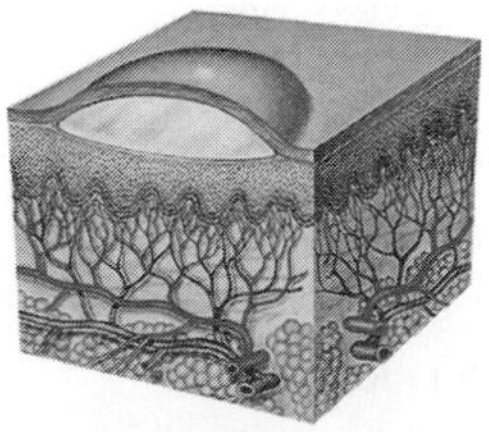

Vesicle

Small (less than 1 cm in diameter), superficial circumscribed elevation; contains serous fluid
Example: Varicella, blister

Pustule

Elevated, superficial, similar to vesicle but filled with purulent fluid
Example: Acne, impetigo, variola

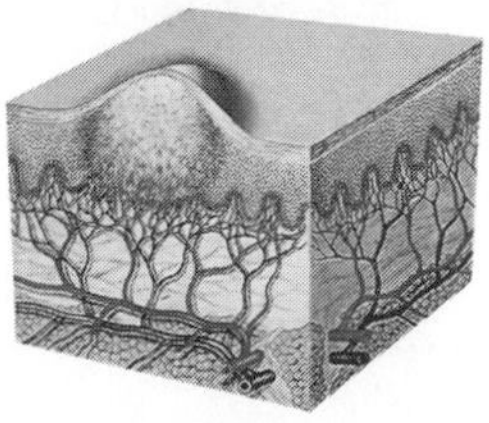

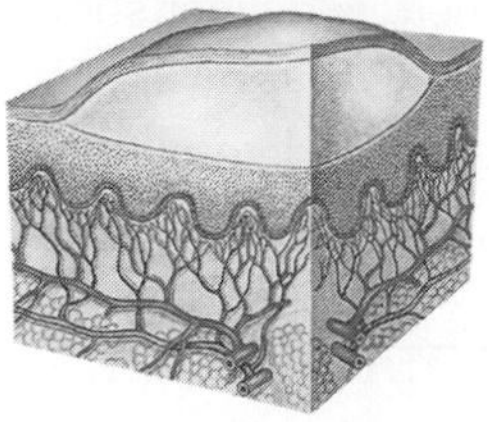

Bulla

Fluid-filled vesicle greater than 1 cm in diameter; a large vesicle; bleb; blister
Example: Blister, pemphigus vulgaris

Illustrations from Seidel HM and others: *Mosby's guide to physical examination,* ed 6, St Louis, 2006, Mosby.

Usual Findings	Comments
Resumes shape immediately with no tenting, wrinkling, or prolonged depression	Good skin turgor indicates adequate hydration and possibly nutrition. Note "tenting" or poor elasticity of the pulled skin (sign of dehydration and/or malnutrition) or obvious pitting of skin on indentation or signs of swelling (signs of edema).

BOX 1-4 | SECONDARY SKIN LESIONS

Mound of keratinized cells; flaky exfoliation; irregular shape; variable thickness and diameter; dry or oily; silver, white, or tan
Example: Psoriasis, exfoliative dermatitis

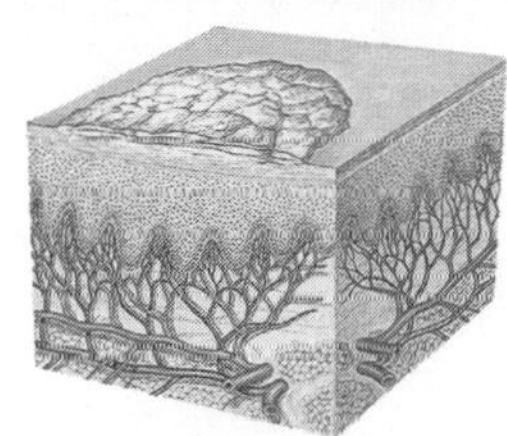

Scale

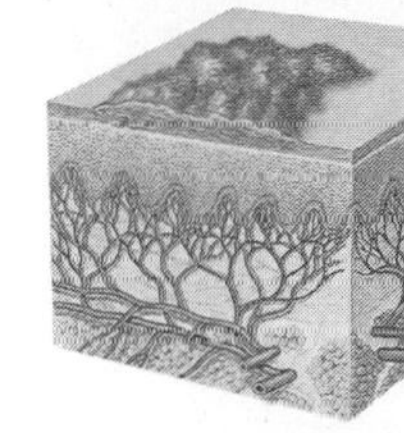

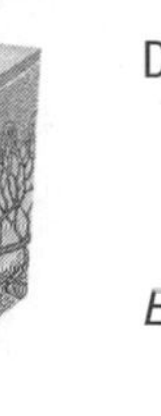

Crust

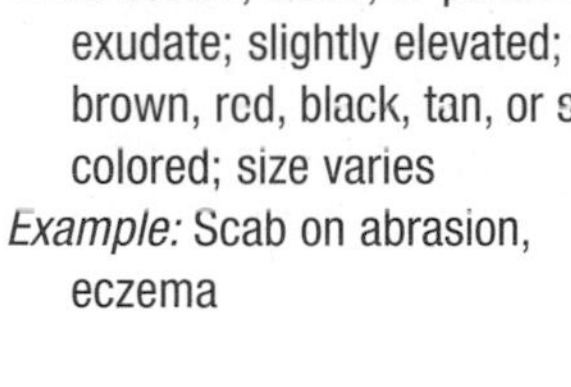

Dried serum, blood, or purulent exudate; slightly elevated; brown, red, black, tan, or straw colored; size varies
Example: Scab on abrasion, eczema

Concave with loss of epidermis and dermis; variable size; exudative; red or reddish blue
Example: Decubiti, stasis ulcers

Ulcer

Fissure

Deep linear split through epidermis into dermis; small; deep; red
Example: Chapping, tinea pedis

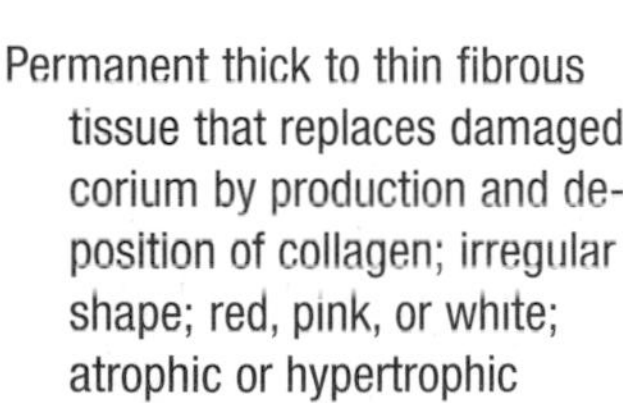

Permanent thick to thin fibrous tissue that replaces damaged corium by production and deposition of collagen; irregular shape; red, pink, or white; atrophic or hypertrophic
Example: Vaccination, healed wound, abrasion, laceration

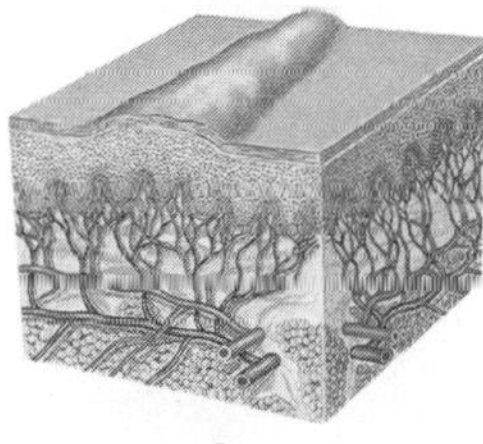

Scar

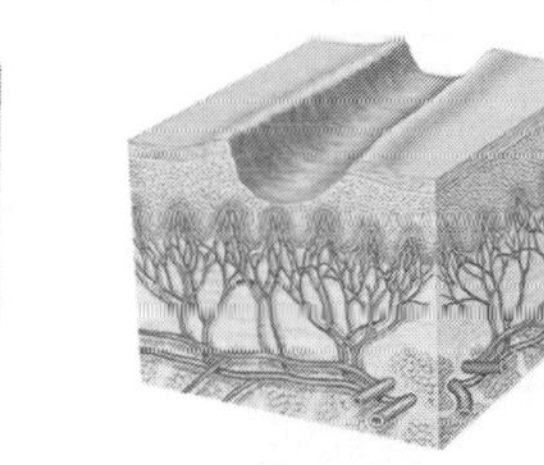

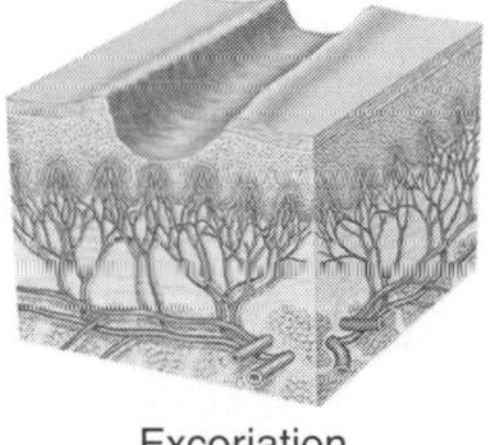

Excoriation

Loss of superficial epidermis, linear or punctate
Example: Scratch, abrasion

Rough, thickened epidermis; accentuated skin markings caused by rubbing or irritation; often involves flexor aspect of extremity
Example: Chronic dermatitis

Lichenification

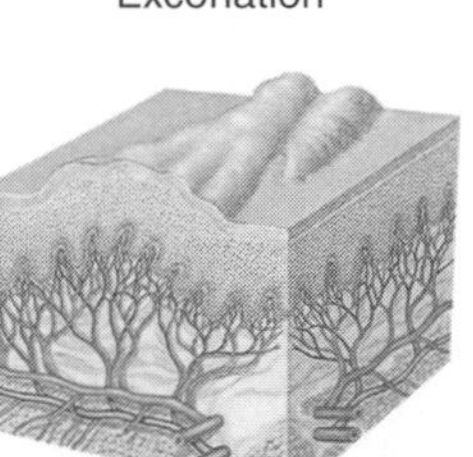

Keloid

Irregularly shaped, elevated, progressively enlarging scar; grows beyond boundaries of wound; caused by excessive collagen formation during healing
Example: Keloid from ear piercing or burn scar

Loss of all or part of epidermis; depressed; moist; glistening; follows rupture of vesicle or bulla; larger than fissure
Example: Varicella; variola following rupture

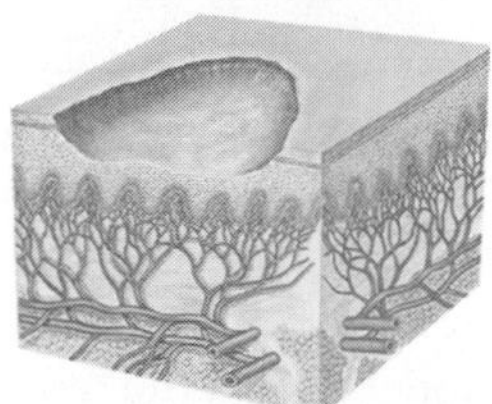

Erosion

Illustrations from Seidel HM and others: *Mosby's guide to physical examination,* ed 6, St Louis, 2006, Mosby.

Continued

Summary of Physical Assessment of the Child–cont'd

Assessment	Procedure
Accessory Structures	
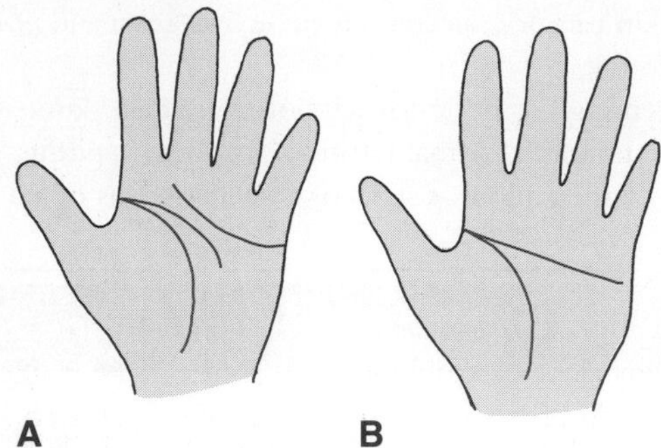 FIGURE **1-8** **A**, Example of normal flexion crease on palm. **B**, Transpalmar crease.	***Hair***—Inspect color, texture, quality, distribution, elasticity, and hygiene. ***Nails***—Inspect color, shape, texture, quality, distribution, elasticity, and hygiene. ***Dermatoglyphics***—Observe flexion creases of palm (Figure 1-8).
Lymph Nodes	
See Figure 1-9.	Palpate using distal portion of fingers. Press gently but firmly in a circular motion. Note size, mobility, temperature, tenderness, and any change in enlarged nodes. ***Submaxillary***—Tilt head slightly downward. ***Cervical***—Tilt head slightly upward. ***Axillary***—Have arms relaxed at side but slightly abducted. ***Inguinal***—Place child supine.
Head	
	Note shape and symmetry. Note head control (especially in infants) and head posture. Evaluate range of motion (ROM).

Usual Findings	Comments
Lustrous, silky, strong, elastic hair Genetic factors influence appearance; for example, a black child's hair is usually coarser, duller, and curlier.	Signs of poor nutrition include stringy, friable, dull, dry, depigmented hair. Note areas of baldness, unusual hairiness, and any evidence of infestation. During puberty, secondary hair growth indicates normal pubertal changes.
Pink, convex, smooth, and flexible, not brittle In dark-skinned child, color is darker.	Note color changes, such as blueness or yellow tint. Observe for uncut or short, ragged nails (nail biting). Report any signs of clubbing (base of the nail becomes swollen and feels springy or floating when palpated), a sign of serious respiratory or cardiac dysfunction.
Three flexion creases	If pattern differs, draw a sketch to describe it. Observe for transpalmar crease (one horizontal crease; see Figure 1-8, *B*), a characteristic of children with Down syndrome.
Generally not palpable, although small, nontender, movable nodes are normal	Note tender, enlarged, warm nodes, which usually indicate infection or inflammation *proximal* to their location.

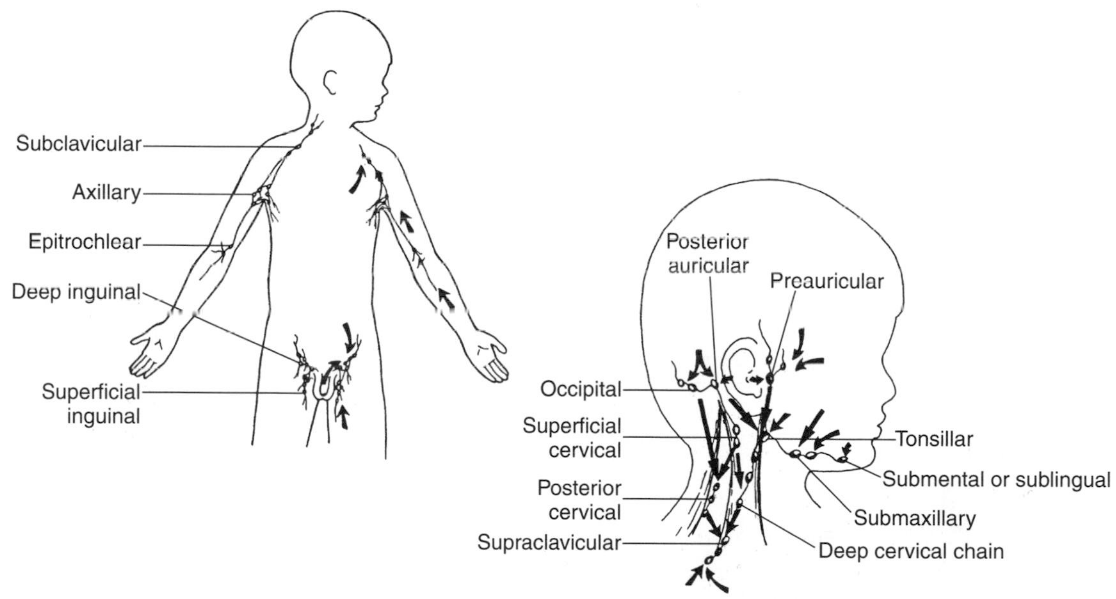

FIGURE **1-9** Locations of superficial lymph nodes. Arrows indicate directional flow of lymph.

Usual Findings	Comments
Even molding of head, occipital prominence Symmetric facial features Head control well established by 6 months of age Head in midline Moves head up, down, and from side to side	Report any deviations from expected findings. Clues to problems include the following: Uneven molding—Premature closure of sutures Asymmetry—Paralysis Head lag—Retarded motor or mental development Head tilt—Poor vision Limited ROM—Torticollis (wryneck)

Continued

Summary of Physical Assessment of the Child—cont'd

Assessment	Procedure

Head—cont'd

Palpate skull for fontanels, nodes, or obvious swellings.

Transilluminate skull in darkened room; firmly place rubber-collared flashlight against skull at various points.

Examine scalp for hygiene, lesions, infestation, signs of trauma, loss of hair, discoloration.

Percuss frontal sinuses in children older than 7 years.

Neck

Inspect size.

Trachea—Palpate for deviation; place thumb and index finger on each side and slide fingers back and forth.

Thyroid—Palpate, noting size, shape, symmetry, tenderness, nodules; place pads of index and middle fingers below cricoid cartilage; feel for isthmus (tissue connecting lobes) rising during swallowing; feel each lobe laterally and posteriorly.

Carotid arteries—Palpate on both sides.

Eyes

Upward palpebral slant

FIGURE **1-10** Upward palpebral slant.

Inspect placement and alignment.

If abnormality is suspected, measure inner canthal distance.

Palpebral slant—Draw imaginary line through two points of medial (inner) canthi (Figure 1-10).

Epicanthal fold—Observe for excess fold from roof of nose to inner termination of eyebrow (Figure 1-11).

Lids—Observe placement, movement, and color (see Figure 1-10).

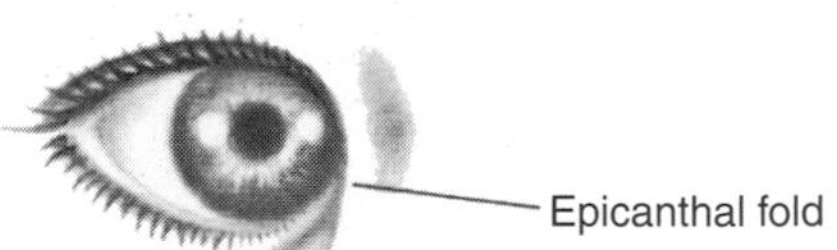

FIGURE **1-11** Epicanthal fold.

Palpebral conjunctiva

Pull lower lid down while child looks up.

Evert upper lid by holding lashes and pulling down and forward.

Observe color.

Bulbar conjunctiva—Observe color.

Lacrimal punctum—Observe color.

Eyelashes and eyebrows—Observe distribution and direction of growth.

Sclera—Observe color (Figure 1-12).

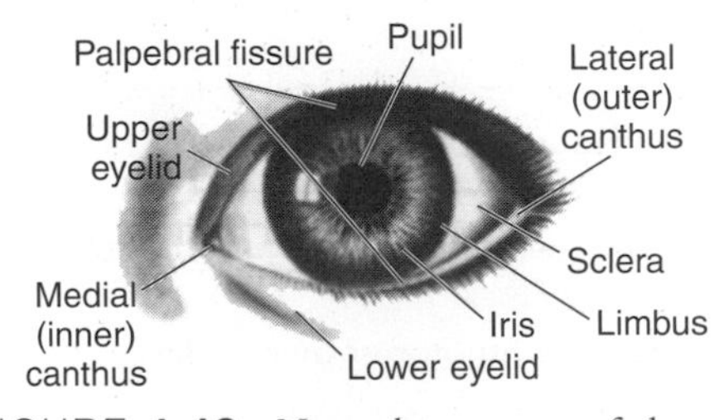

FIGURE **1-12** Normal structures of the eye.

Usual Findings	Comments
Smooth, fused except for fontanels (see p. 22) Posterior fontanel closes by 2 months Anterior fontanel closes by 12-18 months	Resistance to movement and pain—Meningeal irritation
Absence of halo around rubber collar	Halo of light through skull—Loss of cortex (hydrocephaly)
Clean, pink (more deeply pigmented in dark-skinned children)	Ecchymotic areas on scalp—Trauma (possibly abuse) Loss of hair—Trauma (hair pulling), lack of stimulation (lying in same position)
	Painful sinuses—Infection
During infancy, normally short with skinfolds During early childhood, lengthens In midline; rises with swallowing	Note any webbing. Note any deviation, masses, or nodules when palpating neck structures.
In midline; rises with swallowing; lobes equal but often are not palpable	Thyroid is often difficult to palpate. Inquire if child ever received radiation therapy to neck or upper chest area.
Equal bilaterally	Note unequal pulses and protruding neck veins.
Placement is symmetric. Inner canthal distance averages 3 cm (1.2 inches).	Note asymmetry, abnormal spacing (hypertelorism).
Usually palpebral fissures lie horizontally on imaginary line; in Asians, there may be an upward slant.	Presence of upward slant and epicanthal folds in children who are not Asian is significant finding in Down syndrome.
Often present in Asian children	May give false impression of strabismus
When eye is open, falls between upper iris and pupil When eye is closed, sclera, cornea, and palpebral conjunctiva are completely covered. Symmetric blink Color is same as surrounding skin.	Observe for deviations: Ptosis (upper lid covers part of pupil or lower iris) Setting sun sign (upper lid above iris) Inability to completely close eye Entropion (turning in) Asymmetric, excessive, or infrequent blinking Signs of inflammation along lid margin or on lid
Pink and glossy Vertical yellow striations along edge near hair follicle	Note any signs of inflammation. Excessive pallor may indicate anemia.
Transparent and white color of underlying sclera	A reddened conjunctiva may indicate eye strain, fatigue, infection, or irritation such as from excessive rubbing or exposure to environmental irritants.
Same color as lid	Excessive discharge, tearing, pain, redness, or swelling indicates dacryocystitis.
Eyelashes curl away from eye. Eyebrows are above eye; do not meet in midline.	Note inward growth of lashes and unusual hairiness of brows.
White	Note any yellow staining, which may indicate jaundice.

Continued

Summary of Physical Assessment of the Child—cont'd

Assessment	Procedure
Eyes—cont'd	
	Cornea—Check for opacities by shining light toward eye.
	Pupils (see Figure 1-12) Compare size, shape, and movement. Test reaction to light; shine light source toward and away from eye. Test accommodation; have child focus on object from distance and bring object close to face. ***Iris***—Observe shape, color, size, and clarity (see Figure 1-12).
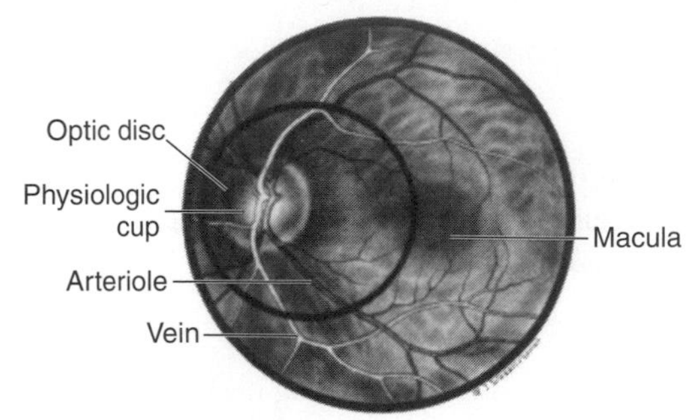 FIGURE **1-13** Structures of the fundus. Interior circle represents approximate size of area seen with ophthalmoscope.	***Lens***—Inspect. ***Fundus*** (Figure 1-13) Examine with ophthalmoscope set at 0; approach the child from a 15-degree angle; change to plus or minus diopters to produce clear focus. Measure structures in relationship to disc's diameter (DD). To facilitate locating macula, have child momentarily look *directly* at light. Assess vision (for visual acuity, see pp. 170-176).
	Use following tests for binocular vision: ***Corneal light reflex test*** (also called *red reflex gemini* or *Hirschberg test*)—Shine a light directly into the eyes from a distance of about 40.5 cm (16 inches). ***Cover test***—Have child fixate on near (33 cm [13 inches]) or distant (50 cm [20 inches]) object; cover one eye, and observe movement of the uncovered eye. ***Alternate cover test***—Same as cover test, except rapidly cover one eye then the other eye several times; observe movement of covered eye when it is uncovered ***Peripheral vision***—Have child look straight ahead; move an object, such as your finger, from beyond child's field of vision into view; ask the child to signal as soon as the object is seen; estimate the angle from straight line of vision to first detection of peripheral vision. ***Color vision***—Use Ishihara or Hardy-Rand-Rittler test.

Usual Findings	Comments
Tiny black marks normal in deeply pigmented children Transparent	Note any opacities or ulcerations.
Round, clear, and equal Pupils constrict when light approaches, dilate when light fades. Pupils constrict as object is brought near face.	***PERRLA*** is common notation for pupils equal, round, react to light and accommodation. Note any asymmetry in size and movement.
Round, equal, clear Color varies from shades of brown, green, or blue.	Note asymmetry in size, lack of clarity, coloboma (cleft at limbus [junction of iris and sclera]), absence of color (a pinkish glow is seen in albinism), or black and white speckling (Brushfield spots are commonly found in Down syndrome).
Should not be seen	Note any opacities.
Red reflex—Brilliant, uniform reflection of red; appears darker color in deeply pigmented children, lighter in infants ***Optic disc***—Creamy pink but lighter than surrounding fundus, round or vertically oval ***Physiologic cup***—Small, pale depression in center of disc ***Blood vessels***—Emanate from disc; veins are darker and about one fourth larger than arteries; narrow band of light, the *arteriolar light reflex*, is reflected from center of arteries, not veins; branches cross each other; may see obvious pulsations ***Macula***—1 DD in size, darker in color than disc or surrounding fundus, located 2 DD temporal to the disc ***Fovea centralis***—Minute, glistening spot of reflected light in center of macula	Visualization of red reflex virtually rules out most serious defects of cornea, lens, and aqueous and vitreous chambers. Observe for abnormalities: Partial red or white reflex Blurring of disc margins Bulging of disc Loss of depression Dilated blood vessels Tortuous vessels Hemorrhages Absence of pulsations Notching or indenting at crossing of vessels
Binocularity is well established by 3-4 months of age.	Refer any child with nonbinocular vision because of malalignment (strabismus) for further evaluation.
Light falls symmetrically within each pupil.	Abnormal if light falls asymmetrically in each pupil
Uncovered eye does not move.	Abnormal if uncovered eye moves when other eye is covered
Neither eye moves when covered or uncovered.	Abnormal if covered eye moves as soon as occluder is removed
In each quadrant, sees object at 50 degrees upward, 70 degrees downward, 60 degrees nasalward, and 90 degrees temporally	Inability to see object until it is brought closer to straight line of vision indicates need for further evaluation
Able to see a letter or figure within the colored dots	Each test consists of cards on which a color field composed of spots of a certain "confusion" color is printed; against the field is a number (Ishihara) or symbol (Hardy-Rand-Rittler) similarly printed in dots but of a color likely to be confused with the field color by the person with a color vision deficit. Counsel the affected child and parents about the practical inconveniences caused by the disorder, the mode of genetic transmission, and its irreversibility.

Continued

Summary of Physical Assessment of the Child–cont'd

Assessment	Procedure
Ears	

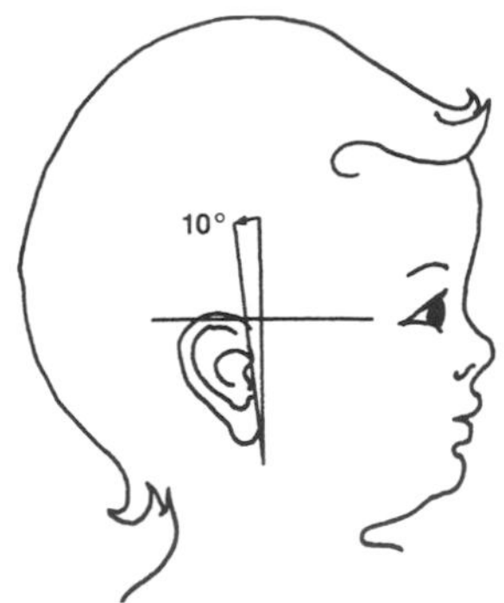

FIGURE **1-14** Placement and alignment of pinna.

Pinnae—Inspect placement and alignment (Figure 1-14).

1. Measure height of pinna by drawing an imaginary line from outer orbit of eye to occiput of skull.
2. Measure angle of pinna by drawing a perpendicular line from the imaginary horizontal line and aligning pinna next to this mark.

Observe the usual landmarks of the pinna.

Note presence of any abnormal openings, tags of skin, or sinuses.

Inspect hygiene (odor, discharge, color).

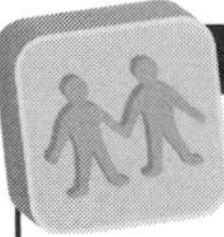

ATRAUMATIC CARE

Reducing Distress from Otoscopy in Young Children

Make examining the ear a game by explaining that you are looking for a "big elephant" in the ear. This kind of fairy tale is an absorbing distraction and usually elicits cooperation. After the ear has been examined, clarify that "looking for elephants" was only pretending and thank the child for letting you look in his or her ear. Another great distraction technique is asking the child to put a finger on the opposite ear to keep the light from getting out.

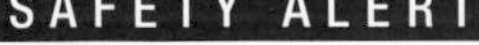

SAFETY ALERT

Sometimes it takes an extra hand to examine a child's ear—one hand to hold the otoscope, a second hand to use the bulb (or a curette), and a third hand to straighten the canal. To gain a third hand, enlist a cooperative child's help. Have the child raise the arm opposite the affected ear up and over the head toward the opposite side. Then ask the child to grasp the upper edge of the earlobe at about the 10 or 1 o'clock position and pull the lobe gently up and back.

Examine external canal and middle ear structures with otoscope (Atraumatic Care box and Safety Alert):

Child younger than 3 years

Position prone with ear to be examined toward ceiling; lean over child, using upper portion of body to restrain arms and trunk and examining hand to restrain the head.

Alternate position: Seat child sideways in parent's lap; have parent hug child securely around trunk and arms and top of head.

Introduce speculum between 3 and 9 o'clock position in a *downward* and *forward* slant.

Pull pinna *down* and *back* to the 6-9 o'clock range (Figure 1-15, *A*).

Child over 3 years

Examine while seated with head tilted slightly away from examiner (if child needs restraining, use one of the previously mentioned positions).

Pull pinna *up* and *back* toward a 10 o'clock position (see Figure 1-15, *B*).

Insert speculum $\frac{1}{4}$-$\frac{1}{2}$ inch; use widest speculum that diameter of canal easily accommodates.

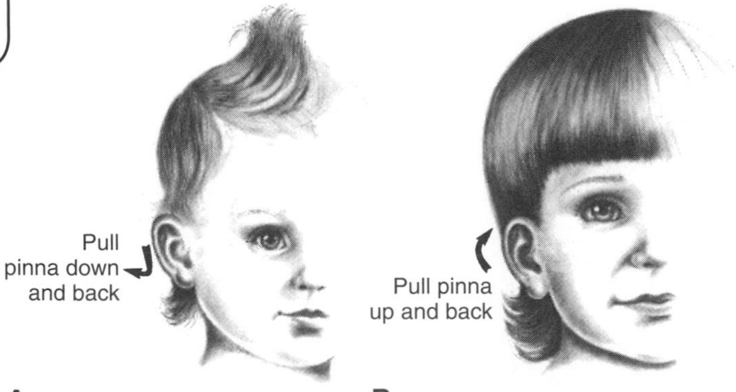

FIGURE **1-15** Positions of eardrum. **A**, Infant. **B**, Child over 3 years of age.

Usual Findings	Comments
Slightly crosses or meets this line	Low-set ears are commonly associated with renal anomalies or mental retardation.
Lies within a 10-degree angle of the vertical line	
Extends slightly forward from the skull	Flattened ears may indicate infrequent change of positioning from a side-lying placement; masses or swelling may make the pinna protrude.
Prominences and depressions symmetric	Abnormal landmarks are often signs of possible middle ear anomalies.
Adherent lobule (normal variation)	If abnormal opening is present, note any discharge.
Soft, yellow cerumen	If ear needs cleaning, discuss hygiene with parent or child. If ear is free of wax, ascertain the method of cleaning, advise against the use of cotton-tipped applicators or sharp or pointed objects in the canal.
External canal—Pink (more deeply colored in dark-skinned child), outermost portion lined with minute hairs, some soft yellow cerumen	Note signs of irritation, infection, foreign bodies, and desiccated, packed wax (may interfere with hearing). If discharge is present, change speculum to examine other ear.
Tympanic membrane (Figure 1-16) Translucent, light pearly pink or gray color Slight redness seen normally in infants and children as a result of crying Light reflex—Cone-shaped reflection, normally points away from face at 5 or 7 o'clock position Bony landmarks present	Note the following: Red, tense, bulging drum Dull, transparent gray color Black areas Absence of light reflex or bony prominences Retraction of drum with abnormal prominence of landmarks

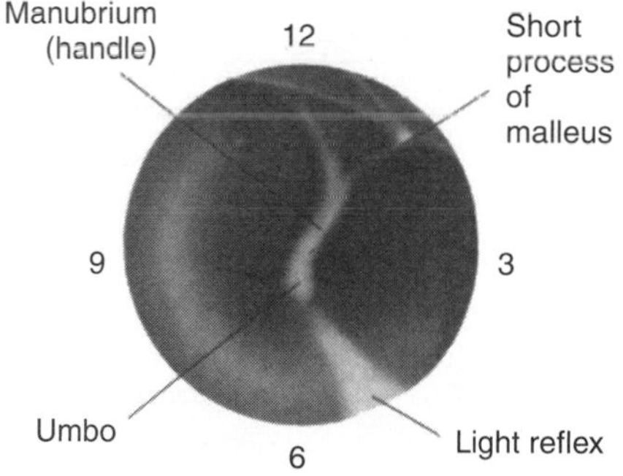

FIGURE **1-16** Landmarks of tympanic membrane with clock superimposed.

Continued

Summary of Physical Assessment of the Child–cont'd

Assessment	Procedure
Ears—cont'd	
	Assess hearing (see also pp. 177-179). ***Rinne test***—Place vibrating stem and tuning fork against mastoid bone until child no longer hears sound; move prongs close to auditory meatus. ***Weber test***—Hold tuning fork in midline of head or forehead.
Nose	
See Figure 1-17.	Inspect size, placement, and alignment; draw imaginary vertical line from center point between eyes to notch of upper lip. ***Anterior vestibule***—Tilt head backward; push tip of nose up, and illuminate cavity with flashlight; to detect perforated septum, shine light into one naris and observe for admittance of light through perforation.

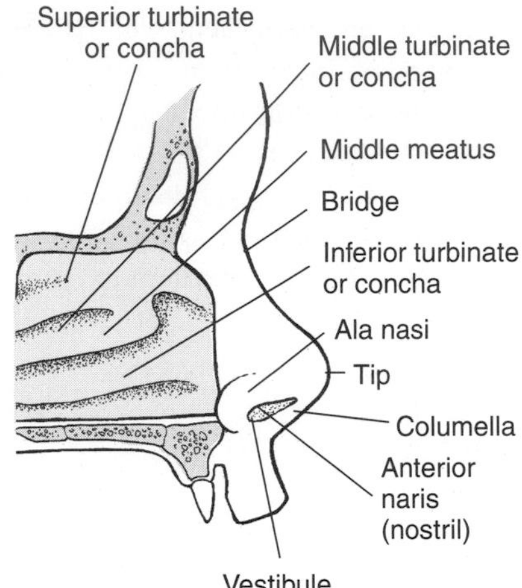

FIGURE **1-17** External landmarks and internal structures of the nose.

Assessment	Procedure
Mouth and Throat	
See Figure 1-18.	***Lips***—Note color, texture, any obvious lesions. Internal structures (Figure 1-18) Ask cooperative child to open mouth wide and say "Ahh"; usually not necessary to use tongue blade (Atraumatic Care box). With young child, place supine with both arms extended along side of head; have parent maintain arm position to immobilize head; may be necessary to use a tongue blade, but avoid eliciting gag reflex by depressing only toward the side of the tongue; use flashlight for good illumination.

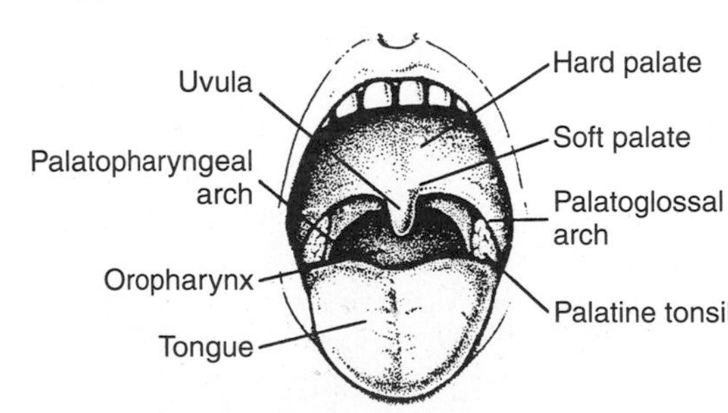

FIGURE **1-18** Internal structures of the mouth.

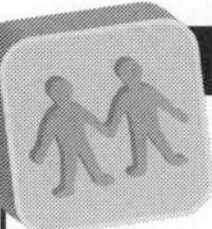

ATRAUMATIC CARE

Encouraging Opening the Mouth for Examination

Perform the examination in front of a mirror.
Let child first examine someone else's mouth, such as the parent, the nurse, or a puppet; then examine child's mouth.
Instruct child to tilt the head back slightly, breathe deeply through the mouth, and hold the breath; this action lowers the tongue to the floor of the mouth without using a tongue blade.

Usual Findings	Comments
Hears sound when prongs are brought close to ear	Rinne and Weber tests distinguish between bone and air conduction; both tests require cooperation and are better suited to children of school age or older.
Hears sound equally in both ears	Note abnormal results: Rinne positive—Sound is not audible through ear. Weber positive—Sound is heard better in *affected* ear.
Both nostrils equal in size Bridge of nose flattened in black or Asian children	Note any deviation to one side, inequality in size of nostrils, or flaring of alae nasi (sign of respiratory distress).
Mucosal lining—Redder than oral membranes, moist, but no discharge	Note the following: Abnormally pale, grayish pink, swollen, and boggy membranes Red, swollen membranes
Turbinate and meatus—Same color as mucosal lining	Any discharge Foreign object in nose
Septum—In midline	Deviated septum Perforated septum
More deeply pigmented than surrounding skin; smooth, moist	Note cyanosis, pallor, lesions, or cracks, especially at corners.
Mucous membranes—Bright pink, glistening, smooth, uniform, and moist	Note lesions, bleeding, sensitivity, odor.
Gingiva—Firm, coral pink, and stippled; margins are "knife-edged"	Note redness, puffiness (especially at margin), tendency to bleed.
Teeth—Number appropriate for age, white, good occlusion of upper and lower jaws General rule for estimating number of teeth in children under 2 years: age (in months) minus 6 (e.g., 12 months minus 6 = 6 teeth)	Note loss of teeth, delayed eruption, malocclusion, obvious discoloration. Compare dental findings with parental report of dental hygiene. Assess need for further dental counseling: Eating habits, such as bottle-feeding or prolonged breast-feeding during day for use as "pacifier" or at bedtime, excessive sugar Toothbrushing Sources of fluoride, need for supplementation Periodic, regular examinations by dentist
Tongue—Rough texture, freely movable, tip extends to lips, no lesions or masses under the tongue	Note smoothness, fissuring, coating on the tongue, excessive redness, swelling, or inability to move the tongue forward to lips; can interfere with speech.
Palate—Intact, slightly arched	Note presence of any clefts.
Uvula—Protrudes from back of soft palate, moves upward during gag reflex	Note if a bifid (divided in midline) uvula is present.

Continued

Summary of Physical Assessment of the Child–cont'd

Assessment	Procedure
Mouth and Throat—cont'd	
Chest	
See Figure 1-19.	Inspect size, shape, symmetry, and movement. Describe findings according to geographic and imaginary landmarks (Figure 1-20). Locate intercostal space (ICS), the space directly below rib, by palpating chest inferiorly from second rib. Other landmarks: Nipples usually at fourth ICS Tip of eleventh rib felt laterally Tip of twelfth rib felt posteriorly Tip of scapula at eighth rib or ICS
	Inspect breast development.

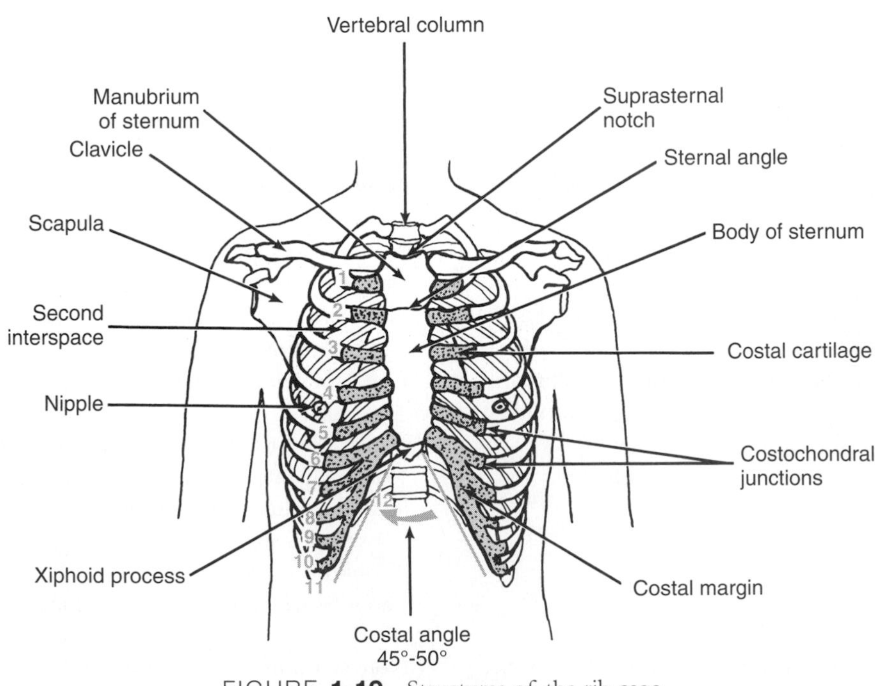

FIGURE **1-19** Structures of the rib cage.

Usual Findings	Comments
Palatine tonsils—Same color as surrounding mucosa, glandular rather than smooth, may be large in prepubertal children	Note exudate and enlargement that could become obstructive.
Posterior pharynx—Same color as surrounding mucosa, smooth, moist	Assess for signs of infection (erythema, edema, white lesions, or exudate).
In infants, shape is almost circular; with growth, the lateral diameter increases in proportion to anteroposterior diameter.	Measurement of chest and palpation of axillary nodes may be done here.
Both sides of chest symmetric Points of attachment between ribs and costal cartilage smooth ***Movement***—During inspiration chest expands, costal angle increases, and diaphragm descends; during expiration, reverse occurs. ***Nipples***—Darker pigmentation, located slightly lateral to mid-clavicular line between fourth and fifth ribs	Note deviations: Barrel-shaped chest Asymmetry Wide or narrow costal angle Bony prominences Pectus carinatum (pigeon breast)—Sternum protrudes outward **Pectus excavatum (funnel chest)**—Lower portion of sternum is depressed Retractions (Figure 1-21) Asymmetric or decreased movement
Breast development depends on age; no masses.	Compare breast development with expected stage for age (see p. 144). Discuss importance of monthly breast self-examination with female adolescents.

Continued

Summary of Physical Assessment of the Child–cont'd

Assessment	Procedure

Chest—cont'd

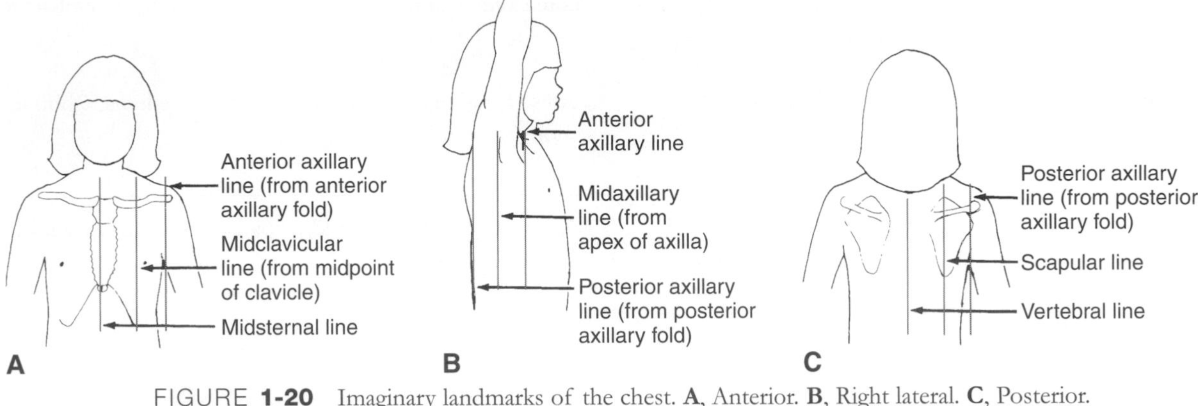

FIGURE **1-20** Imaginary landmarks of the chest. **A**, Anterior. **B**, Right lateral. **C**, Posterior.

Lungs

See Figure 1-22.

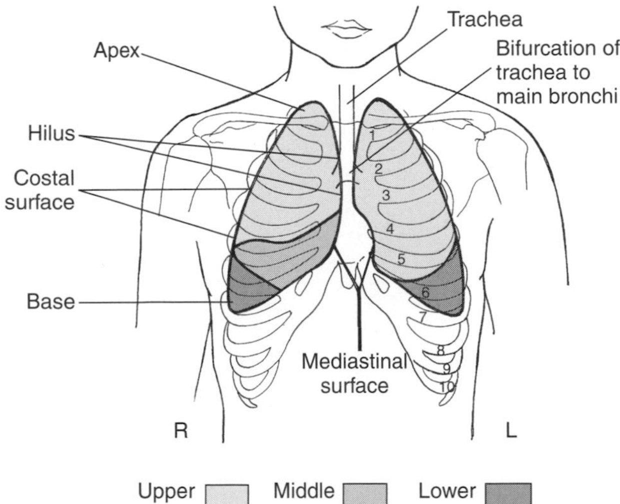

FIGURE **1-22** Location of anterior lobes of lungs within thoracic cavity.

Evaluate respiratory movements for rate, rhythm, depth, quality, and character. (See Atraumatic Care box below)

With child sitting, place each hand flat against back or chest with thumbs in midline along lower costal margins.

Vocal fremitus—Palpate as above, and have child say "99," "eee."

Percuss each side of chest in sequence from apex to base (Figure 1-23):
- For anterior aspects of lungs, child sitting or supine
- For posterior aspects of lungs, child sitting

Auscultate breath and voice sounds for intensity, pitch, quality, and relative duration of inspiration and expiration.

ATRAUMATIC CARE

Encouraging Deep Breaths

Ask child to "blow out" the light on an otoscope or pocket flashlight; discreetly turn off the light on the last try so that the child feels successful.

Place a cotton ball in child's palm; ask child to blow the ball into the air and have parent catch it.

Place a small tissue on the top of a pencil and ask child to blow the tissue off.

Have child blow a pinwheel, a party horn, or bubbles.

Usual Findings	Comments

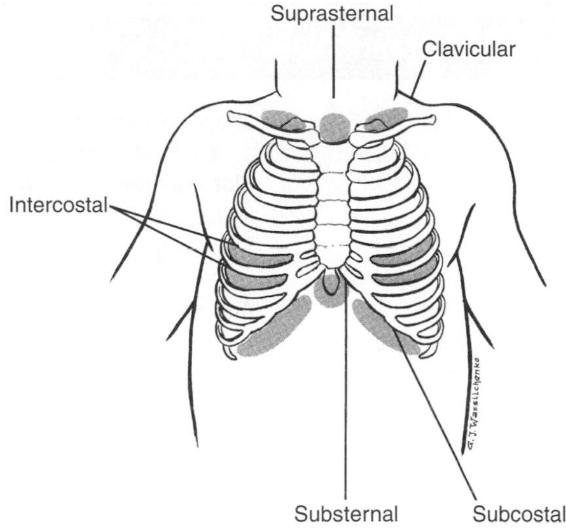

FIGURE **1-21** Location of retractions.

Usual Findings	Comments
Rate expected for age (see inside front cover), regular, effortless, and quiet	Note abnormal rate, irregular rhythm, shallow depth, difficult breathing, or noisy, grunting respirations (Box 1-5).
Moves symmetrically with each breath; posterior base descends 5-6 cm (2-2.3 inches) during deep inspiration	
Vibrations are symmetric and most intense in thoracic area and least intense at base.	Note asymmetric vibrations or sudden absence or decrease in intensity. Note abnormal vibrations, such as pleural friction rub or crepitation.
Lobes are resonant except for (see Figure 1-23): Dullness at fifth interspace right midclavicular line (liver) Dullness from second to fifth interspace over left sternal border to midclavicular line (heart) Tympany below left fifth interspace (stomach)	Note deviation from expected sounds.
Vesicular breath sounds—Heard over entire surface of lungs except upper intrascapular area and beneath manubrium; inspiration louder, longer, and of higher pitch than expiration	Note deviations from expected breath sounds, particularly if diminished; note absence of sounds. Note adventitious sounds.

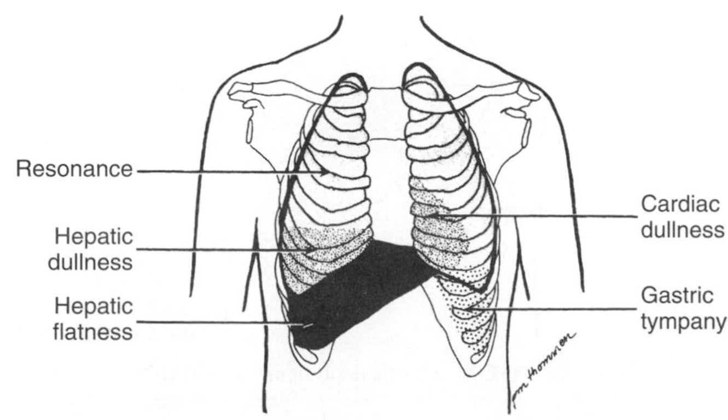

FIGURE **1-23** Percussion sounds in thorax.

Continued

Summary of Physical Assessment of the Child–cont'd

Assessment	Procedure

Lungs—cont'd

BOX 1-5 | Various Patterns of Respiration

Tachypnea—Increased rate
Dradypnea—Decreased rate
Dyspnea—Distress during breathing
Apnea—Cessation of breathing
Hyperpnea—Increased depth
Hypoventilation—Decreased depth (shallow) and irregular rhythm
Hyperventilation—Increased rate and depth
Kussmaul breathing—hyperventilation, gasping, and labored respiration, usually seen in respiratory acidosis (e.g., diabetic coma)
Cheyne-Stokes respiration—Gradually increasing rate and depth with periods of apnea
Biot's breathing—Periods of hyperpnea alternating (similar to Cheyne-Stokes except that the depth remains constant)
Seesaw (paradoxic) respirations—Chest falls on inspiration and rises on expiration
Agonal—Last gasping breaths before death

Heart

See Figure 1-24.

General Instructions

Begin with inspection, followed by palpation, then auscultation.

Percussion is not done because it is of limited value in defining the borders or the size of the heart.

Palpate to determine the location of the apical impulse (AI), the most lateral cardiac impulse that may correspond to the apex.

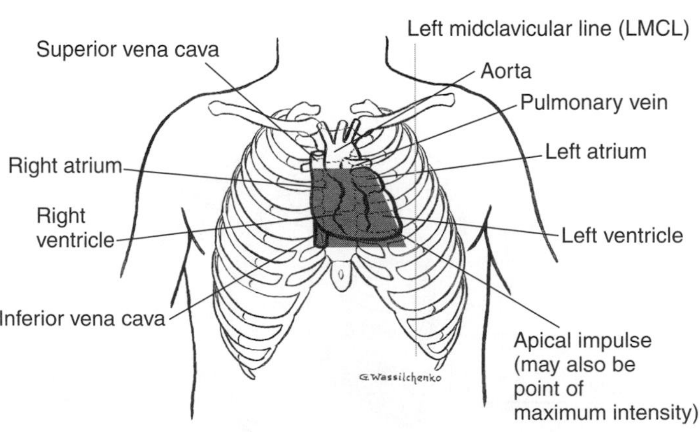

FIGURE **1-24** Position of heart within thorax.

Usual Findings	Comments
Bronchovesicular breath sounds—Heard in upper intrascapular area and manubrium; inspiration and expiration almost equal in duration, pitch, and intensity	***Crackles***—Discrete, noncontinuous crackling sound, heard primarily during inspiration from passage of air through fluid or moisture; if crackles clear with deep breathing, they are not pathologic
Bronchial breath sounds—Heard only over trachea near suprasternal notch; expiration longer, louder, and of higher pitch than inspiration	***Wheezes***—Continuous musical sounds; caused by air passing through narrowed passages, regardless of cause (exudate, inflammation, foreign body, spasm, tumor) ***Audible inspiratory wheeze (stridor)***—Sonorous, musical wheeze heard without a stethoscope; indicates a high obstruction (e.g., epiglottitis) ***Audible expiratory wheeze***—Whistling, sighing wheeze heard without a stethoscope; indicates a low obstruction ***Pleural friction rub***—Crackling, grating sound during inspiration and expiration; occurs from inflamed pleural surfaces; not affected by coughing
Voice sounds—Heard, but syllables are indistinct	Consolidation of lung tissue produces three types of abnormal voice sounds: ***Whispered pectoriloquy***—The child whispers words, and the nurse hears the syllables. ***Bronchophony***—The child speaks words that are not distinguishable, but the vocal resonance is increased in intensity and clarity. ***Egophony***—The child says "ee," which is heard as the nasal sound "ay" through the stethoscope.
Symmetric chest wall AI sometimes apparent (in thin children)	Note obvious bulging. Infant's heart is larger in proportion to chest size and lies more centrally.
Just lateral to the left MCL and fourth ICS in children >7 years of age At the left MCL and fifth ICS in children >7 years of age	Although the AI gives a general idea of the size of the heart (with enlargement, the apex is lower and more lateral), its normal location is quite variable, making it a rather unreliable indicator of heart size; **point of maximum intensity (PMI)**, area of most intense pulsation, usually is located at same site as AI, but it can occur elsewhere. For this reason, the two terms should not be used synonymously. During palpation, may feel abnormal vibrations called **thrills** that are similar to cat's purring; they are produced by blood flowing through narrowed or abnormal opening, such as stenotic valve or septal defect.
Capillary refilling in 1-2 seconds	Refilling taking longer than 2 seconds is abnormal and indicates impaired skin perfusion; cool temperature prolongs capillary refill time.

Continued

Summary of Physical Assessment of the Child–cont'd

Assessment	Procedure

Heart—cont'd

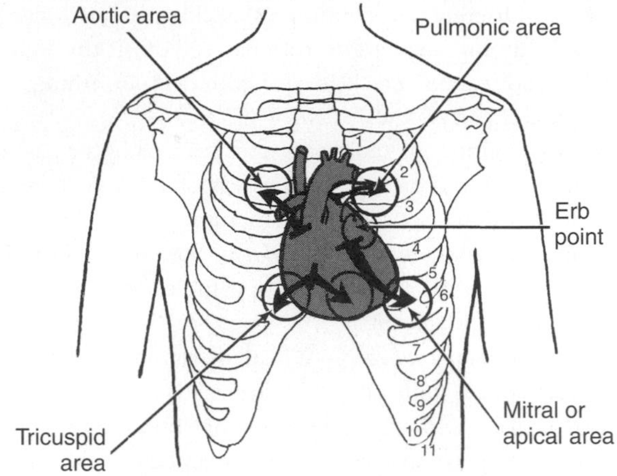

FIGURE **1-25** Directions of heart sounds from anatomic valve sites.

Palpate skin for capillary filling time:
- Lightly press skin on central site, such as forehead, and peripheral site, such as top of hand or foot, to produce slight blanching.
- Assess time it takes for blanched area to return to original color.

Auscultate for heart sounds:
- Listen with child in sitting and reclining positions.
- Use both diaphragm and bell chest pieces.
- Evaluate sounds for quality, intensity, rate, and rhythm (Box 1-6).

Follow sequence (Figure 1-25):

Aortic area—Second right intercostal space close to sternum

Pulmonic area—Second left intercostal space close to sternum

Erb point—Second and third left intercostal spaces close to sternum

Tricuspid area—Fifth right and left intercostal spaces close to sternum

Mitral or apical area—Fifth intercostal space, left midclavicular line (third to fourth intercostal space and lateral to left midclavicular line [MCL] in infants)

BOX 1-6 | VARIOUS PATTERNS OF HEART RATE OR PULSE

Tachycardia—Increased rate

Bradycardia—Decreased rate

Pulsus alternans—Strong beat followed by weak beat

Pulsus bigeminus—Coupled rhythm in which beat is felt in pairs because of premature beat

Pulsus paradoxus—Intensity or force of pulse decreases with inspiration

Sinus arrhythmia—Rate increases with inspiration, decreases with expiration

Water-hammer or Corrigan's pulse—Especially forceful beat caused by a very wide pulse pressure (systolic blood pressure minus diastolic blood pressure)

Dicrotic pulse—Double radial pulse for every apical beat

Thready pulse—Rapid, weak pulse that seems to appear and disappear

Abdomen

General Instructions

Inspection is followed by auscultation, percussion, and palpation, which may distort the normal abdominal sounds.

Palpation may be uncomfortable for the child; deep palpation causes a feeling of pressure, and superficial palpation causes a tickling sensation.

To minimize any discomfort and encourage cooperation, use the following:

Position child supine with legs flexed at hips and knees.

Distract child with statements such as "I am going to guess what you ate by feeling your tummy."

Have child "help" with palpation by placing own hand over examiner's palpating hand.

Have child place own hand on abdomen with fingers spread wide apart and palpate between the fingers.

Usual Findings	Comments
S_1-S_2—Clear, distinct, rate equal to radial pulse; rhythm regular and even ***Aortic area***—S_2 louder than S_1 ***Pulmonic area***—Splitting of S_2 heard best (normally widens on inspiration) ***Erb point***—Frequent site of innocent murmurs ***Tricuspid area***—S_1 louder sound preceding S_2 ***Mitral or apical area***—S_1 heard loudest; splitting of S_1 may be audible ***Quality***—Clear and distinct ***Intensity***—Strong, but not pounding ***Rate***—Same as radial pulse ***Rhythm***—Regular and even	To distinguish S_1 from S_2, palpate for carotid pulse, which is synchronous with S_1. A normal arrhythmia is **sinus arrhythmia,** in which heart rate increases with inspiration and decreases with expiration. Identify abnormal sounds; note presence of adventitious sounds such as pericardial friction rubs (similar to pleural friction rubs but not affected by change in respiration). Record murmurs in relation to the following: Area best heard Timing within S_1-S_2 cycle Change with position Loudness and quality
Usual findings of innocent murmurs: ***Timing within S1 S2 cycle***—Systolic, that is, they occur with or after S_1 ***Quality***—Usually of a low-pitched, musical, or groaning quality ***Loudness***—Grade III or less in intensity and do not increase over time ***Area best heard***—Usually loudest in the pulmonic area with no transmission to other areas of the heart ***Change with position***—Audible in the supine position but absent in the sitting position ***Other physical signs***—Not associated with any physical signs of cardiac disease	Grading of the intensity of heart murmurs: **I**—Very faint, frequently not heard if child sits up **II**—Usually readily heard, slightly louder than grade I, audible in all positions **III**—Loud but not accompanied by a thrill **IV**—Loud, accompanied by a thrill **V**—Loud enough to be heard with the stethoscope barely on the chest, accompanied by a thrill **VI**—Loud enough to be heard with the stethoscope not touching the chest, often heard with the human ear close to the chest, accompanied by a thrill

Continued

Summary of Physical Assessment of the Child–cont'd

Assessment	Procedure
Abdomen—cont'd	
	Inspect contour, size, and tone
	Note condition of skin. Note movement.
	Inspect umbilicus for herniation, fistulas, hygiene, and discharge.
	Observe for hernias (Figure 1-26): ***Inguinal***—Slide little finger into external inguinal ring at base of scrotum; ask child to cough. ***Femoral***—Place finger over femoral canal (located by placing index finger over femoral pulse and middle finger against skin toward midline). Auscultate for bowel sounds and aortic pulsations.
	Percuss the abdomen.
	Palpate abdominal organs (Figure 1-27): Place one hand flat against back, and use palpating hand to "feel" organs between both hands. Proceed from lower quadrants *upward* to avoid missing edge of enlarged organ.

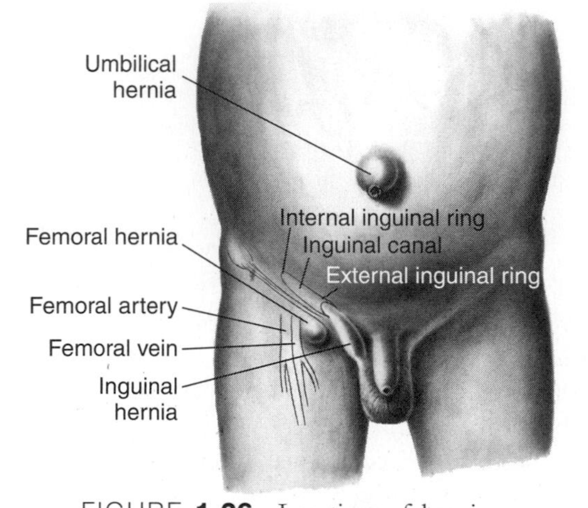

FIGURE **1-26** Locations of hernias.

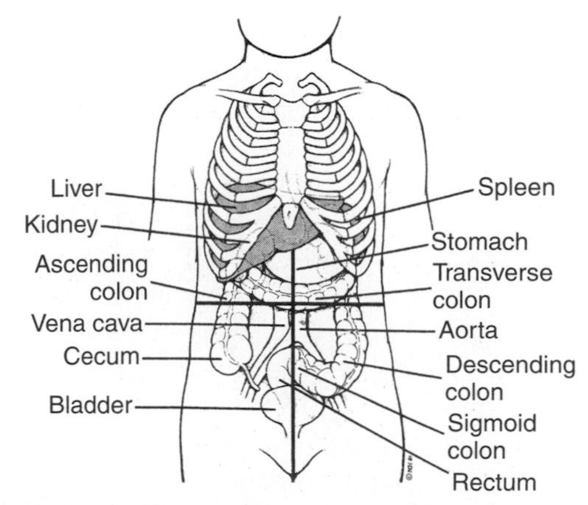

FIGURE **1-27** Locations of structures in abdomen.

Usual Findings	Comments
Infants and young children—Cylindric and prominent in erect position, flat when supine Adolescents—Characteristic adult curves, fairly flat when erect Circumference decreases in relation to chest size with age. Firm tone; muscular in adolescent males	Contour, size, and tone are good indicators of nutritional status and muscular development. Note deviations: Prominent, flabby Distention Concave Tense, boardlike Loose, wrinkled Midline protrusion Silvery, whitish striae Distended veins
Smooth, uniformly taut	
In children under 7 or 8 years, rises with inspiration and synchronous with chest movement In older children, less respiratory movement In thin children, visible pulsations from descending aorta sometimes seen in epigastric region	Paradoxic respirations (chest rises while abdomen falls) Visible peristaltic waves
Flat to slight protrusion; no herniation or discharge	If herniation is present, palpate for abdominal contents. Discuss with parents any home remedies used to reduce the herniation, especially umbilical hernias (e.g., belly binders, taping umbilicus flat).
None	
Bowel sounds—Short, metallic, tinkling sounds like gurgles, clicks, or growls heard every 10-30 seconds ***Aortic pulsations***—Heard in epigastrium, slightly left of midline	Bowel sounds may be stimulated by stroking abdominal wall with a fingertip. Note hyperperistalsis or absence of bowel sounds.
Tympany over stomach on left side and most of abdomen, except for dullness or flatness just below right costal margin (liver)	Note percussion sounds other than those expected.
Liver—1-2 cm below right costal margin in infants and young children	Usually not palpable in older children Considered enlarged if 3 cm below costal margin Normally descends with inspiration; should not be considered a sign of enlargement
Spleen—Sometimes 1-2 cm below left costal margin in infants and young children	Usually not palpable in older children Considered enlarged if more than 2 cm below left costal margin; also descends with inspiration Other structures that sometimes are palpable include kidneys, bladder, cecum, and sigmoid colon; know their location to avoid mistaking them for abnormal masses; most common palpable mass is feces. In sexually active females, consider a palpable mass in the lower abdomen a pregnant uterus.

Continued

Summary of Physical Assessment of the Child–cont'd

Assessment	Procedure
Abdomen—cont'd	
	Use imaginary lines at umbilicus to divide the abdomen into quadrants (see Figure 1-27): Right upper quadrant (RUQ) Right lower quadrant (RLQ) Left upper quadrant (LUQ) Left lower quadrant (LLQ) Palpate femoral pulses simultaneously—Place tips of two or three fingers about midway between iliac crest and pubic symphysis. Elicit abdominal reflex—Scratch skin from side to midline in each quadrant.
Genitalia	
Male See Figure 1-28.	***General Instructions*** Proceed in same manner as examination of other areas; explain procedure and its significance before doing it, such as palpating for testes. Respect privacy at all times. Use opportunity to discuss concerns about sexual development with older child and adolescent. Use opportunity to discuss sexual safety with young children, that this is their private area and if someone touches them in a way that is uncomfortable they should always tell their parent or some other trusted person. If in contact with body substances, wear gloves. ***Penis***—Inspect size.
	Glans and shaft—Inspect for signs of swelling, skin lesions, inflammation. ***Prepuce***—Inspect in uncircumcised male.
	Urethral meatus—Inspect location, and note any discharge.
	Scrotum—Inspect size, location, skin, and hair distribution.
	Testes—Palpate each scrotal sac using thumb and index finger.

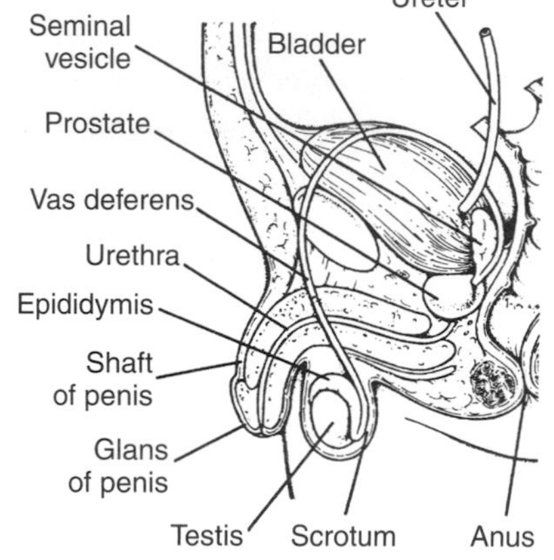

FIGURE **1-28** Major structures of genitalia in circumcised prepubertal male.

Usual Findings	Comments
Equal and strong bilaterally	Note absence of femoral pulse. Normally may be absent in children under 1 year of age
Umbilicus moves toward quadrant that was stroked.	Examination may be anxiety producing for older children and adolescents; may be left for end of physical examination.
Generally, size is insignificant in prepubescent male. Compare growth with expected sexual development during puberty (see p. 143) None	Note large penis, possible sign of precocious puberty. In obese child, penis may be obscured by fat pad over pubic symphysis.
Easily retracted to expose glans and urethral meatus	In infants, prepuce is tight for up to 3 years and should not be retracted. Discuss importance of hygiene.
Centered at tip of glans No discharge	Note location on ventral or dorsal surface of penis, possible sign of ambiguous genitalia, hypospadias, or epispadias. Whenever possible, note strength and direction of urinary stream.
May appear large in infants Hangs freely from perineum behind penis One sac hangs lower than other.	Note scrota that are small, close to perineum, with any degree of midline separation.
Loose, wrinkled skin, usually redder and coarser in adolescents	Well-formed rugae indicate descent of testes.
Compare hair distribution with that expected for pubertal stage; typical mature male pattern forms a diamond shape from umbilicus to anus (see p. 143).	
Small ovoid bodies about 1.5-2 cm long Double in size during puberty	Prevent cremasteric reflex that retracts testes by: Warming hands Having child sit in tailor fashion or squat Blocking pathway of ascent by placing thumb and index finger over upper part of scrotal sac along inguinal canal Note failure to palpate testes after taking these precautions. Discuss testicular self-examination with adolescent male.

Continued

Summary of Physical Assessment of the Child–cont'd

Assessment	Procedure
Genitalia—cont'd	
Female See Figure 1-29.	***External genitalia***—Inspect structures; place young child in semireclining position in parent's lap with knees bent and soles of feet in apposition.
	Labia—Palpate for any masses.
	Urethral meatus—Inspect for location; identified as V-shaped slit by wiping downward from clitoris to perineum.
	Skene glands—Palpate or inspect
	Vaginal orifice—Internal examination usually not performed; inspect for obvious opening.
	Bartholin glands—Palpate or inspect
Anus	
	Anal area—Inspect for general firmness, condition of skin.
	Anal reflex—Elicit by gently pricking or scratching perianal area.
Back and Extremities	
	Inspect curvature and symmetry of spine (Figure 1-30).
	Test for scoliosis: Have child stand erect; observe from behind, and note asymmetry of shoulders and hips. Have child bend forward at the waist until back is parallel to floor; observe from side and note asymmetry or prominence of rib cage.
	Note mobility of spine.
	Inspect each extremity joint for symmetry, size, temperature, color, tenderness, and mobility.
	Test for developmental dysplasia of the hip (see p. 26).

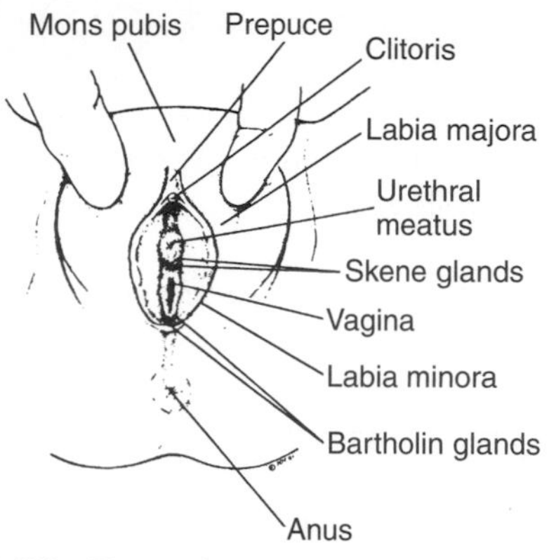

FIGURE **1-29** External structures of genitalia in prepubertal female. Labia are spread to reveal deep structures.

Usual Findings	Comments
Mons pubis—Fat pad over symphysis pubis; covered with hair in adolescence; usual hair distribution is triangular (see p. 145)	
Clitoris—Located at anterior end of labia minora; covered by small flap of skin (prepuce)	Note evidence of enlargement (may be small phallus).
Labia majora—Two thick folds of skin from mons to posterior commissure; inner surface pink and moist	Note any palpable masses (may be testes), evidence of fusion, enlargement, or signs of female circumcision.
Labia minora—Two folds of skin interior to labia majora, usually invisible until puberty; prominent in newborn	
Located posterior to clitoris and anterior to vagina	Note opening from clitoris or inside vagina.
Surround meatus; no lesions	Common sites of cysts and venereal warts (condylomata acuminata)
Located posterior to urethral meatus; may be covered by crescent-shaped or circular membrane **(hymen)**; discharge usually clear or whitish	Note excessive, foul-smelling, or colored discharge.
Surround vaginal opening; no lesions, secrete clear mucoid fluid	
Buttocks—Firm; gluteal folds symmetric	Note evidence of diaper rash; inquire about hygiene and type of diaper (cloth or ultraabsorbent paper; the latter can decrease diaper dermatitis).
Quick contraction of external anal sphincter; no protrusion of rectum	Note: Fissures Polyps Rectal prolapse Hemorrhoids Warts
Rounded or C-shaped in the newborn	Note any abnormal curvatures and presence of masses or lesions.
Cervical secondary curve forms at about 3 months of age. Lumbar secondary curve forms at about 12-18 months, resulting in typical double-S curve Lordosis normal in young children but decreases with age Shoulders, scapula, and iliac crests symmetric	Other signs of scoliosis: Slight limp Crooked hem or waistline Complaint of backache
Flexible, full range of motion, no pain or stiffness	Note stiffness and pain on movement of neck or back; requires immediate evaluation.
Symmetric length Equal size Correct number of digits Nails pink (see assessment of skin, p. 46) Temperature equal, although feet may be cooler than hands Full range of motion	Note any deviations. Note warmth, swelling, tenderness, and immobility of joints.

Continued

Summary of Physical Assessment of the Child–cont'd

Assessment	Procedure
Back and Extremities—cont'd	

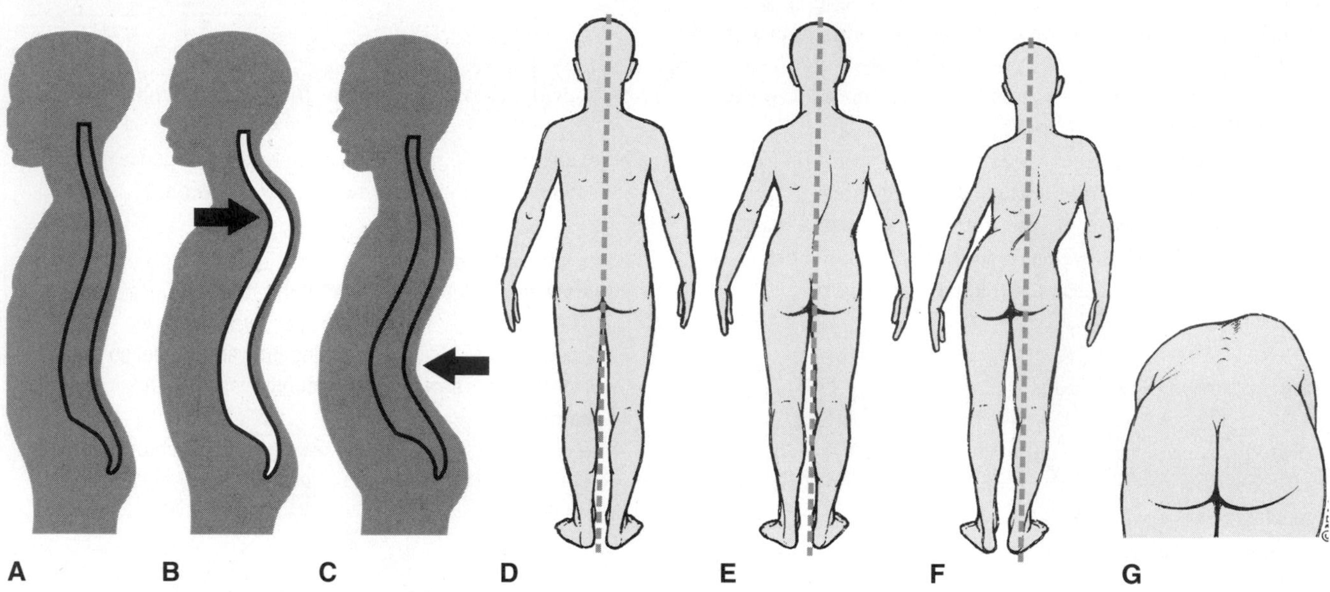

FIGURE **1-30** Defects of spinal column. **A,** Normal spine. **B,** Kyphosis. **C,** Lordosis. **D,** Normal spine in balance. **E,** Mild scoliosis in balance. **F,** Severe scoliosis not in balance. **G,** Rib hump and flank asymmetry seen in flexion caused by rotary component. (Redrawn from Hilt NE, Schmitt EW: *Pediatric orthopedic nursing,* St Louis, 1975, Mosby.)

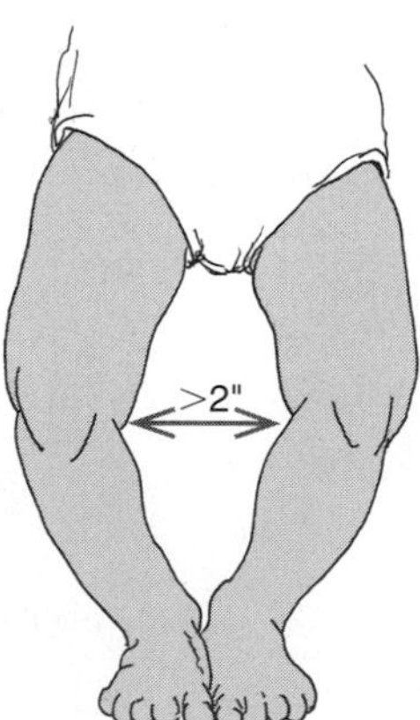

FIGURE **1-31** Genu varum (bowleg).

Assess shape of bones:

- Measure distance between the knees when child stands with malleoli in apposition.
- Measure distance between the malleoli when the child stands with knees together.
- Inspect position of feet; test if foot deformity at birth is result of fetal position or development by scratching outer, then inner, side of sole; if self-correctable, foot assumes right angle to leg.

Inspect gait:

- Have child walk in straight line.
- Estimate angle of gait by drawing imaginary line through center of foot and line of progression.

Plantar reflex—Elicit by stroking lateral sole from heel upward to little toe across to hallux.

Inspect development and tone of muscles.

Test strength:

Arms—Have child raise arms while applying counterpressure with your hands.

Legs—Have child sit with legs dangling; proceed as with arms.

Hands—Have child squeeze your fingers as tightly as possible.

Feet—Have child plantar flex (push soles toward floor) while applying counterpressure to the soles

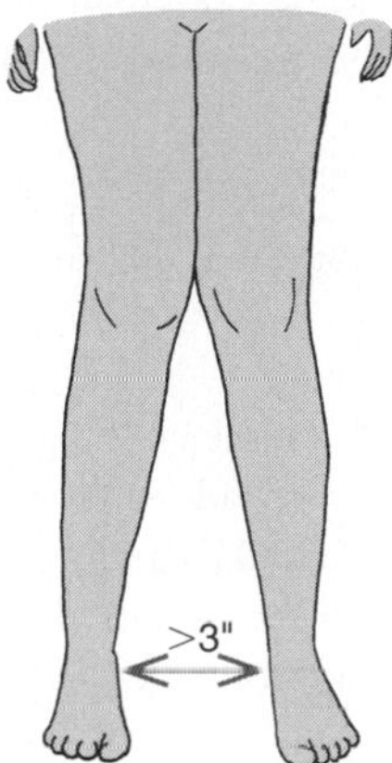

FIGURE **1-32** Genu valgum (knock knee).

BOX 1-7 | TYPES OF FOOT AND ANKLE DEFORMITIES

Pes planus (flatfoot)—Normal finding in infancy; may be result of muscular weakness in older child

Pes valgus—Eversion of entire foot, but sole rests on ground

Pes varus—Inversion of entire foot, but sole rests on ground

Metatarsus valgus—Eversion of forefoot while heel remains straight; also called *toeing out* or *duck walk*

Talipes valgus—Eversion (turning outward) of foot so that only inner side of foot rests on ground

Talipes varus—Inversion (turning inward) of foot so that only outer sole of foot rests on ground

Talipes equinus—Extension or plantar flexion of foot so that only ball and toes rest on ground; commonly combined with talipes varus (most common of clubfoot deformities)

Talipes calcaneus—Dorsal flexion of foot so that only heel rests on ground

Usual Findings	Comments
Less than 5 cm (2 inches) in children over 2 years of age	Greater distance indicates **genu varum (bowleg)** (Figure 1-31).
Less than 7.5 cm (3 inches) in children over 7 years of age	Greater distance indicates **genu valgum (knock knee)** (Figure 1-32).
Held at right angle to leg, pointed straight ahead or turned slightly outward when standing Fat pads on sole give appearance of flat feet; arch develops after child is walking.	Note foot and ankle deformities (Box 1-7).
"Toddling" or broad-based gait normal in young children; gradually assumes graceful gait with feet close together. Feet turn outward less than 30 degrees and inward less than 10 degrees.	Note abnormal gait: Waddling Scissor Toeing-in Broad-based in older children
Flexion of toes in children older than 1 year	Babinski reflex seen in younger children (see p. 27)
Symmetric Increase in tone during muscle contraction Equal bilaterally	Note atrophy, hypertrophy, spasticity, flaccidity, rigidity, or weakness.

Continued

Summary of Physical Assessment of the Child–cont'd

Assessment	Procedure
Neurologic Assessment	
Mental Status	Observe behavior, mood, affect, general orientation to surroundings, level of consciousness (see pp. 100-101).
Motor Functioning	Test muscle strength, tone, and development (see p. 160). Test cerebellar functioning: ***Finger-to-nose test***—With the child's arm extended, have child touch nose with the index finger. ***Heel-to-skin test***—With child standing, have child run the heel of one foot down the shin of the other leg. ***Romberg test***—Have child stand erect with feet together and eyes closed. Have child touch tip of each finger to thumb in rapid succession. Have child pat leg with first one side, then the other side of hand in rapid sequence. Have child tap your hand with ball of foot as quickly as possible.
Sensory Functioning	Test vision and hearing (see pp. 170 and 177). ***Sensory intactness***—Touch skin lightly with a pin, and have child point to stimulated area while keeping eyes closed. Sensory discrimination: Touch skin with pin and cotton; have child describe the sensation as sharp or dull. Touch skin with cold and warm object (e.g., metal and rubber heads of reflex hammer); have child differentiate between temperatures. Using two pins, touch skin simultaneously with both or only one pin; have child discriminate when one or two pins are used.
Reflexes (Deep Tendon)	***Biceps***—Hold the child's arm by placing the partially flexed elbow in your hand with the thumb over the antecubital space; strike your thumbnail with the hammer. ***Triceps***—Bend the arm at the elbow, and rest the palm in your hand; strike the triceps tendon. ***Alternate procedure***—If the child is supine, rest arm over chest and strike the triceps tendon.

Usual Findings	Comments
	Subjective impressions are based on observation throughout the examination. Objective findings can be attained through developmental testing, such as Denver II.
Performs each test successfully with eyes opened and closed	May be difficult to test in children younger than preschool age
During heel-to-shin and Romberg tests, stand close to child to prevent falls. ***Romberg test***—Does not lean to side or fall	Note any awkwardness or lack of coordination in performance. Falling or leaning to one side is abnormal and is called the ***Romberg sign.***
Localizes pinprick	Use sterile pin or other sharp object (e.g., toothpick), being careful not to puncture skin. Compare sensation in symmetric areas at both distal and proximal points.
Able to distinguish types of sensation and temperature	Note difficulty in performing test, especially in older child.
Minimal distance for discrimination on finger is about 2-3 mm.	
Biceps—Partial flexion of forearm ***Triceps***—Partial extension of forearm	Use distraction techniques to prevent child from inhibiting reflex activity: For upper extremity reflexes, ask child to clench teeth or to squeeze thigh with the hand on the side not being tested. Rest upper arm in palm of hand. For lower extremity reflexes, have child lock fingers and pull one hand against the other or grip hands together. Usual grading of reflexes: **Grade 0** 0 Absent **Grade 1** + Diminished **Grade 2** ++ Normal, average **Grade 3** +++ Brisker than normal **Grade 4** ++++ Hyperactive (clonus) Note asymmetric, absent, diminished, or hyperactive reflexes.

Continued

Summary of Physical Assessment of the Child–cont'd

Assessment	Procedure
Neurologic Assessment—cont'd	
	Brachioradialis—Rest the forearm on the lap or abdomen, with the arm flexed at the elbow and palm down; strike the radius about 1 inch (depending on child's size) above the wrist. ***Knee jerk or patellar reflex***—Sit child on the edge of the examining table or on parent's lap with the lower legs flexed at the knee and dangling freely; tap the patellar tendon just below the knee cap. ***Achilles***—Use the same position as for the knee jerk; support the foot lightly in your hand and strike the Achilles tendon. ***Ankle clonus***—See p. 27. ***Kernig's sign***—Flex child's leg at hip and knee while supine; note pain or resistance. ***Brudzinski's sign***—With child supine, flex the head; note pain and involuntary flexion of hip and knees.
Cranial Nerves	(See Assessment of Cranial Nerves, p. 77.)

Usual Findings	Comments
Brachioradialis—Flexion of the forearm and supination (turning upward) of the palm	
Patellar—Partial extension of lower leg	
Achilles—Plantar flexion of foot (foot pointing downward)	
Ankle clonus—Absence of beats	
Kernig's—Absence of pain or resistance	These special reflexes are elicited when meningeal irritation is suspected.
Brudzinski's—Absence of pain or associated movements	Signs of pain, resistance, or associated movements require immediate referral.
	Testing of cranial nerves may be done as part of the neurologic examination or integrated into assessment of each system, such as cranial nerves II, III, IV, and VI with the eye. Cranial nerves can usually be tested in children of preschool age and older. Note inability to perform any of the items correctly.

Temperature Measurement Locations for Infants and Children

Oral

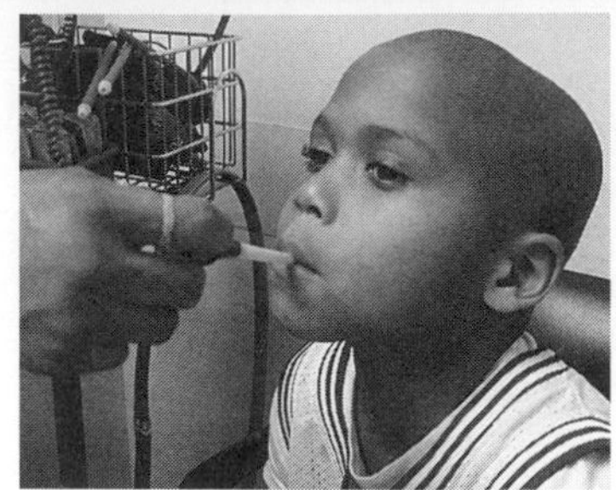

Place tip under tongue in right or left posterior sublingual pocket, not in front of tongue. Have child keep mouth closed, without biting on thermometer.

Pacifier thermometers measure intraoral or supralingual temperature and are available but lack support in the literature.

Several factors affect mouth temperature: eating and mastication, hot and cold beverages, open-mouth breathing, ambient temperature.

Axillary

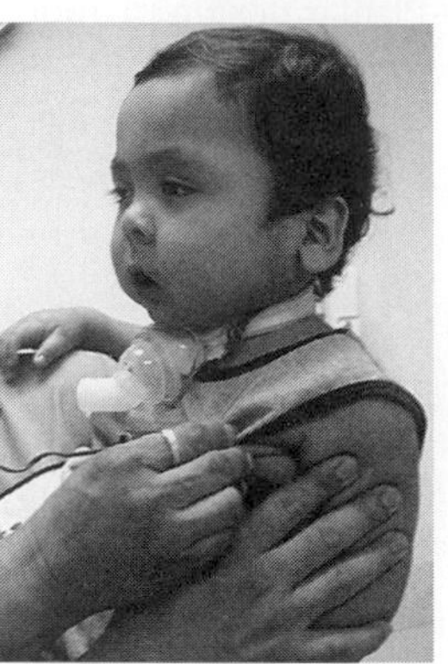

Place tip under arm in center of axilla and keep close to skin, not clothing. Child's arm must be held firmly against side.

May be affected by poor peripheral perfusion (results in lower value), clothing or swaddling, use of radiant warmer, or amount of brown fat in cold-stressed neonate (results in higher value).

Advantage: avoids intrusive procedure and eliminates risk of rectal perforation.

Aural or Ear Based

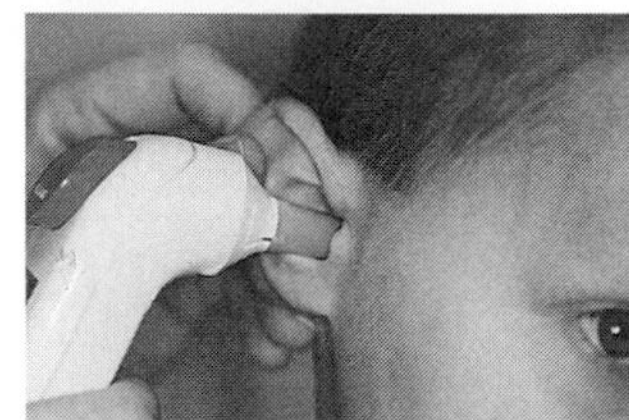

An infrared probe, small enough to be deeply inserted into the canal to allow the sensor to obtain the measurement. The size of the probe (most are 8 mm) may influence accuracy of the result. In young children this may be a problem because of the small diameter of the canal. Proper placement of the ear is controversial with regard to whether the pinna should be pulled as during otoscopy.

Rectal

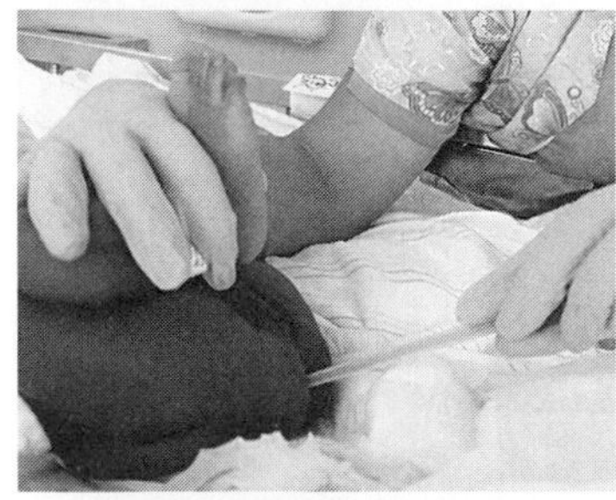

Place well-lubricated tip at maximum 2.5 cm (1 inch) into rectum for children and 1.5 cm for infants; securely hold thermometer close to anus.

Child may be placed in side-lying, supine, or prone position (i.e., supine with knees flexed toward abdomen); cover penis, as procedure may stimulate urination. A small child may be placed prone across parent's lap.

Temporal Artery

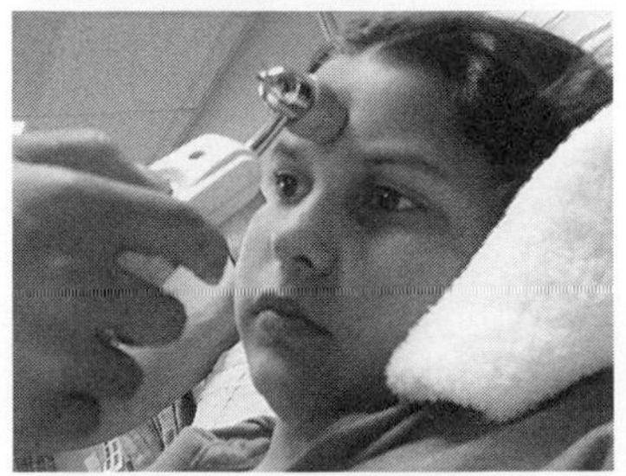

An infrared sensor probe scans across the forehead, capturing the heat from the arterial blood flow. The only artery close enough to the skin's surface to provide access for accurate temperature measurement is the temporal artery.

Adapted from Martin SA, Kline AM: Can there be a standard for temperature measurement in the pediatric intensive care unit? *AACN Clin Issues* 15(2): 254-266, 2004; Falzon A, Grech V, Caruana B, and others: How reliable is axillary temperature measurement? *Acta Pediatr,* 92(3):309-313, 2003.

Assessment of Cranial Nerves

Cranial Nerve	Distribution or Function	Test
I—Olfactory (S)*	Olfactory mucosa of nasal cavity	With child's eyes closed, have child identify odors such as coffee, alcohol, or other smells from a swab; test each nostril separately.
II—Optic (S)	Rods and cones of retina, optic nerve	Check for perception of light, visual acuity, peripheral vision, color vision, and normal optic disc.
III—Oculomotor (M)	Extraocular muscles (EOM) of eye: ***Superior rectus (SR)***—Moves eyeball up and in ***Inferior rectus (IR)***—Moves eyeball down and in ***Medial rectus (MR)***—Moves eyeball nasally ***Inferior oblique (IO)***—Moves eyeball up and out	Have child follow an object (toy) or light in the six cardinal positions of gaze (Figure 1-33).
	Pupil constriction and accommodation	Perform PERRLA (see p. 51).
	Eyelid closing	Check for proper placement of lid (see p. 48).
IV—Trochlear (M)	Superior oblique (SO) muscle—Moves eye down and out	Have child look down and in (see Figure 1-33).
V—Trigeminal (M, S)	Muscles of mastication	Have child bite down hard and open jaw; test symmetry and strength.
	Sensory: Face, scalp, nasal and buccal mucosa	With child's eyes closed, see if child can detect light touch in the mandibular and maxillary regions. Test corneal and blink reflex by touching cornea lightly (approach child from the side so that child does not blink before cornea is touched).
VI—Abducens (M)	Lateral rectus (LR) muscle—Moves eye temporally	Have child look toward temporal side (see Figure 1-33).
VII—Facial (M, S)	Muscles for facial expression	Have child smile, make funny face, or show teeth to see symmetry of expression.
	Anterior two thirds of tongue (sensory)	Have child identify a sweet or salty solution; place each taste on anterior section and sides of protruding tongue; if child retracts tongue, solution will dissolve toward posterior part of tongue.
	Nasal cavity and lacrimal gland, sublingual and submandibular salivary glands	Not tested

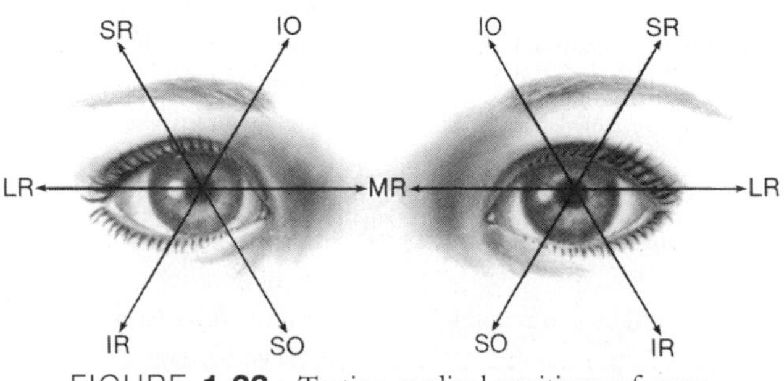

FIGURE **1-33** Testing cardinal positions of gaze.

*S, Sensory; M, motor.

Continued

Assessment of Cranial Nerves—cont'd

Cranial Nerve	Distribution or Function	Test
VIII—Auditory, Acoustic, or Vestibulocochlear (S)	Internal ear Hearing, balance	Test hearing; note any loss of equilibrium or presence of vertigo (dizziness).
IX—Glossopharyngeal (M, S)	Pharynx, tongue	Stimulate the posterior pharynx with a tongue blade; the child should gag.
	Posterior one third of tongue (sensory)	Test sense of sour or bitter taste on posterior segment of tongue.
X—Vagus (M, S)	Muscles of larynx, pharynx, some organs of gastrointestinal system, sensory fibers of root of tongue, heart, lung, and some organs of gastrointestinal system	Note hoarseness of the voice, gag reflex, and ability to swallow. Check that uvula is in midline; when stimulated with a tongue blade, should deviate upward and to the stimulated side.
XI—Accessory (M)	Sternocleidomastoid and trapezius muscles of shoulder	Have child shrug shoulders while applying mild pressure; with the hands placed on shoulders, have child turn head against opposing pressure on either side; note symmetry and strength.
XII—Hypoglossal (M)	Muscles of tongue	Have child move tongue in all directions; have child protrude tongue as far as possible; note any midline deviation. Test strength by placing tongue blade on one side of tongue and having child move it away.

Nursing Assessment of Specific Health Problems

The Child with Acute Respiratory Infection

Acute respiratory infection—An inflammatory process caused by viral, bacterial, or atypical (mycoplasma) infection or aspiration of foreign substances, which involves any or all parts of the respiratory tract

Lower respiratory tract—Consists of the bronchi and bronchioles (which constitute the reactive portion of the airway because of their smooth muscle content and ability to constrict) and the alveoli

Croup syndromes—Consist of the epiglottis, larynx, and trachea (the structurally stable, nonreactive portion of the airway)

Upper respiratory tract (upper airway)—Consists of the nose and pharynx

ASSESSMENT

Assist with diagnostic procedures and tests (e.g., radiography, throat culture, thoracentesis, venipuncture for blood analysis).

Observe for general clinical manifestations of acute respiratory tract infection (Box 1-8).

Identify factors affecting type of illness and response to acute respiratory infection (e.g., age and size of child, ability to resist infection, contact with infected children, coexisting disorders affecting respiratory tract).

Assess respiratory status.

Monitor respirations for rate, depth, pattern, presence of retractions, and flaring nares.

Auscultate lungs.

- Evaluate breath sounds (type and location).
- Detect presence of crackles or wheezes.
- Detect areas of consolidation.
- Evaluate effectiveness of chest physiotherapy.

Observe for presence or absence of retractions, nasal flaring.

Observe color of skin and mucous membranes for pallor and cyanosis.

Observe for presence of hoarseness, stridor, and cough.

Monitor heart rate and regularity.

Observe behavior.

- Restlessness
- Irritability
- Apprehension

Observe for signs of the following:

- Chest pain
- Abdominal pain
- Dyspnea

BOX 1-8 | Signs and Symptoms Associated with Respiratory Infections in Infants and Small Children

Fever

May be absent in newborn infants
Greatest at ages 6 months to 3 years
- Temperature may reach 39.5° to 40.5° C (103° to 105° F), even with mild infections

Often appears as first sign of infection
Child may be listless and irritable, or somewhat euphoric and more active than normal temporarily; some children talk with unaccustomed rapidity
Tendency to develop high temperatures with infection in certain families
- May precipitate febrile seizures
- Febrile seizures uncommon after 3 or 4 years of age

Meningismus

Meningeal signs without infection of the meninges
Occurs with abrupt onset of fever
Accompanied by:
- Headache
- Pain and stiffness in the back and neck
- Presence of Kernig's and Brudzinski's signs

Subsides as temperature drops

Anorexia

Common with most childhood illnesses
Frequently the initial evidence of illness
Almost invariably accompanies acute infections in small children
Persists to a greater or lesser degree throughout febrile stage of illness; often extends into convalescence

Vomiting

Small children vomit readily with illness
A clue to the onset of infection
May precede other signs by several hours
Usually short-lived but may persist during the illness

Diarrhea

Usually mild, transient diarrhea but may become severe
Often accompanies viral respiratory infections
Is frequent cause of dehydration

Abdominal Pain

Common complaint
Sometimes indistinguishable from pain of appendicitis
Mesenteric lymphadenitis may be a cause
Muscle spasms from vomiting may be a factor, especially in nervous, tense children

Nasal Blockage

Small nasal passages of infants easily blocked by mucosal swelling and exudation
Can interfere with respiration and feeding in infants
May contribute to the development of otitis media and sinusitis

Nasal Discharge

Frequent occurrence
May be thin and watery (rhinorrhea) or thick and purulent, depending on the type and/or stage of infection
Associated with itching
May irritate upper lip and skin surrounding the nose

Cough

Common feature
May be evident only during the acute phase
May persist several months after a disease

Respiratory Sounds

Sounds associated with respiratory disease
- Cough
- Hoarseness
- Grunting
- Stridor
- Wheezing

Auscultation
- Wheezing
- Crackles
- Absence of sound

Sore Throat

Frequent complaint of older children
Younger children (unable to describe symptoms) may not complain, even when throat highly inflamed
- Often child will refuse to take oral fluids or solids

Observe for clinical manifestations of respiratory infection (specific).

Upper Respiratory Tract Infections

Nasopharyngitis—Viral infection, *acute rhinitis* or *coryza,* equivalent of the common cold in adults
Edema and vasodilation of mucosa
Younger child
- Fever
- Irritability, restlessness
- Sneezing
- Vomiting and/or diarrhea, sometimes
- Decreased appetite
- Decreased activity

Older child
- Low-grade fever
- Dryness and irritation of nose and throat
- Sneezing, chilly sensations
- Muscular aches

- Irritating nasal discharge
- Cough, sometimes

Pharyngitis—Throat (including the tonsils) is principal anatomic site of pharyngitis (sore throat).

Younger child

- Fever
- General malaise
- Anorexia
- Moderate sore throat
- Headache
- Mild to moderate hyperemia
- Abdominal pain

Older child

- Fever (may reach 40° C [104.0° F])
- Headache
- Anorexia
- Dysphagia
- Vomiting
- Mild to fiery red, edematous pharynx
- Hyperemia of tonsils and pharynx; may extend to soft palate and uvula
- Often abundant follicular exudate that spreads and coalesces to form pseudomembrane on tonsils
- Cervical glands enlarged and tender

Influenza (flu)—Caused by three antigenically distinct orthomyxoviruses: types A and B, which cause epidemic disease; and type C, which is epidemiologically unimportant

May be subclinical, mild, moderate, or severe

Overt illness

- Dry throat and nasal mucosa
- Dry cough
- Tendency toward hoarseness
- Sudden onset of fever and chills
- Flushed face
- Photophobia
- Myalgia
- Hyperesthesia
- Prostration (sometimes)
- Subglottal croup common (especially in infants)

Croup Syndromes

Croup is a general term applied to a symptom complex characterized by hoarseness, a resonant cough described as barking (croupy), varying degrees of inspiratory stridor, and varying degrees of respiratory distress resulting from swelling or obstruction in the region of the larynx.

Acute laryngitis—Infection is usually viral; primary clinical manifestation is hoarseness; common illness of older children and adolescents.

May be accompanied by other upper respiratory symptoms: coryza, sore throat, nasal congestion

May be accompanied by systemic manifestations: fever, headache, myalgia, malaise

Symptoms vary with the infecting virus.

Acute laryngotracheobronchitis (LTB)—Viral infection; most common of the croup syndromes; usually occurs in children age 3 months to 8 years

Onset is slowly progressive.

- (Upper respiratory infection [URI]; several days of coryza)
- URI
- Inspiratory stridor
- Barking (seal-like) cough
- Hoarseness
- Dyspnea
- Suprasternal retractions
- Restlessness
- Irritability
- Low-grade fever
- Nontoxic appearance
- May progress to hypoxia and respiratory failure

Acute spasmodic laryngitis (spasmodic croup)—Viral infection with allergic and psychogenic factors in some cases; distinguished from laryngitis and LTB by characteristic paroxysmal attacks of laryngeal obstruction that occur chiefly at night; usually occurs in children age 3 months to 3 years

Onset is sudden, at night.

- URI
- Croupy cough
- Stridor
- Hoarseness
- Dyspnea
- Restlessness
- Child appears anxious, frightened.
- Symptoms waken child.
- Symptoms disappear during day.
- Tends to recur

Acute epiglottitis (supraglottitis)—Bacterial (usually *Haemophilus influenzae*) infection; serious obstructive inflammatory process that requires immediate attention; occurs principally in children between 2 and 5 years of age but can occur from infancy to adulthood; LTB and epiglottitis do not occur together.

Onset is abrupt, rapidly progressive.

- Sore throat
- Drooling
- Absence of spontaneous cough
- Agitation
- Throat is red, inflamed with distinctive large, cherry-red, edematous epiglottitis (Safety Alert)
- High fever
- Toxic appearance
- Rapid pulse and respirations
- Stridor aggravated when supine
- Child will sit upright, leaning forward, with chin thrust out, mouth open, and tongue protruding; tripod position
- Thick, muffled voice
- Croaking, froglike sound on inspiration
- Anxious and frightened expression
- Suprasternal and substernal retractions possibly visible

- Child seldom struggles to breathe (breathing slowly and quietly provides better air exchange)
- Sallow color of mild hypoxia to frank cyanosis

Acute tracheitis—Bacterial (usually *Staphylococcus aureus*) infection of the mucosa of the upper trachea; is a distinct entity with features of both croup and epiglottitis; may cause airway obstruction severe enough to cause respiratory arrest; occurs in children ages 1 month to 6 years

Onset is moderately progressive.

- Follows previous URI
- Begins with signs and symptoms similar to those of LTB
- Croupy cough
- Stridor unaffected by position
- Copious purulent secretions—may be severe enough to cause respiratory arrest
- Toxic appearance
- High fever
- No response to LTB therapy

Lower Respiratory Tract Infections

Asthmatic bronchitis—Exaggerated response of bronchi to infection; most commonly caused by viruses but may be by any variety of URI pathogens; bronchospasm, exudation, and edema of bronchi are similar to asthma in older children; occurs in late infancy and early childhood.

Previous URI

Wheezing

Productive cough

(See also assessment of bronchial asthma, p. 83.)

Viral-induced bronchitis—Inflammation of large airways (trachea and bronchi); usually occurs in association with viral URI, but other agents (e.g., bacteria, fungi, allergic disorders, airborne irritants) can trigger symptoms; seldom occurs as an isolated entity in childhood; affects children in first 4 years of life.

Persistent dry, hacking cough (worse at night), becoming productive in 2 to 3 days

Tachypnea

Low-grade fever

SAFETY ALERT

Avoid throat examination or culture in suspected epiglottitis because this can precipitate further or complete obstruction. Throat inspection should be attempted only when immediate intubation can be performed if needed.

Respiratory syncytial virus (RSV)/bronchiolitis—Acute viral infection with maximum effect at the bronchiolar level; usually affects children age 2 to 12 months; rare after age 2 years

Begins as simple URI with serous nasal discharge

May be accompanied by mild fever

Gradually causes increasing respiratory distress

Dyspnea

Paroxysmal, nonproductive cough

Tachypnea with flaring nares and retractions

Emphysema

Possible wheezing

Pneumonias

Pneumonia, inflammation of the pulmonary parenchyma, is common throughout childhood but occurs more frequently in infancy and early childhood. Clinically, pneumonia may occur either as a primary disease or as a complication of another illness. Morphologically, the following types of pneumonias are recognized:

Lobar pneumonia—All or a large segment of one or more pulmonary lobes is involved. When both lungs are affected, it is known as *bilateral* or *double pneumonia.*

Bronchopneumonia—Begins in the terminal bronchioles, which become clogged with mucopurulent exudate to form consolidated patches in nearby lobules; also called *lobular pneumonia*

Interstitial pneumonia—The inflammatory process is more or less confined within the alveolar walls (interstitium) and the peribronchial and interlobular tissues.

Pneumonitis is a localized acute inflammation of the lung without the toxemia associated with lobar pneumonia.

The pneumonias are more often classified according to the etiologic agent: viral, atypical (mycoplasma pneumonia), or bacterial pneumonia or pneumonia caused by aspiration of foreign substances. Pneumonia may be caused less often by histomycosis, coccidioidomycosis, and other fungi.

Viral pneumonia—Occurs more frequently than bacterial pneumonia; seen in children of all age-groups; often associated with viral URIs, and RSV accounts for the largest percentage.

Onset may be acute or insidious.

Symptoms variable

Mild—Low-grade fever, slight cough, malaise

Severe—High fever, severe cough, prostration

Cough usually unproductive early in disease

A few wheezes or crackles heard on auscultation

Atypical pneumonia—Etiologic agent is mycoplasma; occurs principally in the fall and winter months; more prevalent in crowded living conditions.

Onset may be sudden or insidious.

General systemic symptoms

- Fever
- Chills (older children)
- Headache
- Malaise
- Anorexia
- Myalgia

Followed by:

- Rhinitis
- Sore throat

- Dry, hacking cough
  - Nonproductive early, then seromucoid sputum, to mucopurulent or blood streaked
  - Fine crepitant crackles over various lung areas

Bacterial pneumonia—Includes pneumococcal, staphylococcal, streptococcal, and chlamydial pneumonias; clinical manifestations differ from other types of pneumonia; individual microorganisms produce a distinct clinical picture.

Onset abrupt

- Usually preceded by viral infection
- Toxic, acutely ill appearance
- Fever, usually high
- Malaise
- Rapid, shallow respirations
- Cough
- Chest pain often exaggerated by deep breathing
- Pain may be referred to abdomen
- Chills
- Meningismus

Pulmonary Tuberculosis

Caused by *Mycobacterium tuberculosis;* other factors that influence development of tuberculosis (TB) include the following: heredity (resistance to the infection may be genetically transmitted); gender (morbidity and mortality higher in adolescent girls); age (lower resistance in infants, higher incidence during adolescence); stress (emotional or physical); nutritional state; and intercurrent infection (especially human immunodeficiency virus [HIV], measles, pertussis).

Extremely variable

May be asymptomatic or produce a broad range of symptoms

- Fever
- Malaise
- Anorexia
- Weight loss
- Cough may or may not be present (progresses slowly over weeks to months).
- Aching pain and tightness in the chest
- Hemoptysis (rare)

With progression

- Respiratory rate increase
- Poor expansion of lung on the affected side
- Diminished breath sounds and crackles
- Dullness to percussion
- Persistence of fever
- Generalized symptoms manifested (especially infants)
- Child develops pallor, anemia, weakness, and weight loss

Aspiration of Foreign Substances

Inflammation of lung tissue can occur as the result of irritation from foreign material (e.g., vomitus, small objects, oral secretions, inhalation of smoke) and aspiration of food. Young children are especially prone to aspiration of foreign substances, and weak and debilitated children are subject to aspiration of food, vomitus, or secretions.

Foreign body (FB) aspiration—Clinical manifestations and changes produced depend on the degree and location of obstruction and type of FB.

- Choking
- Gagging
- Sternal retractions
- Wheezing
- Cough
- Inability to speak or breathe (larynx)
- Decreased airway entry, dyspnea (bronchi)

Signs of acute distress requiring immediate and quick action

- Cannot speak
- Becomes cyanotic
- Collapses

Aspiration pneumonia—May result from aspiration of fluids, food, vomitus, nasopharyngeal secretions, amniotic fluid and debris (during birth process), hydrocarbons, lipids, and talcum powder. Aspiration of fluid or food substances is a particular hazard in children who have difficulty with swallowing; who are unable to swallow because of paralysis, weaknesses, debility, congenital anomalies, or absent cough reflex; or who are force-fed, especially while crying or breathing rapidly. Irritated mucous membranes become a site for secondary bacterial infection.

Inhalation injury—Results from inhalation of smoke (noxious substances are primarily products of incomplete combustion) or other noxious gases

Local injury (smoke)

- Suspected with a history of flames in a closed space whether burns are present or not
- Sooty material around nose, in sputum
- Singed nasal hairs
- Mucosal burns of nose, lips, mouth, throat
- Hoarse voice
- Cough
- Inspiratory and expiratory stridor
- Signs of respiratory distress (tachypnea, tachycardia, diminished or abnormal breath sounds)

Systemic injury

- Gases that are nontoxic to the airways (e.g., carbon monoxide [CO], hydrogen cyanide) can cause injury and death by interfering with or inhibiting cellular respiration.

Mild CO poisoning
- Headache
- Visual disturbances
- Irritability
- Nausea

Severe CO poisoning
- Confusion
- Hallucinations
- Ataxia
- Coma
- Pallor
- Cyanosis
- Possibly bright, cherry-red lips and skin

SAFETY ALERT

SARS

Severe acute respiratory syndrome (SARS) is a respiratory illness that is spread via close person-to-person contact. SARS begins with a fever greater than 38.0° C (100.4° F), headache, general body aches, and mild respiratory symptoms. After 2 to 7 days, SARS patients may develop a dry cough and have trouble breathing. SARS can be fatal and poses a significant risk to others who have been in contact with the patient. Measures should be taken to limit SARS patients from contact with others, and infection control precautions should be used to minimize the potential for transmission. For further information visit the CDC SARS website at *http://www.cdc.gov/ncidod/sars.*

The Child with Asthma

Asthma—A reversible obstructive process characterized by an increased responsiveness and inflammation of the airways, especially the lower airway. It is a complex, chronic disorder involving biochemical, immunologic, infectious, endocrine, and psychologic factors.

Status asthmaticus is an acute, severe, and prolonged asthma attack in which respiratory distress continues despite vigorous therapeutic measures, especially the administration of sympathomimetics.

ASSESSMENT

Obtain a family history, especially regarding presence of atopy in family members.

Obtain a health history, including any evidence of atopy (e.g., eczema, rhinitis); evidence of possible precipitating factor(s); previous episodes of shortness of breath, wheezing, and coughing; and any complaints of prodromal itching at the front of neck or upper part of back.

Observe for manifestations of bronchial asthma.

Cough
- Hacking, paroxysmal, irritative, and nonproductive
- Becomes rattling and productive of frothy, clear, gelatinous sputum

Respiratory-related signs
- Coughing in absence of respiratory infection, especially at night
- Shortness of breath
- Prolonged expiratory phase
- Audible wheeze
- Often appears pale
- May have a malar flush and red ears
- Lips deep, dark, red color
- May progress to cyanosis of nail beds and skin, especially circumoral
- Restlessness
- Apprehension
- Anxious facial expression
- Sweating may be prominent as the attack progresses
- During infancy retractions may occur; clinical symptoms of asthma may be less obvious
- Older children may sit upright with shoulders in a hunched-over position, hands on the bed or chair, and arms braced
- Speaks with panting and short or broken phrases

Chest
- Hyperresonance on percussion
- Coarse, loud breath sounds
- Wheezes throughout the lung fields
- Prolonged expiration
- Crackles
- Generalized inspiratory and expiratory wheezing; increasingly high pitched

With repeated episodes
- Barrel chest
- Elevated shoulders
- Use of accessory muscles of respiration
- Facial appearance—Flattened malar bones, circles beneath the eyes, narrow nose, prominent upper teeth

Observe for manifestations of severe respiratory distress and impending respiratory failure.
- Profuse sweating
- Child sits upright; refuses to lie down
- Suddenly becomes agitated
- Suddenly becomes quiet when previously agitated

Assist with diagnostic procedures and tests (e.g., blood gases, electrolytes, pH; oximetry; urine specific gravity; radiography; pulmonary function tests).

Assess environment for presence of possible allergenic factors.

The Child with Fluid and Electrolyte Disturbance

Dehydration

Isotonic (isoosmotic, isonatremic)—Electrolyte and water deficits present in approximately balanced proportions

Hypertonic (hyperosmotic, hypernatremic)—Water loss in excess of electrolyte loss

Hypotonic (hypoosmotic, hyponatremic)—Electrolyte deficit exceeds water deficit

Fluid excess

Edema—Excess fluid in the interstitial spaces

Water intoxication—Excessive intake of fluid

ASSESSMENT

Take a careful health history, especially regarding current health problem (e.g., length of illness, events that may have precipitated symptoms).

Vomitus—Assess for volume, frequency, and type of vomiting

Sweating—Can be only estimated from frequency of clothing and linen changes

Perform a physical assessment.

Observe for manifestations of fluid and electrolyte disturbances (Table 1-5).

Vital signs—Temperature (normal, elevated, or lowered depending on degree of dehydration), pulse, and blood pressure

Skin—Assess for color, temperature, feel, turgor, and presence or absence of edema

Mucous membranes—Assess for moisture, color, and presence and consistency of secretions; condition of tongue

Fontanel (infants)—Sunken, soft, normal

Behavior—Irritability, lethargy, comatose condition, characteristics of cry (infant), activity level, restlessness

Perform specific assessments.

Intake and output—Accurate measurements of fluid intake and output are vital to the assessment of dehydration. This includes oral and parenteral intake and losses from urine, stools, vomiting, fistulas, nasogastric suction, sweat, and wound drainage.

Body weight—Measure regularly and at same time of day, usually each morning, to detect decreased or increased weight.

Urine—Assess frequency, volume, and color of urine.

Sensory alterations—Assess for presence of thirst.

Stools—Assess frequency, volume, and consistency of stools.

Assist with diagnostic procedures and tests (e.g., urinalysis, blood chemistry, complete blood count [CBC], blood gases).

TABLE 1-5 Signs and Symptoms Related to Fluid and Electrolyte Effects in Children

Significant Variation	Possible Imbalance	Comments
Temperature		
Elevated	Early water depletion Sodium excess	Elevated temperature will increase rate of water loss
Lowered	Fluid volume deficit	Caused by reduced energy output Shock is outcome of severe fluid deficit
Pulse		
Rapid, weak, thready, easily obliterated	Circulatory collapse may result from fluid deficit, hemorrhage, plasma-to-interstitial fluid shift	Pulse rate should include assessment of volume and quality, as well as rate Compare central with peripheral pulses Pulse may be influenced by activity or emotions
Bounding, easily obliterated	Impending circulatory collapse Sodium deficit	
Bounding, not easily obliterated	Fluid volume excess Interstitial fluid-to-plasma shift	
Weak, irregular, rapid	Severe potassium deficit	
Weak, irregular, slowing	Severe potassium excess	
Increased	Sodium excess	

TABLE 1-5 Signs and Symptoms Related to Fluid and Electrolyte Effects in Children—cont'd

Significant Variation	Possible Imbalance	Comments
Pulse—cont'd		
Magnesium deficit		
Decreased	Magnesium excess	
Respiration		
Slow, shallow	Respiratory alkalosis	Rapid respirations increase water loss
Rapid, deep	Metabolic acidosis	Not a reliable sign of respiratory alkalosis in infants
Dyspnea	Fluid volume excess, either general or pulmonary	
Moist crackles	Fluid volume excess Pulmonary edema	
Shallow	Potassium excess or deficit	
Stridor	Severe calcium deficit	
Blood Pressure		
Increased	Fluid volume excess	Blood pressure not a reliable sign in young children
Decreased	Sodium deficit Diminished vascular volume (loss of plasma-to-interstitial fluid shift)	Elasticity of blood vessels may keep blood pressure stable
Skin		
Color		
Pallor	Protein deficit Fluid deficit Fluid compartment shifts	Environmental influences (e.g., a cool room, uncovered infant) and fever may change skin color
Flushed	Sodium excess	
Temperature		
Cold, mottled extremities	Severe fluid volume deficit, even with fever Severe sodium depletion	Caused by decreased peripheral blood flow
Feel		
Dry	Fluid depletion Sodium excess	
Clammy, cold	Sodium deficit Plasma-to-interstitial fluid shift Hypotonic dehydration	
Elasticity		
Poor capillary filling	Fluid volume deficit	
Skin elasticity poor to very poor	Fluid depletion	Pinch of skin from abdomen or inner thigh is lifted and remains raised for several seconds
Pitting Edema		
Slight to severe	Fluid volume excess Plasma-to-interstitial fluid shift	Obese infants may appear normal; loss of foot creases may occur

Continued

TABLE 1-5 Signs and Symptoms Related to Fluid and Electrolyte Effects in Children—cont'd

Significant Variation	Possible Imbalance	Comments
Mucous Membranes		
Dry Longitudinal wrinkles on tongue	Fluid volume depletion	
Sticky; rough, red, dry tongue	Sodium excess Hypertonic dehydration	
Salivation and Tearing		
Absent	Fluid volume deficit	
Fontanels		
Sunken	Fluid volume deficit	
Bulging	Fluid volume excess	
Eyeballs		
Sunken Soft	Fluid volume deficit	
Sensory Alterations		
Tingling in fingers and toes	Calcium deficit Alkalosis	Sensory alterations unreliable in infants and young children who are unable to communicate symptoms
Abdominal cramps	Sodium deficit Potassium excess	
Muscle cramps	Calcium deficit Potassium deficit	
Lightheadedness	Respiratory alkalosis	
Nausea	Calcium excess Potassium excess Potassium deficit	
Thirst	Fluid deficit Sodium excess Calcium excess	May be difficult to assess in infants May be masked by nausea Any condition that reduces intravascular volume will stimulate thirst receptors
Neurologic Signs		
Hypotonia	Potassium deficit Calcium excess	
Flaccid paralysis	Severe potassium deficit Severe potassium excess	
Weakness	Metabolic acidosis	
Hypertonia Positive Chvostek's sign Tremors, cramps, tetany Twitching	Calcium deficit Alkalosis with diminished calcium ionization Calcium deficit Magnesium deficit	Children may develop calcium deficit easily, because growing bones do not readily relinquish calcium to circulation

TABLE 1-5 Signs and Symptoms Related to Fluid and Electrolyte Effects in Children—cont'd

Significant Variation	Possible Imbalance	Comments
Behavior		
Lethargy	Fluid volume deficit	Behavioral changes are among first indications of dehydration as reported by parents
Irritability	Fluid volume deficit	
Comatose condition	Hypotonic fluid deficit Profound acidosis of alkalosis	
Lethargy with hyperirritability on stimulation	Hypertonic fluid deficit	
Extreme restlessness	Potassium excess	
Weight		
Loss	Fluid deficit	
Up to 5% (50 ml/kg)	Mild	
5%-9% (75 ml/kg)	Moderate	
10% or higher (100 ml/kg)	Severe	
	Protein or calorie deficiency	
Gain	Edema, general or pulmonary Ascites	Check for hepatomegaly; children sequester excess fluid in liver
Urine		
Increased (polyuria)	Interstitial fluid-to-plasma shift Increased renal solute load	Normal range Infant: 2-3 ml/kg/hr
Diminished	Mild fluid deficit Moderate-to-severe fluid deficit	Toddler/preschooler: 2 ml/kg/hr School-age child: 1-2 ml/kg/hr
Oliguria	Moderate-to-severe fluid deficit Moderate-to-severe fluid deficit Plasma-to-interstitial fluid shift Sodium deficit Potassium excess Severe sodium excess Renal insufficiency	Adolescent: 0.5-1 ml/kg/hr (varies with intake and other factors)
Specific gravity	Adequate hydration	Used to monitor hydration status in infants
Low (≤1.010)	Fluid excess	Fixed low reading occurs in renal disease
	Renal disease Sodium deficit	
High (≥1.030)	Fluid deficit Sodium excess Glycosuria Proteinuria	

Continued

TABLE 1-5 Signs and Symptoms Related to Fluid and Electrolyte Effects in Children—cont'd

Significant Variation	Possible Imbalance	Comments
Urine—cont'd		
pH		
Acid	Acidosis, metabolic or respiratory	
	Alkalosis accompanied by severe potassium deficit	
	Fluid deficit	
Alkaline	Alkalosis, metabolic or respiratory	
	Hyperaldosteronism	
	Acidosis accompanied by chronic renal infection and renal tubular dysfunction	
	Diuretic therapy with carbonic anhydrase inhibitors	

The Child with Acute Diarrhea (Gastroenteritis)

Acute diarrhea (gastroenteritis)—An inflammation of the stomach and intestines caused by various bacteria, viral, and parasitic pathogens (Table 1-6)

ASSESSMENT

Obtain a careful history of illness including the following:

- Possible ingestion of contaminated food or water
- Possible infection elsewhere (e.g., respiratory or urinary tract infection)

Perform a routine physical assessment.

Observe for manifestations of acute gastroenteritis (see Table 1-6).

Assess state of dehydration (Tables 1-7 and 1-8)

Record fecal output—number, volume, characteristics.

Observe and record presence of associated signs—tenesmus, cramping, vomiting.

Assist with diagnostic procedures (e.g., collect specimens as needed; stools for pH, blood, sugar, frequency; urine for pH, specific gravity, frequency; CBC, serum electrolytes, creatine, blood urea nitrogen [BUN]).

Detect source of infection (e.g., examine other members of household and refer for treatment where indicated).

TABLE 1-6 Infectious Causes of Acute Diarrhea

Agents	Pathology	Characteristics	Comments
Viral			
Rotavirus			
Incubation: 48 hours Diagnosis: enzyme immunoassay (EIA)	Fecal-oral transmission 7 groups (A-G): Most group A virus replicates in mature villous epithelial cells of small intestine; leads to (1) imbalance in ratio of intestinal fluid absorption to secretion and (2) malabsorption of complex carbohydrates	Mild to moderate fever Vomiting followed by the onset of watery stools: Fever and vomiting generally abate in approximately 2 days but diarrhea persists 5-7 days	Most common cause of diarrhea in children <5 years of age Infants 6-12 months are most vulnerable Peak occurrences in winter months Important cause of nosocomial infections Affects all ages; usually milder in children >3 years of age; immunocompromised children at greater risk for complications
Norwalk-like Organisms			
Incubation: 12-48 hours Also called caliciviruses Diagnosis: EIA	Fecal-oral; contaminated water Pathology similar to rotavirus affects villous epithelial cells of small intestine and leads to (1) imbalance in ratio of intestinal fluid absorption to secretion and (2) malabsorption of complex carbohydrates	Abdominal cramps; nausea, vomiting, malaise, low-grade fever, watery diarrhea without blood; duration brief (2-3 days); tends to resemble so-called "food poisoning" symptoms, with nausea predominating	Affects all ages Multiple strains often named for the location of outbreak (e.g., Norwalk, Sapporo, Snow Mountain, Montgomery)
Bacterial			
Escherichia coli			
Incubation: 3-4 days Variable depending on strain Diagnosis: Sorbitol MacConkey Agar (SMAC agar) positive for blood but fecal leukocytes are absent or rare	*E. coli* strains produce diarrhea as result of enterotoxin production, adherence, or invasion (ETEC: enterotoxigenic-producing *E. coli* EHEC: Enterohemorrhagic *E. coli* Enteroaggregative *E. coli*)	Watery diarrhea 1-2 days then severe abdominal cramping and bloody diarrhea Can progress to hemolytic uremic syndrome (HUS)	Foodborne pathogen Traveler's diarrhea Highest incidence in summer Cause of nursery epidemics Symptomatic treatment Antibiotics may worsen course Antimotility agents and opioids should be avoided

Continued

TABLE 1-6 Infectious Causes of Acute Diarrhea—cont'd

Agents	Pathology	Characteristics	Comments
Bacterial—cont'd			
Salmonella *groups*			
Nontyphoidal; gram-negative rods, nonencapsulated nonsporulating Incubation 6-72 hours Diagnosis: gram-stained stool culture	Invasion of mucosa in the small and large intestine; edema of the lamina propria; focal acute inflammation with disruption of the mucosa and micro abscesses	Nausea , vomiting, colicky abdominal pain, bloody diarrhea, fever; symptoms variable: mild to severe May have headache and cerebral manifestations (e.g., drowsiness confusion, meningismus, seizures) Infants may be in afebrile and nontoxic condition May result in life-threatening septicemia and meningitis Nausea and vomiting typically short duration; diarrhea may persist as long as 2-3 weeks Typically shed virus for average of 5 weeks; cases reported up to a year	Incidence highest in warm months: July to November Foodborne outbreaks common Usually transmitted person to person but may transmit via undercooked meats, poultry Poultry and poultry products cause about half the cases In children: pets (e.g., dogs, cats, hamsters, turtles) Communicable as long as organisms are excreted Antibiotics not recommended in uncomplicated cases Antimotility agents also not recommended—prolong transit time and carrier state Incidence has decreased over past 10 years
Salmonella typhi			
Produces enteric fever—systemic syndrome Incubation usually 7-14 days but could be 3-30 days depending on size of inoculum Diagnosis: positive blood cultures; also sometimes positive stool and urine Late stage: positive bone marrow culture	Bloodstream invasion; after ingestion, organism attaches to microvilli of ileal brush borders and bacteria invade the intestinal epithelium via Peyer's patches Next is transported to intestinal lymph nodes and enters bloodstream via thoracic ducts, and circulating organisms reaches reticuloendothelial cells causing bacteremia	Manifestations depend on age Abdominal pain; diarrhea; nausea vomiting, high fever, lethargy Must be treated with antibiotics	Incidence is much lower in developed countries; United States has about 400 cases/year 65% of U.S. cases acquired via international cases Ingestion of foods or water contaminated with human feces is most common mode of transmission

TABLE 1-6 Infectious Causes of Acute Diarrhea—cont'd

Agents	Pathology	Characteristics	Comments
Bacterial—cont'd			
Salmonella typhi—cont'd			Congenital and intrapartum transmission can occur Three vaccines are available
Shigella *groups*			
Gram-negative Nonmotile Anaerobic bacilli Incubation: 1-7 days Diagnosis: stool culture Loaded with polymorphonuclear leukocytes	Enterotoxins: invades the epithelium with superficial mucosal ulcerations	Patients appear sick Symptoms begin with fever, fatigue, anorexia Crampy abdominal pain precede watery or bloody diarrhea Symptoms usually subside in 5-10 days	Most cases in children younger than 9 years with about one third of cases in children ages 1-4 weeks Antibiotics shorten illness and lower mortality All patients are at risk for dehydration Acute symptoms may persist for a week or more Antidiarrheal medications not recommended; may predispose to toxic mega colon
Yersinia *enterocolitis*			
Incubation period: dose-dependent, 1-3 weeks Diagnosis: stool culture serology; enzyme-linked immunosorbent assay (ELISA) Patients have leukocytosis; elevated sedimentation rate	Pathology is poorly understood; believed to involve production of enterotoxin	Mucoid diarrhea, sometimes bloody; abdominal pain suggestive of appendicitis; fever, vomiting	Seen more frequently in the winter months Transmitted by pets and food Antibiotics usually do not alter the clinical course in uncomplicated cases; antibiotics should be used in complicated infections and compromised hosts
Campylobacter jejuni			
Microaerophilic, motile, gram-negative bacilli Incubation period: 1-7 days Ability to cause illness appears dose related	Not fully understood; Possibly (1) adherence to intestinal mucosa by toxin; (2) invasion of the mucosa in the terminal ileum and colon (2) translocation in which the organisms	Fever, abdominal pain, diarrhea, can be bloody; vomiting Watery, profuse, foul-smelling diarrhea Clinically like *Salmonella* or *Shigella* Fecal-oral transmission	Most infections in humans relate to consumption of contaminated foods or water; undercooked meats, particularly chicken

Continued

TABLE 1-6 Infectious Causes of Acute Diarrhea—cont'd

Agents	Pathology	Characteristics	Comments
Bacterial—cont'd			
Campylobacter jejuni—cont'd			
Diagnosis by stool culture, sometimes in the blood Commonly found in GI tract of wild or domestic animals	penetrate the mucosa and replicate in the lamina propria		Also acquired from contaminated household pets (e.g., dogs, cats, hamsters) Bimodal peaks in infants <1 year and again at ages 15-29 Antibiotics do not prolong the carriage of bacteria and may eliminate organism more quickly Erythromycin is the drug of choice Antimotility agents not recommended and tend to prolong symptoms
Vibrio cholerae			
Gram-negative, motile, curved bacillus living in bodies of salt water Incubation 1-3 days Diagnosis by stool culture	Enters via oral route in contaminated food or water; if survives acid stomach environment travels to the small intestine and adheres to the mucosa and produces toxin	Onset abrupt; vomiting, watery diarrhea without cramping or tenesmus Dehydration can occur quickly	More prevalent in developing countries Rehydration most important treatment Antibiotics can shorten diarrhea Despite continued efforts still no vaccine
Clostridium difficile			
Gram-positive anaerobic bacillus Diagnosis by detecting *C. difficile* toxin in stool culture	Produces two important toxins (A and B) Toxin binds to the enterocyte surface receptor resulting in alteration in permeability, protein synthesis, and direct cytotoxicity	Most mild watery diarrhea lasting few days Some prolonged diarrhea and illness May cause pseudomembranous colitis Some individuals are extremely ill with high fever, leukocytosis, hypoalbuminemia	Associated with alteration of normal intestinal flora by antibiotics Adults tend to have more severe symptoms than children Treatment with antibiotics in symptomatic patients—metronidazole Resistant strains have developed Relapse is common

TABLE 1-6 Infectious Causes of Acute Diarrhea—cont'd

Agents	Pathology	Characteristics	Comments
Bacterial—cont'd			
Clostridium perfringens			
Incubation period: 8-24 hours; anaerobic, gram-positive, spore-producing bacilli	Toxins produced in the intestine after ingestion of organism	Acute onset—watery diarrhea, crampy abdominal pain Fever, nausea, and vomiting rare Duration of illness usually 24 hours	Transmitted by contaminated food products, most often meats and poultry Usually self-limiting and medical intervention not needed Oral rehydration usually sufficient Antibiotics serve no purpose and should not be used
Clostridium botulinum			
Incubation period: 12-26 hours (range, 6 hours to 8 days) Gram-positive anaerobic spore-producing bacilli Blood and stool culture should be obtained and transmitted to special laboratory (usually state health department) to detect toxin	Botulism caused by binding of toxin to the neuromuscular junction	Clinical presentation related to age and the strain of the botulism Gastrointestinal—abdominal pain, cramping, and diarrhea Other strains: respiratory, compromise, central nervous system symptoms	Transmitted in contaminated food products Can be acquired via wound infection Treatment involves supportive care and neutralization of the toxin
Staphylococcus			
Incubation period is generally short, 1 to 8 hours Gram-positive nonmotile, aerobic, or facultative anaerobic bacteria Diagnosis by identifying organism in food, blood, pus, aspirate	Direct tissue invasion and production of toxin	Clinical presentation depends on site of entry In food poisoning, profuse diarrhea, nausea, and vomiting	Gastrointestinal illness transmitted in inadequately cooked or refrigerated foods Self-limiting in gastrointestinal illness Symptomatic treatment

TABLE 1-7 Clinical Manifestations of Dehydration

	Isotonic (Loss of Water and Salt)	Hypotonic (Loss of Salt in Excess of Water)	Hypertonic (Loss of Water in Excess of Salt)
Skin			
Color	Gray	Gray	Gray
Temperature	Cold	Cold	Cold or hot
Turgor	Poor	Very poor	Fair
Feel	Dry	Clammy	Thickened, doughy
Mucous membranes	Dry	Slightly moist	Parched
Tearing and salivation	Absent	Absent	Absent
Eyeball	Sunken and soft	Sunken	Sunken
Fontanel	Sunken	Sunken	Sunken
Body temperature	Subnormal or elevated	Subnormal or elevated	Subnormal or elevated
Pulse	Rapid	Very rapid	Moderately rapid
Respirations	Rapid	Rapid	Rapid
Behavior	Irritable to lethargic	Lethargic to comatose; convulsions	Marked lethargy with extreme hyperirritability on stimulation

TABLE 1-8 Signs Associated with Isotonic Dehydration in Infants

	Degree of Dehydration		
	Mild	Moderate	Severe
Fluid volume loss	<50 ml/kg	50-90 ml/kg	≥100 mg/kg
Skin color	Pale	Gray	Mottled
Skin elasticity	Decreased	Poor	Very poor
Mucous membranes	Dry	Very dry	Parched
Urinary output	Decreased	Oliguria	Marked oliguria and azotemia
Blood pressure	Normal	Normal or lowered	Lowered
Pulse	Normal or increased	Increased	Rapid and thready
Capillary filling time	<2 seconds	2-3 seconds	>3 seconds

The Child with Acute Hepatitis

Hepatitis—An acute or chronic inflammation of the liver

Hepatitis of viral origin is caused by at least six types of virus.

- Hepatitis A virus (HAV)
- Hepatitis B virus (HBV)
- Hepatitis C virus (HCV, previously designated parenterally transmitted non-A, non-B hepatitis virus)
- Hepatitis D virus (HDV, occurs in children already infected with HBV)
- Hepatitis E virus (enterically transmitted non-A, non-B hepatitis virus)
- Hepatitis G virus (HGV, bloodborne)

ASSESSMENT

Perform a routine physical assessment.

Take a careful health history, especially regarding:

- Contact with persons known to have hepatitis
- Unsafe sanitation practices (e.g., drinking impure water)
- Eating certain foods (e.g., raw shellfish taken from polluted water)
- Previous blood transfusions
- Ingestion of hepatotoxic drugs (e.g., salicylates, sulfonamides, antineoplastic agents, acetaminophen, anticonvulsants)
- Parenteral administration of illicit drugs, or sexual contact with persons who use these drugs

Observe for manifestations of hepatitis (Table 1-9).

Assist with diagnostic procedures and tests (e.g., blood examination for presence of antibodies, liver function tests).

TABLE 1-9 Comparison of Clinical Features of Hepatitis Types A, B, and C

Characteristics	Type A	Type B	Type C
Onset	Usually rapid, acute	More insidious	Usually insidious
Fever	Common and early	Less frequent	Less frequent
Anorexia	Common	Mild to moderate	Mild to moderate
Nausea and vomiting	Common	Sometimes present	Mild to moderate
Rash	Rare	Common	Sometimes present
Arthralgia	Rare	Common	Rare
Pruritus	Rare	Sometimes present	Sometimes present
Jaundice	Present (many cases anicteric)	Present	Present

The Child with Appendicitis

Appendicitis—An inflammation of the vermiform appendix (blind sac at the end of the cecum)

ASSESSMENT

Take a careful history of illness.

Observe for clinical manifestations of appendicitis:

- Initially abdominal pain is usually colicky, cramping, and located around umbilicus
- Pain progresses and becomes constant
- Right lower quadrant abdominal pain (McBurney point)
- Fever
- Rigid abdomen
- Decreased or absent bowel sounds
- Nausea and vomiting (commonly follows onset of pain)
- Constipation or diarrhea may be present
- Anorexia
- Tachycardia; rapid, shallow breathing
- Pallor
- Lethargy
- Irritability
- Stooped posture

Observe for signs of peritonitis:

- Fever
- Sudden relief from pain (after perforation)
- Subsequent increase in pain, which is usually diffuse and accompanied by rigid guarding of the abdomen
- Progressive abdominal distention
- Tachycardia
- Rapid, shallow breathing
- Pallor
- Chills
- Irritability
- Restlessness

Assist with diagnostic procedures (e.g., white blood count, abdominal radiography).

The Child with Cardiovascular Dysfunction

Cardiac dysfunction—Dysfunction, congenital or acquired, of the heart or the blood vessels

Cardiovascular system—Consists of the heart and blood vessels

ASSESSMENT

Assess general appearance, behavior, and function.

- Inspection

  Nutritional state—Failure to thrive, poor weight gain, poor feeding habits, fatigue during feeding, or sweating during feeding is associated with heart disease.

  Color—Cyanosis is a common feature of congenital heart disease, and pallor is associated with anemia, which frequently accompanies heart disease.

  Chest deformities—An enlarged heart sometimes distorts the chest configuration.

  Unusual pulsations—Visible pulsations are sometimes present.

  Respiratory excursion—The ease or difficulty of respirating (e.g., tachypnea, dyspnea, presence of expiratory grunt, shortness of breath, persistent cough) or frequent respiratory infections.

  Clubbing of fingers—Associated with some types of congenital heart disease.

  Behavior—Assuming knee-chest position or squatting is typical of some types of heart disease; exercise intolerance.
- Palpation and percussion

Chest—Helps discern heart size and other characteristics (e.g., thrills) associated with heart disease.
Abdomen—Hepatomegaly and/or splenomegaly may be evident.
Peripheral pulses—Rate, regularity, and amplitude (strength) may reveal discrepancies.

- Auscultation
  Heart—Detect presence of heart murmurs.
  Heart rate and rhythm—Observe for discrepancies between apical and peripheral pulses.
  Character of heart sounds—Reveals deviations in heart sounds and intensity that help localize heart defects
  Lungs—May reveal crackles, wheezes
  Blood pressure—Deviations present in some cardiac conditions (e.g., discrepancies between upper and lower extremities)

Assist with diagnostic procedures and tests (e.g., electrocardiography, radiography, echocardiography, fluoroscopy, ultrasonography, angiography, blood analysis [blood count, hemoglobin, packed cell volume, blood gases], exercise stress test, cardiac catheterization).

The Child with Congenital Heart Disease

Congenital heart disease—A structural or functional defect of the heart or great vessels present at birth

ASSESSMENT

Perform physical assessment with special emphasis on color, pulse (apical, peripheral), respiration, blood pressure, and examination and auscultation of chest.

Take careful health history, including evidence of poor weight gain, poor feeding, exercise intolerance, unusual posturing, or frequent respiratory tract infections.

Observe child for manifestations of congenital heart disease.

Infants

- ***Cyanosis***—Generalized, especially mucous membranes, lips and tongue, conjunctiva; highly vascularized areas
- Cyanosis during exertion such as crying, feeding, straining, or when immersed in water; peripheral or central
- Dyspnea, especially following physical effort such as feeding, crying, straining
- Fatigue
- Poor growth and development (failure to thrive)
- Frequent respiratory tract infections
- Feeding difficulties
- Hypotonia
- Excessive sweating
- Syncopal attacks such as paroxysmal hyperpnea, anoxic spells

Older children

- Impaired growth
- Delicate, frail body build
- Fatigue
- Effort dyspnea
- Orthopnea
- Digital clubbing
- Squatting for relief of dyspnea
- Headache
- Epistaxis
- Leg fatigue

The Child with Congestive Heart Failure

Congestive heart failure—The inability of the heart to pump an adequate amount of blood to the systemic circulation at normal filling pressures to meet the metabolic demands of the body

ASSESSMENT

Perform a physical assessment.

Perform a cardiac assessment.

Take a careful health history, especially regarding previous cardiac problems.

Observe for manifestations of congestive heart failure.

Impaired myocardial function

- Tachycardia
- Sweating (inappropriate)
- Decreased urine output
- Fatigue
- Weakness
- Restlessness
- Anorexia
- Pale, cool extremities
- Weak peripheral pulses
- Decreased blood pressure
- Gallop rhythm
- Cardiomegaly

Pulmonary congestion

- Tachypnea
- Dyspnea
- Retractions (infants)

- Flaring nares
- Exercise intolerance
- Orthopnea
- Cough, hoarseness
- Cyanosis
- Wheezing
- Grunting

Systemic venous congestion

- Weight gain
- Hepatomegaly
- Peripheral edema, especially periorbital
- Ascites
- Neck vein distention (children)
- Assist with diagnostic procedures and tests (e.g., radiography, electrocardiography, echocardiography).

The Child in Shock (Circulatory Failure)

Shock (circulatory failure)—A clinical syndrome characterized by tissue perfusion that is inadequate to meet the metabolic demands of the body, resulting in cellular dysfunction and eventual organ failure.

STAGES OF SHOCK

Compensated shock—Vital organ function is maintained by intrinsic compensatory mechanisms; blood flow is usually normal or increased but generally uneven or maldistributed in the microcirculation.

Decompensated shock—Efficiency of the cardiovascular system gradually diminishes until perfusion in the microcirculation becomes marginal despite compensatory adjustments.

Irreversible, or terminal, shock—Damage to vital organs such as the heart or brain, of such magnitude that the entire organism will be disrupted regardless of therapeutic intervention; death occurs even if cardiovascular measurements return to normal levels with therapy.

TYPES OF SHOCK

Cardiogenic Shock

Characteristic

- Decreased cardiac output

Most frequent causes

- Following surgery for congenital heart disease
- Primary pump failure—Myocarditis, myocardial trauma, biochemical derangements, congestive heart failure
- Dysrhythmias—Paroxysmal atrial tachycardia, atrioventricular block, and ventricular dysrhythmias; secondary to myocarditis or biochemical abnormalities

Distributive Shock

Characteristics

- Reduction in peripheral vascular resistance
- Profound inadequacies in tissue perfusion
- Increased venous capacity and pooling
- Acute reduction in return blood flow to the heart
- Diminished cardiac output

Most frequent causes

- Anaphylaxis (anaphylactic shock)—Extreme allergy or hypersensitivity to a foreign substance
- Sepsis (septic shock, bacteremic shock, endotoxic shock)—Overwhelming sepsis and circulating bacterial toxins
- Loss of neuronal control (neurogenic shock)—Interruption of neuronal transmission (spinal cord injury)
- Myocardial depression and peripheral dilation—Exposure to anesthesia or ingestion of barbiturates, tranquilizers, narcotics, antihypertensive agents, or ganglionic blocking agents

Hypovolemic Shock

Characteristics

- Reduction in size of vascular compartment
- Falling blood pressure
- Poor capillary filling
- Low central venous pressure (CVP)

Most frequent causes

- Blood loss (hemorrhagic shock)—Trauma, gastrointestinal (GI) bleeding, intracranial hemorrhage
- Plasma loss—Increased capillary permeability associated with sepsis and acidosis, hypoproteinemia, burns, peritonitis
- Extracellular fluid loss—Vomiting, diarrhea, glycosuric diuresis, sunstroke

ASSESSMENT

Maintain vigilance in situations that predispose the patient to shock (e.g., trauma, burns, overwhelming sepsis, diarrhea, vomiting).

Observe for manifestations of shock.

Early clinical signs (compensated shock)

- Apprehension
- Irritability
- Unexplained tachycardia
- Normal blood pressure
- Narrowing pulse pressure
- Thirst
- Pallor
- Diminished urinary output
- Reduced perfusion of extremities

Advanced shock (decompensated shock)

- Confusion and somnolence
- Tachypnea
- Tachycardia
- Moderate metabolic acidosis
- Oliguria

- Cool, pale extremities
- Decreased skin turgor
- Poor capillary filling

Impending cardiopulmonary arrest (irreversible shock)

- Thready, weak pulse
- Hypotension
- Periodic breathing or apnea
- Anuria
- Stupor or coma

Monitor vital signs, CVP, capillary filling, intake and output, and cardiac function, on admission and continuously or very frequently.

Assist with diagnostic procedures and tests (e.g., blood count, blood gases, pH, liver function tests, coagulation studies, renal function tests, cultures, electrolytes, electrocardiography).

The Child with Anemia

Anemia—A condition in which the number of red blood cells (RBCs) and/or the hemoglobin concentration is reduced below normal

ASSESSMENT

Perform a physical assessment.

Take a health history, including a careful dietary history, to identify any deficiencies (e.g., evidence of pica, the eating of nonfood substances such as clay, ice, or paste).

Observe for manifestations of anemia.

General manifestations

- Muscle weakness
- Easy fatigability (frequent resting, shortness of breath, poor sucking in infants)
- Pale skin (waxy pallor seen in severe anemia)
- Pica

Central nervous system manifestations

- Headache
- Dizziness
- Lightheadedness
- Irritability
- Slowed thought processes
- Decreased attention span
- Apathy
- Depression

Shock (blood loss anemia)

- Poor peripheral perfusion
- Skin moist and cool
- Low blood pressure and CVP
- Increased heart rate
- Assist with diagnostic tests (e.g., analysis of blood elements)

The Child with Acute Renal Failure

Acute renal failure (ARF)—A condition that results when the kidneys suddenly are unable to excrete urine of sufficient volume or adequate concentration to maintain normal body fluid balance

ASSESSMENT

Initial Assessment

Perform a physical assessment.

Take a careful health history, especially regarding evidence of glomerulonephritis, obstructive uropathy, and exposure to or ingestion of toxic chemicals (including heavy metals, carbon tetrachloride, or other organic solvents; and nephrotoxic drugs).

Observe for manifestations of acute renal failure.

Specific

- Oliguria
- Anuria uncommon (except in obstructive disorders)

Nonspecific (may develop)

- Nausea
- Vomiting
- Drowsiness
- Edema
- Hypertension
- Cardiac arrhythmia

Ongoing Assessment

Careful monitoring of the following:

- Urinary output (insert Foley catheter)
- Blood pressure, pulse, and respiration
- Cardiac function
- Neurologic function
- Observe for signs of fluid overload
- Manifestations of underlying disorder or pathology

Assist with diagnostic tests (e.g., urinalysis, BUN, nonprotein nitrogen, creatinine, serum electrolytes, CBC, blood gases, and specific tests to determine cause of renal failure).

The Child with Chronic Renal Failure

Chronic renal failure (CRF)—Occurs when the diseased kidneys are unable to maintain the chemical composition of body fluids within normal limits under normal conditions until more than 50% of functional renal capacity is destroyed by disease or injury

The final stage is end-stage renal disease (ESRD), which is irreversible.

Various biochemical substances accumulate in the blood as a result of diminished renal function and produce complications such as the following:

Anemia caused by hematologic dysfunction, including shortened life span of RBCs, impaired RBC production related to decreased production of erythropoietin, prolonged bleeding time, and nutritional anemia

Calcium and phosphorus disturbances resulting in altered bone metabolism, which in turn causes bone demineralization, growth arrest or retardation, bone pain, and deformities known as *renal osteodystrophy*

Growth disturbance, probably caused by such factors as poor nutrition, anorexia, renal osteodystrophy, biochemical abnormalities, corticosteroid treatment, tissue resistance to growth hormone, and mineral and vitamin deficiencies

Hyperkalemia of dangerous levels; occurrence uncommon until the end stage

Metabolic acidosis of a sustained nature because of continual hydrogen ion retention and bicarbonate loss

Retention of waste products, especially BUN and creatinine

Water and sodium retention, which contribute to edema and vascular congestion

ASSESSMENT

Initial Assessment

Perform a routine physical assessment with special attention to measurements of growth parameters.

Take a health history, especially regarding renal dysfunction, eating behavior, frequency of infections, and energy level.

Observe for evidence of manifestations of chronic renal failure.

Early signs

- Loss of normal energy
- Increased fatigue on exertion
- Pallor, subtle (may not be noticed)
- Elevated blood pressure (sometimes)
- Growth delay

As the disease progresses

- Decreased appetite (especially at breakfast)
- Less interest in normal activities
- Increased or decreased urinary output with compensatory intake of fluid
- Pallor more evident
- Sallow, muddy appearance of skin

Possible complaints

- Headache
- Muscle cramps
- Nausea

Other signs and symptoms

- Weight loss
- Facial edema
- Malaise
- Bone or joint pain
- Growth retardation
- Dryness or itching of the skin
- Bruised skin
- Sensory or motor loss (sometimes)
- Amenorrhea (common in adolescent girls)

Uremic syndrome (untreated)

- Gastrointestinal (GI) symptoms
  - Anorexia
  - Nausea and vomiting
- Bleeding tendencies
  - Bruises
  - Bloody, diarrheal stools
  - Stomatitis
  - Bleeding from lips and mouth
- Intractable itching
- Uremic frost (deposits of urea crystals on skin)
- Unpleasant uremic breath odor
- Deep respirations
- Hypertension
- Congestive heart failure
- Pulmonary edema
- Neurologic involvement
  - Progressive confusion
  - Dulled sensorium
  - Coma (ultimately)
  - Tremors
  - Muscular twitching
  - Seizures

Ongoing Assessment

Take a history for new or increasing symptoms.

Carry out frequent physical assessments with particular attention to blood pressure, signs of edema, and neurologic dysfunction.

Assess psychologic responses to the disease and its therapies.

Assist with diagnostic procedures and tests (e.g., urinalysis, CBC, blood chemistry, and renal biopsy).

The Child with Nephrotic Syndrome

Nephrotic syndrome—A clinical state characterized by an increased permeability of the glomerular membrane to protein, which results in massive urinary protein loss

ASSESSMENT

Perform a physical assessment, including assessment of extent of edema.

Take a careful health history, especially relative to recent weight gain or renal dysfunction.

Observe for manifestations of nephrotic syndrome.
- Weight gain
- Edema
- Puffiness of face, especially around the eyes
  - Apparent on arising in the morning
  - Subsides during the day

Abdominal swelling (ascites)

Respiratory difficulty (pleural effusion)

Labial or scrotal swelling

Edema of intestinal mucosa causes:
- Diarrhea
- Anorexia
- Poor intestinal absorption

Extreme skin pallor (often)

Irritability

Easily fatigued

Lethargic

Blood pressure normal or slightly decreased

Susceptibility to infection

Urine alterations
- Decreased volume
- Darkly opalescent
- Frothy

Assist with diagnostic procedures and tests (e.g., urinalysis for protein, casts, and RBCs; blood analysis for serum protein [total, albumin/globulin ratio, cholesterol]; hemoglobin; hematocrit; serum sodium; renal biopsy).

The Child with Neurologic Dysfunction

Cerebral dysfunction—Concerns disorders affecting cerebral structure and function

ASSESSMENT

Initial Assessment

Take a careful history.
- Family history, for evidence of genetic disorders with neurologic manifestations
- Health history, especially for clues regarding the cause of dysfunction (e.g., injury, short febrile illness, encounter with an animal or insect, ingestion of neurotoxic substances, inhalation of chemicals, past illness, or known diabetes mellitus or sickle cell disease)
- Sudden or progressive alterations in movement (e.g., ataxia, seizures) or mental ability
- Headache, nausea, vomiting, double vision, bowel or bladder incontinence in a previously continent child
- Unusual behavior, including nature and frequency

Perform physical assessment with special emphasis on the following:
- Neurologic assessment (see p. 72)
- Assessment of cranial nerves (see p. 77)
- Developmental assessment (see p. 160)

Perform physical evaluation of infant.
- Size and shape of the head
- Spontaneous activity and postural reflex activity
- Sensory responses
- Attitude—Normal flexed posture, extreme extension, opisthotonos, hypotonia
- Symmetry in movement of extremities
- Excessive tremulousness or frequent twitching movements
- Altered expiratory cycle
  - Prolonged apnea
  - Ataxic breathing
  - Paradoxic chest movement
  - Hyperventilation
- Skin and hair texture
- Distinctive facial features
- Presence of a high-pitched, piercing cry
- Abnormal eye movements
- Inability to suck or swallow
- Lip smacking
- Asymmetric contraction of facial muscles
- Yawning (may indicate cranial nerve involvement)
- Muscular activity and coordination
- Level of development

Observe for speed of movement; and presence and location of any tremors, twitching, tics, or other unusual movements.

Observe gait (e.g., ataxia, spasticity, rigidity).

Note any unusual discharge from body orifices.

Note location, extent, and type of any wound.

Assess level of consciousness.*

Full consciousness—Awake and alert; oriented to time, place, and person; behavior appropriate for age

Confusion—Impaired decision making

*Modified from Seidel HM and others, editors: *Mosby's guide to physical examination*, ed 6, St Louis, 2006, Mosby.

Disorientation—Confusion regarding time, place; decreased level of consciousness

Lethargy—Limited spontaneous movement, sluggish speech, drowsiness; falls asleep quickly

Obtundation—Arousable with stimulation

Stupor—Remains in a deep sleep, responsive only to vigorous and repeated stimulation; simple motor or moaning responses to stimuli, responses slow

Coma—No motor or verbal response to noxious or painful stimuli or decerebrate posturing

Persistent vegetative state (PVS)—Permanently lost function of the cerebral cortex; eyes follow objects only by reflex or when attracted to the direction of loud sounds; all four limbs are spastic but can withdraw from painful stimuli; hands show reflexive grasping and groping; the face can grimace; some food may be swallowed; and the child may groan or cry but utters no words.

Observe for evidence of increased intracranial pressure (ICP).

Infants

- Tense, bulging fontanel; lack of normal pulsations
- Separated cranial sutures
- Macewen's (cracked-pot) sign
- Irritability
- High-pitched cry
- Increased frontooccipital circumference (FOC)
- Distended scalp veins
- Changes in feeding
- Cries when disturbed
- Setting-sun sign

Children

- Headache
- Nausea
- Forceful vomiting, often without nausea
- Diplopia, blurred vision
- Seizures

Personality and behavior signs

- Irritability, restlessness
- Indifference, drowsiness, or lack of interest
- Decline in school performance
- Diminished physical activity and motor performance
- Increased devoted sleeping
- Significant
- Memory loss if pressure is markedly increased
- Inability to follow simple commands
- Progression to lethargy and drowsiness

Late signs

- Decreased motor response to command
- Decreased sensory response to painful stimuli
- Alterations in pupil size and reactivity
- Sometimes decerebrate or decorticate posturing
- Cheyne-Stokes respirations
- Papilledema
- Decreased consciousness
- Coma

Assist with diagnostic procedures and tests (e.g., lumbar puncture, subdural tap, ventricular puncture, electroencephalography, radiography, magnetic resonance imaging (MRI), computed tomography (CT), nuclear brain scan, echoencephalography, positron emission transaxial tomography, real-time ultrasonography, digital subtraction angiography; blood biochemistry [pH, blood gases, ammonia, glucose], and any special tests).

Ongoing Assessment (Extent of Assessment Depends on Condition)

Monitor vital signs, especially noting changes in:

- Temperature, pulse, blood pressure
- Respirations—Regular or irregular, deep or shallow, pattern of breathing, odor of breath

Eye movements

- Position of globes—Divergence, conjugate deviation, skewed
- Movement of globes—Extraocular palsy, nystagmus, fixed gaze
- Pupil size—Dilated, pinpoint, unequal
- Pupil reaction—Sluggish, absent, different
- Doll's head maneuver (only if cervical spine injury has been ruled out)

Motor function

- Voluntary movements of extremities (e.g., purposeful or random)
- Changes in muscular tone
- Changes in position of body and/or head
- Tremor, twitching
- Seizure activity (e.g., generalized or partial)
- Signs of meningeal irritation (e.g., nuchal rigidity or opisthotonos)
- Spontaneous—Normal but reduced, involuntary, evoked
- Evoked—Purposeful, reflex withdrawal
- Paresis—Decorticate, decerebrate; any lateralized difference in function
- Crying and speech—Present or absent, conversant or confused, monosyllabic, jargon, type of cry (piercing, difficult to hear)
- Level of consciousness
- Monitor ICP device
- Monitor CVP device
- Monitor fluid intake and output
- Weigh daily or as ordered to detect fluid accumulation or reduction
- Headache (if information can be elicited)—Presence or absence, type and location, continuous or intermittent
- In infants:
  - Measure FOC
  - Assess status of fontanel—Size and tension

The Child with Seizures

Epilepsy—A chronic seizure disorder with recurrent and unprovoked seizures, which requires long-term treatment. Not every seizure is epileptic.

Seizures—Brief malfunctions of the brain's electrical system resulting from cortical neuronal discharge. Seizures may manifest as **convulsions** (involuntary muscular contraction and relaxation); changes in behavior, sensations, or perception; visual and auditory hallucinations; and altered consciousness or unconsciousness.

ASSESSMENT

Obtain a health history, especially regarding prenatal, perinatal, and neonatal events; any instances of infection, apnea, colic, or poor feeding; and any information regarding previous accidents or serious illnesses.

Obtain a history of seizure activity including the following:

- Description of child's behavior during seizure
- Age of onset
- Time when seizure occurred—Time of day, while awake or during sleep, relationship to meals
- Any triggering factors that might have precipitated seizure (e.g., fever, infection); falls that may have caused trauma to the head; anxiety; fatigue; activity (e.g., hyperventilation); environmental events (e.g., exposure to strong stimuli such as bright, flashing lights or loud noises)
- Sensory phenomena child experiences
- Duration, progression, and any postictal feelings or behaviors

Perform a physical and neurologic assessment.

Observe seizure manifestations (Box 1-9).

Assist with diagnostic procedures and tests (e.g., electroencephalography, tomography, skull radiography, echoencephalography, brain scan; blood chemistry, serum glucose, BUN, ammonia; and specific tests for metabolic disorders).

Observe Seizure

Describe the following:

- Only what is actually observed
- Order of events (before, during, and after)

Duration of seizure

- Tonic-clonic: from first signs of event until jerking stops
- Absence: from loss of consciousness until patient regains consciousness
- Complex partial: from first sign of unresponsiveness, motor activity, or automatisms until there is responsiveness to environment

Onset

Time of onset

Significant preseizure events—Bright lights, noise, excitement, emotional outbursts

Behavior

- Change in facial expression, such as fear
- Cry or other sound
- Stereotypic or automatous movements
- Random activity (wandering)

Position of head, body, extremities

- Unilateral or bilateral posturing of one or more extremities
- Body deviation to side

Movement

Change of position, if any

Site of commencement—Hand, thumb, mouth, generalized

Tonic phase, if present—Length, parts of body involved

Clonic phase—Twitching or jerking movements, parts of body involved, sequence of parts involved, generalized, change in character of movements

Lack of movement or muscle tone of any body part or entire body

Face

Color change—Pallor, cyanosis, flushing

Perspiration

Mouth—Position, deviation to one side, teeth clenched, tongue bitten, frothing at mouth, flecks of blood or bleeding

Lack of expression

Eyes

Position—Straight ahead, deviation upward, deviation outward, conjugate or divergent

Pupils (if able to assess)—Change in size, equality, reaction to light, and accommodation

Respiratory Effort

Presence and length of apnea

Presence of stertor

Other

Involuntary urination

Involuntary defecation

Observe Postictally

Duration of postictal period

Method of termination

State of consciousness—Unresponsiveness, drowsiness, confusion

Orientation to time, persons

Sleeping but able to be aroused

Motor ability

- Any change in motor power
- Ability to move all extremities
- Any paresis or weakness
- Ability to whistle (if appropriate to age)

Speech—Changes, peculiarities, type and extent of any difficulties
Sensations
- Complaint of discomfort or pain
- Any sensory impairment of hearing, vision
- Recollection of preseizure sensations, warning of attack
- Awareness that attack was beginning
- Recall of words spoken to child

BOX 1-9 | Classification and Clinical Manifestations of Seizures

Partial Seizures

Simple Partial Seizures with Motor Signs

Characteristics
- Localized motor symptoms
- Somatosensory, psychic, and autonomic symptoms
- Combination of these
- Abnormal discharges remain unilateral

Manifestations
- Aversive seizure (most common motor seizure in children)
  Eye or eyes and head turn away from the side of the focus
  Awareness of movement or loss of consciousness
- Rolandic (Sylvian) seizure
  Tonic-clonic movements involving the face
  Salivation
  Arrested speech
  Most common during sleep
- Jacksonian march (rare in children)
  Orderly, sequential progression of clonic movements beginning in a foot, hand, or face and moving or "marching" to adjacent body parts

Simple Partial Seizures with Sensory Signs

Characterized by various sensations, including:
- Numbness, tingling, prickling, paresthesia, or pain originating in one area (e.g., face, extremities) and spreading to other parts of the body
- Visual sensations or formed images
- Motor phenomena such as posturing or hypertonia
- Uncommon in children under 8 years of age

Complex Partial Seizures (Psychomotor Seizures)

Observed more often in children from 3 years through adolescence

Characteristics
- May begin with an aura
- Period of altered behavior
- Amnesia for event (no recollection of behavior)
- Inability to respond to environment
- Impaired consciousness during event
- Drowsiness or sleep usually follows seizure
- Confusion and amnesia may be prolonged
- Complex sensory phenomena (aura)
  Most frequent sensation is strange feeling in the pit of the stomach that rises toward the throat
  Often accompanied by:
  - Odd or unpleasant odors or tastes
  - Complex auditory or visual hallucinations
  - Ill-defined feelings of elation or strangeness (e.g., déjà vu, a feeling of familiarity in a strange environment)

  May be strong feelings of fear and anxiety, distorted sense of time and self
  Small children may emit a cry or attempt to run for help

Patterns of motor behavior
- Stereotypic
- Similar with each subsequent seizure
- May suddenly cease activity, appear dazed, stare into space, become confused and apathetic, and become limp or stiff or display some form of posturing
- May be confused
- May perform purposeless, complicated activities in a repetitive manner (automatisms), such as walking, running, kicking, laughing, or speaking incoherently, most often followed by postictal confusion or sleep; may be oropharyngeal activities, such as smacking, chewing, drooling, swallowing, and nausea or abdominal pain followed by stiffness, a fall, and postictal sleep; rarely manifests as rage or temper tantrums; aggressive acts uncommon during seizure

Generalized Seizures

Tonic-Clonic Seizures (Formerly Known as Grand Mal)

Most common and most dramatic of all seizure manifestations
Occur without warning
Tonic phase: lasts approximately 10 to 20 seconds
- Manifestations
  Eyes roll upward
  Immediate loss of consciousness
  If standing, falls to floor or ground
  Stiffens in generalized, symmetric tonic contraction of entire body musculature
  Arms usually flexed
  Legs, head, and neck extended
  May utter a peculiar piercing cry
  Apneic, may become cyanotic
  Increased salivation and loss of swallowing reflex

Clonic phase: lasts about 30 seconds but can vary from only a few seconds to a half hour or longer
- Manifestations
  Violent jerking movements as the trunk and extremities undergo rhythmic contraction and relaxation
  May foam at the mouth
  May be incontinent of urine and feces
  As event ends, movements become less intense, occur at longer intervals, then cease entirely

Continued

BOX 1-9 | Classification and Clinical Manifestations of Seizures—cont'd

Generalized Seizures—cont'd

Tonic-Clonic Seizures—cont'd

Status epilepticus: series of seizures at intervals too brief to allow the child to regain consciousness between the time one event ends and the next begins
- Requires emergency intervention
- Can lead to exhaustion, respiratory failure, and death

Postictal state
- Appears to relax
- May remain semiconscious and difficult to rouse
- May awaken in a few minutes
- Remains confused for several hours
- Poor coordination
- Mild impairment of fine motor movements
- May have visual and speech difficulties
- May vomit or complain of severe headache
- When left alone, usually sleeps for several hours
- On awakening is fully conscious
- Usually feels tired and complains of sore muscles and headache
- No recollection of entire event

Absence Seizures (Formerly Called Petit Mal or Lapses)

Characteristics
- Onset usually between 4 and 12 years of age
- More common in girls than in boys
- Usually cease at puberty
- Brief loss of consciousness
- Minimal or no alteration in muscle tone
- May go unrecognized because little change in child's behavior
- Abrupt onset; child suddenly develops 20 or more attacks daily
- Event often mistaken for inattentiveness or daydreaming
- Events can be precipitated by hyperventilation, hypoglycemia, stresses (emotional, physiologic), fatigue, or sleeplessness

Manifestations
- Brief loss of consciousness
- Appear without warning or aura
- Usually last about 5 to 10 seconds
- Slight loss of muscle tone may cause child to drop objects
- Able to maintain postural control; seldom falls
- Minor movements such as lip smacking, twitching of eyelids or face, or slight hand movements
- Not accompanied by incontinence
- Amnesia for episode
- May need to reorient self to previous activity

Atonic and Akinetic Seizures (Also Known as Drop Attacks)

Characterized by:
- Onset usually between 2 and 5 years of age
- Sudden, momentary loss of muscle tone and postural control
- Events recur frequently during the day, particularly in the morning hours and shortly after awakening

Manifestations
- Loss of tone causes child to fall to floor violently

  Unable to break fall by putting out hand

  May incur a serious injury to the face, head, or shoulder
- Loss of consciousness only momentary

Myoclonic Seizures

A variety of convulsive episodes

May be isolated as benign essential myoclonus

May occur in association with other seizure forms

Characterized by:
- Sudden, brief contractures of a muscle or group of muscles
- Occur singly or repetitively
- No postictal state
- May or may not be symmetric
- May or may not involve loss of consciousness

Infantile Spasms

Also called *infantile myoclonus, massive spasms, hypsarrhythmia, salaam episodes,* or *infantile myoclonic spasms*

Most commonly occur during the first 6 to 8 months of life

Twice as common in males as in females

Child may have numerous seizures during the day without postictal drowsiness or sleep

Outlook for normal intelligence poor

Manifestations
- Possible series of sudden, brief, symmetric, muscular contractions
- Head flexed, arms extended, and legs drawn up
- Eyes may roll upward or inward
- May be preceded or followed by a cry or giggling
- May or may not be loss of consciousness
- Sometimes flushing, pallor, or cyanosis

Infants who are able to sit but not stand
- Sudden dropping forward of the head and neck with trunk flexed forward and knees drawn up (the salaam or jackknife seizure)

Less often: alternate clinical forms observed
- Extensor spasms rather than flexion of arms, legs, and trunk and head nodding
- Lightning events involving a single, momentary, shocklike contraction of the entire body

The Child with a Head Injury

Head injury—A pathologic process involving the scalp, skull, meninges, or brain as a result of mechanical force

Concussion—A transient and reversible neuronal dysfunction, with instantaneous loss of awareness and responsiveness, that results from trauma to the head

Contusion—Petechial hemorrhages or localized bruising along superficial aspects of the brain at the site of impact (coup injury) or a lesion remote from the site of direct trauma (contrecoup injury)

ASSESSMENT

Assess airway, breathing, and circulation.

Examine head for evidence of injury—bruises, lacerations, swelling, depression, drainage or bleeding from any orifice.

Perform a physical assessment of body for evidence of associated injuries, especially spinal cord injury.

Obtain a history of event and subsequent management.

Observe for manifestations of head injury.

Minor Injury

May or may not lose consciousness
Transient period of confusion
Somnolence
Listlessness
Irritability
Pallor
Vomiting (one or more episodes)

Signs of Progression

Altered mental status (e.g., difficulty rousing child)
Mounting agitation
Development of focal lateral neurologic signs
Marked changes in vital signs

Severe Injury

Signs of increased ICP (see p. 101)
- Increased head size (infant)
- Bulging fontanel (infant)

Retinal hemorrhage
Extraocular palsies (especially cranial nerve VI)
Hemiparesis
Quadriplegia
Elevated temperature
Unsteady gait
Papilledema

Associated Signs

Scalp trauma
Other injuries (e.g., to extremities)
- Observe for additional neurologic data
- Bruises and wounds—Location, extent, type
- Unusual behavior—Note nature and frequency, related circumstances
- Incontinence in toilet-trained child (bowel, bladder); spontaneous or associated with other phenomena (e.g., seizure activity)

Assist with diagnostic procedures and tests. (See assessment of the child with neurologic dysfunction, pp. 100-101.)

Ongoing Assessment

Perform frequent neurologic (Figure 1-34) assessment including the following:
- Level of consciousness
- Position and movement
- Presence of headache

NEUROLOGIC ASSESSMENT

Pupils	Right	Size	
		Reaction	
	Left	Size	
		Reaction	

++ = Brisk
+ = Sluggish
– = No reaction
C = Eye closed by swelling

GLASGOW COMA SCALE

Eyes open	Spontaneously	4	
	To speech	3	
	To pain	2	
	None	1	
Best motor response	Obeys commands	6	
	Localizes pain	5	
	Flexion withdrawal	4	
	Flexion abnormal	3	
	Extension	2	
	None	1	

Usually record best arm or age-appropriate response

	≥2 years			<2 years
Best response to auditory and/or visual stimulus	Orientation	5		5 Smiles, listens, follows
	Confused	4		4 Cries, consolable
	Inappropriate words	3		3 Inappropriate persistent cry
	Incomprehensible words	2		2 Agitated, restless
	None	1		1 No response
	Endotracheal tube or trach	T		

COMA SCALE TOTAL	

Pupil scale (mm): 1, 2, 3, 4, 5, 6, 7, 8

HAND GRIP
Equal
Unequal
R_____L
Weakness

LOC
Alert/oriented ×4
Sleepy
Irritable
Comatose
Disoriented
Combative
Lethargic
Awake
Sleeping
Drowsy
Agitated

MUSCLE TONE
Normal
Arching
Spastic
Flaccid
Weak
Decorticate
Decerebrate
Other ________

EYE MOVEMENT
Normal
Nystagmus
Strabismus
Other ________

FONTANEL/WINDOW
Soft
Flat
Sunken
Tense
Bulging
Closed
Other ________

MOOD/AFFECT
Happy
Content
Quiet
Withdrawn
Sad
Flat
Hostile

FIGURE **1-34** Pediatric Glasgow Coma Scale.

- Young child—Fussy and restless when handled; rolls head from side to side
- Older child—Self-report
- Presence of vertigo
- Child assumes a position and vigorously resists efforts to be moved; forcible movement causes child to vomit and display spontaneous nystagmus.
- Seizures (relatively common in head injury) (see pp. 102-104)
- Presence of drainage from any orifice—Amount and characteristics
- Signs of increased ICP (see p. 101)
- Observe for bleeding from nose or ears.
- Test rhinorrhea for glucose (suggests leaking of cerebrospinal fluid [CSF]).

Assist with diagnostic tests (CT scan, MRI, skull x-ray films).

The Child with Acute Bacterial Meningitis

Acute bacterial meningitis—A bacterial infection of the meninges and CSF

ASSESSMENT

Obtain a health history, especially regarding a previous infection, injury, or exposure.

Perform a physical assessment.

Observe for the following manifestations of bacterial meningitis.

Children and adolescents

- Usually abrupt onset
- Fever
- Chills
- Headache
- Vomiting
- Alterations in sensorium
- Seizures (often the initial sign)
- Irritability
- Agitation
- May develop:
  - Photophobia
  - Delirium
  - Hallucinations
  - Aggressive behavior
  - Drowsiness
  - Stupor
  - Coma
- Nuchal rigidity
  - May progress to opisthotonos
- Positive Kernig's and Brudzinski's signs (see p. 75)
- Hyperactive but variable reflex responses
- Signs and symptoms peculiar to individual organisms
  - Petechial or purpuric rashes (meningococcal infection), especially when associated with a shocklike state
  - Joint involvement (meningococcal and *H. influenzae* infection)
  - Chronically draining ear (pneumococcal meningitis)

Infants and young children

- Classic picture rarely seen in children between 3 months and 2 years of age
- Fever
- Poor feeding
- Vomiting
- Marked irritability
- Restlessness
- Frequent seizures (often accompanied by a high-pitched cry)
- Bulging fontanel
- Nuchal rigidity may or may not be present.
- Brudzinski's and Kernig's signs may occur late.
- Subdural empyema (*H. influenzae* infection)

Neonates: specific signs

- Extremely difficult to diagnose
- Manifestations vague and nonspecific
- Well at birth but within a few days begins to look and behave poorly
- Refuses feedings
- Poor sucking ability
- Vomiting or diarrhea
- Poor tone
- Lack of movement
- Poor cry
- Full, tense, and bulging fontanel may appear late in course of illness
- Neck usually supple

Nonspecific signs that may be present in neonates

- Hypothermia or fever (depending on the maturity of the infant)
- Jaundice
- Irritability
- Drowsiness
- Seizures
- Respiratory irregularities or apnea
- Cyanosis
- Weight loss

Assist with diagnostic procedures and tests (e.g., lumbar puncture, spinal fluid examination, cultures).

The Child with Diabetes Mellitus

Diabetes mellitus (DM)—A chronic disorder involving primarily carbohydrate metabolism and characterized by a partial or complete deficiency of the hormone insulin. DM can be classified into the following three major groups:

Maturity-onset diabetes of youth—Transmitted as an autosomal-dominant disorder that is characterized by impaired insulin secretion with minimal or no defects in insulin action

Type 1 (previously called insulin-dependent diabetes mellitus [IDDM])—Characterized by destruction of the pancreatic beta cells, which produce insulin; this usually leads to absolute insulin deficiency.

Type 2 (previously called non–insulin-dependent diabetes mellitus [NIDDM])—Usually arises because of insulin resistance, in which the body fails to use insulin properly, combined with relative (not absolute) insulin deficiency

ASSESSMENT

Perform a physical assessment.

Obtain a family history, especially regarding other members who have diabetes.

Obtain a health history, especially relative to weight loss, frequency of drinking and voiding, increased appetite, diminished activity level, behavior changes, and other manifestations of type 1 diabetes mellitus as follows:

- The three polys (cardinal signs of diabetes)
  - Polyphagia
  - Polyuria
  - Polydipsia
- Weight loss
- Child may start bed-wetting
- Irritability and "not himself" or "not herself"
- Shortened attention span
- Temper tantrums in young children
- Appears overly tired
- Dry skin
- Blurred vision
- Poor wound healing
- Flushed skin
- Headache
- Frequent infections, including perineal yeast infections and/or thrush
- Hyperglycemia (Table 1-10)
  - Elevated blood glucose levels
  - Glucosuria
- Diabetic ketosis
  - Ketones as well as glucose in urine
  - No noticeable dehydration
- Diabetic ketoacidosis
  - Dehydration
  - Electrolyte imbalance
  - Acidosis
  - Progresses to coma, death

Perform or assist with diagnostic procedures and tests (e.g., fasting blood sugar, serum insulin levels, urine for ketones, blood glucose, serum islet cell antibody level).

TABLE 1-10 Comparison of Manifestations of Hypoglycemia and Hyperglycemia

Variable	Hypoglycemia	Hyperglycemia
Onset	Rapid (minutes)	Gradual (days)
Mood	Labile, irritable, nervous, weepy, combative	Lethargic
Mental status	Difficulty concentrating, speaking, focusing, coordinating	Dulled sensorium Confused
Inward feeling	Shaky feeling, hunger Headache Dizziness	Thirst Weakness Nausea and vomiting Abdominal pain
Skin	Pallor Sweating	Flushed Signs of dehydration
Mucous membranes	Normal	Dry, crusty
Respirations	Shallow	Deep, rapid (Kussmaul's)
Pulse	Tachycardia	Less rapid, weak
Breath odor	Normal	Fruity, acetone
Neurologic	Tremors Late: hyperreflexia, dilated pupils, seizure	Diminished reflexes Paresthesia

Continued

TABLE 1-10 Comparison of Manifestations of Hypoglycemia and Hyperglycemia—cont'd

Variable	Hypoglycemia	Hyperglycemia
Ominous signs	Shock, coma	Acidosis, coma
Blood		
Glucose	Low: below 60 mg/dl	High: 240 mg/dl or more
Ketones	Negative or trace	High or large
Osmolarity	Normal	High
pH	Normal	Low (7.25 or less)
Hematocrit	Normal	High
HCO_3	Normal	Less than 15 mEq/L
Urine		
Output	Normal	Polyuria (early) to oliguria (late)
Glucose	Negative	High
Acetone	Negative or trace	High

The Child with a Fracture

Fracture—A break in the continuity of a bone caused when the resistance of the bone yields to a stress or force exerted on it

Comminuted fracture—Small fragments of bone are broken from fractured shaft and lie in surrounding tissue (rare in children).

Complete fracture—Fracture fragments are separated.

Complicated fracture—Bone fragments cause damage to other organs or tissues (e.g., lung, bladder).

Incomplete fracture—Fracture fragments remain attached.

Open or compound fracture—Fracture has an open wound through which the bone has protruded.

Simple or closed fracture—Fracture does not produce a break in the skin.

Most frequent fractures in children:

Bends—A child's flexible bone can be bent 45 degrees or more before breaking. However, if bent, the bone will straighten slowly, but not completely, to produce some deformity but without the angulation that exists when the bone breaks. Bends occur more commonly in the ulna and fibula, often associated with fractures of the radius and tibia.

Buckle fracture—Compression of the porous bone produces a *buckle* or *torus* fracture. This appears as a raised or bulging projection at the fracture site. Torus fractures occur in the most porous portion of the bone near the metaphysis (the portion of the bone shaft adjacent to the epiphysis) and are more common in young children.

Greenstick fracture—Occurs when a bone is angulated beyond the limits of bending; the compressed side bends and the tension side fails, causing an incomplete fracture similar to the break observed when a green stick is broken.

Complete fracture—Divides the bone fragments; they often remain attached by a periosteal hinge, which can aid or hinder reduction.

ASSESSMENT

Obtain a history of event, previous injury, and experience with health personnel.

Observe for manifestations of fracture.

Signs of injury

Generalized swelling

Pain or tenderness

Diminished functional use of affected part (Strongly suspect fracture in small child who refuses to walk or move an upper extremity.)

Bruising

Severe muscular rigidity

Crepitus (grating sensation at fracture site)

Assess for location of fracture. Observe for deformity, instruct child to point to painful area.

Assess for circulation and sensation distal to fracture site.

Assist with diagnostic procedures and tests (e.g., radiography, tomography).

ASSESSMENT OF THE EXTREMITY IN A CAST OR TRACTION

Assess the 5 *P*s:

- Pain and point of tenderness
- Pulselessness—distal to the fracture site (late and ominous sign)
- Pallor
- Paresthesia—sensation distal to the fracture site
- Paralysis—movement distal to the fracture site

The Child Who Is Maltreated

Child maltreatment—A broad term that includes intentional physical abuse or neglect, emotional abuse or neglect, and sexual abuse of children, usually by an adult

Emotional abuse—The deliberate attempt to destroy or significantly impair a child's self-esteem or competence

Emotional neglect—Failure to meet the child's needs for affection, attention, and emotional nurturance

Physical abuse—The deliberate infliction of physical injury

Physical neglect—The deprivation of necessities, such as food, clothing, shelter, supervision, medical care, and education

Munchausen syndrome by proxy—Physical abuse inflicted on a child, usually by the mother, to fabricate or induce an illness that requires medical care for the child

Sexual abuse—Contacts or interactions between a child and an adult when the child is being used for the sexual stimulation of that adult or another person

ASSESSMENT

Perform a physical assessment with special attention to manifestations of potential abuse or neglect (Box 1-10).

Obtain a history of event, being alert for discrepancies in descriptions by caregiver and observations.

- Note sequence of events, including times, especially time lapse between occurrence of injury and initiation of treatment.
- Interview child when appropriate, including verbal quotations and information from drawings or other play activities.
- Interview parents, witnesses, and other significant persons, including their verbal quotations.

Observe parent child interactions (e.g., verbal interactions, eye contact, touching, evidence of parental concern).

Observe or obtain information regarding names, ages, and conditions of other children in the home (if possible).

Perform a developmental test.

Assist with diagnostic procedures and tests (e.g., radiology, collection of specimens for examination).

BOX 1-10 | Clinical Manifestations of Potential Child Maltreatment

Physical Neglect

Suggestive Physical Findings

Failure to thrive
Signs of malnutrition, such as thin extremities, abdominal distention, lack of subcutaneous fat
Poor personal hygiene
Unclean and/or inappropriate dress
Evidence of poor health care, such as delayed immunization, untreated infections, frequent colds
Frequent injuries from lack of supervision

Suggestive Behaviors

Dull and inactive; excessively passive or sleepy
Self-stimulatory behaviors, such as finger-sucking or rocking
Begging or stealing food
Absenteeism from school
Drug or alcohol addiction
Vandalism or shoplifting

Emotional Abuse and Neglect

Suggestive Physical Findings

Failure to thrive
Feeding disorders
Enuresis
Sleep disorders

Suggestive Behaviors

Self-stimulatory behaviors such as biting, rocking, sucking
During infancy, lack of social smile and stranger anxiety
Withdrawal
Unusual fearfulness
Antisocial behavior, such as destructiveness, stealing, cruelty
Extremes of behavior, such as overcompliant and passive or aggressive and demanding
Lags in emotional and intellectual development, especially language
Suicide attempts

Physical Abuse

Suggestive Physical Findings

Bruises and welts (may be in various stages of healing)
On face, lips, mouth, back, buttocks, thighs, or areas of torso
Regular patterns descriptive of object used, such as belt buckle, hand, wire hanger, chain, wooden spoon, squeeze or pinch marks
Burns on soles of feet, palms of hands, back, or buttocks
Patterns descriptive of object used, such as round cigar or cigarette burns, sharply demarcated areas from immersion in scalding water, rope burns on wrists or ankles from being bound, burns in the shape of an iron, radiator, or electric stove burner
Absence of "splash" marks and presence of symmetric burns
Fractures and dislocations
Skull, nose, or facial structures
Injury may denote type of abuse, such as spiral fracture or dislocation from twisting of an extremity or whiplash from shaking the child
Multiple new or old fractures in various stages of healing
Lacerations and abrasions on backs of arms, legs, torso, face, or external genitalia

Continued

BOX 1-10 | Clinical Manifestations of Potential Child Maltreatment—cont'd

Physical Abuse—cont'd

Suggestive Physical Findings—cont'd

Unusual symptoms, such as abdominal swelling, pain, and vomiting from punching
Descriptive marks such as from human bites or pulling out of hair
Chemical
Unexplained repeated poisoning, especially drug overdose
Unexplained sudden illness, such as hypoglycemia from insulin administration

Suggestive Behaviors

Wariness of physical contact with adults
Apparent fear of parents or of going home
Lying very still while surveying environment
Inappropriate reaction to injury, such as failure to cry from pain
Lack of reaction to frightening events
Apprehensiveness when hearing other children cry
Indiscriminate friendliness and displays of affection
Superficial relationships
Acting-out behavior, such as aggression, to seek attention
Withdrawal behavior

Sexual Abuse

Suggestive Physical Findings

Bruises, bleeding, lacerations or irritation of external genitalia, anus, mouth, or throat
Torn, stained, or bloody underclothing
Pain on urination or pain, swelling, and itching of genital area
Penile discharge
Sexually transmitted disease, nonspecific vaginitis, or venereal warts
Difficulty in walking or sitting
Unusual odor in the genital area
Recurrent urinary tract infections
Presence of semen
Pregnancy in young adolescent

Suggestive Behaviors

Sudden emergence of sexually related problems, including excessive or public masturbation, age-inappropriate sexual play, promiscuity, or overtly seductive behavior
Withdrawn behavior, excessive daydreaming
Preoccupation with fantasies, especially in play
Poor relationships with peers
Sudden changes, such as anxiety, loss or gain of weight, clinging behavior
In incestuous relationships, excessive anger at mother for not protecting daughter
Regressive behavior, such as bed-wetting or thumb sucking
Sudden onset of phobias or fears, particularly fears of the dark, men, strangers, or particular settings or situations (e.g., undue fear of leaving the house or staying at the daycare center or the baby-sitter's house)
Running away from home
Substance abuse, particularly of alcohol or mood-elevating drugs
Profound and rapid personality changes, especially extreme depression, hostility, and aggression (often accompanied by social withdrawal)
Rapidly declining school performance
Suicidal attempts or ideation

The Child with Burns

Burns—The destruction of skin caused by thermal, chemical, electric, or radioactive agents

Burn severity criteria

Minor burns—Partial-thickness burns of less than 10% of body surface area (BSA)

Moderate burns—Partial-thickness burns of 10% to 20% of BSA (age-related; see Major, or critical, burns)

Major, or critical, burns

- Burns complicated by respiratory tract injury
- Partial-thickness burns of 20% or more of BSA
- Burns of face, hands, feet, or genitalia, even if they appear to be partial thickness
- All full-thickness burns
- Any child younger than 2 years of age, unless the burn is very small and very superficial (20% or more of BSA considered critical in child younger than 2 years of age)
- Electric burns that penetrate
- Deep chemical burns
- Respiratory tract damage
- Burns complicated by fractures or soft tissue injury
- Burns complicated by concurrent illness, such as obesity, diabetes, epilepsy, or cardiac or renal disease

ASSESSMENT

Initial Assessments

Assess respiratory status.

Assess for extent of burn injury based on percentage of BSA involved (Figure 1-35).

Assess for depth of burn injury.

Superficial (first-degree) burns

- Dry, red surface
- Blanches on pressure and refills
- Minimal or no edema
- Painful; sensitive to touch

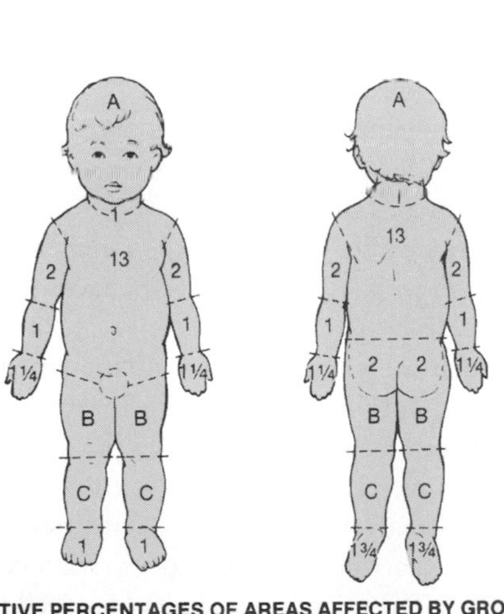

RELATIVE PERCENTAGES OF AREAS AFFECTED BY GROWTH

AREA	BIRTH	AGE 1 YR	AGE 5 YR
A = ½ of head	9½	8½	6½
B = ½ of one thigh	2¾	3¼	4
C = ½ of one leg	2½	2½	2¾

A

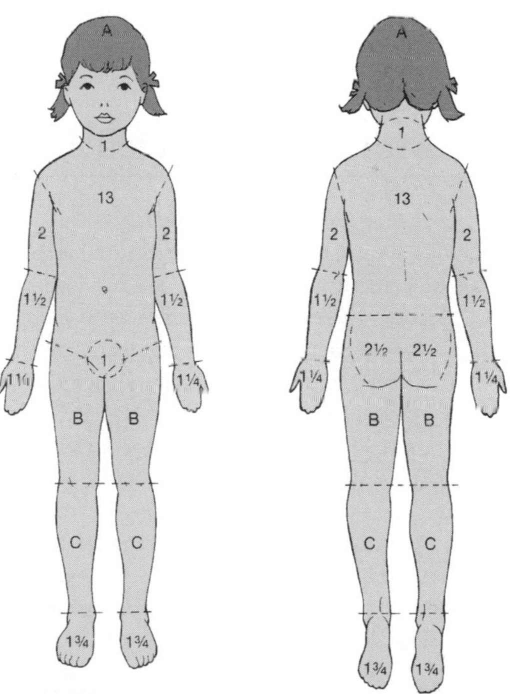

RELATIVE PERCENTAGES OF AREAS AFFECTED BY GROWTH

AREA	AGE 10 YR	AGE 15 YR	ADULT
A = ½ of head	5½	4½	3½
B = ½ of one thigh	4½	4½	4¾
C = ½ of one leg	3	3¼	3½

B

FIGURE **1-35** Estimation of distribution of burns in children. **A,** Children from birth to age 5 years. **B,** Older children.

Partial-thickness (second-degree) burns
- Blistered, moist
- Serous drainage
- Edema
- Mottled pink or red
- Blanches on pressure and refills
- Very painful; sensitive to touch

Full-thickness (third-degree) burns
- Tough, leathery
- Dull, dry surface
- Marbled, pale white, brown, tan, red, or black
- Does not blanch on pressure
- Edema
- Variable pain, often severe

Assess for evidence of associated injuries.
- Check eyes for injury or irritation.
- Check nasopharynx for edema or redness.
- Check for singed hair, including nasal hair.
- Assess for other injuries (e.g., bruises, fractures, internal injuries).

Observe for evidence of respiratory distress.
Assess need for pain medication.
Weigh child on admission; take vital signs.
Assess level of consciousness (see p. 100).
Obtain history of burn injury, especially time of injury, nature of burning agent, duration of contact, whether injury occurred in an enclosed area, any medication given.
Obtain pertinent history relative to preburn condition—weight, preexisting illnesses, any allergies, tetanus immunization.
Assist with diagnostic procedures and tests (e.g., blood count, urinalysis, wound cultures, hematocrit).

Ongoing Assessments

Monitor vital signs, including blood pressure.
Measure intake and output.
Monitor intravenous (IV) infusion; observe for evidence of overhydration.
Assess circulation of areas peripheral to burns.
Assess for evidence of healing, stability of temporary cover or graft, infection.
Observe for evidence of complications—pneumonia, wound sepsis, Curling (stress) ulcer, central nervous system (CNS) dysfunction (hallucinations, personality changes, delirium, seizures, alterations in sensorium), hypertension.

The Child with Attention Deficit Hyperactivity Disorder

Attention deficit hyperactivity disorder (ADHD)—An illness consisting of three primary characteristics: inappropriate degrees of inattention, impulsivity, and hyperactivity. The goals of treatment for ADHD include pharmacologic therapy with CNS stimulants such as methylphenidate (Ritalin, Metadate) and dextroamphetamine (Dexedrine),* home behavior management to reduce impulsive behavior and increase attentiveness, a structured school environment to increase educational success and decrease frustration with learning, and psychologic counseling for the child and family. Coexisting problems sometimes seen in the child with ADHD include speech disorders, anxiety, depression, mood disorders, hearing and vision problems, oppositional defiant disorder, and learning disorders.

ASSESSMENT

Perform a comprehensive age-appropriate physical assessment.
Perform a developmental assessment.
Obtain a developmental history for evidence of:
- Aggressive behavior in early childhood
- History of excessive fussiness and irritability as infant and toddler
- History of destructive behavior as small child
- History of disciplinary problems in early childhood

Obtain a family history.
- Some evidence suggests one parent may have had similar problems as child; therefore a history of parents' childhoods is imperative.
- Note if other children in the family have been diagnosed with ADHD or have behaviors consistent with ADHD.
- Inquire about family daily routines, including mealtimes, time set aside for school work and play time (to rule out the environment as a potential cause for distractions related to learning).

Assist with diagnostic test (e.g., electroencephalogram [EEG], blood lead levels, and thyroid levels to rule out potential organic causes of seizures, lead poisoning, and hyperthyroidism; neurologic evaluation; hearing and vision screening).
Evaluate the effectiveness of therapies prescribed (e.g., structured environment at school and home, pharmacotherapy, family and child psychotherapy).
Perform and/or assist with psychometric testing.

*Note that pharmacotherapy is not limited to these medications.

The Child with Poisoning

Poisoning—The condition or physical state produced when a substance, in relatively small amounts, is applied to body surfaces, ingested, injected, inhaled, or absorbed and subsequently causes structural damage or disturbance of function

ASSESSMENT

Perform a physical assessment with particular attention to vital signs, breath odor, state of consciousness, skin changes, and neurologic signs.

Obtain a careful and detailed history regarding what, when, and how much of a toxic substance has entered the body.

Look for evidence of poison (e.g., container, plant, vomitus).

Observe for evidence of ingestion, inhalation, or absorption of toxic substances.

Skin manifestations

- Pallor
- Redness
- Evidence of burning
- Pain

Mucous membrane manifestations

- Evidence of irritation
- Red discoloration
- White discoloration
- Swelling

Gastrointestinal manifestations

- Salivation
- Dry mouth
- Nausea and vomiting
- Diarrhea
- Abdominal pain
- Anorexia

Cardiovascular manifestations

- Arrhythmias
- Delayed capillary refill
- Decreased blood pressure
- Increased, weak pulse
- Pallor
- Cool, clammy skin
- Evidence of shock

Respiratory manifestations

- Gagging, choking, coughing
- Increased, shallow respirations
- Bradypnea
- Unexplained cyanosis
- Grunting

Renal manifestations

- Oliguria
- Hematuria

Metabolic and autonomic manifestations

- Sweating
- Hyperthermia
- Hypothermia
- Metabolic acidosis

Neuromuscular manifestations

- Weakness
- Involuntary movements
- Teeth gnashing
- Ataxia
- Dilated pupils
- Constricted pupils
- Seizures

Altered sensorium

- Anxiety, agitation
- Hallucinations
- Loss of consciousness
- Dizziness
- Confusion
- Lethargy, stupor
- Coma

Observe for clinical manifestations characteristic of specific poison.

Assist with diagnostic tests (e.g., blood levels of toxins, radiograph to determine presence of masses of undissolved tablets remaining in GI tract).

Observe for latent symptoms of poisoning.

The Child with Inhaled or Ingested Poisoning

Lead poisoning—The chronic ingestion or inhalation of lead-containing substances, resulting in physical and mental dysfunction

ASSESSMENT

Perform a physical assessment.

Obtain a history of possible sources of lead in the child's environment.

Ingested

- Lead-based paint*
    - Interior: walls, windowsills, floors, furniture
    - Exterior: door frames, fences, porches, siding
- Plaster, caulking
- Unglazed pottery
- Colored newsprint
- Painted food wrappers
- Cigarette butts and ashes
- Water from leaded pipes, water fountains
- Foods or liquids from cans soldered with lead
- Household dust
- Soil, especially along heavily trafficked roadways
- Food grown in contaminated soil
- Urban playgrounds
- Folk remedies
- Pewter vessels or dishes
- Food or drinks stored in lead crystal
- Lead bullets
- Lead fishing sinkers
- Lead curtain weights
- Hobby materials (e.g., leaded paint or solder for stained glass windows)

Inhaled

- Sanding and scraping of lead-based painted surfaces*
- Burning of leaded objects
    - Automobile batteries
    - Logs made of colored newspaper
- Automobile exhaust
- Cigarette smoke
- Sniffing leaded gasoline
- Dust
    - Poorly cleaned urban housing
    - Contaminated clothing and skin of household members working in smelting factories or construction

Obtain a history of pica, or look for evidence of this behavior during assessment.

*Most common sources

Obtain a dietary history, especially regarding intake of iron and calcium.

Observe for manifestations of lead poisoning.

General signs
- Anemia
- Acute crampy abdominal pain
- Vomiting
- Constipation
- Anorexia
- Headache
- Fever
- Lethargy
- Impaired growth

CNS signs (early)
- Hyperactivity
- Aggression
- Impulsiveness
- Decreased interest in play
- Lethargy
- Irritability
- Loss of developmental progress
- Hearing impairment
- Learning difficulties
- Short attention span
- Distractibility
- Mild intellectual deficits

CNS signs (late)
- Mental retardation
- Paralysis
- Blindness
- Convulsions
- Coma
- Death

Signs of gasoline sniffing
- Irritability
- Tremor
- Hallucinations
- Confusion
- Lack of impulse control
- Depression
- Impaired perception and coordination
- Sleep disturbances

Assist with diagnostic procedures and tests (e.g., blood-lead concentration, erythrocyte-protoporphyrin level, bone radiography, urinalysis, hemoglobin and CBC, lead mobilization test).

The Child with a Communicable Disease

Communicable disease—An illness caused by a specific infectious agent or its toxic products through a direct or indirect mode of transmission of that agent from a reservoir

Disease

Chickenpox (Varicella) (Figure 1-36)

Cause: Varicella-zoster virus (VZV)

Source: Respiratory secretions, to a lesser degree, skin lesions (scabs not infectious)

Transmission: Direct contact, droplet (airborne) spread, and contaminated objects

Incubation period: 2-3 weeks, usually 13-17 days

Period of communicability: 1 day before eruption of lesions (prodromal period) to the time when all lesions have crusted

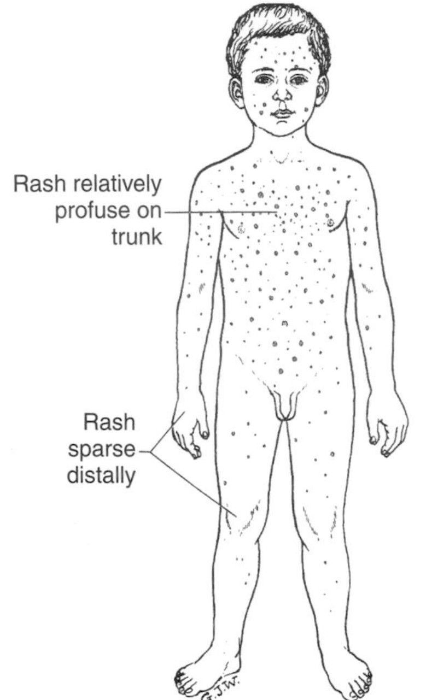

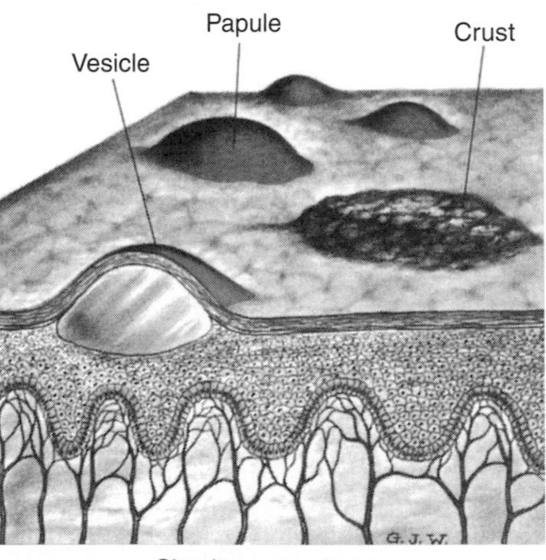

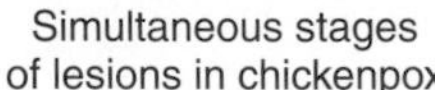
Simultaneous stages of lesions in chickenpox

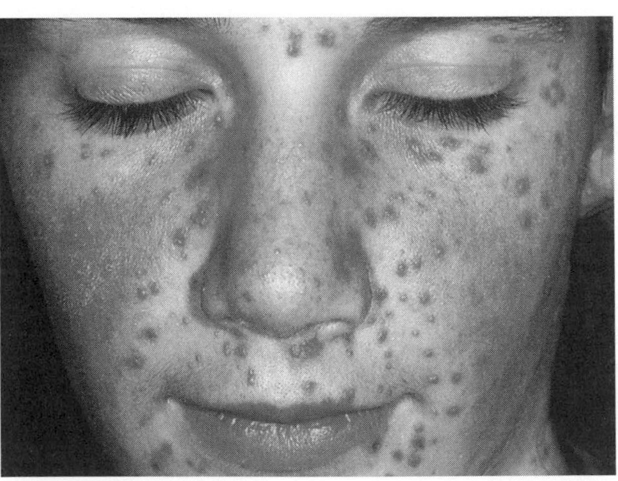

FIGURE **1-36** Chickenpox (varicella). (Clinical view from Habif TP: *Clinical dermatology: a color guide to diagnosis and therapy,* ed 4, St Louis, 2004, Mosby.)

Clinical Manifestations	Nursing Considerations
Prodromal stage: Slight fever, malaise, and anorexia for first 24 hours; rash highly pruritic; begins as macule, rapidly progresses to papule and then vesicle (surrounded by erythematous base, breaks easily and forms crusts); all three stages (papule, vesicle, crust) present in varying degrees at one time **Distribution:** Centripetal, spreading to face and proximal extremities but sparse on distal limbs and less on areas not exposed to heat (e.g., from clothing or sun) **Constitutional signs and symptoms:** Fever, irritability from pruritus	Maintain strict isolation in hospital. Isolate child in home until vesicles have dried, and isolate high-risk children from infected children. Administer skin care: give bath and change clothes and linens daily; administer topical application of calamine lotion; keep child's fingernails short and clean; apply mittens if child scratches. Administer antihistamines and antiviral agents. If older child, reason with child regarding danger of scar formation from scratching. Avoid use of aspirin; use of acetaminophen controversial.

Continued

The Child with a Communicable Disease–cont'd

Disease

Diphtheria

Cause: *Corynebacterium diphtheriae*

Source: Respiratory secretions, skin, and other lesions

Transmission: Direct contact with infected person, a carrier, or contaminated articles

Incubation period: Usually 2-5 days, possibly longer

Period of communicability: Variable; until virulent bacilli are no longer present (identified by three negative cultures); usually 2 weeks but as long as 4 weeks

Erythema Infectiosum (Fifth Disease) (Figure 1-37)

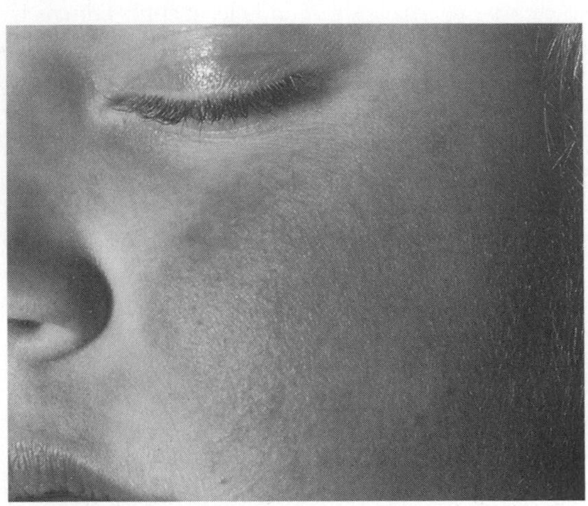

FIGURE **1-37** Erythema infectiosum. (From Habif TP: *Clinical dermatology: a color guide to diagnosis and therapy,* ed 4, St Louis, 2004, Mosby.)

Exanthema subitum (roseola) (Figure 1-38)

Cause: Human herpesvirus type 6 (HHV-6)

Source: Unknown

Transmission: Unknown (occurs between 6 months and 3 years of age)

Incubation period: Usually 5-15 days

Period of communicability: Unknown

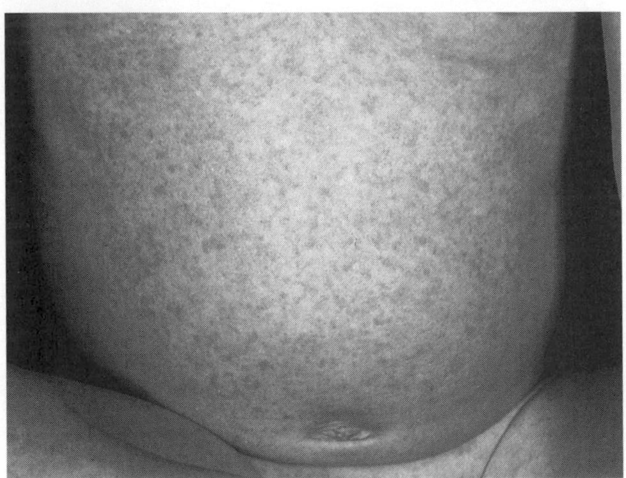

FIGURE **1-38** Roseola infantum. (From Habif TP: *Clinical dermatology: a color guide to diagnosis and therapy,* ed 4, St Louis, 2004, Mosby.)

Clinical Manifestations	Nursing Considerations
Vary according to anatomic location of pseudomembrane **Nasal:** Resembles common cold, serosanguineous mucopurulent nasal discharge without constitutional symptoms; may be frank epistaxis **Tonsillar or pharyngeal:** Malaise; anorexia; sore throat; low-grade fever; smooth, adherent, white or gray membrane; lymphadenitis **Laryngeal:** Fever, hoarseness, cough, with or without previous signs listed; potential airway obstruction, apprehension, dyspnea, cyanosis	Maintain strict isolation in hospital. Participate in sensitivity testing; have epinephrine available. Administer antibiotics; observe for signs of sensitivity to penicillin. Administer complete care to maintain bed rest. Use suctioning as needed to maintain patent airway. Observe respirations for signs of obstruction. Administer humidified oxygen if prescribed.
Rash appears in three stages. I—Erythema on face, chiefly on cheeks, "slapped face" appearance; disappears by 1-4 days II—About 1 day after rash appears on face, maculopapular red spots appear, symmetrically distributed on upper and lower extremities; rash progresses from proximal to distal surfaces and may last a week or more. III—Rash subsides but reappears if skin is irritated or traumatized (sun, heat, cold, friction). In child with aplastic crisis, rash is usually absent and prodromal illness includes fever, myalgia, lethargy, nausea, vomiting, and abdominal pain.	Isolation of child not necessary, except hospitalized child (immunosuppressed or with aplastic crisis) suspected of human papillomavirus (HPV) infection is placed on respiratory isolation. Pregnant women: need not be excluded from workplace where HPV infection is present; explain low risk of fetal death to those in contact with affected children.
Persistent high fever (greater than 38.9° C [102° F]) for 3-4 days in child who appears well Precipitous drop in fever to normal with appearance of rash (a typical exanthema subitum can occur without rash) **Rash:** Discrete rose-pink macules or maculopapules appearing first on trunk, then spreading to neck, face, and extremities; nonpruritic, fades on pressure; appears 2-3 days after onset of fever and lasts 1-2 days **Associated signs and symptoms:** Cervical or postauricular lymphadenopathy, injected pharynx, cough, coryza	Administer antipyretics as needed. If child is prone to seizures, discuss appropriate precautions, possibility of recurrent febrile seizures.

Continued

The Child with a Communicable Disease–cont'd

Disease

Measles (rubeola) (Figure 1-39)

Cause: Virus

Source: Respiratory secretions, blood, and urine

Transmission: Usually by direct contact with droplets from infected person

Incubation period: 10-20 days

Period of communicability: From 4 days before to 5 days after rash appears, but mainly during prodromal (catarrhal) stage

First day of rash

Third day of rash

Koplik spots on buccal mucosa (see inset)

Confluent maculopapules

Rash discrete

Discrete maculopapules

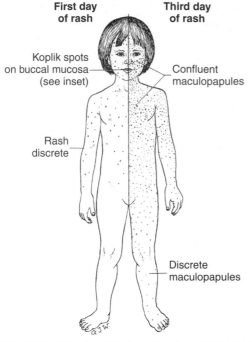

FIGURE **1-39** Measles. (Clinical view from Seidel HM, Ball JW, Dains JE and others: *Mosby's guide to physical examination,* ed 4, St Louis, 1999, Mosby.)

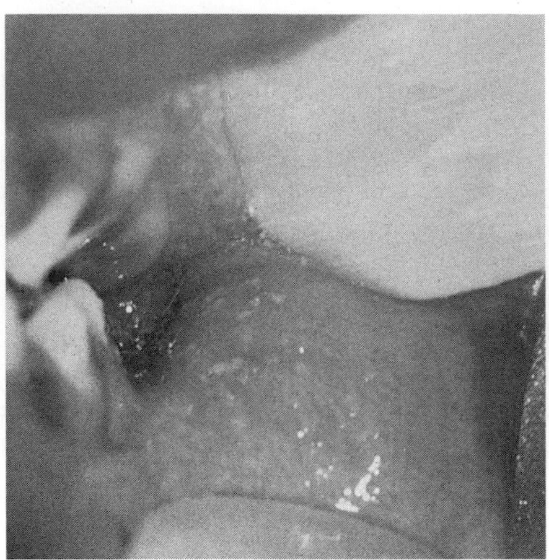

Koplik's spots

FIGURE **1-40** Koplik's spots. (From Zitelli BJ, Davis HW: Atlas of pediatric physical diagnosis, ed 3, St Louis, 1997, Mosby.)

Mumps

Cause: Paramyxovirus

Source: Saliva

Transmission: Direct contact or droplet spread from an infected person

Incubation period: 14-21 days

Period of communicability: Most communicable immediately before and after swelling begins

Pertussis (whooping cough)

Cause: Bordetella pertussis

Source: Respiratory secretions

Transmission: Direct contact or droplet spread from infected person; indirect contact with freshly contaminated articles

Incubation period: 5-21 days, usually 10

Period of communicability: Greatest during catarrhal stage before onset of paroxysms and may extend to fourth week after onset of paroxysms

Clinical Manifestations	Nursing Considerations
Prodromal (catarrhal) stage: Fever and malaise, followed in 24 hours by coryza, cough, conjunctivitis, Koplik's spots (small, irregular red spots with a minute, bluish-white center first seen on buccal mucosa opposite molars 2 days before rash; Figure 1-40); symptoms gradually increase in severity until second day after rash appears, when they begin to subside. **Rash:** Appears 3-4 days after onset of prodromal stage; begins as erythematous maculopapular eruption on face and gradually spreads downward; more severe in earlier sites (appears confluent) and less intense in later sites (appears discrete); after 3-4 days assumes brownish appearance, and fine desquamation occurs over areas of extensive involvement. Constitutional signs and symptoms: Anorexia, malaise, generalized lymphadenopathy	Isolation until fifth day of rash; if hospitalized, institute respiratory precautions. Maintain bed rest during prodromal stage; provide quiet activity. **Fever:** Instruct parents to administer antipyretics; avoid chilling; if child is prone to seizures, institute appropriate precautions. (Fever spikes to 40° C [104° F] between fourth and fifth days.) **Eye care:** Dim lights if photophobia present; clean eyelids with warm saline solution to remove secretions or crusts; keep child from rubbing eyes; examine cornea for signs of ulceration. **Coryza/cough:** Use cool-mist vaporizer; protect skin around nares with layer of petrolatum; encourage fluids and soft, bland foods. **Skin care:** Keep skin clean; use tepid baths as necessary.
Prodromal stage: Fever, headache, malaise, and anorexia for 24 hours, followed by jaw or ear pain that is aggravated by chewing **Parotitis:** By third day, parotid gland(s) (either unilateral or bilateral) enlarge and reach maximum size in 1-3 days; accompanied by pain and tenderness.	Isolation during period of communicability; institute respiratory precautions during hospitalization. Maintain bed rest during prodromal phase until swelling subsides. Give analgesics for pain. Encourage fluids and soft, bland foods; avoid foods requiring chewing. Apply hot or cold compresses to neck, whichever is more comforting. To relieve orchitis, provide warmth and local support with tight-fitting underpants. (Stretch bathing suit works well.)
Catarrhal stage: Begins with signs and symptoms of upper respiratory tract infection, such as coryza, sneezing, lacrimation, cough, and low-grade fever; symptoms continue for 1-2 weeks, when dry, hacking cough becomes more severe. **Paroxysmal stage:** Cough most often occurs at night and consists of short, rapid coughs followed by sudden inspiration associated with a high-pitched crowing sound or whoop; during paroxysm cheeks become flushed or cyanotic, vomiting frequently follows attack; stage generally lasts 4-6 weeks, followed by convalescent stage.	Isolation during catarrhal stage; if hospitalized, institute respiratory precautions. Maintain bed rest as long as fever is present. Provide restful environment and reduce factors that promote paroxysms (e.g., dust, smoke, sudden changes in temperature, chilling, activity, excitement); keep room well ventilated. Encourage fluids; offer small amounts of fluids frequently; refeed child after vomiting. Provide high humidity (humidifier or tent); suction as needed. Observe for signs of airway obstruction (e.g., increased restlessness, apprehension, retractions, cyanosis).

Continued

The Child with a Communicable Disease–cont'd

Disease

Poliomyelitis

Cause: Enteroviruses, three types: type 1—most frequent cause of paralysis, both epidemic and endemic; type 2—least frequently associated with paralysis; type 3—second most frequently associated with paralysis

Source: Feces and oropharyngeal secretions

Transmission: Direct contact with person with apparent or inapparent active infection; spread is via fecal-oral and pharyngeal-oropharyngeal routes

Incubation period: Usually 7-14 days, with range of 5-35 days

Period of communicability: Not exactly known; virus is present in throat and feces shortly after infection and persists for about 1 week in throat and 4-6 weeks in feces

Rubella (German measles) (Figure 1-41)

Cause: Rubella virus

Source: Respiratory secretions; virus also present in blood, stool, and urine

Transmission: Direct contact and spread via infected person; indirectly via articles freshly contaminated with nasopharyngeal secretions, feces, or urine

Incubation period: 14-21 days

Period of communicability: 7 days before to about 5 days after appearance of rash

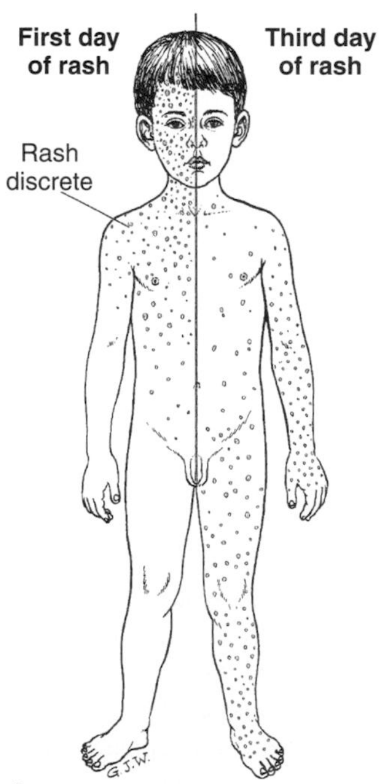

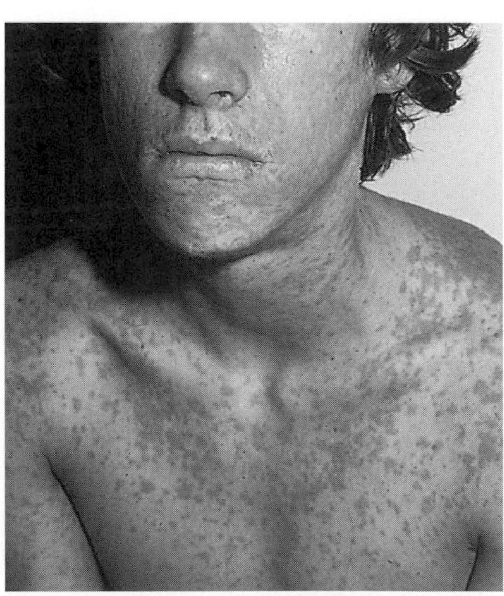

FIGURE **1-41** Rubella (German measles). **A,** progression of rash. **B,** Clinical view. (From Zitelli BJ, Davis HW: *Atlas of pediatric physical diagnosis,* ed 4, St Louis, 2002, Mosby; courtesy Dr. Michael Sherlock.)

Clinical Manifestations	Nursing Considerations
May be manifested in three different forms: **Abortive or inapparent:** Fever, uneasiness, sore throat, headache, anorexia, vomiting, abdominal pain; lasts a few hours to a few days **Nonparalytic:** Same manifestations as abortive but more severe, with pain and stiffness in neck, back, and legs **Paralytic:** Initial course similar to nonparalytic type, followed by recovery, then signs of CNS paralysis	Maintain complete bed rest. Administer mild sedatives as necessary to relieve anxiety and promote rest. Participate in physiotherapy procedures (use of moist hot packs and range-of-motion exercises). Position child to maintain body alignment and prevent contractures or decubiti; use footboard. Encourage child to move; administer analgesics for maximum comfort during physical activity. Observe for respiratory paralysis (difficulty in talking, ineffective cough, inability to hold breath, shallow and rapid respirations); report such signs and symptoms to practitioner; have tracheostomy tray at bedside.
Prodromal stage: Absent in children, present in adults and adolescents; consists of low-grade fever, headache, malaise, anorexia, mild conjunctivitis, coryza, sore throat, cough, and lymphadenopathy; lasts for 1-5 days, subsides 1 day after appearance of rash **Rash:** First appears on face and rapidly spreads downward to neck, arms, trunk, and legs; by end of first day body is covered with a discrete, pinkish-red maculopapular exanthema; disappears in same order as it began and is usually gone by third day **Constitutional signs and symptoms:** Occasionally low-grade fever, headache, malaise, and lymphadenopathy	Reassure parents of benign nature of illness in affected child. Employ comfort measures as necessary. Isolate child from pregnant women.

Continued

The Child with a Communicable Disease–cont'd

Disease

Scarlet fever (Figure 1-42)

Cause: Group A β-hemolytic streptococci

Source: Respiratory secretions

Transmission: Direct contact with infected person or droplet spread; indirectly by contact with contaminated articles or ingestion of contaminated milk or other food

Incubation period: 2-4 days, with range of 1-7 days

Period of communicability: During incubation period and clinical illness approximately 10 days; during first 2 weeks of carrier phase, although may persist for months

First day of rash

Third day of rash

Flushed cheeks

Circumoral pallor

White strawberry tongue (see inset)

Red strawberry tongue (see inset)

Increased density on neck

Increased density in axilla

Transverse lines (Pastia sign)

Positive blanching test (Schultz-Charlton)

Increased density in groin

G.J.W.

First day

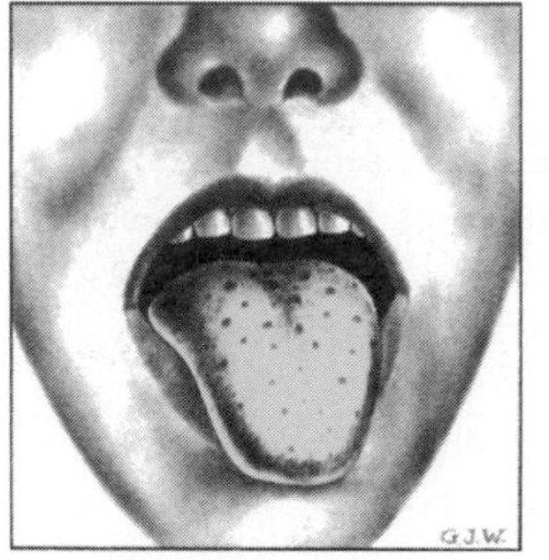

White strawberry tongue

Third day

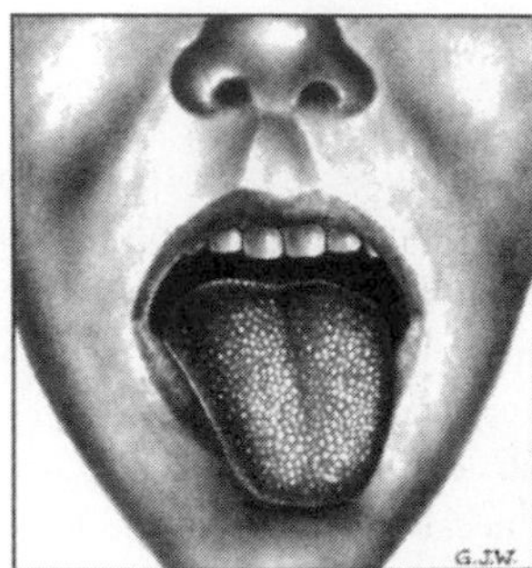

Red strawberry tongue

FIGURE **1-42** Scarlet fever.

The Child with Anorexia Nervosa*

1. Refusal to maintain body weight at or above a minimally normal weight for age and height (e.g., weight loss leading to maintenance of body weight less than 85% of that expected; or failure to make expected weight gain during period of growth, leading to body weight less than 85% of that expected).
2. Intense fear of gaining weight or becoming fat, even though underweight.
3. Disturbance in the way in which one's body weight or shape is experienced, undue influence of body weight or shape on self-evaluation, or denial of the seriousness of the current low body weight.
4. In postmenarcheal females, amenorrhea (i.e., the absence of at least three consecutive menstrual cycles). A woman is considered to have amenorrhea if her periods occur only after hormone (e.g., estrogen) administration.

Specify type:

Restricting type: During the current episode of anorexia nervosa, the person has not regularly engaged in binge-eating or purging behavior (i.e., self-induced vomiting or the misuse of laxatives, diuretics, or enemas).

Binge-eating/purging type: During the current episode of anorexia nervosa, the person has regularly engaged in binge-eating or purging behavior (i.e., self-induced vomiting or the misuse of laxatives, diuretics, or enemas).

*From American Psychiatric Association (APA): *Diagnostic and statistical manual of mental disorders,* ed 4, text revision (DSM-IV-TR), Washington, DC, 2000, APA.

Clinical Manifestations	Nursing Considerations
Prodromal stage: High fever, vomiting, headache, chills, malaise, abdominal pain **Enanthema:** Tonsils enlarged, edematous, reddened, and covered with patches of exudate; in severe case appearance resembles membrane seen in diphtheria; pharynx is edematous and beefy red; during first 1-2 days tongue is coated and papillae become red and swollen (white strawberry tongue); by fourth or fifth day white coat sloughs off, leaving prominent papillae (red strawberry tongue); palate is covered with erythematous punctate lesions. **Exanthema:** Rash appears within 12 hours after prodromal signs; red, pinhead-sized punctate lesions rapidly become generalized but are absent on face, which becomes flushed with striking circumoral pallor; rash is more intense in folds of joints; by end of first week desquamation begins (fine, sandpaper-like on torso; sheet like sloughing on palms and soles), which may be complete by 3 weeks or longer.	Institute respiratory precautions until 24 hours after initiation of treatment. Ensure compliance with oral antibiotic therapy. (Intramuscular benzathine penicillin G [Bicillin] may be given if compliance is questionable.) Maintain bed rest during febrile phase; provide quiet activity during convalescent period. Relieve discomfort of sore throat with analgesics, gargles, lozenges, antiseptic throat sprays, and inhalation of cool mist. Encourage fluids during febrile phase; avoid irritating liquids (citrus juices) or rough foods; when child is able to eat, begin with soft diet. Advise parents to consult practitioner if fever persists after beginning therapy.

The Child with Bulimia Nervosa*

1. Recurrent episodes of binge eating. An episode of binge eating is characterized by both of the following:
   a. Eating, in a discrete period of time (e.g., within any 2-hour period), an amount of food that is definitely larger than most people would eat during a similar period of time and under similar circumstances
   b. A sense of lack of control over eating during the episode (e.g., a feeling that one cannot stop eating or control what or how much one is eating)
2. Recurrent inappropriate compensatory behavior in order to prevent weight gain, such as self-induced vomiting; misuse of laxatives, diuretics, enemas, or other medications; fasting; or excessive exercise.
3. The binge eating and inappropriate compensatory behaviors both occur, on average, at least twice a week for 3 months.
4. Self-evaluation is unduly influenced by body shape and weight.
5. The disturbance does not occur exclusively during episodes of anorexia nervosa.

Specify type:

Purging type: During the current episode of bulimia nervosa, the person has regularly engaged in self-induced vomiting or the misuse of laxatives, diuretics, or enemas.

Nonpurging type: During the current episode of bulimia nervosa, the person has used other inappropriate compensatory behaviors, such as fasting or excessive exercise, but has not regularly engaged in self-induced vomiting or the misuse of laxatives, diuretics, or enemas.

*From American Psychiatric Association (APA): *Diagnostic and statistical manual of mental disorders,* ed 4, text revision (DSM-IV-TR), Washington, DC, 2000, APA.

Family Assessment

Family assessment involves the collection of data about:

Family structure—The composition of the family (who lives in the home) and those social, cultural, religious, and economic characteristics that influence the child's and family's overall psychobiologic health

Family function—How the family members behaves toward one another, the roles family members assume, and the quality of their relationships

In its broadest sense, "family" refers to all those individuals who are significant to the nuclear unit, including relatives, friends, and other social groups, such as the school and church. The more common method of eliciting information on family structure and function is by interviewing family members. However, several family assessment tools can be used to collect and graphically record data about family composition, environment, and relationships. These tools include screening questionnaires and diagrams.

Indications for Comprehensive Family Assessment

Children receiving comprehensive well-child care
Children experiencing major stressful life events, such as chronic illness, disability, parental divorce, foster care, or death of a family member
Children requiring extensive home care
Children with developmental delays
Children with repeated injuries and those with suspected child abuse
Children with behavioral or physical problems that suggest family dysfunction as the cause

Cultural Considerations

Who is considered "family"?
Who makes the decisions for the family?
What family members will be involved?
Who helps the family when someone is ill?
What support services are available through the family's cultural community?

Family Assessment Interview

GENERAL GUIDELINES FOR FAMILY INTERVIEW

Schedule the interview with the family at a time that is most convenient for all parties; include as many family members as possible; clearly state the purpose of the interview.
Begin the interview by asking each person's name and relationship to others in the family.
Restate the purpose and the objective of the interview.
Keep the initial conversation general to put members at ease and to learn the "big picture" of the family.
Identify major concerns, and reflect these back to the family to be certain that all parties perceive the same message.
Terminate the interview with a summary of what was discussed and a plan for additional sessions if needed.

STRUCTURAL ASSESSMENT AREAS

Family Composition

Immediate members of the household (names, ages, relationships)
Significant extended family members
Previous marriages, separations, deaths of spouses, or divorces

Home and Community Environment

Type of dwelling, number of rooms, occupants
Sleeping arrangements
Number of floors, accessibility of stairs, elevators
Adequacy of utilities
Safety features (fire escape, smoke detector, guardrails on windows, use of car restraint) and firearms
Environmental hazards (e.g., chipped paint, poor sanitation, pollution, heavy street traffic)
Availability and location of health facilities, schools, play areas
Relationship with neighbors
Recent crises or changes in home
Child's reaction and adjustment to recent stresses

Occupation and Education of Family Members

Types of employment
Work schedules
Work satisfaction
Exposure to environmental or industrial hazards
Sources of income and adequacy

Effect of illness on financial status
Highest degree or grade level attained

Cultural and Religious Traditions

Religious beliefs and practices
Cultural or ethnic beliefs and practices
Language spoken in home

Assessment questions

- Does the family identify with a particular religious or ethnic group? Are both parents from that group?
- How is religious or ethnic background part of family life?
- What special religious or cultural traditions are practiced in the home (e.g., food choices and preparation)?
- Where were family members born, and how long have they lived in the United States?
- What language does the family speak most frequently?
- Do they speak or understand English?
- What do they believe causes health or illness?
- What religious or ethnic beliefs influence the family's perception of illness and its treatment?
- What methods are used to prevent and treat illness?
- How does the family know when a health problem needs medical attention?
- Who is the person the family contacts when a member is ill?
- Does the family rely on cultural or religious healers or remedies? If so, ask them to describe the type of healer or remedy.
- Who does the family go to for support (clergy, medical healer, relatives)?
- Does the family experience discrimination because of their race, beliefs, or practices? Ask them to describe.

FUNCTIONAL ASSESSMENT AREAS

Family Interactions and Roles

Interactions refer to ways family members relate to one another.

Chief concern is amount of intimacy and closeness among the members, especially spouses.

Roles refer to behaviors of people as they assume a different status or position.

Observations

- Family members' responses to one another (cordial, hostile, cool, loving, patient, short-tempered)
- Obvious roles of leadership vs submission
- Support and attention shown to various members

Assessment questions

- What activities do the family members perform together?
- Whom do family members talk to when something is bothering them?
- What are members' household chores?
- Who usually oversees what is happening with the children, such as at school or concerning their health?
- How easy or difficult is it for the family to change or to accept new responsibilities for household tasks?

POWER, DECISION MAKING, AND PROBLEM SOLVING

Power refers to an individual member's control over others in family; manifested through family decision making and problem solving.

Chief concern is clarity of boundaries of power between parents and children.

One method of assessment involves offering a hypothetical conflict or problem, such as a child failing school, and asking family members how they would handle the situation.

Assessment questions

- Who usually makes the decisions in the family?
- If one parent makes a decision, can the child appeal to the other parent to change it?
- What input do children have in making decisions or discussing rules?
- Who makes and enforces the rules?
- What happens when a rule is broken?

Communication

Concerned with clarity and directness of communication patterns

Observations

- Who speaks to whom
- Whether one person speaks for or interrupts another
- Whether members appear disinterested when certain individuals speak
- Whether there is agreement between verbal and nonverbal messages
- Further assessment, such as periodically asking family members if they understood what was just said and to repeat the message

Assessment questions

- How often do family members wait until others are through talking before "having their say"?
- Do parents or older siblings tend to lecture and preach?
- Do parents tend to talk down to the children?

Expression of Feelings and Individuality

Concerned with personal space and freedom to grow within limits and structure needed for guidance.

Observing patterns of communication offers clues to how freely feelings are expressed.

Assessment questions include:

- Is it acceptable for family members to get angry or sad?
- Who gets angry most of the time? What does this person do?
- If someone is upset, how do other family members try to comfort this person?
- Who comforts specific family members?
- When someone wants to do something, such as try out for a new sport or get a job, what is the family's response (offer assistance, discouragement, or no advice)?

Assessment of Temperament

Temperament is the *behavioral style* or the *how* rather than the what or why of behavior. Nine temperament variables have been identified.*

1. ***Activity level***—The activity level of the child
   Scored in terms of movement during bathing, eating, playing, dressing, handling, reaching, crawling, walking, and sleep-wake cycles
   High activity refers to high motor activity, such as preference for running or inability to sit still.
   Low activity refers to low motor activity, such as preference for reading or quiet games and ability to sit still for prolonged periods.
2. ***Rhythmicity***—The predictability and/or unpredictability of the child's functions
   Scored in terms of sleep-wake cycles, hunger, feeding pattern, and elimination schedule
   High rhythmicity refers to a child with regular bodily habits.
   Low rhythmicity refers to a child with irregular bodily habits.
3. ***Approach-withdrawal***—The initial response of the child to a new stimulus
   Scored in terms of response to new food, toy, person, or experience, such as first day at school
   Approach refers to predominantly positive response, such as smiling, verbalizations, and reaching for the stimulus.
   Withdrawal refers to predominantly negative response, such as fussing, crying, and moving away from or refusing the stimulus.
4. ***Adaptability***—The child's ability to adapt or adjust the routine to fit a new situation
   Scored in terms of ease of adjusting to new or altered situation (similar to approach-withdrawal) but is concerned with more than the nature of the initial response
   High adaptability refers to the ability to settle in easily.
   Low adaptability refers to the inability to adjust easily.
5. ***Intensity***—The energy level of response, irrespective of its quality or direction
   Scored in terms of reactions to sensory stimuli, environmental objects, and social contacts
   High intensity refers to behavioral reactions such as loud crying or laughing in response to a stimulus, such as receiving a new toy.
   Low intensity refers to behavioral reactions such as whimpering or failing to react to a stimulus.
6. ***Threshold***—How much stimulus is required before the child reacts to a given situation
   Scored in terms of level of sensory stimuli needed before child responds
   Low threshold indicates high intensity to slight stimulus, such as waking up to soft sounds.
   High threshold indicates low intensity to moderate to strong stimulus, such as lack of discomfort with a wet diaper.
7. ***Mood***—The amount of happy, joyful behavior in contrast to unhappy, crying, whining behavior
   Scored in terms of response to sensory stimuli, environmental objects, and social contacts
   Positive mood refers to child who is generally pleasant and cooperative.
   Negative mood refers to child who is generally fussy and complaining.
8. ***Attention-persistence***—The length of time that a given activity is pursued by the child and the continuation of an activity in spite of obstacles
   Scored in terms of the child's ability to pursue an activity, such as read a book, or try to master a skill without giving up
   Long attention–high persistence refers to a child who can pay attention for prolonged periods and continues working on a project or playing despite obstacles, such as a parent telling him or her to stop or someone interrupting activity.
   Short attention–low persistence refers to a child who has difficulty paying attention and gives up easily.
9. ***Distractibility***—The effectiveness of outside stimuli in diverting the child's behavior or attention
   Low distractibility refers to the child who is not easily distracted.
   High distractibility refers to the child who is easily distracted.

The three most common patterns of child temperament, which describe most but not all children, are given in Table 1-11.

Approximately one third of children do not fall into these categories but are characterized by a variety of combinations of temperament variables.

*From Chess S, Thomas A: Dynamics of individuality: individual behavioral development. In Levine MD and others, editors: *Developmental-behavioral pediatrics*, ed 2, Philadelphia, 1992, Saunders.

TABLE 1-11 Three Common Patterns of Child Temperament

	Temperament Variables					
Pattern (% of Children)	Activity	Rhythmicity	Approach or Withdrawal	Adaptability	Intensity	Mood
Easy (40%)	Moderate	High	Approach	High	Low	Positive
Difficult (10%)	High	Low	Withdrawal	Low	High	Negative
Slow to warm up (15%)	Low	Moderate	Withdrawal	Low	Low	Negative

Nutritional Assessment

A nutritional assessment is an essential part of a complete health appraisal. Its purpose is to evaluate the child's nutritional status—the condition of health as it relates to the state of balance between nutrient intake and nutrient expenditure or need. A thorough nutritional assessment includes information about dietary intake, clinical assessment of nutritional status, anthropometric measures, sociodemographic data, and biochemical status.

Information about dietary intake usually begins with a dietary history (see next section) and may be coupled with a more detailed account of actual food intake. Two methods of recording food intake are a food diary and a food frequency record. The *food diary* is a record of every food and liquid consumed for a certain number of days, usually 2 weekdays and 1 weekend day (see p. 131). A *food frequency record* provides information about the number of times in a day or week items from MyPyramid for Kids (see p. 132) are consumed.

Clinical assessment of nutritional status provides information regarding signs of adequate nutrition and deficient or excess nutrition. The overview on pp. 134-135 also identifies specific nutrients that may be responsible for abnormal clinical findings. In addition, measurement of height, weight, head circumference, skinfold thickness, and arm circumference is assessed. Techniques for measurement are on p. 38, and expected norms are on pp. 147-158.

A number of biochemical tests are available for studying nutritional status. Common laboratory procedures related to nutritional status include measurement of hemoglobin, hematocrit, transferrin, albumin, creatinine, and nitrogen. (See Common Laboratory Tests in Unit 6.)

Dietary History

What are the family's usual mealtimes?
Do family members eat together or at separate times?
Who does the family grocery shopping and meal preparation?
How much money is spent to buy food each week?
How are most foods cooked—baked, broiled, boiled, microwaved, stir-fried, deep-fried, other?
How often does the family or your child eat out?
- What kinds of restaurants do you go to?
- What kinds of food does your child typically eat at restaurants?

Does your child eat breakfast regularly?
Where does your child eat lunch?
What are your child's favorite foods, beverages, and snacks?
- What are the average amounts eaten per day?
- What foods are artificially sweetened?
- What are your child's snacking habits?
- When are sweet foods usually eaten?
- What are your child's toothbrushing habits?

What special cultural practices are followed?
- What ethnic foods are eaten?
- Are there dietary restrictions? What foods and beverages does your child dislike?

How would you describe your child's usual appetite (hearty eater, picky eater)?
What are your child's feeding habits (breast, bottle, cup, spoon, eats by self, needs assistance, any special devices)?
Does your child take vitamins or other supplements; do they contain iron or fluoride? How often are they given?
Are there any known or suspected food allergies; is your child on a special diet?
Has your child lost or gained weight recently?
Are there any feeding problems (excessive fussiness, spitting up, colic, difficulty sucking or swallowing); any dental problems or appliances, such as braces, that affect eating?
What types of exercise does your child do regularly?
Is there a family history of cancer, diabetes, heart disease, high blood pressure, or obesity?

Cultural Considerations

What are the common foods eaten by the child and family?
Are there dietary patterns that may be contraindicated in the plan of care?
What foods are thought to promote health?
Are there religious food prescriptions and restrictions?

Additional Questions for Infant Feeding

What was your infant's birth weight; when did it double? Triple?
Was your infant premature?
Are you breast-feeding or have you breast-fed your infant? For how long?
If you use a formula, what is the brand?
- How long has your infant been taking it?
- How many ounces does your infant drink a day? Per feeding?

Are you giving your infant cow's milk (whole, low-fat, skim)?
- When did you start?
- How many ounces does your infant drink a day?

Do you give your infant extra fluids (water, juice)?
If your infant takes a bottle to bed at naptime or nighttime, what is in the bottle?
- Is liquid or powder formula used, and how is it prepared?
- How much juice does your infant take a day?

At what age did you start feeding cereal, vegetables, meat or other protein sources, fruit or juice, finger food, and table food?
Do you make your own baby food or use commercial foods, such as infant cereal?
Does your infant take a vitamin or mineral supplement? If so, what type? How much is given?
Has your infant shown an allergic reaction to any food(s)? If so, list the foods and describe the reaction.
Does your infant spit up frequently, have unusually loose stools, or have hard, dry stools? If so, how often?
How often do you feed your infant?
How would you describe your infant's appetite?

Food Diary

TOTAL FOOD INTAKE						COMMENTS
Meals and Snacks		Description of Food Items				
Time	Place	Food	Amount	Type of Preparation	With Whom Eaten?	Any Related Factors? (Associated Activity, Place Person, Money, Feelings, Hunger, Child's Disposition at Meals, etc.)

From Williams S: *Handbook of maternal and infant nutrition,* Berkeley, Calif, 1976, SRW Productions.

Food Frequency Record*

Food Group	Number of Servings†	Serving Size‡	Food Group	Number of Servings†	Serving Size‡
Breads, Cereals, Rice, Pasta			***Milk, Cheese, Yogurt***		
Bread, tortilla			Milk		
Cooked pasta, rice, hot cereal			Cheese		
Dry cereal			Yogurt		
Crackers			Pudding		
Muffins			Ice cream		
Other			Other		
Vegetables			***Other Protein Foods***		
Yellow or orange			Meat		
Green, leafy			Fish		
Other			Poultry		
			Egg		
			Peanut butter		
			Legumes (dried beans, peas)		
			Nuts		
			Other		
Fruits, Juice			***Fats, Oils, Sweets***		
Citrus (orange, grapefruit, tangerine)			Butter, oil, margarine, mayonnaise, salad dressing		
Noncitrus			Soda, punch		
Other			Cakes, cookies, etc.		
			Candy		

*For comparison of actual intake with recommended intake, see MyPyramid for Kids, Figure 2-1.
†Per day, week.
‡In cup, tablespoon, or ounce portions.

Clinical Assessment of Nutritional Status

Evidence of Adequate Nutrition	Evidence of Deficient or Excess Nutrition	Deficiency or Excess*
General Growth		
Within 5th and 95th percentiles for height, weight, and head circumference	Below 5th or above 95th percentiles for weight	Protein, calories, fats, and other essential nutrients, especially vitamin A, pyridoxine, niacin, calcium, iodine, manganese, zinc
Steady gain with expected growth spurts during infancy and adolescence	Absence of or delayed growth spurts; poor weight gain	Excess vitamins A, D
	Sudden drop in height or weight percentiles	
	Recent excess weight loss or gain	
Sexual development appropriate for age	Delayed sexual development	
Skin		
Smooth, slightly dry to touch	Hardening and scaling	Vitamin A
Elastic and firm	Seborrheic dermatitis	Excess niacin
Absence of lesions	Dry, rough, petechiae	Riboflavin
Color appropriate to genetic background	Delayed wound healing	Vitamin C
	Scaly dermatitis on exposed surfaces	Riboflavin, vitamin C, zinc
	Wrinkled, flabby	Niacin
	Crusted lesions around orifices, especially nares	Protein and calories
		Zinc
	Pruritus	Excess vitamin A, riboflavin, niacin
	Poor turgor	Water, sodium
	Edema	Protein, thiamin
		Excess sodium
	Yellow tinge (jaundice)	Vitamin B_{12}
		Excess vitamin A, niacin
	Depigmentation	Protein, calories
	Pallor (anemia)	Pyridoxine, folic acid, vitamin B_{12}, C, E (in premature infants), iron
		Excess vitamin C, zinc
	Paresthesia	Excess riboflavin
Hair		
Lustrous, silky, strong, elastic	Stringy, friable, dull, dry, thin	Protein, calories
	Alopecia	Protein, calories, zinc
	Depigmentation	Protein, calories, copper
	Raised areas around hair follicles	Vitamin C
Head		
Even molding, occipital prominence, symmetric facial features	Softening of cranial bones, prominence of frontal bones, skull flat and depressed toward middle	Vitamin D
Fused sutures after 18 months	Delayed fusion of sutures	Vitamin D
	Hard tender lumps in occiput	Excess vitamin A
	Headache	Excess thiamin
Neck		
Thyroid not visible, palpable in midline	Thyroid enlarged; may be grossly visible	Iodine

*Nutrients listed are deficient unless specified as excess.

Continued

Clinical Assessment of Nutritional Status—cont'd

Evidence of Adequate Nutrition	Evidence of Deficient or Excess Nutrition	Deficiency or Excess*
Eyes		
Clear, bright	Hardening and scaling of cornea and conjunctiva	Vitamin A
Good night vision	Night blindness	Vitamin A
Conjunctiva—Pink, glossy	Burning, itching, photophobia, cataracts, corneal vascularization	Riboflavin
Ears		
Tympanic membrane—Pliable	Calcified (hearing loss)	Excess vitamin D
Nose		
Smooth, intact nasal angle	Irritation and cracks at nasal angle	Riboflavin Excess vitamin A
Mouth		
Lips—Smooth, moist, darker color than skin	Fissures and inflammation at corners	Riboflavin Excess vitamin A
Gums—Firm, coral pink, stippled	Spongy, friable, swollen, bluish red or black, bleed easily	Vitamin C
Mucous membranes—Bright pink, smooth, moist	Stomatitis	Niacin
Tongue—Rough texture, no lesions, taste sensation	Glossitis	Niacin, riboflavin, folic acid
	Diminished taste sensation	Zinc
Teeth—Uniform white, smooth, intact	Brown mottling, pits, fissures	Excess fluoride
	Defective enamel	Vitamins A, C, D, calcium, phosphorus
	Caries	Excess simple carbohydrates or sugars
Chest		
In infants, shape almost circular	Depressed lower portion of rib cage	Vitamin D
In children, lateral diameter increases in proportion to anteroposterior diameter	Sharp protrusion of sternum	Vitamin D
Smooth costochondral junctions	Enlarged costochondral junctions	Vitamins C, D
Breast development—Normal for age	Delayed development	(See General Growth, p. 133, especially zinc.)
Cardiovascular System		
Pulse and blood pressure (BP) within normal limits	Palpitations	Thiamin
	Rapid pulse	Potassium Excess thiamin
	Arrhythmias	Magnesium, potassium Excess niacin, potassium
	Increased BP	Excess sodium
	Decreased BP	Thiamin; excess niacin
Abdomen		
In young children, cylindric and prominent	Distended, flabby, poor musculature	Protein, calories
In older children, flat	Prominent, large	Excess calories
Normal bowel habits	Pot belly, constipation	Vitamin D
	Diarrhea (excess juices may cause diarrhea)	Niacin Excess vitamin C
	Constipation (lack of fiber may cause constipation)	Excess calcium, potassium

Clinical Assessment of Nutritional Status–cont'd

Evidence of Adequate Nutrition	Evidence of Deficient or Excess Nutrition	Deficiency or Excess*
Musculoskeletal System		
Muscles—Firm, well-developed, equal strength bilaterally	Flabby, weak, generalized wasting	Protein, calories
	Weakness, pain, cramps	Excess thiamin
	Muscle twitching, tremors	Thiamin, sodium, chloride, potassium, phosphorus, magnesium
	Muscular paralysis	Excess potassium
Spine—Cervical and lumbar curves (double S curve)	Kyphosis, lordosis, scoliosis	Vitamin D
Extremities—Symmetric; legs straight with minimum bowing	Bowing of extremities, knock knees	Vitamin D, calcium, phosphorus
	Epiphyseal enlargement	Vitamins A, D
	Bleeding into joints and muscles, joint swelling, pain	Vitamin C
Joints—Flexible, full range of motion, no pain or stiffness	Thickening of cortex of long bones with pain and fragility; hard, tender lumps in extremities	Excess vitamin A
	Osteoporosis of long bones	Calcium; excess vitamin D
Neurologic System		
Behavior—Alert, responsive, emotionally stable	Listless, irritable, lethargic, apathetic (sometimes apprehensive, anxious, drowsy, mentally slow, confused)	Thiamin, niacin, pyridoxine, vitamin C, potassium, magnesium, iron, protein, calories
	Masklike facial expression, blurred speech, involuntary laughing	Excess vitamins A, D, thiamin, folic acid, calcium
		Excess manganese
Absence of tetany and convulsions	Convulsions	Thiamin, pyridoxine, vitamin D, calcium, magnesium
		Excess phosphorus (in relation to calcium)
Intact peripheral nervous system	Peripheral nervous system toxicity (unsteady gait, numb feet and hands, fine motor clumsiness)	Excess pyridoxine
Intact reflexes	Diminished or absent tendon reflexes	Thiamin, vitamin E

Recommended Dietary Allowances

DIETARY REFERENCE INTAKES

		Weight		Height			Fat-Soluble Vitamins			
Category	Age (yr) or Condition	kg	lb	cm	in	Protein RDA (g/d)	Vitamin A RDA (mcg/d)[a]	Vitamin D AI (mcg/d)[b]	Vitamin E RDA (mg/d)[c]	Vitamin K AI (mcg/d)
Infants[f]	0.0-0.5	6	13	62	24		400	5	4	2
	0.5-1	9	20	71	28		500	5	5	2.5
Children	1-3	12	27	86	34	1.10	300	5	6	30
	4-8	20	44	115	45	0.95	400	5	7	55
Males	9-13	36	79	144	57	0.95	600	5	11	60
	14-18	61	134	174	68	0.85	900	5	15	75
	19-30	70	154	177	70	0.80	900	5	15	120
Females	9-13	37	81	144	57	0.95	600	5	11	60
	14-18	54	119	163	64	0.85	700	5	15	75
	19-30	57	126	163	64	0.80	700	5	15	90
Pregnant	≤18					+25 g/d	750	5	15	75
Lactating	≤18					+25 g/d	1200	5	19	75

Modified from the *Dietary reference intake series*, National Academy of Science, National Academies Press, 1997, 1998, 2000, 2001; and American Academy of Pediatrics: *Pediatric nutrition handbook,* ed 5, Washington, DC, 2004, National Academies Press.

AI, Adequate intake; *RDA,* recommended dietary allowance.

[a]Retinol equivalent (RAE). 1 RAE = 1 mcg retinol.

[b]Cholecaciferol. 1 mcg cholecalciferol = 40 IU vitamin D. Assumes an absence of adequate exposure to sunlight.

[c]Expressed as α-tocopherol.

[d]Expressed as niacin equivalents (NE); except for infants <6 months of age, expressed as preformed niacin. 1 mg niacin = 60 mg tryptophan.

[e]Expressed as dietary folate equivalents (DFE); 1 DFE = 1 mcg food folate = 0.6 mcg folic acid from fortified food or as a supplement consumed with food = 5 mcg of a supplement taken on an empty stomach.

[f]For all nutrients, values for infants are Adequate Intake (AI).

[g]In view of evidence linking folate intake with neural tube defects in the fetus, it is recommended that all women capable of becoming pregnant consume 400 mcg from supplements or fortified foods in addition to intake of food folate from the diet.

[h]It is assumed all women will continue consuming 400 mcg from supplements or fortified food until their pregnancy is confirmed and they enter prenatal care, which ordinarily occurs after the end of the preconceptional period—the critical time for formation of the neural tube.

Water-Soluble Vitamins							Minerals							
Vitamin C RDA (mg/d)	Thiamin RDA (mg/d)	Riboflavin RDA (mg/d)	Niacin RDA (mg/d)[d]	Vitamin B_6 RDA (mg/d)	Folate RDA (mcg/d)[e]	Vitamin B_{12} RDA (mcg/d)	Calcium AI (mg/d)	Phosphorus RDA (mg/d)	Magnesium RDA (mg/d)	Iron RDA (mg/d)	Zinc RDA (mg/d)	Iodine RDA (mcg/d)	Selenium RDA (mcg/d)
40	0.2	0.3	2	0.1	65	0.4	210	100	30	0.27	2	110	15
50	0.3	0.4	4	0.3	80	0.5	270	275	75	11	3	130	20
15	0.5	0.5	6	0.5	150	0.9	500	460	80	7	3	90	20
25	0.6	0.6	8	0.6	200	1.2	800	500	130	10	5	90	30
45	0.9	0.9	12	1	300	1.8	1300	1250	240	8	8	120	40
75	1.2	1.3	16	1.3	400	2.4	1300	1250	410	11	11	150	55
90	1.2	1.3	16	1.3	400	2.4	1000	700	400	8	11	150	55
45	0.9	0.9	12	1	300	1.8	1300	1250	240	8	8	120	40
65	1	1	14	1.2	400	2.4	1300	1250	360	15	9	150	55
75	1.1	1.1	14	1.3	400[g]	2.4	1000	700	310	18	8	150	55
80	1.4	1.4	18	1.9	600[h]	2.6	1300	1250	400	27	13	220	60
115	1.4	1.6	17	2	500	2.8	1300	1250	360	10	14	290	70

ESTIMATED SAFE AND ADEQUATE DAILY DIETARY INTAKES OF SELECTED VITAMINS AND MINERALS*

		Vitamins		Trace Elements†				
Category	Age (yr)	Biotin (mcg)	Pantothenic Acid (mg)	Copper (mg)	Manganese (mg)	Fluoride (mg)	Chromium (mcg)	Molybdenum (mcg)
Infants‡	0-0.5	10	2	0.4-0.6	0.3-0.6	0.1-0.5	10-40	15-30
	0.5-1	15	3	0.6-0.7	0.6-1	0.2-1	20-60	20-40
Children and adolescents	1-3	20	3	0.7-1	1-1.5	0.5-1.5	20-80	25-50
	4-6	25	3-4	1-1.5	1.5-2	1-2.5	30-120	30-75
	7-10	30	4-5	1-2	2-3	1.5-2.5	50-200	50-150
	11+	30-100	4-7	1.5-2.5	2-5	1.5-2.5	50-200	75-250
Adults		30-100	4-7	1.5-3	2-5	1.5-4	50-200	75-250

From Food and Nutrition Board, National Research Council: *Recommended dietary allowances*, ed 10, Washington, DC, 1989, National Academy of Sciences.

*Because there is less information on which to base allowances, these figures are not given in the main table of recommended dietary allowances and are provided here in the form of ranges of recommended intakes.

†Because the toxic levels for many trace elements may be only several times usual intakes, the upper levels for the trace elements given in this table should not be habitually exceeded.

‡For all nutrients, values for infants are Adequate Intake (AI).

ESTIMATED SODIUM, CHLORIDE, AND POTASSIUM MINIMUM REQUIREMENTS OF HEALTHY PERSONS*

Age	Weight (kg)*	Sodium (mg)*†	Chloride (mg)*†	Potassium (mg)‡
0-5 mo	4.5	120	180	500
6-11 mo	8.9	200	300	700
1 yr	11	225	350	1000
2-5 yr	16	300	500	1400
6-9 yr	25	400	600	1600
10-18 yr	50	500	750	2000
>18 yr§	70	500	750	2000

From Food and Nutrition Board, National Research Council: *Recommended dietary allowances,* ed 10, Washington, DC, 1989, National Academy of Sciences.

*No allowance has been included for large, prolonged losses from the skin through sweat.

†There is no evidence that higher intakes confer any health benefit.

‡Desirable intakes of potassium may considerably exceed these values (≈3500 mg for adults).

§No allowance included for growth. Values for those younger than 18 years of age assume a growth rate at the 50th percentile reported by the NCHS and averaged for males and females.

MEDIAN HEIGHTS AND WEIGHTS AND ESTIMATED ENERGY REQUIREMENTS (EERS)*

		Weight		Height		
Category	**Age (yr) or Condition**	**kg**	**lb**	**cm**	**in**	**Energy EER (kcal/day) (male/female)**
Infants	0-0.5	6	13	60	24	570/520
	0.5-1	9	20	71	28	743/676
Children	1-3	12	27	86	34	1046/992
	4-8	20	44	115	45	1742/1642
Males	9-13	36	79	144	57	2279
	14-18	61	134	174	68	3152
	19-30	70	154	177	70	3067
Females	9-13	37	81	144	57	2071
	14-18	54	119	163	64	2368
	19-30	57	126	163	64	2403
Pregnant	First trimester					2368
	Second trimester					2708
	Third trimester					2820
Lactating	First 6 months					2698
	Second 6 months					2768

Modified from the Dietary reference intake series, National Academy of Science, National Academies Press, 1997, 1998, 2000, 2001; and American Academy of Pediatrics: *Pediatric nutrition handbook,* ed 5, Washington, DC, 2004, National Academies Press.
*The estimated energy requirement (EER) represents an average dietary energy intake that will maintain energy balance in a healthy individual based on gender and age.

Sleep Assessment

A sleep history is usually taken during the general health history. However, when sleep problems are identified, a more detailed history of sleep and awake patterns is needed for planning appropriate intervention (see p. 140). The following information includes a summary of a comprehensive sleep history.

Assessment of Sleep Problems in Children*

GENERAL HISTORY OF CHIEF COMPLAINT

Ask parents or child to describe sleep problems; record in their words.

Inquire about onset, duration, character, frequency, and consistency of sleep problems:

Circumstances surrounding onset (e.g., birth of sibling, start of toilet training, death of significant other, move from crib to bed)

Circumstances that aggravate problem (e.g., overtiredness, family conflict, disrupted routine [visitors])

Remedies used to correct problem, and results of interventions

24-HOUR SLEEP HISTORY*

Time and regularity of meals[†]
- Family members present
- Activities afterward, especially evening meal

Time of night and day sleep periods
- Hours of sleep and waking
- Hours of being put to bed and taken out of bed
- How bedtime is decided (when child looks tired or at a time decided by parent; do both parents agree on bedtime?)

*Modified from Ferber R: Assessment procedures for diagnosis of sleep disorders in children. In Noshpitz J, editor: *Sleep disorders for the clinician*, London, 1987, Butterworths, pp 185-193.
†A convenient point to start the 24-hour history is the evening meal.

Prebedtime or prenap rituals (bath, bottle- or breast-feeding, snack, television, active or quiet playing, story)
- Mood before nap or bedtime (wide awake, sleepy, happy, cranky)
- Which parent(s) participates in nap or bedtime rituals?

Nap and bedtime rituals
- Where is child allowed to fall asleep? (own bed or crib, couch, parent's bed, someone's lap, other)
- Is child helped to fall asleep? (rocked; walked; patted; given pacifier or bottle; placed in room with light; television, radio, or tape recorder on; other)
- Are patterns consistent each time, or do they vary?
- Does child awake if sleep aids are changed or taken away? (placed in own bed, television turned off, other)
- Does child verbally insist that parents stay in room?
- Child's behaviors if refuses to go to sleep or stay in room
- If child complains of fears, how convincing are the fears?

Sleep environment
- Number of bedrooms
- Location of bedrooms, especially in relation to parent's (parents') room
- Sensory features (light on, door open or closed, noise level, temperature)

Night wakings
- Time, frequency, and duration
- Child's behavior (calls out; cries; comes out of room; appears frightened, confused, or upset)
- Parental responses (let child cry, go in immediately, take to own bed, feed, pick up, rock, give pacifier, talk, scold, threaten, other)
- Conditions that reestablish sleep
  - Do they always work?
  - How long do the interventions take to work?
  - Which parent intervenes?
  - Do both parents use same or different approach?

Daytime sleepiness
- Occurrence of falling asleep at inappropriate times (circumstances, suddenness and irresistibility of onset, length of sleep, mood on awakening)
- Signs of fatigue (yawning or lying down, as well as overactivity, impulsivity, distractibility, irritability, temper tantrums)

PAST SLEEP HISTORY

Sleep patterns since infancy, especially ages when started to sleep through the night, stopped daytime naps, began later bedtime

Response to changes in sleep arrangements (crib to bed, different room or house, other)

Sleep behaviors (restlessness, snoring, sleepwalking, nightmares, partial wakings [young child may wake confused, crying, and thrashing but does not respond to parent; falls asleep without intervention if not excessively disturbed])

Parental perception of child's sleep habits (good or poor sleeper, light or deep sleeper, needs little sleep)

Family history of sleep problems (sibling behavior imitated by child; some sleep disorders [e.g., narcolepsy, enuresis] tend to recur in families)

Growth Measurements

This section primarily includes reference data for evaluating and recording a child's growth. It begins with a comparison of the general trends in physical growth throughout childhood and a chart illustrating the sequence of tooth eruption and shedding (Figure 1-43). Included next is a summary of pubertal sexual development (Figures 1-44 through 1-48). The remainder of the section consists of tables and charts of height, weight, head circumference, triceps skinfold measurements, and midarm circumference for girls and boys at different ages (Figures 1-49 through 1-65).

General Trends in Physical Growth During Childhood

Age	Weight*	Height*
Infants		
Birth to 6 months	Weekly gain: 140-200 g (5-7 ounces) Birth weight doubles by end of first 6 months†	Monthly gain: 2.5 cm (1 inch)
6-12 months	Weekly gain: 85-140 g (3-5 ounces) Birth weight triples by end of first year†	Monthly gain: 1.25 cm (0.5 inch) Birth length increases by approximately 50% by end of first year
Toddlers	Birth weight quadruples by age 2½ years Yearly gain: 2-3 kg (4.4-6.6 pounds)	Height at 2 years is approximately 50% of eventual adult height Gain during second year: about 12 cm (4.8 inches) Gain during third year: about 6-8 cm (2.4-3.2 inches)
Preschoolers	Yearly gain: 2-3 kg (4.4-6.6 pounds)	Birth length doubles by 4 years of age Yearly gain: 6-8 cm (2.4-3.2 inches)
School-age children	Yearly gain: 2-3 kg (4.4-6.6 pounds)	Yearly gain after age 6 years: 5 cm (2 inches) Birth length triples by about 13 years of age
Pubertal growth spurt		
Females (10-14 years)	Weight gain: 7-25 kg (15-55 pounds) Mean: 17.5 kg (38.1 pounds)	Height gain: 5-25 cm (2-10 inches); approximately 95% of mature height achieved by onset of menarche or skeletal age of 13 years Mean: 20.5 cm (8.2 inches)
Males (12-16 years)	Weight gain: 7-30 kg (15-65 pounds) Mean: 23.7 kg (52.1 pounds)	Height gain: 10-30 cm (4-12 inches); approximately 95% of mature height achieved by skeletal age of 15 years Mean: 27.5 cm (11 inches)

*Yearly height and weight gains for each age-group represent averaged estimates from a variety of sources.

†A study (Jung E, Czajka-Narins DM: Birth weight doubling and tripling times: an updated look at the effects of birth weight, sex, race, and type of feeding, *Am J Clin Nutr* 42:182-189, 1985) has shown the mean doubling time for birth weight to be 4.7 months and mean tripling time to be 14.7 months.

Sequence of Tooth Eruption and Shedding

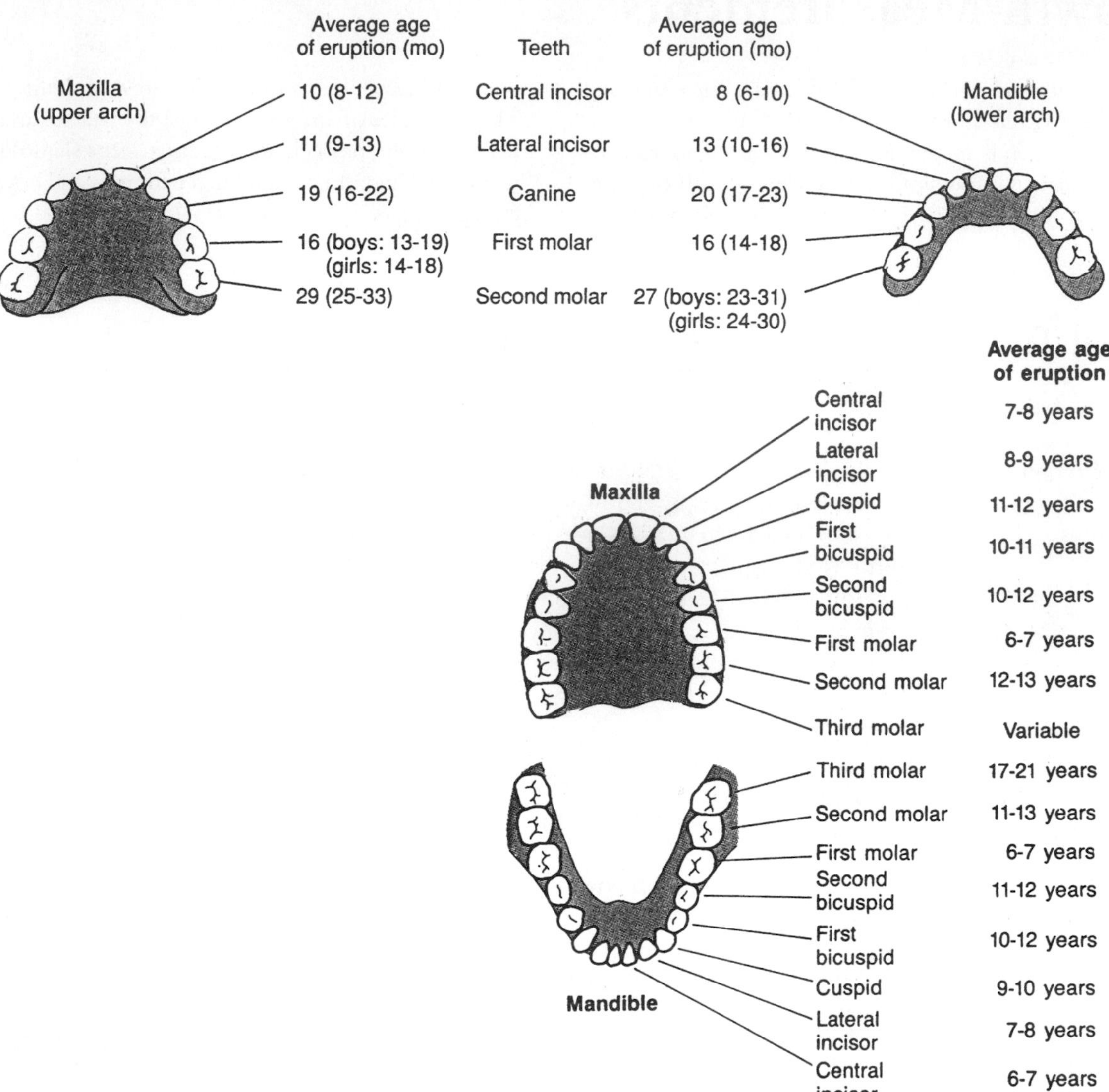

FIGURE **1-43** **A**, Sequence of eruption of primary teeth. Range represents ± standard deviation, or 67% of subjects studied. **B**, Sequence of eruption of secondary teeth. (Data from McDonald RE, Avery DR: *Dentistry for the child and adolescent*, ed 6, St Louis, 1994, Mosby.)

Sexual Development in Adolescent Males

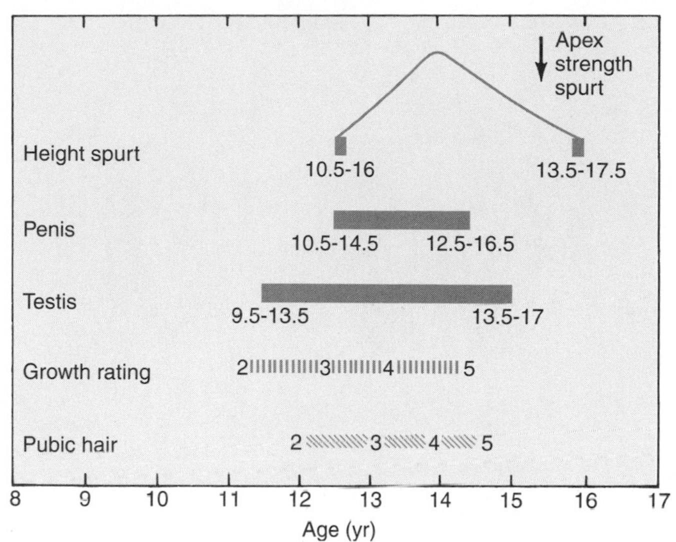

FIGURE **1-44** Approximate timing of developmental changes in boys. Numbers across from growth rating and pubic hair indicate stages of development. Range of ages during which some of the changes occur is indicated by inclusive numbers. (From Marshall WA, Tanner JM: Variations in the pattern of pubertal changes in boys, *Arch Dis Child* 45[239]:13-23, 1970.)

Stage 1 prepubertal)

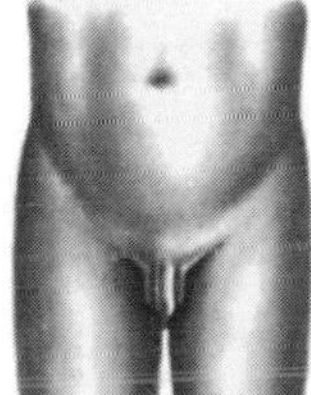

No pubic hair; essentially the same as during childhood; no distinction between hair on pubis and over the abdomen

Stage 2 (pubertal)

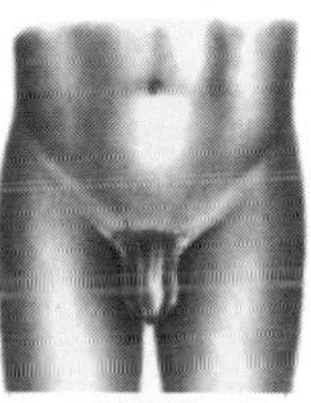

Initial enlargement of scrotum and testes; reddening and textural changes of scrotal skin; sparse growth of long, straight, downy, and slightly pigmented hair at base of penis

Stage 3

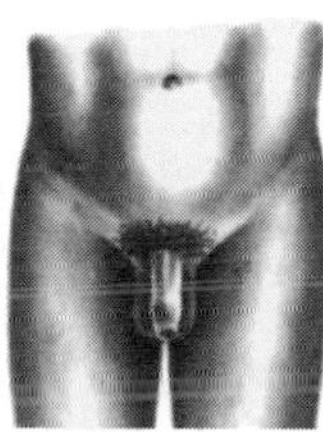

Initial enlargement of penis, mainly in length; testes and scrotum further enlarged hair darker, coarser, and curly and spread sparsely over entire pubis

Stage 4

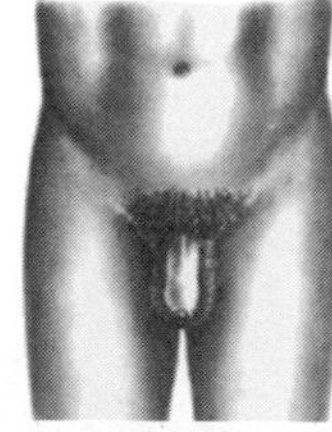

Increased size of penis with growth in diameter and development of glans; glans larger and broader; scrotum darker; pubic hair more abundant with curling but restricted to pubic area

Stage 5

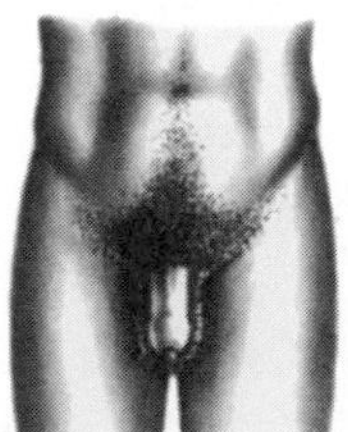

Testes, scrotum, and penis adult in size and shape; hair adult in quantity and type with spread to inner surface of thighs

FIGURE **1-45** Developmental stages of secondary sex characteristics and genital development in boys. Average age span is 12 to 16 years. (Modified from Marshall WA, Tanner JM: Variations in the pattern of pubertal changes in boys, *Arch Dis Child* 45[239]:13-23, 1970; Tanner JM: *Growth at adolescence,* Springfield, Ill, 1995, CC Thomas.)

Sexual Development in Adolescent Females

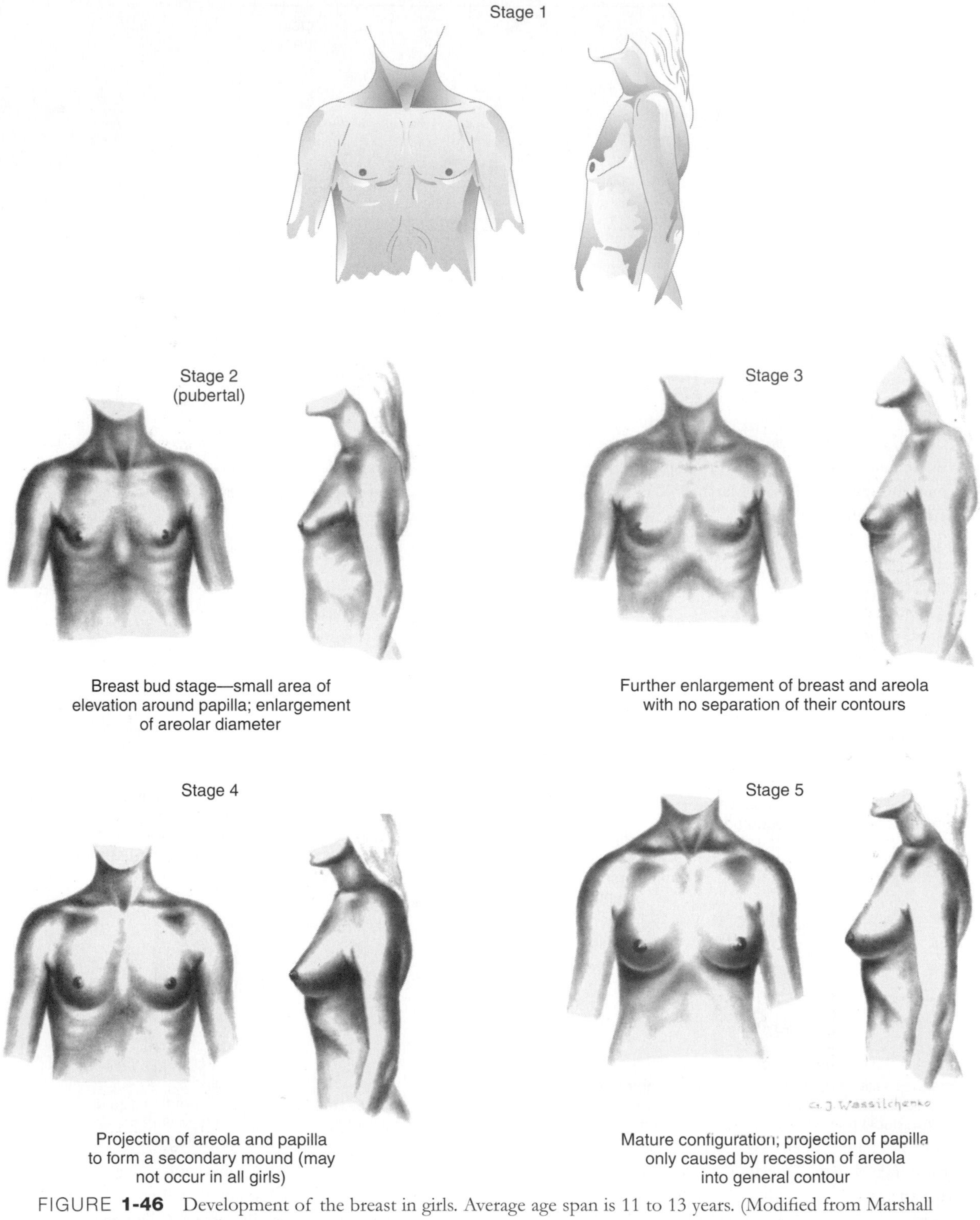

Stage 1

Stage 2
(pubertal)

Breast bud stage—small area of elevation around papilla; enlargement of areolar diameter

Stage 3

Further enlargement of breast and areola with no separation of their contours

Stage 4

Projection of areola and papilla to form a secondary mound (may not occur in all girls)

Stage 5

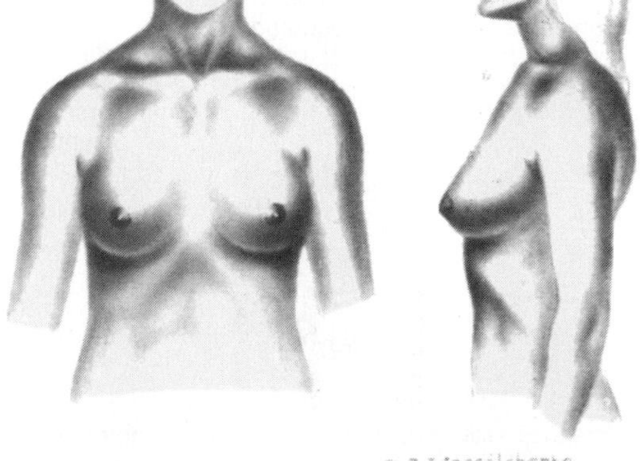

Mature configuration; projection of papilla only caused by recession of areola into general contour

FIGURE **1-46** Development of the breast in girls. Average age span is 11 to 13 years. (Modified from Marshall WA, Tanner JM: Variations in pattern of pubertal changes in girls, *Arch Dis Child* 44[235]:291-303, 1969; Tanner JM: *Growth at adolescence,* Springfield, Ill, 1995, CC Thomas.)

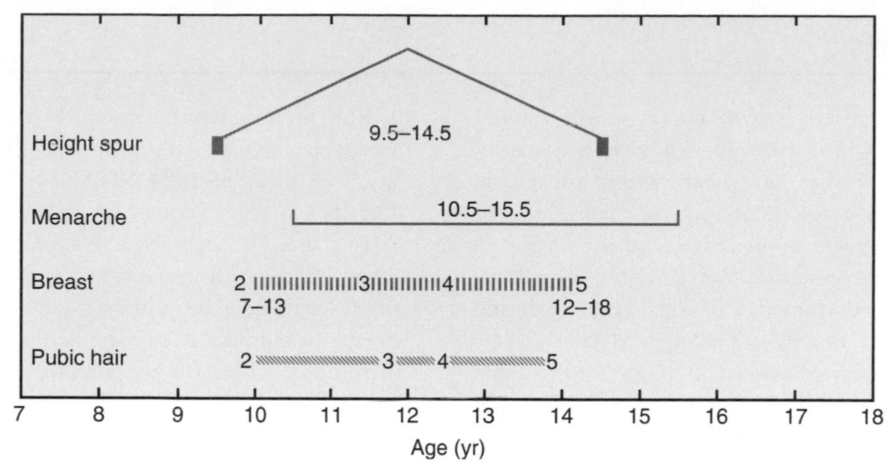

FIGURE **1-47** Approximate timing of developmental changes in girls. Numbers across from breast and pubic hair indicate stages of development. Range of ages during which some of the changes occur is indicated by inclusive numbers. (From Marshall WA, Tanner JM: Variations in the pattern of pubertal changes in girls, *Arch Dis Child,* 44[235]:291-303, 1969.)

Stage 1 (prepubertal)

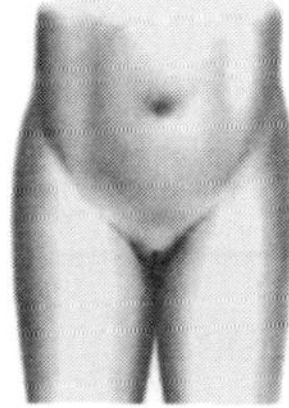

No pubic hair; essentially the same as during childhood; no distinction between hair on pubis and over the abdomen

Stage 2

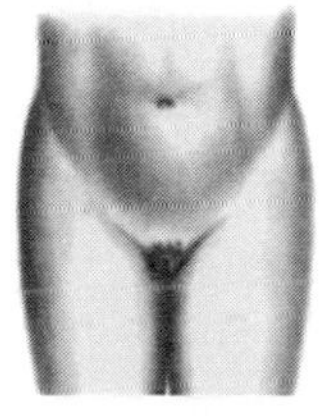

Sparse growth of long, straight, downy, and slightly pigmented hair extending along labia; between stages 2 and 3 begins to appear on pubis

Stage 3

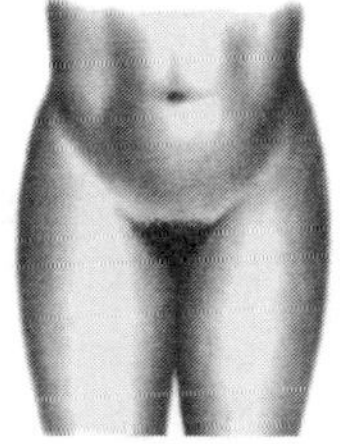

Hair darker, coarser, and curly and spread sparsely over entire pubis in the typical female triangle

Stage 4

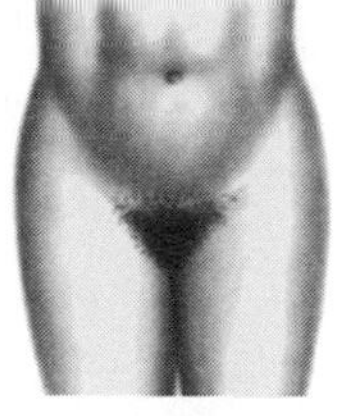

Pubic hair denser, curled, and adult in distribution but less abundant and restricted to the pubic area

Stage 5

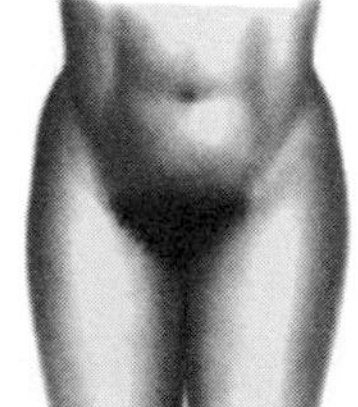

Hair adult in quantity, type, and pattern with spread to inner aspect of thighs

FIGURE **1-48** Growth of pubic hair in girls. Average age span for stages 2 through 5 is 11 to 14 years. (Modified from Marshall WA, Tanner JM: Variations in the pattern of pubertal changes in girls, *Arch Dis Child* 44[235]:291-303, 1969; Tanner JM: *Growth at adolescence,* Springfield, Ill, 1955, CC Thomas.)

Growth Charts

The most commonly used growth charts in the United States are from the National Center for Health Statistics (NCHS). The growth charts have been revised to include the body mass index–for-age (BMI-for-age) charts, 3rd and 97th smoothed percentiles for all charts, and the 85th percentile for the weight-for-stature and BMI-for-age charts. The data were collected from five national surveys during the period from 1963 to 1994. The revised charts have eliminated the disjunctions between the curves for infants and other children and have been extended for children and adolescents to 20 years (NCHS, 2000).*

The weight-for-age percentile distributions are now continuous between the infant and the older child charts at 24 to 36 months. The length-for-age to stature-for-age and the weight-for-length to weight-for-stature curves are parallel in the overlapping ages of 24 to 36 months. The revised weight-for-stature charts provide a smoother transition from the weight-for-length charts for preschool-age children.

The most prominent change to the complement of growth charts for older children and adolescents is the addition of the BMI-for-age growth curves. The BMI-for-age charts were developed with national survey data (1963 to 1994), excluding data from the 1988-1994 NHANES III survey for children older than 6 years because an increase in body weight and BMI occurred between NHANES III and previous national surveys. Without this exclusion, the 85th and 95th percentile curves would have been higher, and fewer children and adolescents would have been classified as at risk or overweight. Therefore the BMI-for-age growth curves do not represent the current population of children over 6 years of age.

The gender-specific BMI-for-age charts for ages 2 to 20 years replace the 1977 NCHS weight-for-stature charts that were limited to prepubescent boys under 11½ years of age and statures less than 145 cm and to prepubescent girls under 19 years of age and statures less than 137 cm. BMI-for-age may be used to identify children and adolescents at the upper end of the distribution who are either overweight (≥95th percentile) or at risk for overweight (≥85th and <95th percentiles). The formulas for determining BMI are available at *http://www.cdc.gov* and below.

Versions of the Growth Charts

Three different versions of the charts are available at *http://www.cdc.gov/growthcharts.* The first set contains all nine smoothed percentile lines (3rd, 5th, 10th, 25th, 50th, 75th, 90th, 95th, 97th), and the second and third sets contain seven smoothed percentile lines. The second set contains the 5th and 95th percentile lines, and the third set contains the 3rd and 97th percentile lines at the extremes of the distribution. In addition, the charts for weight-for-stature and BMI-for-age contain the 85th percentile. In all the growth charts, age is truncated to the nearest full month; for example, 1 month (1-1.9 months), 11 months (11 to 11.9 months), and 23 months (23-23.9 months).

The three sets of charts are provided to meet the needs of various users. Set 1 shows all the major percentile curves but may have limitations when the curves are close together, especially at the youngest ages. Most users in the United States may wish to use the format shown in set 2 for the majority of routine clinical applications (see pp. 150-158). Pediatric endocrinologists and others dealing with special populations, such as children with failure to thrive, may wish to use the format for set 3.

Body Mass Index Formula

ENGLISH FORMULA

BMI = [(Weight in pounds ÷ Height in inches) ÷ Height in inches] × 703

Fractions and ounces must be entered as decimal values.*

Example: A 33-pound, 4-ounce child is 37⅝ inches tall.
33.25 pounds divided by 37.625 inches,
divided by 37.625 inches multiplied by 703 = 16.5

Fraction	Ounces	Decimal	Fraction	Ounces	Decimal
1/8	2	0.125	5/8	10	0.625
1/4	4	0.25	3/4	12	0.75
3/8	6	0.375	7/8	14	0.875
1/2	8	0.5			

METRIC FORMULA

BMI = Weight in kilograms ÷ [Height in meters]^2

or

BMI = [(Weight in kilograms ÷ Height in cm) ÷ Height in cm] × 10,000

Example: A 16.9-kg child is 105.2 cm tall.
16.9 divided by 105.2 cm divided by 105.2 cm
multiplied by 10,000 = 15.3

*Kuczmarski RJ and others: *CDC growth charts: United States. Advance data from vital and health statistics, no 314*, Hyattsville, Md, June 8, 2000, NCHS.

Head Circumference Charts

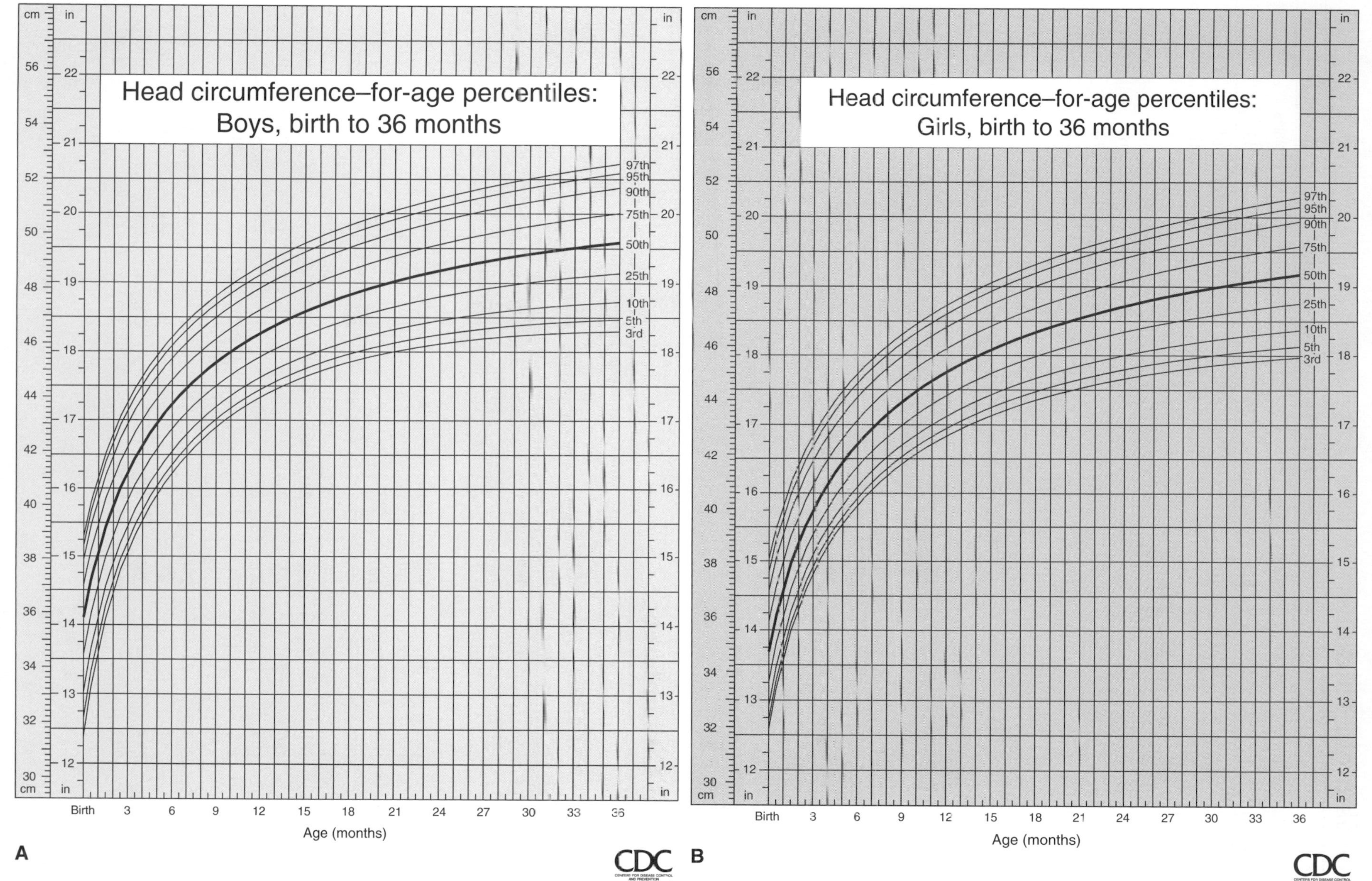

FIGURE **1-49** Head circumference–for-age percentiles, birth to 36 months. **A**, Boys. **B**, Girls. (CDC growth charts: United States, developed by the National Center for Health Statistics in collaboration with the National Center for Chronic Disease Prevention and Health Promotion, 2000.)

Triceps Skinfold Thickness

	Triceps Skinfold Percentiles (mm)									
	Males					Females				
Age-Group (Years)	5	25	50	75	95	5	25	50	75	95
1-1.9	6	8	10	12	16	6	8	10	12	16
2-2.9	6	8	10	12	15	6	9	10	12	16
3-3.9	6	8	10	11	15	7	9	11	12	15
4-4.9	6	8	9	11	14	7	8	10	12	16
5-5.9	6	8	9	11	15	6	8	10	12	18
6-6.9	5	7	8	10	16	6	8	10	12	16
7-7.9	5	7	9	12	17	6	9	11	13	18
8-8.9	5	7	8	10	16	6	9	12	15	24
9-9.9	6	7	10	13	18	8	10	13	16	22
10-10.9	6	8	10	14	21	7	10	12	17	27
11-11.9	6	8	11	16	24	7	10	13	18	28
12-12.9	6	8	11	14	28	8	11	14	18	27
13-13.9	5	7	10	14	26	8	12	15	21	30
14-14.9	4	7	9	14	24	9	13	16	21	28
15-15.9	4	6	8	11	24	8	12	17	21	32
16-16.9	4	6	8	12	22	10	15	18	22	31
17-17.9	5	6	8	12	19	10	13	19	24	37
18-18.9	4	6	9	13	24	10	15	18	22	30
19-24.9	4	7	10	15	22	10	14	18	24	34

From Frisancho A: New norms of upper limb fat and muscle areas for assessment of nutritional status, *Am J Clin Nutr* 34:2540-2545, 1981.

Upper Arm Circumference

	Arm Circumference Percentiles (mm)									
	Males					Females				
Age-Group (Years)	5	25	50	75	95	5	25	50	75	95
1-1.9	142	150	159	170	183	138	148	156	164	177
2-2.9	141	153	162	170	185	142	152	160	167	184
3-3.9	150	160	167	175	190	143	158	167	175	189
4-4.9	149	162	171	180	192	149	160	169	177	191
5-5.9	153	167	175	185	204	153	165	175	185	211
6-6.9	155	167	179	188	228	156	170	176	187	211
7-7.9	162	177	187	201	230	164	174	183	199	231
8-8.9	162	177	190	202	245	168	183	195	214	261
9-9.9	175	187	200	217	257	178	194	211	224	260
10-10.9	181	196	210	231	274	174	193	210	228	265
11-11.9	186	202	223	244	280	185	208	224	248	303
12-12.9	193	214	232	254	303	194	216	237	256	294
13-13.9	194	228	247	263	301	202	223	243	271	338
14-14.9	220	237	253	283	322	214	237	252	272	322
15-15.9	222	244	264	284	320	208	239	254	279	322
16-16.9	244	262	278	303	343	218	241	258	283	334
17-17.9	246	267	285	308	347	220	241	264	295	350
18-18.9	245	276	297	321	379	222	241	258	281	325
19-24.9	262	288	308	331	372	221	247	265	290	345

From Frisancho A: New norms of upper limb fat and muscle areas for assessment of nutritional status, *Am J Clin Nutr* 34:2540-2545, 1981.

Height and Weight Measurements for Boys in the United States

	Height by Percentiles						Weight by Percentiles					
	5		50		95		5		50		95	
Age*	**cm**	**inches**	**cm**	**inches**	**cm**	**inches**	**kg**	**lb**	**kg**	**lb**	**kg**	**lb**
Birth	46.4	18¼	50.5	20	54.4	21½	2.54	5½	3.27	7¼	4.15	9¼
3 months	56.7	22¼	61.1	24	65.4	25¾	4.43	9¾	5.98	13¼	7.37	16¼
6 months	63.4	25	67.8	26¾	72.3	28½	6.20	13¾	7.85	17¼	9.46	20¾
9 months	68	26¾	72.3	28½	77.1	30¼	7.52	16½	9.18	20¼	10.93	24
1	71.7	28¼	76.1	30	81.2	32	8.43	18½	10.15	22½	11.99	26½
1½	77.5	30½	82.4	32½	88.1	34¾	9.59	21¼	11.47	25¼	13.44	29½
2†	82.5	32½	86.8	34¼	94.4	37¼	10.49	23¼	12.34	27¼	15.50	34¼
2½†	85.4	33½	90.4	35½	97.8	38½	11.27	24¾	13.52	29¾	16.61	36½
3	89	35	94.9	37¼	102	40¼	12.05	26½	14.62	32¼	17.77	39¼
3½	92.5	36½	99.1	39	106.1	41¾	12.84	28¼	15.68	34½	18.98	41¾
4	95.8	37¾	102.9	40½	109.9	43¼	13.64	30	16.69	36¾	20.27	44¾
4½	98.9	39	106.6	42	113.5	44¾	14.45	31¾	17.69	39	21.63	47¾
5	102	40¼	109.9	43¼	117	46	15.27	33¾	18.67	41¼	23.09	51
6	107.7	42½	116.1	45¾	123.5	48½	16.93	37¼	20.69	45½	26.34	58
7	113	44½	121.7	48	129.7	51	18.64	41	22.85	50¼	30.12	66½
8	118.1	46½	127	50	135.7	53½	20.40	45	25.30	55¾	34.51	76
9	122.9	48½	132.2	52	141.8	55¾	22.25	49	28.13	62	39.58	87¼
10	127.7	50¼	137.5	54¼	148.1	58¼	24.33	53¾	31.44	69¼	45.27	99¾
11	132.6	52¼	143.3	56½	154.9	61	26.80	59	35.30	77¾	51.47	113½
12	137.6	54¼	149.7	59	162.3	64	29.85	65¾	39.78	87¾	58.09	128
13	142.9	56¼	156.5	61½	169.8	66¾	33.64	74¼	44.95	99	65.02	143¼
14	148.8	58½	163.1	64¼	176.7	69½	38.22	84¼	50.77	112	72.13	159
15	155.2	61	169	66½	181.9	71½	43.11	95	56.71	125	79.12	174½
16	161.1	63½	173.5	68¼	185.4	73	47.74	105¼	62.10	137	85.62	188¾
17	164.9	65	176.2	69¼	187.3	73¾	51.50	113½	66.31	146¼	91.31	201¼
18	165.7	65¼	176.8	69½	187.6	73¾	53.97	119	68.88	151¾	95.76	211

Modified from NCHS (NCHS), Health Resources Administration, Department of Health, Education and Welfare, Hyattsville, Md. Conversion of metric data to approximate inches and pounds by Ross Laboratories.

*Years unless otherwise indicated.

†Height data include some recumbent length measurements, which make values slightly higher than if all measurements had been of stature (standing height).

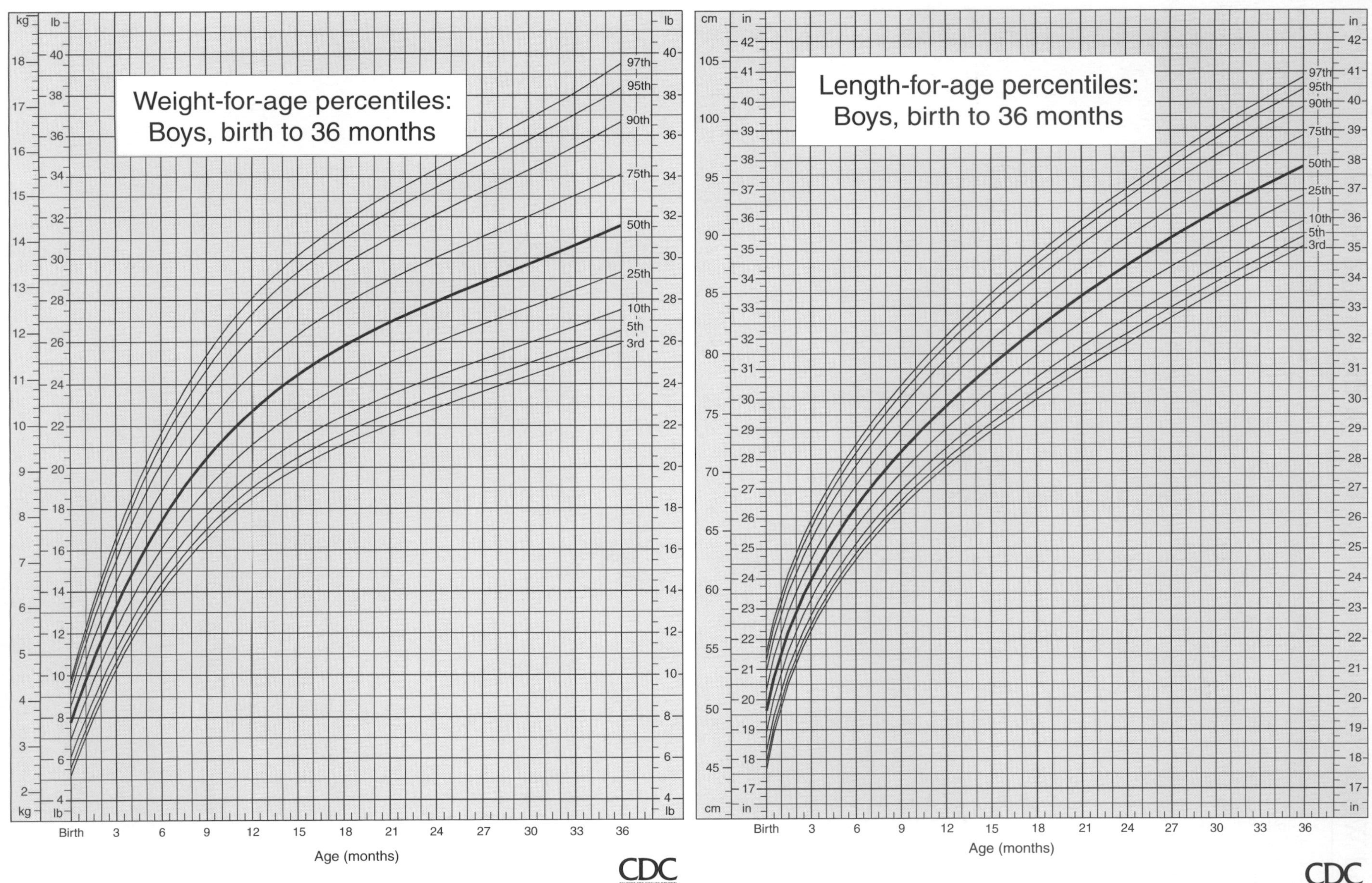

FIGURE **1-50** Weight-for-age percentiles, boys, birth to 36 months, Centers for Disease Control and Prevention (CDC) growth charts: United States. (Developed by the National Center for Health Statistics in collaboration with the National Center for Chronic Disease Prevention and Health Promotion [2000].)

FIGURE **1-51** Length-for-age percentiles, boys, birth to 36 months, CDC growth charts: United States. (Developed by the National Center for Health Statistics in collaboration with the National Center for Chronic Disease Prevention and Health Promotion [2000].)

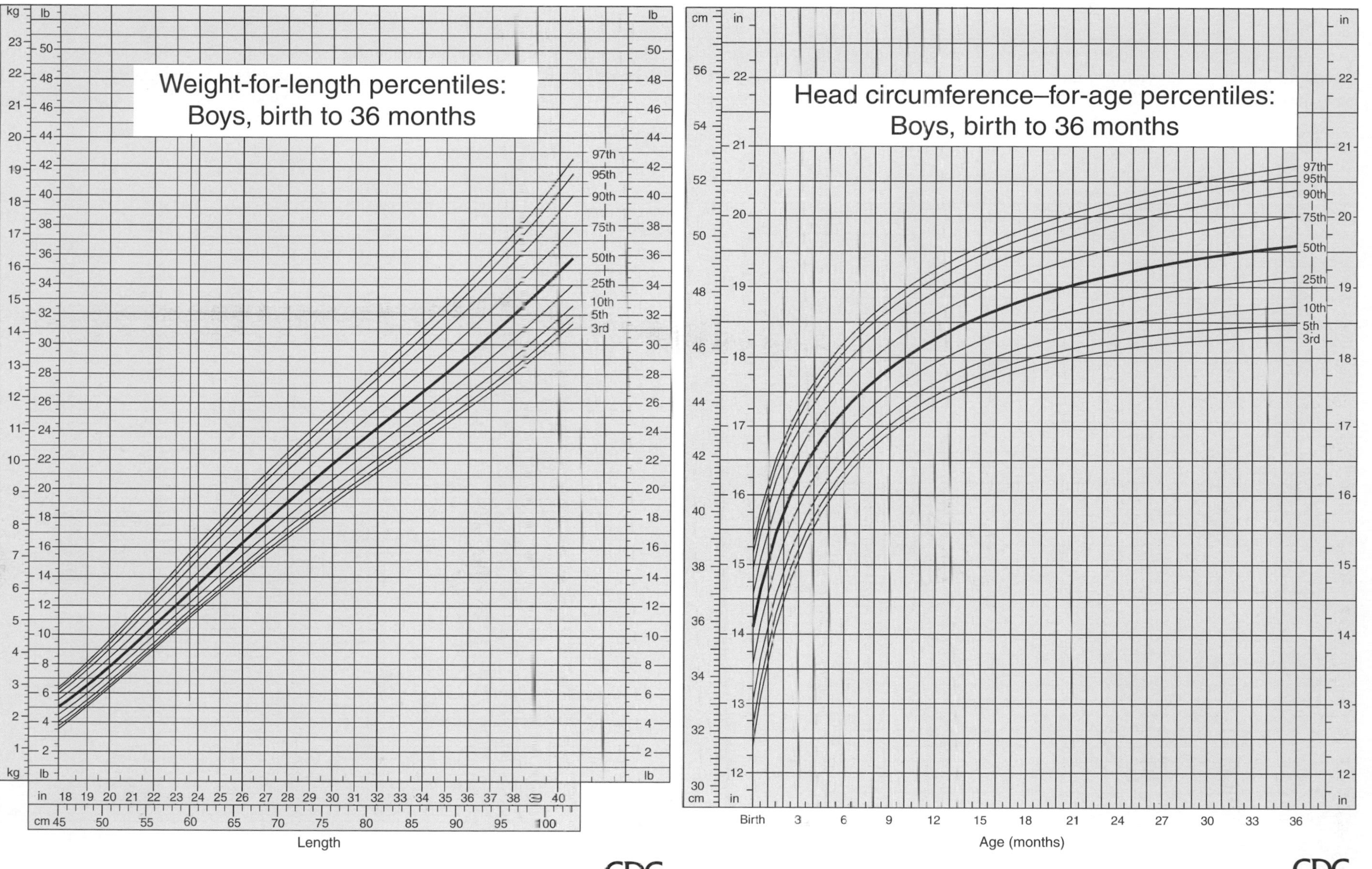

FIGURE **1-52** Weight-for-length percentiles, boys, birth to 36 months, CDC growth charts: United States. (Developed by the National Center for Health Statistics in collaboration with the National Center for Chronic Disease Prevention and Health Promotion [2000].)

FIGURE **1-53** Head circumference–for–age percentiles, boys, birth to 36 months, CDC growth charts: United States. (Developed by the National Center for Health Statistics in collaboration with the National Center for Chronic Disease Prevention and Health Promotion [2000].)

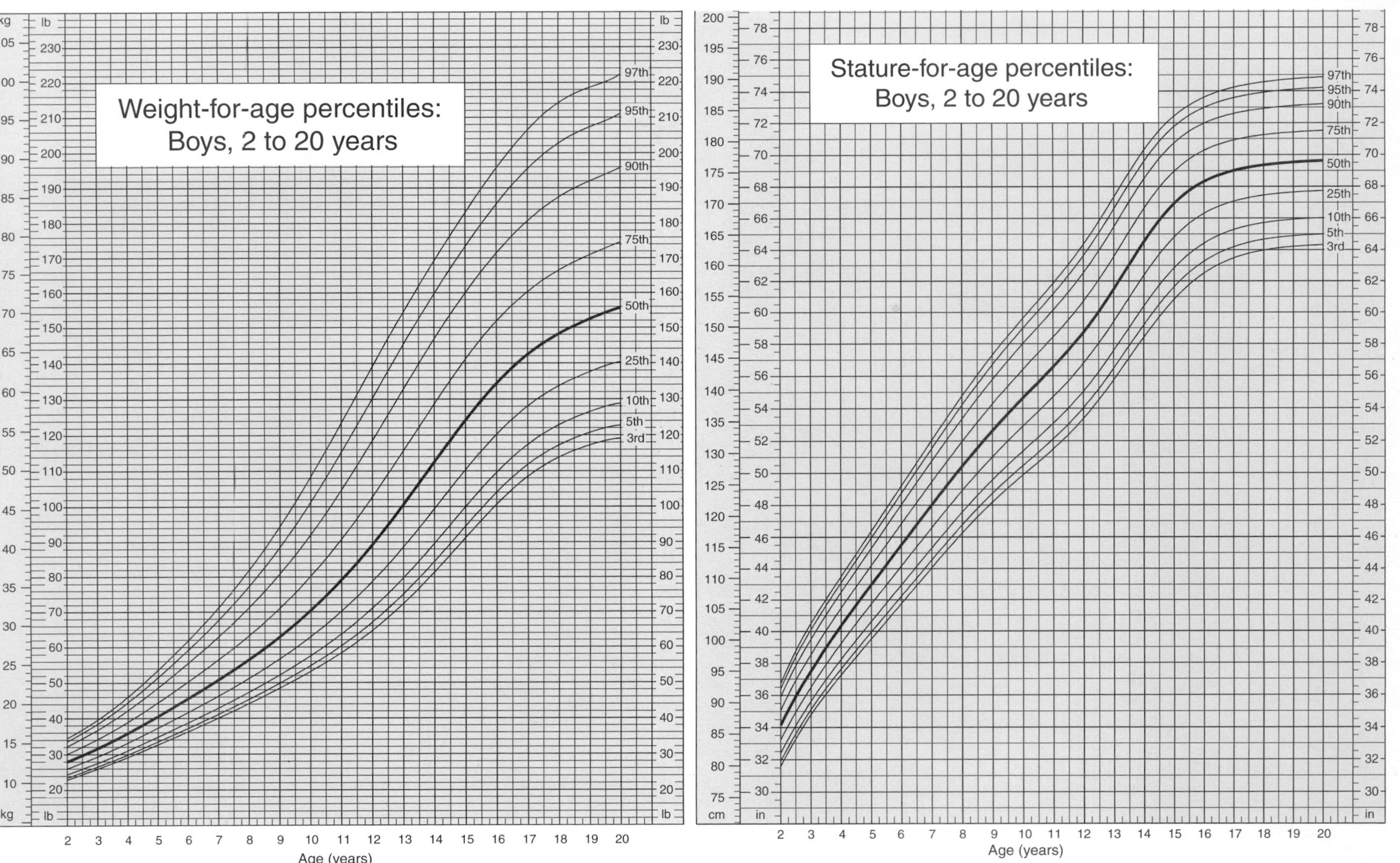

FIGURE **1-54** Weight-for-age percentiles, boys, 2-20 years, CDC growth charts: United States. (Developed by the National Center for Health Statistics in collaboration with the National Center for Chronic Disease Prevention and Health Promotion [2000].)

FIGURE **1-55** Stature-for-age percentile, boys, 2-20 years, CDC growth charts: United States. (Developed by the National Center for Health Statistics in collaboration with the National Center for Chronic Disease Prevention and Health Promotion [2000].)

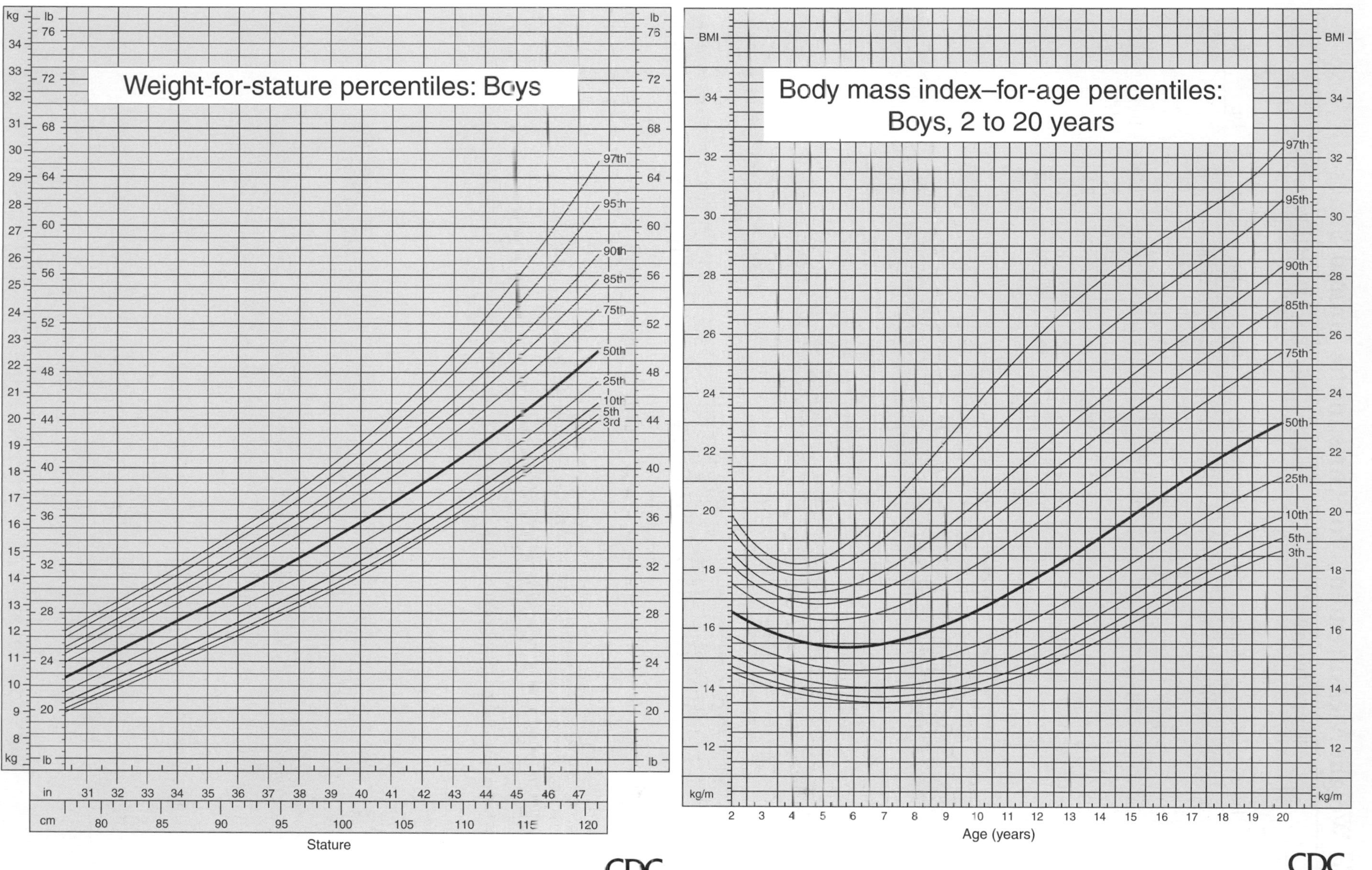

FIGURE **1-56** Weight-for-stature percentiles, boys, CDC growth charts: United States. (Developed by the National Center for Health Statistics in collaboration with the National Center for Chronic Disease Prevention and Health Promotion [2000].)

FIGURE **1-57** Body mass index–for–age percentiles, boys, 2-20 years, CDC growth charts: United States. (Developed by the National Center for Health Statistics in collaboration with the National Center for Chronic Disease Prevention and Health Promotion [2000].)

Height and Weight Measurements for Girls in the United States

	Height by Percentiles						Weight by Percentiles					
	5		50		95		5		50		95	
Age*	cm	inches	cm	inches	cm	inches	kg	lb	kg	lb	kg	lb
Birth	45.4	17¾	49.9	19¾	52.9	20¾	2.36	5¼	3.23	7	3.81	8½
3 months	55.4	21¾	59.5	23½	63.4	25	4.18	9¼	5.4	12	6.74	14¾
6 months	61.8	24¼	65.9	26	70.2	27¾	5.79	12¾	7.21	16	8.73	19¼
9 months	66.1	26	70.4	27¾	75	29½	7	15½	8.56	18¾	10.17	22½
1	69.8	27½	74.3	29¼	79.1	31¼	7.84	17¼	9.53	21	11.24	24¾
1½	76.0	30	80.9	31¾	86.1	34	8.92	19¾	10.82	23¾	12.76	28¼
2†	81.6	32¼	86.8	34¼	93.6	36¼	9.95	22	11.8	26	14.15	31¼
2½†	84.6	33¼	90	35½	96.6	38	10.8	23¾	13.03	28¾	15.76	34¾
3	88.3	34¾	94.1	37	100.6	39½	11.61	25½	14.1	31	17.22	38
3½	91.7	36	97.9	38½	104.5	41¼	12.37	27¼	15.07	33¼	18.59	41
4	95	37½	101.6	40	108.3	42¾	13.11	29	15.96	35¼	19.91	44
4½	98.1	38½	105	41¼	112	44	13.83	30½	16.81	37	21.24	46¾
5	101.1	39¾	108.4	42¾	115.6	45½	14.55	32	17.66	39	22.62	49¾
6	106.6	42	114.6	45	122.7	48¼	16.05	35½	19.52	43	25.75	56¾
7	111.8	44	120.6	47½	129.5	51	17.71	39	21.84	48¼	29.68	65½
8	116.9	46	126.4	49¾	136.2	53½	19.62	43¼	24.84	54¾	34.71	76½
9	122.1	48	132.2	52	142.9	56¼	21.82	48	28.46	62¾	40.64	89½
10	127.5	50¼	138.3	54½	149.5	58¾	24.36	53¾	32.55	71¾	47.17	104
11	133.5	52½	144.8	57	156.2	61½	27.24	60	36.95	81½	54.0	119
12	139.8	55	151.5	59¾	162.7	64	30.52	67¼	41.53	91½	60.81	134
13	145.2	57¼	157.1	61¾	168.1	66¼	34.14	75¼	46.1	101¾	67.3	148¼
14	148.7	58½	160.4	63¼	171.3	67½	37.76	83¼	50.28	110¾	73.08	161
15	150.5	59¼	161.8	63¾	172.8	68	40.99	90¼	53.68	118¼	77.78	171½
16	151.6	59¾	162.4	64	173.3	68¼	43.41	95¾	55.89	123¼	80.99	178½
17	152.7	60	163.1	64¼	173.5	68¼	44.74	98¾	56.69	125	82.46	181¾
18	153.6	60½	163.7	64½	173.6	68¼	45.26	99¾	56.62	124¾	82.47	181¾

Modified from NCHS (NCHS), Health Resources Administration, Department of Health, Education and Welfare, Hyattsville, Md. Conversion of metric data to approximate inches and pounds by Ross Laboratories.

*Years unless otherwise indicated.

†Height data include some recumbent length measurements, which make values slightly higher than if all measurements had been of stature.

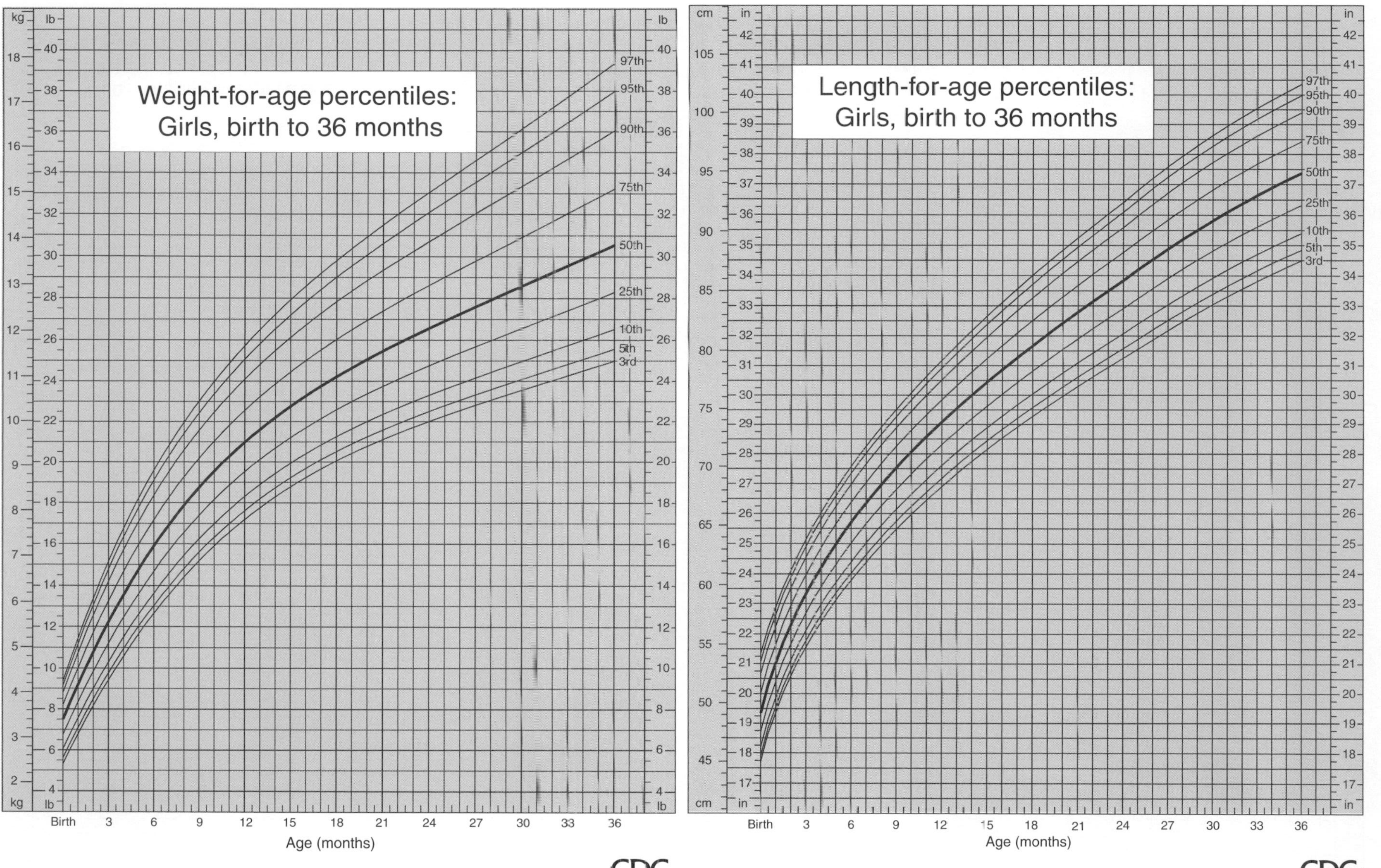

FIGURE **1-58** Weight-for-age percentiles, girls, birth to 36 months, CDC growth charts: United States. (Developed by the National Center for Health Statistics in collaboration with the National Center for Chronic Disease Prevention and Health Promotion [2000].)

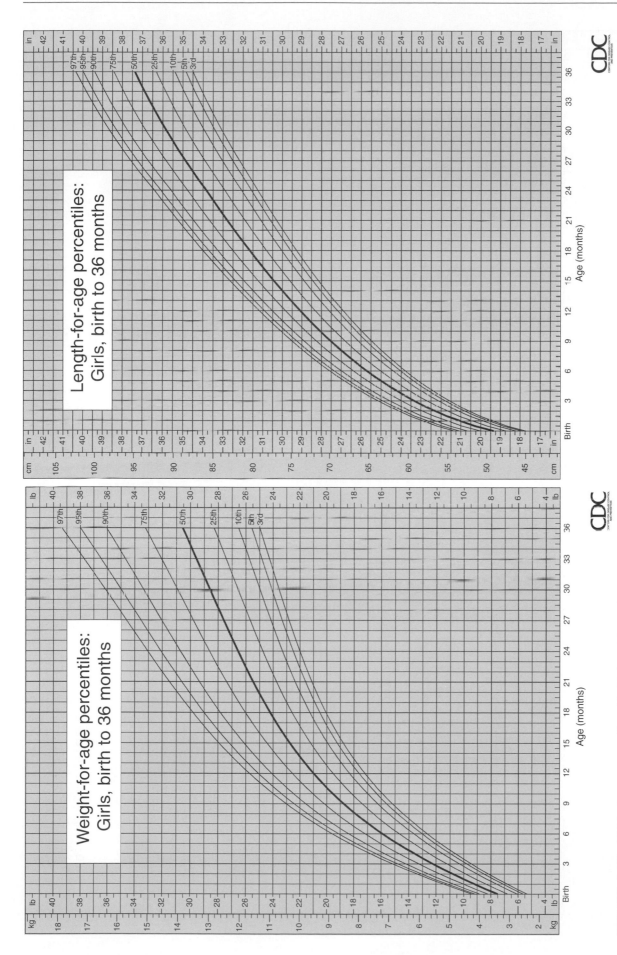

FIGURE **1-59** Length-for-age percentiles, girls, birth to 36 months, CDC growth charts: United States. (Developed by the National Center for Health Statistics in collaboration with the National Center for Chronic Disease Prevention and Health Promotion [2000].)

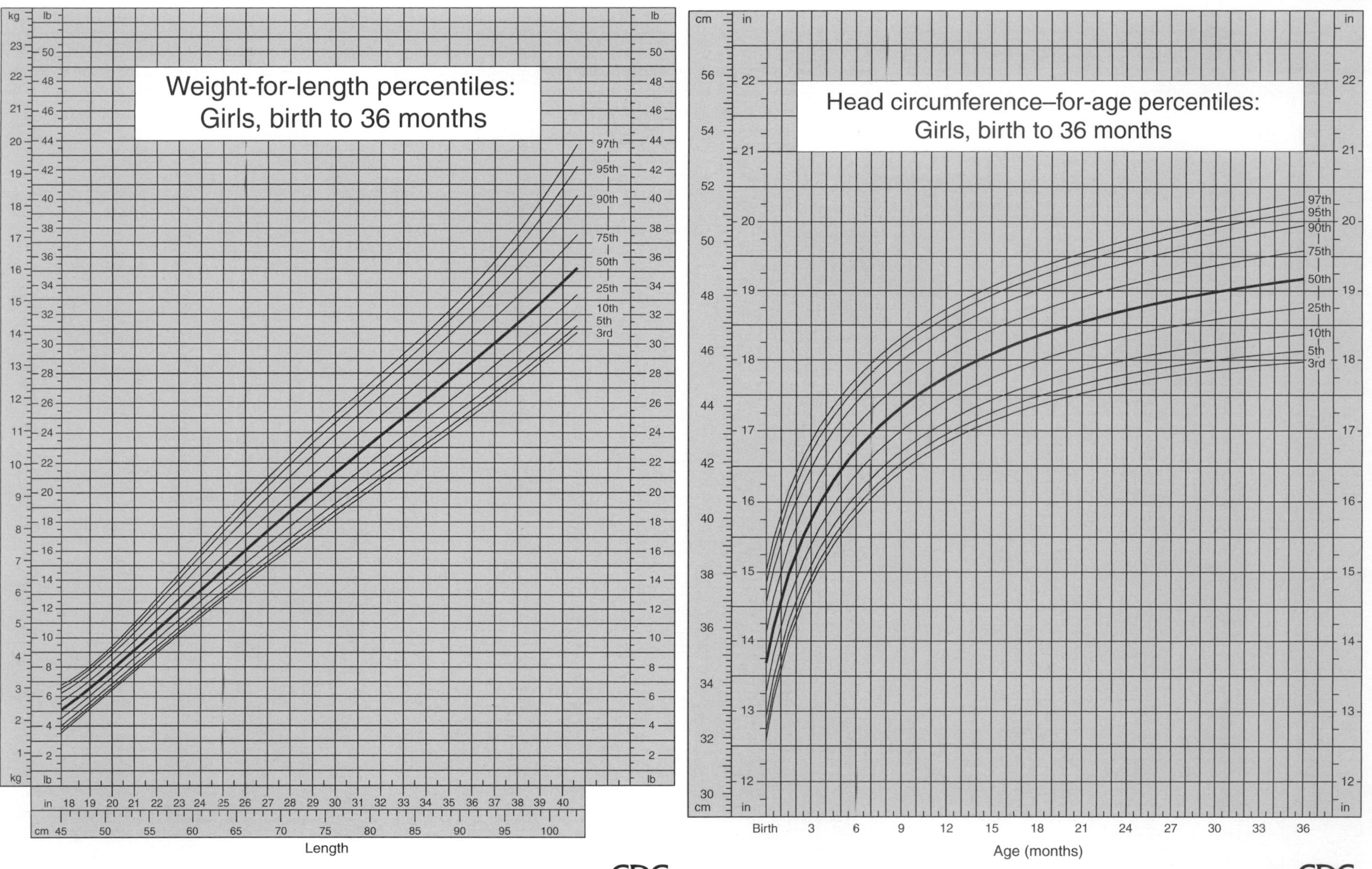

FIGURE **1-60** Weight-for-length percentiles, girls, birth to 36 months, CDC growth charts: United States. (Developed by the National Center for Health Statistics in collaboration with the National Center for Chronic Disease Prevention and Health Promotion [2000].)

FIGURE **1-61** Head circumference–for-age percentiles, girls, birth to 36 months, CDC growth charts: United States. (Developed by the National Center for Health Statistics in collaboration with the National Center for Chronic Disease Prevention and Health Promotion [2000].)

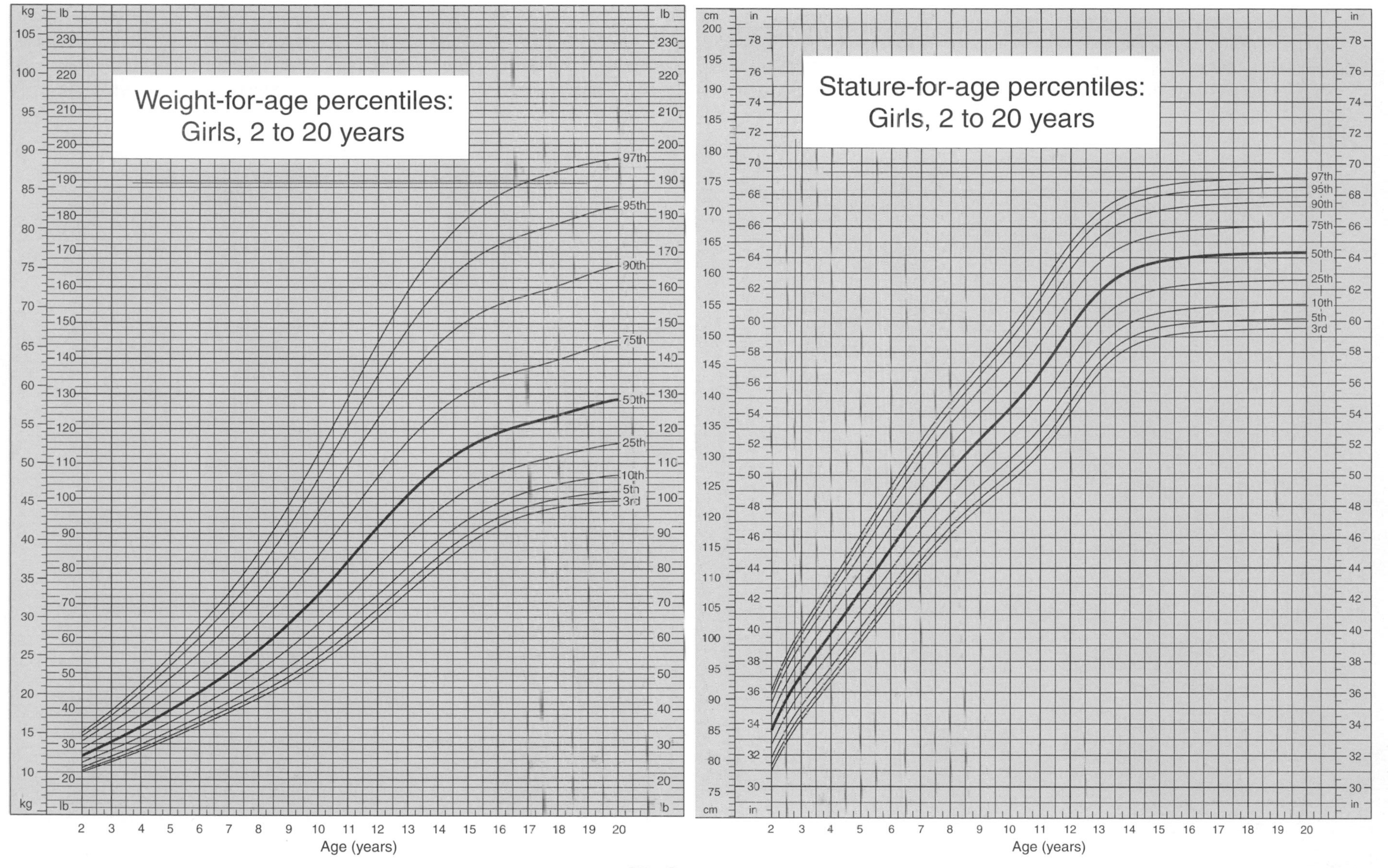

FIGURE **1-62** Weight-for-age percentiles, girls, 2-20 years, CDC growth charts: United States. (Developed by the National Center for Health Statistics in collaboration with the National Center for Chronic Disease Prevention and Health Promotion [2000].)

FIGURE **1-63** Stature-for-age percentiles, girls, 2-20 years, CDC growth charts: United States. (Developed by the National Center for Health Statistics in collaboration with the National Center for Chronic Disease Prevention and Health Promotion [2000].)

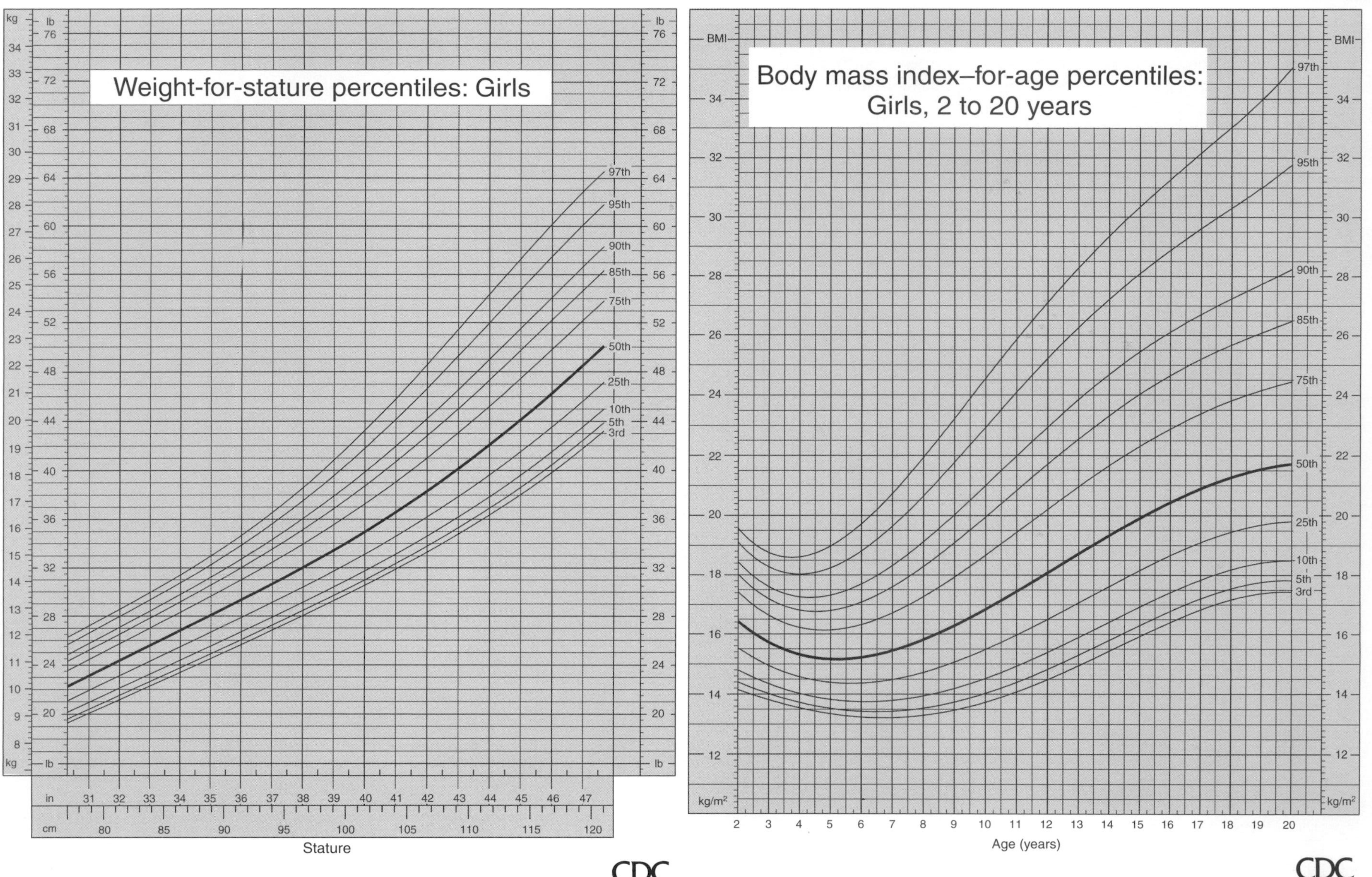

FIGURE **1-64** Weight-for-stature percentiles, girls, CDC growth charts: United States. (Developed by the National Center for Health Statistics [NCHS] in collaboration with the National Center for Chronic Disease Prevention and Health Promotion [2000].)

FIGURE **1-65** Body mass index–for-age percentiles, girls, 2-20 years, CDC growth charts: United States. (Developed by the National Center for Health Statistics in collaboration with the National Center for Chronic Disease Prevention and Health Promotion [2000].)

Growth Standards of Healthy Chinese Children

	Weight (kg)		Height (cm)		Head Circumference (cm)	
Age	**Boys**	**Girls**	**Boys**	**Girls**	**Boys**	**Girls**
Birth	3.27	3.17	50.6	50	34.3	33.7
1 mo	4.97	4.64	56.5	55.5	38.1	37.3
2 mo	5.95	5.49	59.6	58.4	39.7	38.7
3 mo	6.73	6.23	62.3	60.9	41	40
4 mo	7.32	6.69	64.4	62.9	42	41
5 mo	7.70	7.19	65.9	64.5	42.9	41.9
6 mo	8.22	7.62	68.1	66.7	43.9	42.8
8 mo	8.71	8.14	70.6	69	44.9	43.7
10 mo	9.14	8.57	72.9	71.4	45.7	44.5
12 mo	9.56	9.04	75.6	74.1	46.3	45.2
15 mo	10.15	9.54	78.3	76.9	46.8	45.6
18 mo	10.67	10.08	80.7	79.4	47.3	46.2
21 mo	11.18	10.56	83	81.7	47.8	46.7
24 mo	11.95	11.37	86.5	85.3	48.2	47.1
2.5 yr	12.84	12.28	90.4	89.3	48.8	47.7
3 yr	13.63	13.16	93.8	92.8	49.1	48.1
3.5 yr	14.45	14	97.2	96.3	49.4	48.5
4 yr	15.26	14.89	100.8	100.1	49.7	48.9
4.5 yr	16.07	15.63	103.9	103.1	50	49.1
5 yr	16.88	16.46	107.2	106.5	50.2	49.4
5.5 yr	17.65	17.18	110.1	109.2	50.5	49.6
6 yr	19.25	18.67	114.7	113.9	50.8	50
7 yr	21.01	20.35	120.6	119.3	51.1	50.2
8 yr	23.08	22.43	125.3	124.6	51.4	50.6
9 yr	25.33	24.57	130.6	129.5	51.7	50.9
10 yr	27.15	27.05	134.4	134.8	51.9	51.3
11 yr	30.13	30.51	139.2	140.6	52.3	51.7
12 yr	33.05	34.74	144.2	146.6	52.7	52.3
13 yr	36.90	38.52	149.8	150.7	53	52.8

Data from Beijing Children's Hospital China, 1987.

Assessment of Development

Denver II*

The Denver II is a major revision and a restandardization of the Denver Developmental Screening Test (DDST) and the revised Denver Development Screening Test (DDST-R). It differs from the earlier screening tests in items included as well as in the form, the interpretation, and the referral (Figures 1-66 and 1-67). Like the other tests, it assesses gross motor, language, fine motor, adaptive, and personal-social development in children from 1 month to 6 years of age.

ITEM DIFFERENCES

The previous total of 105 items has been increased to 125, including an increase from 21 DDST items to 39 Denver II language items.

Previous items that were difficult to administer and/or interpret have been either modified or eliminated. Many items that were previously tested by parental report now require observation by the examiner.

Each item was evaluated to determine if significant differences existed on the basis of gender, ethnic group, maternal education, and place of residence. Items for which clinically significant differences existed were replaced or, if retained, are discussed in the *Technical Manual.* When evaluating children delayed on one of these items, the examiner can look up norms for the subpopulations to determine if the delay may be a result of sociocultural differences.

TEST FORM DIFFERENCES

The age scale is similar to the American Academy of Pediatrics suggested periodicity schedule for health maintenance visits. This facilitates use of the Denver II at these times.

In children born prematurely, the age is adjusted only until the child is 2 years old.

The items on the test form are arranged in the same format as the DDST-R.

The norms for the distribution bars were updated with the new standardization data but retained the 25th, 50th, 75th, and 90th percentile divisions.

The test form contains a place to rate the child's behavioral characteristics (compliance, interest in surroundings, fearfulness, attention span).

INTERPRETATION AND REFERRAL

Explain to the parents that the Denver II is not an intelligence test but a systematic appraisal of the child's present development. Stress that the child is not expected to perform each item.

To determine relative areas of advancement and areas of delay, sufficient items should be administered to establish the basal and ceiling levels in each sector.

By scoring appropriate items as "pass," "fail," "refusal," or "no opportunity" and relating such scores to the age of the child, each item can be interpreted as described in Box 1-11.

To identify cautions, all items intersected by the age line are administered.

To screen solely for developmental delays, only the items located totally to the *left* of the child's age line are administered.

Criteria for referral are based on the availability of resources in the community.

BOX 1-11 | DENVER II SCORING

Interpretation of Denver II Scores

Advanced: Passed an item completely to the *right* of the age line (passed by less than 25% of children at an age older than the child)

OK: Passed, failed, or refused an item intersected by the age line between the 25th and 75th percentiles

Caution: Failed or refused items intersected by the age line on or between the 75th and 90th percentiles

Delay: Failed an item completely to the *left* of the age line; refusals to the left of the age line may also be considered delays, because the reason for the refusal may be inability to perform the task

Interpretation of Test

Normal: No delays and a maximum of one caution

Suspect: One or more delays and/or two or more cautions

Untestable: Refusals on one or more items completely to the left of the age line or on more than one item intersected by the age line in the 75th to 90th percentile area

Recommendations for Referral for Suspect and Untestable Tests

Rescreen in 1 to 2 weeks to rule out temporary factors

If rescreen is suspect or subject is untestable, use clinical judgment based on the following: number of cautions and delays; which items are cautions and delays; rate of past development; clinical examination and history; and availability of referral resources

*To ensure that the Denver II is administered and interpreted in the prescribed manner, it is recommended that those intending to administer it receive the appropriate training, which can be obtained with the forms and instructional manual from Denver Developmental Materials, PO Box 371075, Denver, CO 80237-5075, (303)355-4729 or (800)419-4729.

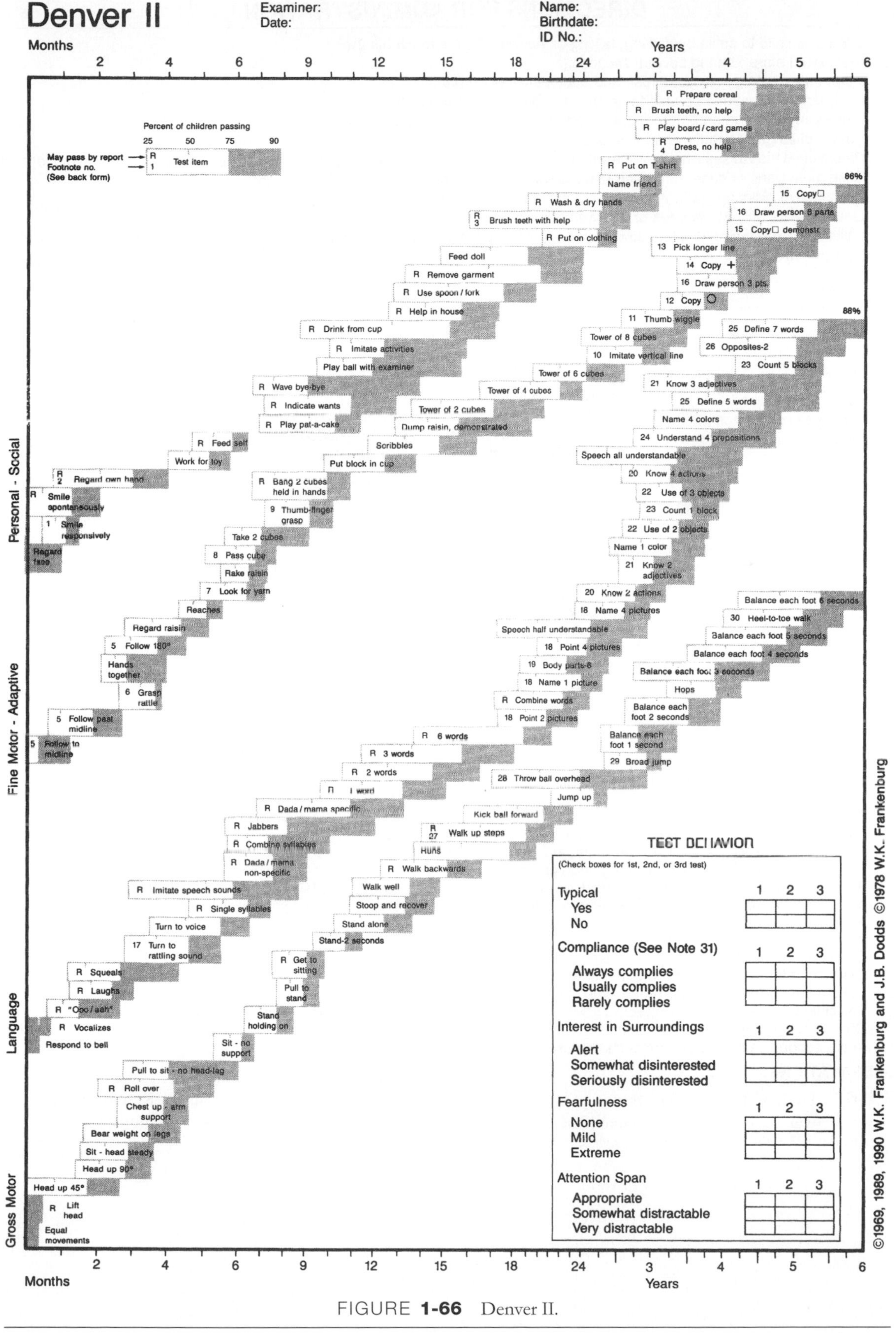

FIGURE **1-66** Denver II.

DIRECTIONS FOR ADMINISTRATION

1. Try to get child to smile by smiling, talking or waving. Do not touch him/her.
2. Child must stare at hand several seconds.
3. Parent may help guide toothbrush and put toothpaste on brush.
4. Child does not have to be able to tie shoes or button/zip in the back.
5. Move yarn slowly in an arc from one side to the other, about 8" above child's face.
6. Pass if child grasps rattle when it is touched to the backs or tips of fingers.
7. Pass if child tries to see where yarn went. Yarn should be dropped quickly from sight from tester's hand without arm movement.
8. Child must transfer cube from hand to hand without help of body, mouth, or table.
9. Pass if child picks up raisin with any part of thumb and finger.
10. Line can vary only 30 degrees or less from tester's line.
11. Make a fist with thumb pointing upward and wiggle only the thumb. Pass if child imitates and does not move any fingers other than the thumb.

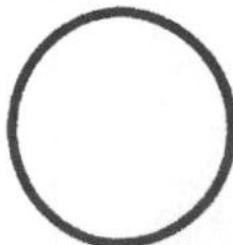

12. Pass any enclosed form. Fail continuous round motions.

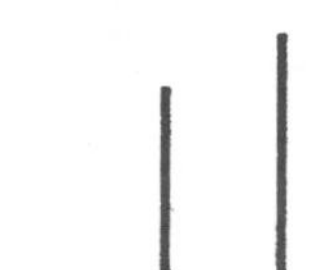

13. Which line is longer? (Not bigger.) Turn paper upside down and repeat. (pass 3 of 3 or 5 of 6)

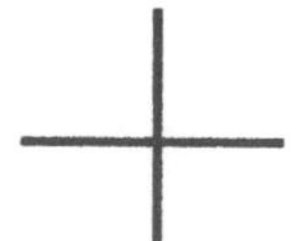

14. Pass any lines crossing near midpoint.

15. Have child copy first. If failed, demonstrate.

When giving items 12, 14, and 15, do not name the forms. Do not demonstrate 12 and 14.

16. When scoring, each pair (2 arms, 2 legs, etc.) counts as one part.
17. Place one cube in cup and shake gently near child's ear, but out of sight. Repeat for other ear.
18. Point to picture and have child name it. (No credit is given for sounds only.)
    If less than 4 pictures are named correctly, have child point to picture as each is named by tester.

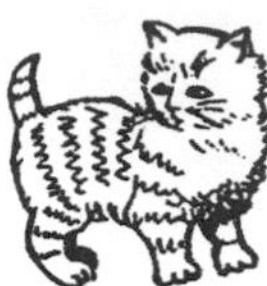
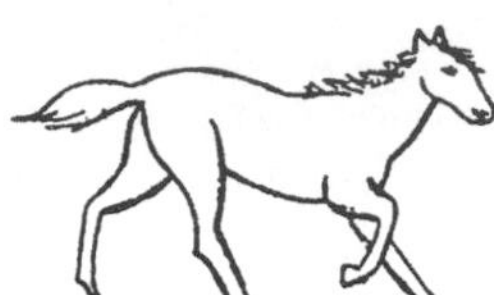
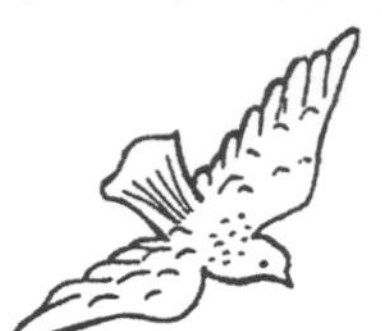
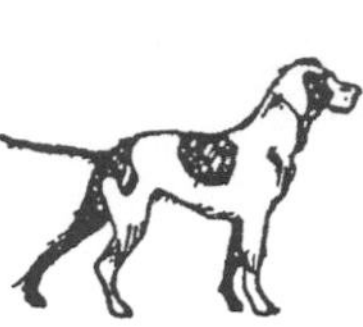
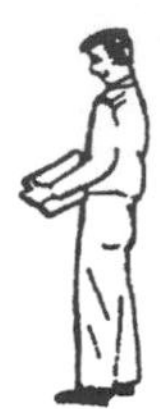

19. Using doll, tell child: Show me the nose, eyes, ears, mouth, hands, feet, tummy, hair. Pass 6 of 8.
20. Using pictures, ask child: Which one flies?... says meow?... talks?... barks?... gallops? Pass 2 of 5, 4 of 5.
21. Ask child: What do you do when you are cold?... tired?... hungry? Pass 2 of 3, 3 of 3.
22. Ask child: What do you do with a cup? What is a chair used for? What is a pencil used for?
    Action words must be included in answers.
23. Pass if child correctly places and says how many blocks are on paper. (1, 5).
24. Tell child: Put block **on** table; **under** table; **in front of** me, **behind** me. Pass 4 of 4.
    (Do not help child by pointing, moving head or eyes.)
25. Ask child: What is a ball?... lake?... desk?... house?... banana?... curtain?... fence?... ceiling? Pass if defined in terms of use, shape, what it is made of, or general category (such as banana is fruit, not just yellow). Pass 5 of 8, 7 of 8.
26. Ask child: If a horse is big, a mouse is __? If fire is hot, ice is __? If the sun shines during the day, the moon shines during the __? Pass 2 of 3.
27. Child may use wall or rail only, not person. May not crawl.
28. Child must throw ball overhand 3 feet to within arm's reach of tester.
29. Child must perform standing broad jump over width of test sheet (8 1/2 inches).
30. Tell child to walk forward, ∞∞∞∞→ heel within 1 inch of toe. Tester may demonstrate.
    Child must walk 4 consecutive steps.
31. In the second year, half of normal children are non-compliant.

OBSERVATIONS:

FIGURE **1-67** Directions for administration of numbered items on Denver II. (From Frankenburg WK, and others. *The Denver II training manual,* Denver, Denver Developmental Materials, Inc.)

Revised Denver Prescreening Developmental Questionnaire*

The Revised Prescreening Developmental Questionnaire (R-PDQ) is a revision of the original PDQ. Advantages of the R-PDQ include the addition and arrangement of items to be more age-appropriate, simplified parent scoring, and easier comparison with DDST norms for professionals. The R-PDQ is a parent-answered prescreen consisting of 105 questions from the DDST, although only a subset of questions are asked for each age-group. The form may need to be read to less educated caregivers.

Preparation and scoring of the R-PDQ include the following:

1. Calculate the child's age as detailed in the Denver II manual, and choose the appropriate form* for the child: orange (0-9 months), purple (9-24 months), gold (2-4 years), or white (4-6 years). (See sample of 0 to 9 month form, Figure 1-68.)
2. Give the appropriate form to the child's caregiver, and have person note relationship to the child. Have the caregiver answer questions until (1) three "no's" are circled (they do not have to be consecutive), or (2) all the questions on both sides of the form have been answered.
3. Check form to see that all appropriate questions have been answered.
4. Review "yes" and "no" responses. Ensure that the child's caregiver understood each question and scored the items correctly. Give particular attention to the scoring of questions that require verbal responses by the child and that require the child to draw.
5. Identify delays (items passed by 90% of children at a younger age than the child being screened). Ages at which 90% of children in the DDST sample passed the items are indicated in parentheses in the "For Office Use" column. These ages are shown in months and weeks up to 24 months and in years and months after 24 months. Highlight delays by circling the 90% age in parentheses to the right of the item that the child was not able to perform.
6. Children who have no delays are considered to be developing normally.
7. If a child has one delay, give the caregiver age-appropriate developmental activities to pursue with the child† and schedule the child for rescreening with the R-PDQ 1 month later. If on rescreening 1 month later the child has one or more delays, schedule second-stage screening with the Denver II as soon as possible.
8. If a child has two or more delays on the first-stage screening with the R-PDQ, schedule a second-stage screening with the Denver II as soon as possible. If on second-stage screening with the Denver II the child receives other than normal results, schedule the child for a diagnostic evaluation.

*Forms and complete instructions are available from Denver Developmental Materials, Inc., PO Box 371075, Denver, CO 80237-5075, USA; (303)355-4729 or (800)419-4729.

†Suggested Denver Developmental Activities are available from Denver Developmental Materials, Inc.

0-9 MONTHS (R-PDQ)

REVISED DENVER PRESCREENING DEVELOPMENTAL QUESTIONNAIRE

Child's Name ____________________

Person Completing R-PDQ: ____________________

Relation to Child: ____________________

For Office Use

Today's Date: ____ yr ____ mo ____ day

Child's Birthdate: ____ yr ____ mo ____ day

Subtract to get Child's Exact Age: ____ yr ____ mo ____ day

R-PDQ Age: (____ yr ____ mo ____ completed wks)

CONTINUE ANSWERING UNTIL **3 "NOs"** ARE CIRCLED

			For Office Use
1. Equal Movements When your baby is lying on his/her back, can (s)he move each of his/her arms as easily as the other and each of the legs as easily as the other? Answer **No** if your child makes jerky or uncoordinated movements with one or both of his/her arms or legs.	**Yes**	**No**	(0) FMA
2. Stomach Lifts Head When your baby is on his/her stomach on a flat surface, can (s)he lift his/her head off the surface?	**Yes**	**No**	(0-3) GM
3. Regards Face When your baby is lying on his/her back, can (s)he look at you and watch your face?	**Yes**	**No**	(1) PS
4. Follows To Midline When your child is on his/her back, can (s)he follow your movement by turning his/her head from one side to facing directly forward?	**Yes**	**No**	(1-1) FMA
5. Responds To Bell Does your child respond with eye movements, change in breathing or other change in activity to a bell or rattle sounded outside his/her line of vision?	**Yes**	**No**	(1-2) L
6. Vocalizes Not Crying Does your child make sounds other than crying, such as gurgling, cooing, or babbling?	**Yes**	**No**	(1-3) L
7. Smiles Responsively When you smile and talk to your baby, does (s)he smile back at you?	**Yes**	**No**	(1-3) PS
8. Follows Past Midline When your child is on his/her back, does (s)he follow your movement by turning his/her head from one side ***almost all the way to the other side?***	**Yes**	**No**	(2-2) FMA
9. Stomach, Head Up 45° When your baby is on his/her stomach on a flat surface, can (s)he lift his/her head 45°?	**Yes**	**No**	(2-2) GM
10. Stomach, Head Up 90° When your baby is on his/her stomach on a flat surface, can (s)he lift his/her head 90°?	**Yes**	**No**	(3) GM
11. Laughs Does your baby laugh out loud without being tickled or touched?	**Yes**	**No**	(3-1) L
12. Hands Together Does your baby play with his/her hands by touching them together?	**Yes**	**No**	(3-3) FMA
13. Follows 180° When your child is on his/her back, does (s)he follow your movement from one side ***all the way*** to the other side?	**Yes**	**No**	(4) FMA
14. Grasps Rattle ***It is important that you follow instructions carefully.*** Do ***not*** place the pencil in the palm of your child's hand. When you touch the pencil to the back or tips of your baby's fingers, does your baby grasp the pencil for a few seconds?	**Yes**	**No**	(4) FMA

TRY THIS   **NOT** THIS

(Please turn page)

FIGURE **1-68** Revised Denver Prescreening Developmental Questionnaire. (The first page is reprinted with permission from William K. Frankenburg, MD, Copyright 1975, 1986, WK Frankenburg, MD.)

Assessment of Language and Speech

Major Development Characteristics of Language and Speech

Age (yr)	Normal Language Development	Normal Speech Development	Intelligibility
1	Says two or three words with meaning	Omits most final and some initial consonants	Usually no more than 25% intelligible to unfamiliar listener
	Imitates sounds of animals	Substitutes consonants *m, w, p, b, k, g, n, t, d,* and *h* for more difficult sounds	Height of unintelligible jargon at age 18 months
2	Uses two- or three-word phrases Has vocabulary of about 300 words Uses "I," "me," "you"	Uses above consonants with vowels, but inconsistently and with much substitution Omission of final consonants Articulation lags behind vocabulary	At age 2 years, 50% intelligible in context
3	Says four- or five-word sentences Has vocabulary of about 900 words Uses "who," "what," and "where" in asking questions Uses plurals, pronouns, and prepositions	Masters *b, t, d, k,* and *g*; sounds *r* and *l* may still be unclear, omits or substitutes *w* Repetitions and hesitations common	At age 3 years, 75% intelligible
4-5	Has vocabulary of 1500-2100 words Able to use most grammatic forms correctly, such as past tense of verb with "yesterday" Uses complete sentences with nouns, verbs, prepositions, adjectives, adverbs, and conjunctions	Masters *f* and *v*; may still distort *r, l, s, z, sh, ch, y,* and *th* Little or no omission of initial or final consonants	Speech is 100% intelligible, although some sounds are still imperfect
5-6	Has vocabulary of 3000 words Comprehends "if," "because," and "why"	Masters *r, l,* and *th*; may still distort *s, z, sh, ch,* and *j* (usually mastered by age 7½-8 years)	

Assessment of Communication Impairment

Key questions for language disorders

1. How old was your child when he or she spoke his or her first words?
2. How old was your child when he or she began to put words into sentences?
3. Does your child have difficulty in learning new vocabulary words?
4. Does your child omit words from sentences (i.e., do sentences sound telegraphic?) or use short or incomplete sentences?
5. Does your child have trouble with grammar, such as using the verbs *is, am, are, was*, and *were?*
6. Can your child follow two or three directions given at once?
7. Do you have to repeat directions or questions?
8. Does your child respond appropriately to questions?
9. Does your child ask questions beginning with *who, what, where*, and *why?*
10. Does it seem that your child has made little or no progress in speech and language in the last 6 to 12 months?

Key questions for speech impairment

1. Does your child ever stammer or repeat sounds or words?
2. Does your child seem anxious or frustrated when trying to express an idea?
3. Have you noted certain behaviors, such as blinking, jerking the head, or attempting to rephrase thoughts with different words when your child stammers?
4. What do you do when any of these occurs?
5. Does your child omit sounds from words?
6. Does it seem like your child uses *t, d, k*, or *g* in place of most other consonants when speaking?
7. Does your child omit sounds from words or replace the correct consonant with another one (e.g., *rabbit* with *wabbit*)?
8. Do you have any difficulty in understanding your child's speech?
9. Has anyone else ever remarked about having difficulty in understanding your child?
10. Has there been any recent change in the sound of your child's voice?

Clues for Detecting Communication Impairment

LANGUAGE DISABILITY

Assigning meaning to words

- First words not uttered before second birthday
- Vocabulary size reduced for age or fails to show steady increase
- Difficulty in describing characteristics of objects, although may be able to name them
- Infrequent use of modifier words (adjectives, adverbs)
- Excessive use of jargon past age 18 months

Organizing words into sentences

- First sentences not uttered before third birthday
- Short and incomplete sentences
- Tendency to omit words (articles, prepositions)
- Misuse of the *be, do*, and *can* verb forms
- Difficulty understanding and producing questions
- Plateaus at an early developmental level; uses easy speech patterns

Altering word forms

- Omission of endings for plurals and tenses
- Inappropriate use of plurals and tense endings
- Inaccurate use of possessive words

SPEECH IMPAIRMENT

Dysfluency (stuttering)

- Noticeable repetition of sounds, words, or phrases after age 4 years
- Obvious frustration when attempting to communicate
- Demonstration of struggling behavior while talking (head jerks, blinks, retrials, circumlocution)
- Embarrassment about own speech

Articulation deficiency

- Intelligibility of conversational speech absent by age 3 years
- Omission of consonants at beginning of words by age 3 years and at end of words by age 4 years
- Persisting articulation faults after age 7 years
- Omission of a sound where one should occur
- Distortion of a sound
- Substitution of an incorrect sound for a correct one

Voice disorders

- Deviations in pitch (too high or too low, especially for age and gender); monotone
- Deviations in loudness
- Deviations in quality (hypernasality, hyponasality)

Guidelines for Referral Regarding Communication Impairment

2 years of age
- Failure to speak any meaningful words spontaneously
- Consistent use of gestures rather than vocalizations
- Difficulty in following verbal directions
- Failure to respond consistently to sound

3 years of age
- Speech is largely unintelligible
- Failure to use sentences of three or more words
- Frequent omission of initial consonants
- Use of vowels rather than consonants

5 years of age
- Stutters or has any other type of dysfluency
- Sentence structure noticeably impaired
- Substitutes easily produced sounds for more difficult ones
- Omits word endings (plurals, tenses of verbs, etc.)

School age
- Poor voice quality (monotonous, loud, or barely audible)
- Vocal pitch inappropriate for age and gender
- Any distortions, omissions, or substitutions of sounds after age 7 years
- Connected speech characterized by use of unusual confusions or reversals

General
- Any child with signs that suggest a hearing impairment
- Any child who is embarrassed or disturbed by own speech
- Parents who are excessively concerned or who pressure the child to speak at a level above that appropriate for age

Denver Articulation Screening Examination

The Denver Articulation Screening Examination (DASE) (Figure 1-69) is designed to reliably discriminate between significant developmental delays and normal variations in the acquisition of speech sounds in children from 2½ to 6 years of age. It uses the *imitative* method for assessing speech sounds. A complete instructional manual is available.*

General guidelines include the following:

1. Tell the child to repeat a word, such as *car.* Give child several examples to ensure understanding. Beginning with the first word, *table,* have the child repeat all 22 words after you. Score the child's pronunciation of the *underlined* sounds or blends in each word. (There are 30 articulated sound elements for testing.)
2. If the child is shy or hard to test, use the simple line drawings to illustrate each word.
3. To determine test results, match the raw score line (number of correct sounds) with the column denoting child's age. A child is considered to be the closest *previous* age-group shown on the percentile rank chart. The child's percentile rank is at the point where the line and column meet. Percentiles above the heavy line are *abnormal,* and those below are *normal.*
4. Rate the child's spontaneous speech in terms of intelligibility:
   a. Easy to understand
   b. Understandable half the time
   c. Not understandable
   d. Cannot evaluate (if the child does not speak in sentences or phrases during the interview)
5. Rate the child's total test results as follows:
   a. **Normal**—Normal on DASE *and* intelligibility
   b. **Abnormal**—Abnormal on DASE *and/or* intelligibility
6. Rescreen children with abnormal results within 2 weeks.

*Available from Denver Developmental Materials, Inc, PO Box 371075, Denver, CO 80237-5075, (303)355-4729 or (800)419-4729.

DENVER ARTICULATION SCREENING EXAM
for children 2½ to 6 years of age

Instructions: Have child repeat each word after you. Circle the underlined sounds that he pronounces correctly. Total correct sounds is the Raw Score. Use charts on reverse side to score results.

Name:

Hosp. No.:

Address:________________________
____

Date: ________ Child's age: ________ Examiner: ________ Raw score: ____
Percentile: ______ Intelligibility: ________ Result: ________

1. table	6. zipper	11. sock	16. wagon	21. leaf
2. shirt	7. grapes	12. vacuum	17. gum	22. carrot
3. door	8. flag	13. yarn	18. house	
4. trunk	9. thumb	14. mother	19. pencil	
5. jumping	10. toothbrush	15. twinkle	20. fish	

Intelligibility: (circle one)
1. Easy to understand
2. Understandable ½ the time
3. Not understandable
4. Can't evaluate

Comments:

Date: ________ Child's age: ________ Examiner: ________ Raw score: ____
Percentile: ______ Intelligibility: ________ Result: ________

1. table	6. zipper	11. sock	16. wagon	21. leaf
2. shirt	7. grapes	12. vacuum	17. gum	22. carrot
3. door	8. flag	13. yarn	18. house	
4. trunk	9. thumb	14. mother	19. pencil	
5. jumping	10. toothbrush	15. twinkle	20. fish	

Intelligibility: (circle one)
1. Easy to understand
2. Understandable ½ the time
3. Not understandable
4. Can't evaluate

Comments:

Date: ________ Child's age: ________ Examiner: ________ Raw score ____
Percentile: ______ Intelligibility: ________ Result: ________

1. table	6. zipper	11. sock	16. wagon	21. leaf
2. shirt	7. grapes	12. vacuum	17. gum	22. carrot
3. door	8. flag	13. yarn	18. house	
4. trunk	9. thumb	14. mother	19. pencil	
5. jumping	10. toothbrush	15. twinkle	20. fish	

Intelligibility: (circle one)
1. Easy to understand
2. Understandable ½ the time
3. Not understandable
4. Can't evaluate

A

FIGURE **1-69** **A**, Denver Articulation Screening Examination for children 2½ to 6 years of age. (From AF Drumwright, University of Colorado Medical Center, 1971.)

To score DASE words: Note raw score for child's performance. Match raw score line (extreme left of chart) with column representing child's age (to the closest previous age group). Where raw score line and age column meet number in that square denotes percentile rank of child's performance when compared to other children that age. Percentiles above heavy line are ABNORMAL percentiles, below heavy line are NORMAL.

PERCENTILE RANK (years)

Raw Score	2.5	3.0	3.5	4.0	4.5	5.0	5.5	6
2	1							
3	2							
4	5							
5	9							
6	16							
7	23							
8	31	2						
9	37	4	1					
10	42	6	2					
11	48	7	4					
12	54	9	6	1	1			
13	58	12	9	2	3	1	1	
14	62	17	11	5	4	2	2	
15	68	23	15	9	5	3	2	
16	75	31	19	12	5	4	3	
17	79	38	25	15	6	6	4	
18	83	46	31	19	8	7	4	
19	86	51	38	24	10	9	5	1
20	89	58	45	30	12	11	7	3
21	92	65	52	36	15	15	9	4
22	94	72	58	43	18	19	12	5
23	96	77	63	50	22	24	15	7
24	97	82	70	58	29	29	20	15
25	99	87	78	66	36	34	26	17
26	99	91	84	75	46	43	34	24
27		94	89	82	57	54	44	34
28		96	94	88	70	68	59	47
29		98	98	94	84	84	77	68
30		100	100	100	100	100	100	100

To score intelligibility:

	NORMAL	ABNORMAL
2½ years	Understandable half the time, or, "easy"	Not understandable
3 years and older	Easy to understand	Understandable half time Not understandable

Test result: 1. NORMAL on DASE and Intelligibility = NORMAL

2. ABNORMAL on DASE and/or Intelligibility = ABNORMAL

*If abnormal on initial screening, rescreen within 2 weeks.
If abnormal again, child should be referred for complete speech evaluation.

B

FIGURE **1-69, cont'd** B, Percentile rank.

Assessment of Vision

Major Developmental Characteristics of Vision

Birth
- Visual acuity 20/100 to 20/400 (Table 1-12)*
- Pupillary and corneal (blink) reflexes present
- Able to fixate on moving object in range of 45 degrees when held 20 to 25 cm (8 to 10 inches) away
- Cannot integrate head and eye movements well (doll's eye reflex—eyes lag behind if head is rotated to one side)

4 weeks of age
- Can follow in range of 90 degrees
- Can watch parent intently as he or she speaks to infant
- Tear glands begin to function
- Visual acuity is hyperoptic because of less spherical eyeball than in adult

6 to 12 weeks of age
- Has peripheral vision to 180 degrees
- Binocular vision begins at age 6 weeks, is well established by age 4 months
- Convergence on near objects begins by age 6 weeks, is well developed by age 3 months
- Doll's eye reflex disappears

12 to 20 weeks of age
- Recognizes feeding bottle
- Able to fixate on a 1.25-cm (0.5-inch) block
- Looks at hand while sitting or lying on back
- Able to accommodate to near objects

20 to 28 weeks of age
- Adjusts posture to see an object
- Able to rescue a dropped toy
- Develops color preference for yellow and red
- Able to discriminate among simple geometric forms
- Prefers more complex visual stimuli
- Develops hand-eye coordination

28 to 44 weeks of age
- Can fixate on very small objects
- Depth perception begins to develop.
- Lack of binocular vision indicates strabismus.

44 to 52 weeks of age
- Visual acuity 20/40 to 20/60
- Visual loss may develop if strabismus is present.
- Can follow rapidly moving objects

Clues for Detecting Visual Impairment

REFRACTIVE ERRORS

Myopia

Nearsightedness—Ability to see objects clearly at close range but not at a distance

Pathophysiology—Results from eyeball that is too long, causing image to fall in front of retina

Clinical manifestations
- Rubs eyes excessively
- Tilts head or thrusts head forward
- Has difficulty in reading or performing other close work
- Holds books close to eyes
- Writes or colors with head close to table
- Clumsy; walks into objects
- Blinks more than usual or is irritable when doing close work
- Is unable to see objects clearly
- Does poorly in school, especially in subjects that require demonstration, such as arithmetic
- Dizziness
- Headache
- Nausea following close work

Treatment—Corrected with biconcave lenses that focus image on retina

Hyperopia

Farsightedness—Ability to see objects at a distance but not at close range

Pathophysiology—Results from eyeball that is too short, causing image to focus beyond retina

Clinical manifestations
- Because of accommodative ability, child can usually see objects at all ranges.
- Most children normally hyperopic until about 7 years of age

Treatment—If correction is required, use convex lenses to focus rays on retina.

Astigmatism

Unequal curvatures in refractive apparatus

Pathophysiology—Results from unequal curvatures in cornea or lens that cause light rays to bend in different directions

Clinical manifestations
- Depend on severity of refractive error in each eye
- May have clinical manifestations of myopia

Treatment—Corrected with special lenses that compensate for refractive errors

*Measurement of visual acuity varies according to testing procedures.

TABLE 1-12 Eye Examination Guidelines*

Function	Recommended Tests	Referral Criteria	Comments
Ages 3-5 Years			
Distance visual acuity	Snellen letters Snellen numbers Tumbling E HOTV Picture test Allen figures LEA symbols	1. Fewer than four of six correct at 20-ft line with either eye tested at 10-ft monocularly (i.e., less than 10/20 or 20/40) or 2. Two-line difference between eyes, even within the passing range (i.e., 10/12.5 and 10/20 or 20/25 and 20/40)	1. Tests are listed in decreasing order of cognitive difficulty; the highest test that the child is capable of performing should be used; in general, the tumbling E or the HOTV test should be used for children 3-5 years of age and Snellen letters or numbers for children age 6 years and older. 2. Testing distance of 10 ft is recommended for all visual acuity tests. 3. A line of figures is preferred over single figures. 4. The nontested eye should be covered by an occluder held by the examiner or by an adhesive occluder patch applied to eye; the examiner must ensure that it is not possible to peek with the nontested eye.
Ocular alignment	Cross-cover test at 10 ft (3 m) Random dot E stereo test at 40 cm Simultaneous red reflex test (Bruckner test)	Any eye movement Fewer than four of six correct Any asymmetry of pupil color, size, brightness	Child must be fixing on a target while cross-cover test is performed Direct ophthalmoscope used to view both red reflexes simultaneously in a darkened room from 2 to 3 feet away; detects asymmetric refractive errors as well
Ocular media clarity (cataracts, tumors, etc.)	Red reflex	White pupil, dark spots, absent reflex	Direct ophthalmoscope, darkened room View eyes separately at 12 to 18 inches; white reflex indicates possible retinoblastoma

From American Academy of Pediatrics: Eye examination in infants, children, and young adults by pediatricians, *Pediatrics* 111(4):902-907, 2003.

*Assessing visual acuity (vision screening) represents one of the most sensitive techniques for the detection of eye abnormalities in children. The American Academy of Pediatrics Section on Ophthalmology, in cooperation with the American Association for Pediatric Ophthalmology and Strabismus and the American Academy of Ophthalmology, has developed these guidelines to be used by physicians, nurses, educational institutions, public health departments, and other professionals who perform vision evaluation services.

Continued

TABLE 1-12 Eye Examination Guidelines—cont'd

Function	Recommended Tests	Referral Criteria	Comments
6 Years and Older			
Distance visual acuity	Snellen letters Snellen numbers Tumbling E HOTV Picture test Allen figures LEA symbols	1. Fewer than four of six correct on 15-ft line with either eye tested at 10 ft monocularly (i.e., less than 10/15 or 20/30) or 2. Two-line difference between eyes, even within the passing range (i.e., 10/10 and 10/15 or 20/20 and 20/30)	1. Tests are listed in decreasing order of cognitive difficulty; the highest test that the child is capable of performing should be used; in general, the tumbling E or the HOTV test should be used for children 3-5 years or age and Snellen letters or numbers for children 6 years and older. 2. Testing distance of 10 ft is recommended for all visual acuity tests. 3. A line of figures is preferred over single figures. 4. The nontested eye should be covered by an occluder held by the examiner or by an adhesive occluder patch applied to eye; the examiner must ensure that it is not possible to peek with the nontested eye.
Ocular alignment	Cross-cover test at 10 ft (3 m) Random dot E stereo test at 40 cm Simultaneous red reflex test (Bruckner test)	Any eye movement Fewer than four of six correct Any asymmetry of pupil color, size, brightness	Child must be fixing on a target while cross-cover test is performed Direct ophthalmoscope used to view both red reflexes simultaneously in a darkened room from 2 to 3 feet away; detects asymmetric refractive errors as well
Ocular media clarity (cataracts, tumors, etc)	Red reflex	White pupil, dark spots, absent reflex	Direct ophthalmoscope, darkened room View eyes separately at 12 to 18 inches; white reflex indicates possible retinoblastoma

Anisometropia

Different refractive strengths in each eye

Pathophysiology—May develop amblyopia because weaker eye is used less

Clinical manifestations

- Depend on severity of refractive error in each eye
- May have clinical manifestations of myopia

Treatment—Treated with corrective lenses, preferably contact lenses, to improve vision in each eye so they work as a unit

AMBLYOPIA

Lazy eye—Reduced visual acuity in one eye

Pathophysiology

- Condition results when one eye does not receive sufficient stimulation (e.g., from refractive errors, cataract, or strabismus).
- Each retina receives different images, resulting in diplopia (double vision).
- Brain accommodates by suppressing less intense image.
- Visual cortex eventually does not respond to visual stimulation, with loss of vision in that eye.

Clinical manifestation—Poor vision in affected eye

Treatment—Preventable if treatment of primary visual defect, such as anisometropia or strabismus, begins before 6 years of age

STRABISMUS

"Squint" or cross-eye—Malalignment of eyes

Esotropia—Inward deviation of eye

Exotropia—Outward deviation of eye

Pathophysiology

- May result from muscle imbalance or paralysis, from poor vision, or as congenital defect.
- Because visual axes are not parallel, brain receives two images and amblyopia can result.

Clinical manifestations

- Squints eyelids together or frowns
- Has difficulty focusing from one distance to another
- Inaccurate judgment in picking up objects
- Unable to see print or moving objects clearly
- Closes one eye to see
- Tilts head to one side
- If combined with refractive errors, may see any of the manifestations listed for refractive errors
- Diplopia
- Photophobia
- Dizziness
- Headache
- Cross-eye

Treatment

- Depends on cause of strabismus
- May involve occlusion therapy (patching stronger eye) or surgery to increase visual stimulation to weaker eye
- Early diagnosis essential to prevent vision loss

CATARACTS

Opacity of crystalline lens

Pathophysiology—Prevents light rays from entering eye and being refracted on retina

Clinical manifestations

- Gradually less able to see objects clearly
- May lose peripheral vision
- Nystagmus (with complete blindness)
- Gray opacities of lens
- Strabismus
- Absence of red reflex

Treatment

- Requires surgery to remove cloudy lens and replace lens (intraocular lens implant, removable contact lens, prescription glasses)
- Must be treated early to prevent blindness from amblyopia

GLAUCOMA

Increased intraocular pressure

Pathophysiology

- Congenital type results from defective development of some component related to flow of aqueous humor.
- Increased pressure on optic nerve causes eventual atrophy and blindness.

Clinical manifestations

- Mostly seen in acquired types; loses peripheral vision
- May bump into objects not directly in front
- Sees halos around objects
- May complain of mild pain or discomfort (severe pain, nausea, vomiting, if sudden rise in pressure)
- Redness
- Excessive tearing (epiphora)
- Photophobia
- Spasmodic winking (blepharospasm)
- Corneal haziness
- Enlargement of eyeball (buphthalmos)

Treatment

- Requires surgical treatment (goniotomy) to open outflow tracts
- May require more than one procedure

Special Tests of Visual Acuity and Estimated Visual Acuity at Different Ages

Test	Description	Birth	4 Months	1 Year	Age of 20/20 Vision (months)
Optokinetic nystagmus	A striped drum is rotated or a striped tape is moved in front of infant's eyes. Presence of nystagmus indicates vision. Acuity is assessed by using progressively smaller stripes.	20/400	20/200	20/60	20-30
Forced-choice preferential looking*	Either a homogeneous field or a striped field is presented to infant; an observer monitors the direction of the eyes during presentation of pattern. Acuity is assessed by using progressively smaller striped fields.	20/400	20/200	20/50	18-24
Visually evoked potentials	Eyes are stimulated with bright light or pattern, and electrical activity to visual cortex is recorded through scalp electrodes. Acuity is assessed by using progressively smaller patterns.	20/100 to 20/200	20/80	20/40	6-12

Data from Hoyt C, Nickel B, Billson F: Ophthalmological examination of the infant: development aspects, *Surv Ophthalmol* 26:177-189, 1982.
*One type of preferential looking test is the *Teller Acuity Card Test,* in which a set of rectangular cards containing different black-and-white patterns or grading is presented to the child as an observer looks through a central peephole in the card. The observer, who is hidden from view, observes the variety of visual cues, such as fixation, eye movements, head movements, or pointing. The finest grading the child is judged to be able to see is taken as the acuity estimate. The test is appropriate for children from birth to 24-36 months of age (Teller D and others: Assessment of visual acuity in infants and children: the acuity card procedure, *Dev Med Child Neurol* 28:779-789, 1986).

Denver Eye Screening Test

The Denver Eye Screening Test (DEST) (Figure 1-70) tests visual acuity in children age 3 years or older by using a single card for the letter E (20/30) from a distance of 15 feet. A complete instructional manual is available.

General guidelines include the following:

1. Mark a distance of 15 feet for testing.
2. Use the large E (20/100) to explain and to demonstrate the testing procedure to the child. (See procedure for Snellen E below.)
3. Use the small E for actual testing. Test each eye separately using the occluder.
4. Consider the results *abnormal* if the child fails to correctly identify the direction of the small E over three trials.
5. Test children from 2½ to 3 years of age or those untestable with the letter E using the picture (Allen) cards. (Cooperative children as young as 2 years can also be tested.)
6. Show each card to the child at close range to make certain he or she can identify it.
7. Present the pictures at a distance of 15 feet for actual testing. Test each eye separately if possible.
8. Consider the results *abnormal* if the child fails to correctly name three of the seven cards in three to five trials.
9. Screen children from 6 to 30 months of age by testing for the following:
   a. Fixation (ability to follow a moving light source or spinning toy)
   b. Squinting (observation of the child's eyes or report by parent)
   c. Strabismus (report by parent and performance on cover and pupillary light reflex tests; see pp. 48-49)
10. Consider the results *abnormal* if failure to fixate occurs, if a squint is present, and/or if the child fails two of the three procedures for strabismus.
11. Retest all children with abnormal findings. Refer those with a repeat failure.

DENVER EYE SCREENING TEST

Name:
Hospital No:
Ward:
Address:

	1ST SCREENING: DATE:						RESCREENING: DATE:					
	Right Eye			Left Eye			Right Eye			Left Eye		
Vision Tests	Normal	Abnormal	Untestable	Normal	Abnormal	Untestable	Normal	Abnormal	Untestable	Normal	Abnormal	Untestable
1. E (3 years and above—3 to 5 trials)	3P	3F	U	3P	3F	U	3P	3F	U	3P	3F	U
2. Picture card ($2^1/_2$ to $2^{11}/_{12}$ years—3 to 5 trials)	3P	3F	U	3P	3F	U	3P	3F	U	3P	3F	U
3. Fixation (6 months to $2^5/_{12}$ years)	P	F	U	P	F	U	P	F	U	P	F	U
4. Squinting		Yes			Yes			Yes			Yes	
Tests for Nonstraight Eyes	Normal		Abnormal		Untestable		Normal		Abnormal		Untestable	
1. Do your child's eyes turn in or out, or are they ever not straight?	No		Yes		U		No		Yes		U	
2. Cover test	P		F		U		P		F		U	
3. Pupillary light reflex	P		F		U		P		F		U	
Total Test Rating (Both Eyes)												
Normal (passed vision test plus no squint, plus passed 2 of 3 tests for nonstraight eyes)	Normal						Normal					
Abnormal (abnormal on any vision test, squinting on 2 of 3 procedures for nonstraight eyes)	Abnormal						Abnormal					
Untestable (untestable on any vision test or untestable on 2 of 3 tests for nonstraight eyes)	Untestable						Untestable					
Future Rescreening Appointment for Total Test Rating (Abnormal or Untestable)	Date:						Date:					

FIGURE **1-70** Denver Eye Screening Test. (From Frankenburg WK, Dodds JB. Denver Developmental Materials, Inc. Denver, 1969.)

Snellen Screening*

PREPARATION

1. Hang the Snellen chart (Figure 1-71) on a light-colored wall so that the 20- to 30-foot lines are at eye level when children 6 to 12 years old are tested in the standing position.
2. Secure the chart to the wall with double-stick tape on the back side of all four corners. If the chart must be reversed for use of the letter or E chart, secure it at the top and bottom with tacks. Make sure that the chart does not swing when in place.
3. The illumination intensity on the chart should be 10 to 30 foot-candles, without any glare from windows or light fixtures. The illumination should be checked with a light meter.
4. Mark an exact 20-foot distance from the chart. Mark the floor with a piece of tape or "footprints" positioned so that the heels touch the 20-foot line.

PROCEDURE

1. Place the child at the 20-foot mark, with the heel edging the line if child is standing or with the back of the chair placed at the marker if the child is seated.
2. If the E chart is used, accustom the child to identifying which direction the legs of the E are pointing. Use a demonstration E card for this purpose.

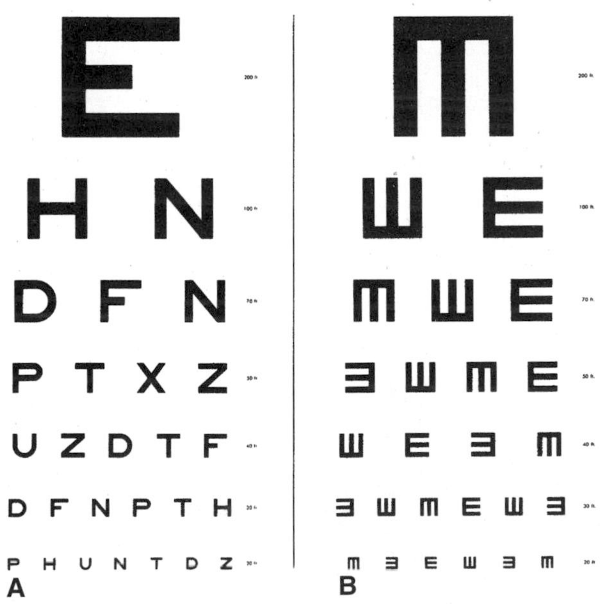

FIGURE **1-71** Snellen chart. **A**, Letter (alphabet) chart. **B**, Symbol E chart.

3. Teach the child to use the occluder to cover one eye. Instruct child to keep both eyes open during the test. Provide a clean cover card for each child, and discard after use.
4. If the child wears glasses, test only with glasses on.
5. Test both eyes together, then right eye, then left eye.
6. Begin with the 40- or 30-foot line, and proceed with test to include the 20-foot line.
7. With a child suspected to have low vision, begin with the 20-foot line and proceed until the child can no longer correctly read three out of four or four out of six symbols on a line.
8. Use covers on the Snellen chart to expose only one symbol or one line at a time. When screening kindergarten-age or older children, expose one line, but a pointer may be used to point to one symbol at a time.

RECORDING AND REFERRAL

1. Record the last line the child read correctly (three out of four or four out of six symbols).
2. Record visual acuity as a fraction. The numerator represents the distance from the chart, and the denominator represents the last line read correctly. For example, 20/30 means that the child read the 30-foot line at a 20-foot distance.
3. Observe the child's eyes during testing, and record any evidence of squinting, head tilting, thrusting the head forward, excessive blinking, tearing, or redness.
4. Make referrals only after a second screening has been made on children who are potential candidates for referral.
5. The following children should be referred for a complete eye examination:
   a. Three-year-old children with vision in either eye of 20/50 or less (inability to correctly identify one more than half the symbols on the 40-foot line) *or* a two-line difference in visual acuity between the eyes in the passing range; for example, 20/20 in one eye and 20/40 in the other
   b. All other ages and grades with vision in either eye of 20/40 or less (inability to correctly identify one more than half the symbols on the 30-foot line)
   c. All children who consistently show any of the signs of possible visual disturbances, regardless of visual acuity

*Modified from recommendations of Prevent Blindness America: *Guide to testing distance visual acuity*, Schaumburg, Ill, 1995, Prevent Blindness America.

Assessment of Hearing

Major Developmental Characteristics of Hearing

Birth
- Responds to loud noise with startle reflex
- Responds to sound of human voice more readily than to any other sound
- Becomes quiet with low-pitched sounds, such as lullaby, metronome, or heartbeat

2 to 3 months of age
- Turns head to side when sound is made at level of ear

3 to 4 months of age
- Locates sound by turning head to side and looking in same direction

4 to 6 months of age
- Can localize sounds made below ear, which is followed by localization of sound made above ear; will turn head to side and then look up or down
- Begins to imitate sounds

6 to 8 months of age
- Locates sounds by turning head in a curving arc
- Responds to own name

8 to 10 months of age
- Localizes sounds by turning head diagonally and directly toward sound

10 to 12 months of age

Knows several words and their meanings, such as "no" and the names of family members

Learns to control and adjust own response to sound, such as listening for sound to occur again

18 months of age
- Begins to discriminate between harshly dissimilar sounds, such as the sounds of a doorbell and a train

24 months of age
- Refines gross discriminative skills

36 months of age
- Begins to distinguish more subtle differences in speech sounds, such as between *e* and *er*

48 months of age
- Begins to distinguish between similar sounds such as *f* and *th* or between *f* and *s*
- Listening becomes considerably refined
- Able to be tested with an audiometer

Assessment of Child for Hearing Impairment

Family history
- Genetic disorders associated with hearing impairment
- Family members, especially siblings, with hearing disorders

Prenatal history
- Miscarriages
- Illnesses during pregnancy (rubella, syphilis, diabetes)
- Drugs taken
- Exposure to childhood diseases
- Eclampsia

Delivery
- Duration of labor, type of delivery
- Fetal distress
- Presentation (especially breech)
- Drugs used
- Blood incompatibility

Birth history
- Birth weight <1500 g
- Hyperbilirubinemia at level exceeding indications for exchange transfusion
- Severe asphyxia
- Prematurity
- Congenital perinatal viral infection (cytomegalovirus, rubella, herpes, syphilis, toxoplasmosis)
- Congenital anomalies involving head and neck

Past health history
- Immunizations
- Serious illness (e.g., bacterial meningitis)
- Seizures
- High unexplained fevers
- Ototoxic drugs
- Hyperbilirubinemia (if preterm)
- No history (adopted child)
- Colds, ear infections, allergies
- Treatment of ear problems
- Visual difficulties
- Exposure to excessive noise (e.g., monitor alarms, gunshot)

Hearing
- Parental concerns regarding hearing loss (what cues, at what age)
- Response to name calling, loud noises, sounds of different frequencies (crinkling paper, whisper, bell, rattle)
- Results of previous audiometric testing

Speech development
- Age of babbling, first meaningful words, phrases
- Intelligibility of speech
- Present vocabulary

Motor development
- Age of sitting, standing, walking
- Level of independence in self-care, feeding, toileting, grooming

Adaptive behavior
- Play activities
- Socialization with other children
- Behaviors: temper tantrums, stubbornness, self-vexation, vibratory stimulus
- Educational achievement
- Recent behavioral and/or personality changes

Clues for Detecting Hearing Impairment

Orientation response
- Lack of startle or blink reflex to a loud sound
- Persistence of Moro reflex beyond 4 months of age (associated with mental retardation)
- Failure to be awakened by loud environmental noises during early infancy
- Failure to localize a source of sound by 6 months of age
- General indifference to sound
- Lack of response to the spoken word; failure to follow verbal directions
- Response to loud noises as opposed to the voice

Vocalizations and sound production
- Monotone quality, unintelligible speech, lessened laughter
- Normal quality in central auditory loss
- Lessened experimental sound play and squealing
- Normal use of jargon during early infancy in central auditory loss, with persistent use later
- Absence of babble or inflections in voice by age 7 months
- Failure to develop intelligible speech by age 24 months
- Vocal play, head banging, or foot stamping for vibratory sensation
- Yelling or screeching to express pleasure, annoyance, or need
- Asking to have statements repeated or answering them incorrectly

Visual attention
- Augmented visual alertness and attentiveness
- Responding more to facial expression than to verbal explanation
- Being alert to gestures and movement
- Use of gestures rather than verbalization to express desires, especially after age 15 months
- Marked imitativeness in play

Social rapport and adaptations
- Less interest and involvement in vocal nursery games
- Intense preoccupation with things rather than persons
- Avoidance of social interactions; often puzzled and unhappy in such situations
- Inquiring, sometimes confused facial expression
- Suspicious alertness, sometimes interpreted as paranoia, alternating with cooperation
- Marked reactivity to praise, attention, and physical affection
- Shows less interest than peers in casual conversation
- Is often inattentive unless the environment is quiet and the speaker is close to the child
- Is more responsive to movement than to sound
- Intently observes the speaker's face, responding more to facial expression than verbalization
- Often asks to have statements repeated
- May not follow directions exactly

Emotional behavior
- Use of tantrums to call attention to self or needs
- Frequently stubborn because of lack of comprehension
- Irritable at not making self understood
- Shy, timid, and withdrawn
- Often appears dreamy, in a world of his or her own, or markedly inattentive

Selected Hearing and Tympanic Membrane Compliance Tests*

Description	Comments
Clinical Hearing Tests	
In newborns elicit the startle reflex and observe other neonatal responses to loud noises, such as facial grimaces, blinking, gross motor movement, quiet if crying or crying if quiet, opening the eyes, or ceasing sucking activity. During infancy note child's reaction to a noise. Stand approximately 18 inches away from infant, to the side, and out of child's peripheral field of vision. With the room silent and infant sitting in parent's lap, distracted by some object, make a voice sound such as *ps* or *phth* (high pitched) or *oo* (low pitched), ring a bell or a rattle, or rustle tissue paper.	An objective sign of alerting to sound may be an increase in heart rate or respiratory rate. Absence of alerting behaviors suggests hearing loss. Eliciting the startle reflex is used only in infants from birth to 4 months. Test is usually inadequate for children beyond infancy because of their tendency to ignore sounds or be distracted. Compare response of localizing sound with expected age response.
Tympanometry	
Tympanometry measures tympanic membrane compliance (or mobility) and estimates middle ear air pressure. A soft rubber cuff is pressed over the external canal to produce an airtight seal; an automatic reading of air pressure registers on the machine.	Detects middle ear disease and abnormalities but does not indicate the degree of hearing loss or the interpretation of sound. Difficult to perform in young children because of inability to maintain an adequate seal or excessive movement by the child.
Conduction Tests	
Rinne test—Stem of tuning fork is placed against the mastoid bone until the sound ceases to be audible. Tuning fork is then moved so that the prongs are held near, but not touching, the auditory meatus. Child should again hear the sound **(Rinne positive).** If sound is not again audible **(Rinne negative),** some abnormality is interfering with the conduction of air through the external and middle chambers.	Requires the cooperation and ability of the child to signal when the sound is no longer audible and when it is again heard; not useful for most children before preschool age.
Weber test—Stem of tuning fork is held in the midline of the head. Child should hear the sound equally in both ears **(Weber positive).** With air conductive loss, child will hear the sound better in the affected ear **(Weber negative).**	Often not suitable for young children because of their difficulty in discriminating among *better, more,* and *less.*
Audiometry	
Electrical audiometer measures the threshold of hearing for pure-tone frequencies and loudness. A sound is transmitted to the child's ear and reduced until child indicates the sound is no longer heard; this procedure is repeated for several sounds covering the range found in conversation. In an air conduction audiogram the sounds are transmitted through earphones. In a bone conduction audiogram the sounds are passed through a plaque placed over the mastoid bone.	Audiometry provides valuable information regarding the severity of the hearing loss, the sound cycles involved, and the possible location of the defect. It requires specialized training of personnel, expensive equipment, and cooperation from the child in terms of confirming the perception of sound. For children ages 2 years to approximately 5 years, play audiometry can be used; it is based on behavior modification and involves reinforcement for correct response.

*Any child who is suspected of a hearing loss because of poor performance using screening tests is referred for special audiometric or ABR testing.

Continued

Selected Hearing and Tympanic Membrane Compliance Tests–cont'd

Description	Comments
Otoacoustic Emissions (OAES)	
Special OAE analyzer delivers a rapid series of clicks to the ear through a probe fitted with a tympanometry tip that is inserted closely in the external auditory canal. The presence of OAEs, defined as sound energy emitted by the cochlea that is believed to be generated by movement of the outer hairs of the organ of Corti, is usually associated with normal or near-normal cochlear sensitivity; with hearing losses of 40 db or more, it is unlikely that the emissions are present.[†]	Preferred method of screening neonates for sensorineural hearing loss (ototoxicity and noise-induced hearing loss). Requires specialized equipment. Minimal training is required. Infants must be in a quiet sleep for testing. Results do not indicate severity of cochlear damage; should be followed by ABR (see below).
Auditory Brainstem Response (ABR)	
Through electrode wires attached to the infant's or child's scalp, electrical or brain wave potentials generated within the auditory system are transmitted to a computer for analysis. After repetitive acoustic stimulation, the waveforms from a normal sleeping or quiet infant consist of several peaks and valleys that reflect activations of neural structures of the brain.	Requires expensive equipment and specialized training of personnel.

[†]Callison DM: Early identification and intervention of hearing-impaired infants, *J Otolaryngol Clin North Am* 32(6):1009-1018, 1999.

Summary of Growth and Development

This summary of growth and development offers a broad overview of the significant physical, psychosocial, and mental achievements during childhood. It begins with a comparison of cognitive and personality development throughout the life span according to different theorists. Following are summaries of the specific developmental milestones associated with each major age-group of children.

Personality, Moral, and Cognitive Development

Stage and Age	Psychosexual Stages (Freud)	Psychosocial Stages (Erikson)	Cognitive Stages (Piaget)	Moral Judgment Stages (Kohlberg)
I Infancy (Birth–1 year)	Oral sensory	Trust vs mistrust	Sensorimotor (birth to 18 months)	
II Toddlerhood (1-3 years)	Anal-urethral	Autonomy vs shame and doubt	Preoperational thought, preconceptual phase (transductive reasoning; e.g., specific to specific) (2-4 years)	Preconventional (premoral) level Punishment and obedience orientation
III Early Childhood (3-6 years)	Phallic-locomotion	Initiative vs guilt	Preoperational thought, intuitive phase (transductive reasoning) (4-7 years)	Preconventional (premoral) level Naive instrumental orientation
IV Middle Childhood (6-12 years)	Latency	Industry vs inferiority	Concrete operations (inductive reasoning and beginning logic)	Conventional level Good-boy, nice-girl orientation Law-and-order orientation
V Adolescence (13-18 years)	Genitality	Identity and repudiation vs identity confusion	Formal operations (deductive and abstract reasoning)	Postconventional or principled level Social-contract orientation Universal ethical principle orientation (no longer included in revised theory)
VI Early Adulthood		Intimacy and solidarity vs isolation		
VII Young and Middle Adulthood		Generativity vs self-absorption		
VIII Later Adulthood	Ego integrity vs despair			

Growth and Development During Infancy

Physical	Gross Motor	Fine Motor
1 Month		
Weight gain of 150-210 g (5-7 ounces) weekly for first 6 months Height gain of 2.5 cm (1 inch) monthly for first 6 months Head circumference increases by 2 cm (0.75 inch) monthly for first 3 months Primitive reflexes present and strong Doll's eye reflex and dance reflex fading Obligatory nose breathing (most infants)	Assumes flexed position with pelvis high but knees not under abdomen when prone (at birth, knees flexed under abdomen)* Can turn head from side to side when prone; lifts head momentarily from bed* Has marked head lag, especially when pulled from lying to sitting position Holds head momentarily parallel and in midline when suspended in prone position Assumes asymmetric tonic neck reflex position when supine When infant is held in standing position, body limp at knees and hips In sitting position back is uniformly rounded, head control is absent	Hands predominantly closed Grasp reflex strong Hand clenches on contact with rattle
2 Months		
Posterior fontanel closed Crawling reflex disappears	Assumes less flexed position when prone—hips flat, legs extended, arms flexed, head to side* Less head lag when pulled to sitting position Can maintain head in same plane as rest of body when held in ventral suspension When infant is prone, can lift head almost 45 degrees off table When infant is held in sitting position, head is held up but bobs forward Assumes asymmetric tonic neck reflex position intermittently	Hands frequently open Grasp reflex fading
3 Months		
Primitive reflexes fading	Able to hold head more erect when sitting but still bobs forward Has only slight head lag when pulled to sitting position Assumes symmetric body positioning Able to raise head and shoulders from prone position to a 45- to 90-degree angle from table; bears weight on forearms When infant is held in standing position, able to bear slight fraction of weight on legs Regards own hand	Actively holds rattle but will not reach for it* Grasp reflex absent Hands kept loosely open Clutches own hand; pulls at blankets and clothes
4 Months		
Drooling begins Moro, tonic neck, and rooting reflexes have disappeared*	Has almost no head lag when pulled to sitting position* Balances head well in sitting position* Back less rounded, curved only in lumbar area Able to sit erect if propped up Able to raise head and chest off surface to angle of 90 degrees Assumes predominant symmetric position Rolls from back to side*	Inspects and plays with hands; pulls clothing or blanket over face in play* Tries to reach object with hand but overshoots Grasps object with both hands Plays with rattle placed in hand, shakes it, but cannot pick it up if dropped Can carry objects to mouth

*Milestones that represent essential integrative aspects of development that lay the foundation for the achievement of more advanced skills.
†Degree of visual acuity varies according to vision measurement procedure used.

Sensory	Vocalization	Socialization and Cognition
Able to fixate on moving object in range of 45 degrees when held at a distance of 20-25 cm (8-10 inches) Visual acuity approaches 20/100† Follows light to midline Quiets when hears a voice	Cries to express displeasure Makes small, throaty sounds Makes comfort sounds during feeding	Is in sensorimotor phase—stage I, use of reflexes (birth–1 month), and stage II, primary circular reactions (1-4 months) Watches parent's face intently as she or he talks to infant
Binocular fixation and convergence to near objects beginning When infant is supine, follows dangling toy from side to point beyond midline Visually searches to locate sounds Turns head to side when sound is made at level of ear	Vocalizes, distinct from crying* Crying becomes differentiated Coos Vocalizes to familiar voice	Demonstrates social smile in response to various stimuli*
Follows object to periphery (180 degrees)† Locates sound by turning head to side and looking in same direction* Begins to have ability to coordinate stimuli from various sense organs	Squeals to show pleasure* Coos, babbles, chuckles Vocalizes when smiling "Talks" a great deal when spoken to Less crying during periods of wakefulness	Displays considerable interest in surroundings Ceases crying when parent enters room Can recognize familiar faces and objects, such as feeding bottle Shows awareness of strange situations
Able to accommodate to near objects Binocular vision fairly well established Can focus on a 1.25-cm (½-inch) block Beginning eye-hand coordination	Makes consonant sounds *n, k, g, p, b* Laughs aloud* Vocalization changes according to mood	Is in stage III, secondary circular reactions Demands attention by fussing; becomes bored if left alone Enjoys social interaction with people Anticipates feeding when sees bottle or mother if breast-feeding Shows excitement with whole body, squeals, breathes heavily Shows interest in strange stimuli Begins to show memory

Continued

Growth and Development During Infancy–cont'd

Physical	Gross Motor	Fine Motor
5 Months		
Beginning signs of tooth eruption Birth weight doubles	No head lag when pulled to sitting position When infant is sitting, able to hold head erect and steady Able to sit for longer periods when back is well supported Back straight When infant is prone, assumes symmetric positioning with arms extended Can turn over from abdomen to back* When infant is supine, puts feet to mouth	Able to grasp objects voluntarily* Uses palmar grasp, bidextrous approach Plays with toes Takes objects directly to mouth Holds one cube while regarding a second one
6 Months		
Growth rate may begin to decline Weight gain of 90-150 g (3-5 ounces) weekly for next 6 months Height gain of 1.25 cm (0.5 inch) monthly for next 6 months Teething may begin with eruption of two lower central incisors* Chewing and biting occur*	When infant is prone, can lift chest and upper abdomen off table, bearing weight on hands When infant is about to be pulled to a sitting position, lifts head Sits in highchair with back straight Rolls from back to abdomen When infant is held in standing position, bears almost all of weight Hand regard absent	Resecures a dropped object Drops one cube when another is given Grasps and manipulates small objects Holds bottle Grasps feet and pulls to mouth
7 Months		
Eruption of lower central incisors Parachute reflex appears	When infant is supine, spontaneously lifts head off table Sits, leaning forward on hands* When infant is prone, bears weight on one hand Sits erect momentarily Bears full weight on feet When infant is held in standing position, bounces actively	Transfers objects from one hand to the other* Has unidextrous approach and grasp Holds two cubes more than momentarily Bangs cube on table Rakes at a small object
8 Months		
Begins to show regular patterns in bladder and bowel elimination	Sits steadily unsupported* Readily bears weight on legs when supported; may stand holding on to furniture Adjusts posture to reach an object	Has beginning pincer grasp using index, fourth, and fifth fingers against lower part of thumb Releases objects at will Rings bell purposely Retains two cubes while regarding third cube Secures an object by pulling on a string Reaches persistently for toys out of reach

*Milestones that represent essential integrative aspects of development that lay the foundation for the achievement of more advanced skills.

Sensory	Vocalization	Socialization and Cognition
Visually pursues a dropped object Is able to sustain visual inspection of an object Can localize sounds made below the ear	Squeals Makes vowel cooing sounds interspersed with consonant sounds (e.g., *ah-goo*)	Smiles at mirror image Pats bottle or breast with both hands More enthusiastically playful but may have rapid mood swings Is able to discriminate strangers from family Vocalizes displeasure when object is taken away Discovers parts of body
Adjusts posture to see an object Prefers more complex visual stimuli Can localize sounds made above the ear Will turn head to the side, then look up or down	Begins to imitate sounds* Babbling resembles one-syllable utterances—*ma, mu, da, di, hi** Vocalizes to toys, mirror image Takes pleasure in hearing own sounds (self-reinforcement)	Recognizes parents; begins to fear strangers Holds arms out to be picked up Has definite likes and dislikes Begins to imitate (cough, protrusion of tongue) Excites on hearing footsteps Laughs when head is hidden in a towel Briefly searches for a dropped object (object permanence beginning)* Frequent mood swings—From crying to laughing with little or no provocation
Can fixate on very small objects* Responds to own name Localizes sound by turning head in an arc Beginning awareness of depth and space Has taste preferences	Produces vowel sounds and chained syllables—*baba, dada, kaka** Vocalizes four distinct vowel sounds "Talks" when others are talking	Increasing fear of strangers; shows signs of fretfulness when parent disappears* Imitates simple acts and noises Tries to attract attention by coughing or snorting Plays peek-a-boo Demonstrates dislike of food by keeping lips closed Exhibits oral aggressiveness in biting and mouthing Demonstrates expectation in response to repetition of stimuli
	Makes consonant sounds *t, d,* and *w* Listens selectively to familiar words Utterances signal emphasis and emotion Combines syllables, such as *dada,* but does not ascribe meaning to them	Increasing anxiety over loss of parent, particularly mother, and fear of strangers Responds to word "no" Dislikes dressing, diaper change

Continued

Growth and Development During Infancy—cont'd

Physical	Gross Motor	Fine Motor
9 Months		
Eruption of upper central incisor may begin	Creeps on hands and knees Sits steadily on floor for prolonged time (10 minutes) Recovers balance when leans forward but cannot do so when leaning sideways Pulls self to standing position and stands holding on to furniture*	Uses thumb and index finger in crude pincer grasp* Preference for use of dominant hand now evident Grasps third cube Compares two cubes by bringing them together
10 Months		
Labyrinth-righting reflex is strongest—infant in prone or supine position is able to raise head	Can change from prone to sitting position Stands while holding on to furniture, sits by falling down Recovers balance easily while sitting While child is standing, lifts one foot to take a step	Crude release of an object beginning Grasps bell by handle
11 Months		
Eruption of lower lateral incisors may begin	When child is sitting, pivots to reach toward back to pick up an object Cruises or walks holding on to furniture or with both hands held*	Explores objects more thoroughly (e.g., clapper inside bell) Has neat pincer grasp Drops object deliberately for it to be picked up Puts one object after another into a container (sequential play) Able to manipulate an object to remove it from tight-fitting enclosure
12 Months		
Birth weight tripled* Birth length increased by 50%* Head and chest circumference equal (head circumference 46 cm [18 inches]) Has total of six to eight deciduous teeth Anterior fontanel almost closed Landau reflex fading Babinski reflex disappears Lumbar curve develops; lordosis evident during walking	Walks with one hand held* Cruises well May attempt to stand alone momentarily; may attempt first step alone* Can sit down from standing position without help	Releases cube in cup Attempts to build two-block tower but fails Tries to insert a pellet into a narrow-necked bottle but fails Can turn pages in a book, many at a time

*Milestones that represent essential integrative aspects of development that lay the foundation for the achievement of more advanced skills.

Sensory	Vocalization	Socialization and Cognition
Localizes sounds by turning head diagonally and directly toward sound Depth perception increasing	Responds to simple verbal commands Comprehends "no-no"	Parent (usually mother) is increasingly important for own sake Shows increasing interest in pleasing parent Begins to show fears of going to bed and being left alone Puts arms in front of face to avoid having it washed
	Says "dada," "mama" with meaning Comprehends "bye-bye" May say one word (e.g., "hi," "bye," "no")	Inhibits behavior to verbal command of "no-no" or own name Imitates facial expressions; waves bye-bye Extends toy to another person but will not release it Develops object permanence* Repeats actions that attract attention and cause laughter Pulls clothes of another to attract attention Plays interactive games such as pat-a-cake Reacts to adult anger; cries when scolded Demonstrates independence in dressing, feeding, locomotive skills, and testing of parents Looks at and follows pictures in a book
	Imitates definite speech sounds	Experiences joy and satisfaction when a task is mastered Reacts to restrictions with frustration Rolls ball to another on request Anticipates body gestures when a familiar nursery rhyme or story is being told (e.g., holds toes and feet in response to "This little piggy went to market") Plays games such as up-down, so big, or peek-a-boo Shakes head for "no"
Discriminates simple geometric forms (e.g., circle) Amblyopia may develop with lack of binocularity Can follow rapidly moving object Controls and adjusts response to sound; listens for sound to recur	Says three to five words besides "dada," "mama"* Comprehends meaning of several words (comprehension always precedes verbalization) Recognizes objects by name Imitates animal sounds Understands simple verbal commands (e.g., "Give it to me," "Show me your eyes")	Shows emotions such as jealousy, affection (may give hug or kiss on request), anger, fear Enjoys familiar surroundings and explores away from parent Is fearful in strange situation; clings to parent May develop habit of security blanket or favorite toy Has increasing determination to practice locomotor skills Searches for an object even if it has not been hidden but searches only where object was last seen*

Growth and Development During Toddler Years

Physical	Gross Motor	Fine Motor
15 Months		
Steady growth in height and weight Head circumference 48 cm (19 inches) Weight 11 kg (24 pounds) Height 78.7 cm (31 inches)	Walks without help (usually since age 13 months) Creeps up stairs Kneels without support Cannot walk around corners or stop suddenly without losing balance Assumes standing position without support Cannot throw ball without falling	Constantly casting objects to floor Builds tower of two cubes Holds two cubes in one hand Releases a pellet into a narrow-necked bottle Scribbles spontaneously Uses cup with lid well but rotates spoon
18 Months		
Physiologic anorexia from decreased growth needs Anterior fontanel closed Physiologically able to control sphincters	Runs clumsily, falls often Walks up stairs with one hand held Pulls and pushes toys Jumps in place with both feet Seats self on chair Throws ball overhand without falling	Builds tower of three or four cubes Release, prehension, and reach well developed Turns pages in a book two or three at a time In drawing, makes stroke imitatively Manages spoon without rotation
24 Months		
Head circumference 49-50 cm (19.5-20 inches) Chest circumference exceeds head circumference. Lateral diameter of chest exceeds anteroposterior diameter. Usual weight gain of 1.8-2.7 kg (4-6 pounds) Usual gain in height of 10-12.5 cm (4-5 inches) Adult height approximately double height at 2 years May have achieved readiness for beginning daytime control of bowel and bladder Primary dentition of 16 teeth	Goes up and down stairs alone with 2 feet on each step Runs fairly well, with wide stance Picks up object without falling Kicks ball forward without overbalancing	Builds tower of six or seven cubes Aligns two or more cubes like a train Turns pages of book one at a time In drawing, imitates vertical and circular strokes Turns doorknob, unscrews lid
30 Months		
Birth weight quadrupled Primary dentition (20 teeth) completed May have daytime bowel and bladder control	Jumps with both feet Jumps from chair or step Stands on one foot momentarily Takes a few steps on tiptoe	Builds tower of eight cubes Adds chimney to train of cubes Good hand-finger coordination; holds crayon with fingers rather than fist Moves fingers independently In drawing, imitates vertical and horizontal strokes, makes two or more strokes for cross

Sensory	Vocalization	Socialization
Able to identify geometric forms; places round object into appropriate hole Binocular vision well developed Displays an intense and prolonged interest in pictures	Uses expressive jargon Says four to six words, including names Asks for objects by pointing Understands simple commands May use head-shaking gesture to denote "no" Uses "no" even while agreeing to the request	Tolerates some separation from parent Less likely to fear strangers Beginning to imitate parents, such as cleaning house (sweeping, dusting), folding clothes, mowing lawn Feeds self using covered cup with little spilling May discard bottle Manages spoon but rotates it near mouth Kisses and hugs parents, may kiss pictures in a book Expressive of emotions, has temper tantrums
	Says 10 or more words Points to a common object, such as shoe or ball, and to two or three body parts	Great imitator (domestic mimicry) Manages spoon well Takes off gloves, socks, and shoes and unzips Temper tantrums may be more evident Beginning awareness of ownership ("my toy") May develop dependency on transitional objects, such as security blanket
Accommodation well developed In geometric discrimination, able to insert square block into oblong space	Has vocabulary of approximately 300 words Uses two- to three-word phrases Uses pronouns "I," "me," "you" Understands directional commands Gives first name; refers to self by name Verbalizes need for toileting, food, or drink Talks incessantly	Stage of parallel play Has sustained attention span Temper tantrums decreasing Pulls people to show them something Increased independence from mother Dresses self in simple clothing
	Gives first and last names Refers to self by appropriate pronoun Uses plurals Names one color	Separates more easily from mother In play, helps put things away, can carry breakable objects, pushes with good steering Begins to note gender differences; knows own gender May attend to toilet needs without help except for wiping

Growth and Development During Preschool Years

Physical	Gross Motor	Fine Motor	Language
3 Years			
Usual weight gain of 1.8-2.7 kg (4-6 pounds) Average weight of 14.6 kg (32 pounds) Usual gain in height of 6.75-7.5 cm (2.5-3 inches) Average height of 95 cm (37.25 inches) May have achieved nighttime control of bowel and bladder	Rides tricycle Jumps off bottom step Stands on one foot for a few seconds Goes up stairs using alternate feet, may still come down using both feet on step Broad jumps May try to dance, but balance may not be adequate	Builds tower of nine or 10 cubes Builds bridge with three cubes Adeptly places small pellets in narrow-necked bottle In drawing, copies a circle, imitates a cross, names what has been drawn, cannot draw stick figure but may make circle with facial features	Has vocabulary of about 900 words Uses primarily "telegraphic" speech Uses complete sentences of three or four words Talks incessantly regardless of whether anyone is paying attention Repeats sentence of six syllables Asks many questions Begins to sing songs
4 Years			
Average weight of 16.7 kg (36.75 pounds) Average height of 103 cm (40.5 inches) Length at birth is doubled Maximum potential for development of amblyopia	Skips and hops on one foot Catches ball reliably Throws ball overhand Walks down stairs using alternate footing	Uses scissors successfully to cut out picture following outline Can lace shoes but may not be able to tie bow In drawing, copies a square, traces a cross and diamond, adds three parts to stick figure	Has vocabulary of 1500 words or more Uses sentences of four or five words Questioning is at peak Tells exaggerated stories Knows simple songs May be mildly profane if associates with older children Obeys prepositional phrases, such as "under," "on top of," "beside," "in back of," or "in front of" Names one or more colors Comprehends analogies, such as, "If ice is cold, fire is________"
5 Years			
Average weight of 18.7 kg (41.25 pounds) Average height of 110 cm (43.25 inches) Eruption of permanent dentition may begin Handedness is established (about 90% are right handed)	Skips and hops on alternate feet Throws and catches ball well Jumps rope Skates with good balance Walks backward with heel to toe Balances on alternate feet with eyes closed	Ties shoelaces Uses scissors, simple tools, or pencil very well In drawing, copies a diamond and triangle; adds seven to nine parts to stick figure; prints a few letters, numbers, or words, such as first name	Has vocabulary of about 2100 words Uses sentences of six to eight words, with all parts of speech Names coins (e.g., nickel, dime) Names four or more colors Describes drawing or comment and enumeration Knows names of days of week, months, and other time-associated words Knows composition of articles, such as, "A shoe is made of ____" Can follow three commands in succession

Socialization	Cognition	Family Relationships
Dresses self almost completely if helped with back buttons and told which shoe is right or left Has increased attention span Feeds self completely Can prepare simple meals, such as cold cereal and milk Can help set table; can dry dishes without breaking any May have fears, especially of dark and of going to bed Knows own gender and gender of others Play is parallel and associative; begins to learn simple games but often follows own rules; begins to share	Is in preconceptual phase Is egocentric in thought and behavior Has beginning understanding of time; uses many time-oriented expressions; talks about past and future as much as about present; pretends to tell time Has improved concept of space as demonstrated in understanding of prepositions and ability to follow directional command Has beginning ability to view concepts from another perspective	Attempts to please parents and conform to their expectations Is less jealous of younger sibling; may be opportune time for birth of additional sibling Is aware of family relationships and gender-role functions Boys tend to identify more with father or other male figure Has increased ability to separate easily and comfortably from parents for short periods
Very independent Tends to be selfish and impatient Aggressive physically as well as verbally Takes pride in accomplishments Has mood swings Shows off dramatically, enjoys entertaining others Tells family tales to others with no restraint Still has many fears Play is associative: Imaginary playmates are common Uses dramatic, imaginative, and imitative devices Sexual exploration and curiosity demonstrated through play, such as being "doctor" or "nurse"	Is in phase of intuitive thought Causality is still related to proximity of events Understands time better, especially in terms of sequence of daily events Judges everything according to one dimension, such as height, width, or order Immediate perceptual clues dominate judgment Is beginning to develop less egocentrism and more social awareness May count correctly but has poor mathematic concept of numbers Obeys because parents have set limits, not because of understanding of right and wrong	Rebels if parents expect too much, such as impeccable table manners Takes aggression and frustration out on parents or siblings Dos and don'ts become important May have rivalry with older or younger siblings; may resent older sibling's privileges and younger sibling's invasion of privacy and possessions May "run away" from home Identifies strongly with parent of opposite gender Is able to run simple errands outside the home
Less rebellious and quarrelsome than at age 4 years More settled and eager to get down to business Not as open and accessible in thoughts and behavior as in earlier years Independent but trustworthy; not foolhardy; more responsible Has fewer fears; relies on outer authority to control world Eager to do things right and to please; tries to "live by the rules" Has better manners Cares for self totally except for teeth, occasionally needs supervision in dress or hygiene Not ready for concentrated close work or small print because of slight farsightedness and still unrefined eye-hand coordination Play is associative; tries to follow rules but may cheat to avoid losing	Begins to question what parents think by comparing them with age-mates and other adults May note prejudice and bias in outside world Is more able to view another's perspective but tolerates differences rather than understanding them May begin to show understanding of conservation of numbers through counting objects regardless of arrangement Uses time-oriented words with increased understanding Very curious about factual information regarding world	Gets along well with parents May seek out parent more often than at age 4 years for reassurance and security, especially when entering school Begins to question parents' thinking and principles Strongly identifies with parent of same gender, especially boys with their fathers Enjoys activities such as sports, cooking, shopping with parent of same gender

Growth and Development During School-Age Years

Physical and Motor	Mental	Adaptive	Personal-Social
6 Years			
Growth and weight gain continue slowly Weight: 16-23.6 kg (35.5-53 pounds); height: 106.6-123.5 cm (42-48 inches) Central mandibular incisors erupt Loses first tooth Gradual increase in dexterity Active age; constant activity Often returns to finger feeding More aware of hand as a tool Likes to draw, print, and color Vision reaches maturity	Develops concept of numbers Counts 13 pennies Knows whether it is morning or afternoon Defines common objects such as fork and chair in terms of their use Obeys triple commands in succession Knows right and left hands Says which is pretty and which is ugly of a series of drawings of faces Describes the objects in a picture rather than simply enumerating them Attends first grade	At table, uses knife to spread butter or jam on bread At play, cuts, folds, and pastes paper toys, sews crudely if needle is threaded Takes bath without supervision; performs bedtime activities alone Reads from memory; enjoys oral spelling game Likes table games, checkers, simple card games Giggles a lot Sometimes steals money or attractive items Has difficulty owning up to misdeeds Tries out own abilities	Can share and cooperate better Has great need for children of own age Will cheat to win Often engages in rough play Often jealous of younger brother or sister Does what adults are seen doing May have occasional temper tantrums Is a boaster Is more independent, probably influence of school Has own way of doing things Increases socialization
7 Years			
Begins to grow at least 5 cm (2 inches) a year Weight: 17.7-30 kg (39-66.5 pounds); height: 111.8-129.7 cm (44-51 inches) Maxillary central incisors and lateral mandibular incisors erupt Jaw begins to expand to accommodate permanent teeth More cautious in approaches to new performances Repeats performances to master them	Notes that certain parts are missing from pictures Can copy a diamond Repeats three numbers backward Develops concept of time; reads ordinary clock or watch correctly to nearest quarter hour; uses clock for practical purposes Attends second grade More mechanical in reading; often does not stop at the end of a sentence, skips words such as "it," "the," and "he"	Uses table knife for cutting meat; may need help with tough or difficult pieces Brushes and combs hair acceptably without help May steal Likes to help and have a choice Is less resistant and stubborn	Is becoming a real member of the family group Takes part in group play Boys prefer playing with boys; girls prefer playing with girls Spends a lot of time alone; does not require a lot of companionship
8 to 9 Years			
Continues to grow at least 5 cm (2 inches) a year Weight: 19.6-39.6 kg (43-87 pounds); height: 117-141.8 cm (46-56 inches) Lateral incisors (maxillary) and mandibular cuspids erupt Movement fluid, often graceful and poised Always on the go; jumps, chases, skips	Gives similarities and differences between two things from memory Counts backward from 20 to 1; understands concept of reversibility Repeats days of the week and months in order; knows the date Describes common objects in detail, not merely their use	Makes use of common tools such as hammer, saw, or screwdriver Uses household and sewing utensils Helps with routine household tasks such as dusting, sweeping Assumes responsibility for share of household chores Looks after all of own needs at table	Is easy to get along with at home Likes the reward system Dramatizes Is more sociable Is better behaved Is interested in boy-girl relationships but will not admit it Goes about home and community freely, alone, or with friends

Growth and Development During School-Age Years—cont'd

Physical and Motor	Mental	Adaptive	Personal-Social
8 to 9 Years—cont'd			
Increased smoothness and speed in fine motor control; uses cursive writing Dresses self completely Likely to overdo; hard to quiet down after recess More limber; bones grow faster than ligaments	Makes change out of a quarter Attends third and fourth grades Reads more; may plan to wake up early just to read Reads classic books but also enjoys comics More aware of time; can be relied on to get to school on time Can grasp concepts of parts and whole (fractions) Understands concepts of space, cause and effect, nesting (puzzles), conservation (permanence of mass and volume) Classifies objects by more than one quality; has collections Produces simple paintings or drawings	Buys useful articles; exercises some choice in making purchases Runs useful errands Likes pictorial magazines Likes school; wants to answer all the questions Is afraid of failing a grade; is ashamed of bad grades Is more critical of self Takes music and sport lessons	Likes to compete and play games Shows preference in friends and groups Plays mostly with groups of own gender but is beginning to mix Develops modesty Compares self with others Enjoys Scouts, group sports
10 to 12 Years			
Boys: Slow growth in height and rapid weight gain; may become obese in this period *Girls:* Pubescent changes may begin to appear; body lines soften and round out Weight: 24.3-58 kg (54-128 pounds); height: 127.5-162.3 cm (50-64 inches) Posture is more similar to an adult's; will overcome lordosis Remainder of teeth will erupt and tend toward full development (except wisdom teeth)	Writes brief stories Attends fifth to seventh grades Writes occasional short letters to friends or relatives on own initiative Uses telephone for practical purposes Responds to magazine, radio, or other advertising Reads for practical information or own enjoyment—Stories or library books of adventure or romance, or animal stories	Makes useful articles or does easy repair work Cooks or sews in small way Raises pets Washes and dries own hair Is responsible for a thorough job of cleaning hair but may need reminding to do so Is sometimes left alone at home for an hour or so Is successful in looking after own needs or those of other children left in his or her care	Loves friends; talks about them constantly Chooses friends more selectively; may have a best friend Enjoys conversation Develops beginning interest in opposite gender Is more diplomatic Likes family; family really has meaning Likes mother and wants to please her in many ways Demonstrates affection Likes father, who is adored and idolized Respects parents

Growth and Development During Adolescence

Early Adolescence (11-14 years)	Middle Adolescence (14-17 years)	Late Adolescence (17-20 years)
Growth		
Rapidly accelerating growth Reaches peak velocity Secondary sex characteristics appear	Growth decelerating in girls Stature reaches 95% of adult height Secondary sex characteristics well advanced	Physically mature Structure and reproductive growth almost complete
Cognition		
Explores newfound ability for limited abstract thought Clumsy groping for new values and energies Comparison of "normality" with peers of same gender	Developing capacity for abstract thinking Enjoys intellectual powers, often in idealistic terms Concern with philosophic, political, and social problems	Established abstract thought Can perceive and act on long-range operations Able to view problems comprehensively Intellectual and functional identity established
Identity		
Preoccupied with rapid bodily changes Trying out of various roles Measurement of attractiveness by acceptance or rejection of peers Conformity to group norms	Modifies bodily image Very self-centered; increased narcissism Tendency toward inner experience and self-discovery Has a rich fantasy life Idealistic Able to perceive future implications of current behavior and decisions; variable application	Bodily image and gender role definition nearly secured Mature sexual identity Phase of consolidation of identity Stability of self-esteem Comfortable with physical growth Social roles defined and articulated
Relationships with Parents		
Defining independence-dependence boundaries Strong desire to remain dependent on parents while trying to detach No major conflicts over parental control	Major conflicts over independence and control Low point in parent-child relationship Greatest push for emancipation; disengagement Final and irreversible emotional detachment from parents; mourning	Emotional and physical separation from parents completed Independence from family with less conflict Emancipation nearly secured
Relationships with Peers		
Seeks peer affiliations to counter instability generated by rapid change Upsurge of close idealized friendships with members of the same gender Struggle for mastery takes place within peer group	Strong need for identity to affirm self-image Behavioral standards set by peer group Acceptance by peers extremely important—Fear of rejection Exploration of ability to attract the opposite gender	Peer group recedes in importance in favor of individual friendship Testing of male-female relationships against possibility of permanent alliance Relationships characterized by giving and sharing

Growth and Development During Adolescence—cont'd

Early Adolescence (11-14 years)	Middle Adolescence (14-17 years)	Late Adolescence (17-20 years)
Sexuality		
Self-exploration and evaluation Limited dating, usually group Limited intimacy	Multiple plural relationships Decisive turn toward heterosexuality (if homosexual, knows by this time) Exploration of "self appeal" Feeling of "being in love" Tentative establishment of relationships	Forms stable relationships and attachment to another Growing capacity for mutuality and reciprocity Dating as a male-female pair Intimacy involves commitment rather than exploration and romanticism
Psychologic Health		
Wide mood swings Intense daydreaming Anger outwardly expressed with moodiness, temper outbursts, and verbal insults and name calling	Tendency toward inner experiences; more introspective Tendency to withdraw when upset or feelings are hurt Vacillation of emotions in time and range Feelings of inadequacy common; difficulty in asking for help	More constancy of emotion Anger more apt to be concealed

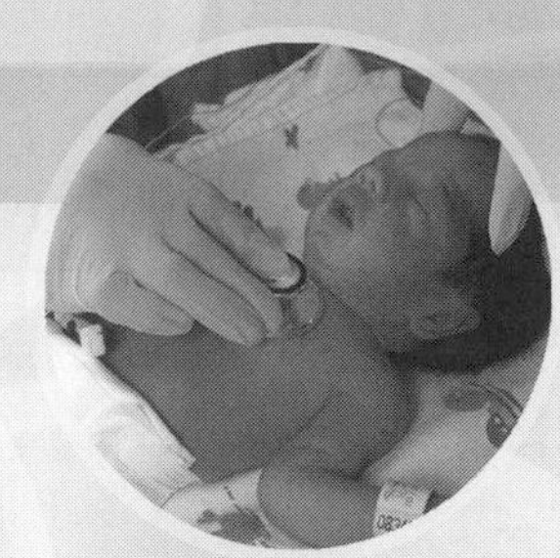

Health Promotion

RELATED TOPICS

Atraumatic care: Injections, 285
Nutritional assessment, 129
Patient and family education: Applying a topical anesthetic, 546-548
Play during hospitalization, 255
Preparing children for procedures based on developmental characteristics, 253
Procedures related to administration of medications, 282
Sleep assessment, 139

Symbol ▶ indicates material that may be photocopied and distributed to families.

Recommendations for Child Preventive Care

CHILD PREVENTIVE CARE TIMELINE

Clinical Preventive Services for Normal-Risk Children

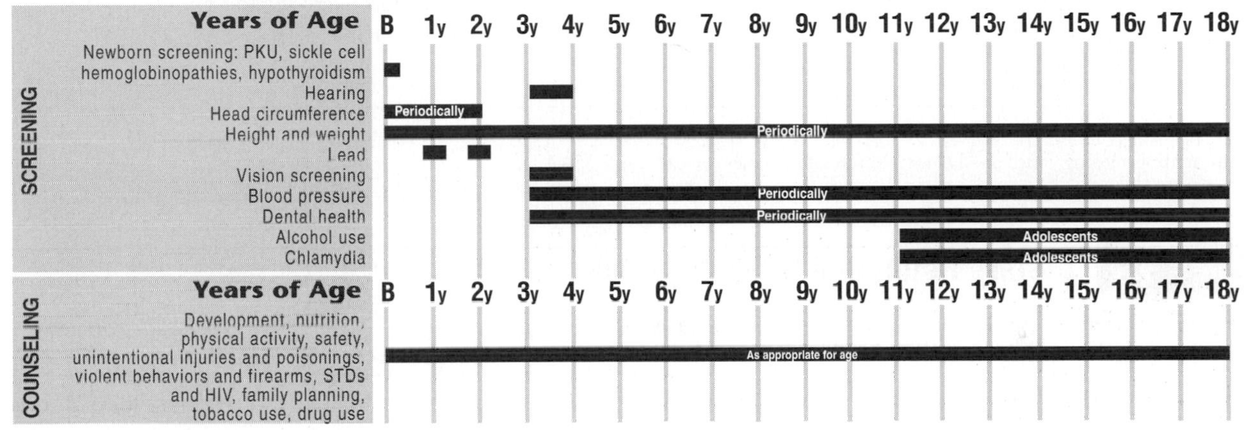

*For immunization schedules, see pp. 213-214.

The information on immunizations is based on recommendations issued by the Advisory Committee on Immunization Practices, the American Academy of Pediatrics, and the American Academy of Family Physicians.

Nutrition

Dietary Reference Intakes

The Institute of Medicine (IOM) has developed guidelines for nutritional intake that encompass the Recommended Dietary Allowances (RDAs) yet extend their scope to include additional parameters related to nutritional intake. The Dietary Reference Intakes (DRIs)* are composed of four categories. These include estimated average requirements (EARs) for age and gender categories, tolerable upper-limit (UL) nutrient intakes that are associated with a low risk of adverse effects, adequate intakes (AIs) of nutrients, and new standard RDAs. The new guidelines present information about lifestyle factors that may affect nutrient function, such as caffeine intake and exercise, and about how the nutrient may be related to chronic disease. See Table 2-1.

*For information on the DRIs go to IOM website: *http://www.iom.edu.* At this site either use the site's search engine for DRIs or go to the IOM site map: Ongoing Studies—Dietary Reference Intakes, or call (202) 334-1732.

TABLE 2-1 Dietary Reference Intakes (DRIs)

DRI Populations and Life Stage Groups	Recommended Dietary Allowance (RDA)	Estimated Average Requirements (EARS)	Adequate Intake (AI)	Tolerable Upper Intake Level (UL)
• Pregnancy and lactation • Birth to 6 months • 7-12 mo • 1-3 yr • 4-8 yr • 9-13 yr • 14-18 yr • 19-30 yr • 31-50 yr • 51-70 yr • >70 yr	Average daily dietary intake level sufficient to meet the nutrient requirement of most healthy individuals in a given gender group or life stage. May be used to evaluate nutrient intake of a given population—e.g., vegetarian.	Daily nutrient intake value estimated to meet the requirement of half the healthy persons in a given life stage or gender group (used to assess dietary adequacy and is the basis for RDAs).	Recommended intake value based on observed or experimentally determined approximations of nutrient intake by a group of healthy persons, which are assumed to be adequate when an RDA cannot be determined. In healthy breastfed infants (0-6 mo) AI is the mean intake.	Highest level of daily nutrient intake likely to pose no risk of adverse effects for most individuals in the general population. Risk increases as intake above the UL increases. May be used to set limits on nutrient supplementation, especially for vitamins and minerals that could be harmful.
Clinical Applications				
Folate				
• Pregnant 19- to 30-year-old women	600 mcg/d	520 mcg/d	400 mcg/d*	1000 mcg/d
Iron				
• 4- to 8-year-old boy	10 mg/d	4.1 mg/d	10 mg/d	40 mg/d
Vitamin C				
• 16-year-old girl	65 mg/d	56 mg/d	65 mg/d	1800 mg/d

Portions adapted from *Dietary Reference Intakes (DRIs):* Food and Nutrition Board, Institute of Medicine, National Academy of Sciences, 2004, *http://www.nap.edu; Dietary Reference Intakes: An Update,* International Food Information Council Foundation, 2005, *http://ific.org.*
See also Unit 1 for select DRI values.
*Women of childbearing age and with expectation of becoming pregnant should consume 400 mcg/d from supplements or fortified foods, or both, in addition to intake of folate from a varied diet.

Dietary Guidelines for Children (American Heart Association)

The American Heart Association dietary guidelines (Table 2-2). may also be used to encourage healthy dietary intakes designed to decrease obesity and cardiovascular risk factors and subsequent cardiovascular disease, which is now known to occur in young children as well as adults.

MyPyramid for Kids

MyPyramid, developed by the U.S. Department of Agriculture, replaces the Food Guide Pyramid as a guide for adult and childhood nutrition. This interactive dietary guide aims to simplify food choices designed to decrease fat and empty calorie intake and increase consumption of grains and vegetables. MyPyramid for Kids incorporates examples of exercise for children as well as suggested serving sizes. The Internet version of MyPyramid for Kids *(http://www.mypyramid.gov)* offers an interactive game for children (Blast Off). See also Figure 2-1.

TABLE 2-2 Daily Estimated Calories and Recommended Servings for Grains, Fruits, Vegetables, and Dairy Products by Age and Gender

	1 year	2-3 years	4-8 years	9-13 years	14-18 years
Kilocalories*					
Female	900 kcal	1000 kcal	1200 kcal	1600 kcal	1800 kcal
Male	900 kcal	1000 kcal	1400 kcal	1800 kcal	2200 kcal
Fat (% of total kcal)	30%-40%	30%-35%	25%-35%	25%-35%	25%-35%
Milk or dairy†	2 cups‡	2 cups	2 cups	3 cups	3 cups
Lean meat or beans					
Female	1½ oz	2 oz	3 oz	5 oz	5 oz
Male	1½ oz	2 oz	4 oz	5 oz	6 oz
Fruits§					
Female	1 cup	1 cup	1½ cups	1½ cups	1½ cups
Male	1 cup	1 cup	1½ cups	1½ cups	2 cups
Vegetables§					
Female	¾ cup	1 cup	1 cup	2 cups	2½ cups
Male	¾ cup	1 cup	1½ cups	2½ cups	3 cups
Grains¶					
Female	2 oz	3 oz	4 oz	5 oz	6 oz
Male	2 oz	3 oz	5 oz	6 oz	7 oz

Data from American Heart Association, *http://www.americanheart.org/presenter.jhtml?identifier53033999;* and American Heart Association, Giddings SS, Dennison BA, and others: Dietary recommendations for children and adolescents: a guide for practitioners, *Pediatrics* 117(2):544-559, 2006.

Estimates are based on sedentary lifestyle. Increased physical activity requires additional calories by 0-200 kcal/day for moderately active children and 200-400 kcal/day for very physically active children.

*For children 2 years and older. Nutrient and energy contributions from each group are calculated according to the nutrient-dense forms of food in each group (e.g., lean meats and fat-free milk).

†Milk listed is fat-free except for children <2 years of age. If 1%, 2%, or whole-fat milk is substituted, this will use, for each cup, 19, 39, or 63 kcal of discretionary calories and add 2.6, 5.1, or 9 g of fat, of which 1.3, 2.6, or 4.6 g are saturated fat.

‡For 1-year-old children, calculations are based on 2%-fat milk. If 2 cups of whole milk are substituted, 48 kcal of discretionary calories will be used. The American Academy of Pediatrics recommends that low-fat or reduced fat milk not be started before 2 years of age.

§Serving sizes are ¼ cup for age 1 year, ⅓ cup for 2-3 years of age, and ½ cup for ≥4 years of age. A variety of vegetables should be selected from each subgroup over the week.

¶Half of all grains should be whole grains.

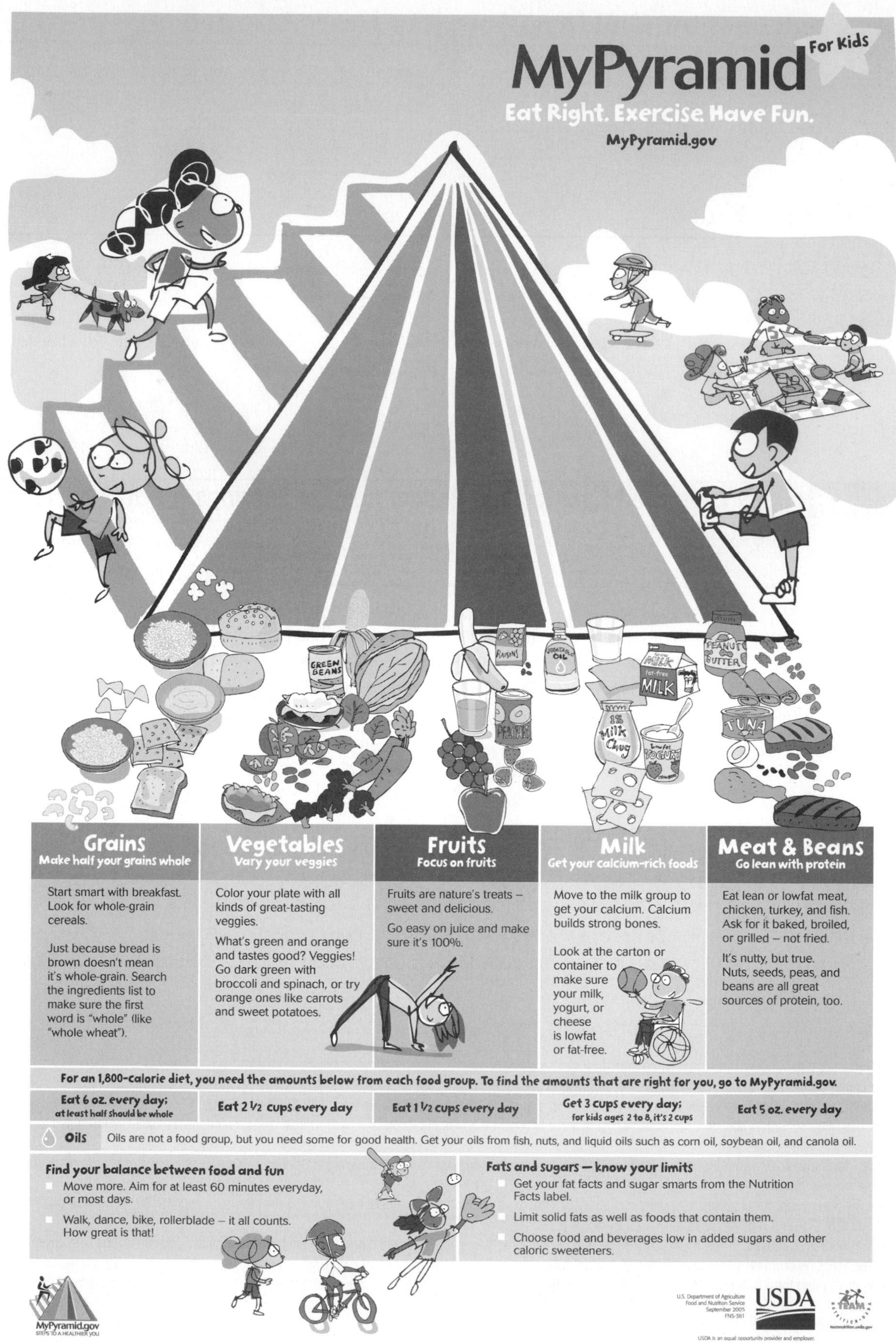

FIGURE **2-1** MyPyramid for Kids. (From Food and Nutrition Service, U.S. Department of Agriculture: *MyPyramid for kids* (FNS-381), Washington, DC, September 2005, The Service, available online at *http://www.mypyramid.gov.*)

COMMUNITY FOCUS

Fluoride Supplementation*

Age	Fluoride Concentration in Local Water Supply (in ppm)		
	<0.3	0.3-0.6	>0.6
Birth to 6 mo	0	0	0
6 mo to 3 yr	0.25†	0	0
3 to 6 yr	0.50	0.25	0
6 to at least 16 yr	1	0.50	0

From American Academy of Pediatric Dentistry: *Reference manual 2005-2006: guideline on fluoride therapy,* Chicago, 2003, The Academy, p 90, retrieved July 12, 2007, from *http://www.aapd.org/media/Policies_Guidelines/G_FluorideTherapy.pdf.*

*Must know fluoride concentration in patient's drinking water before prescribing fluoride supplements.

†All values are milligrams of fluoride supplement per day.

COMMUNITY FOCUS

Nutrition: Iron Absorption

To ensure that children receive an adequate supply of iron from foods, consider the following factors that may increase or decrease iron absorption.

Increase

Acidity (low pH)—Administer iron between meals (gastric hydrochloric acid)
Ascorbic acid (vitamin C)—Administer iron with juice, fruit, or multivitamin preparation
Vitamin A
Calcium
Tissue need
Meat, fish, poultry
Cooking in cast iron pots

Decrease

Alkalinity (high pH)—Avoid antacid preparations.
Phosphates—Milk is unfavorable vehicle for iron administration.
Phytates—Found in cereals
Oxalates—Found in many fruits and vegetables (plums, currants, green beans, spinach, sweet potatoes, tomatoes)
Tannins—Found in tea, coffee
Tissue saturation
Malabsorptive disorders
Disturbances that cause diarrhea or steatorrhea
Infection

Normal and Special Infant and Child Formulas*

Formula (Manufacturer)	Protein Source	Carbohydrate Source	Fat Sources	Indications for Use	Comments (Nutritional Considerations)
Human and Cow's Milk Formulas					
Human breast milk	Mature human milk; whey/casein ratio—60:40	Lactose	Mature human milk	For all full-term infants except those with galactosemia; may also be used for low-birth-weight infants	Recommended sole form of feeding for first 12 months; nutritionally complete; supplement with 200 IU vitamin D daily unless consuming at least 500 ml of vitamin D–fortified milk
Evaporated cow's milk formulas	Milk protein; whey/casein ratio—18:82	Lactose, sucrose	Butterfat	For full-term infants with no special nutritional requirements	Supplement with iron and vitamin C; A and D if not fortified; fluoride if fluoridated water is not used for formula preparation (after 6 months)
Commercial Infant Formulas					
Enfamil Gentlease Lipil (Mead Johnson)	Whey/casein ratio—60:40	Corn syrup, ¼ carbohydrates from lactose	Palm, soy, coconut, high-oleic safflower oils	For full-term infants with gas or fussiness	Contains DHA and ARA†; iron fortified; reduced lactose
Similac (Ross)	Nonfat cow's milk; whey/casein ratio—48:52	Lactose	Soy, coconut, high-oleic safflower oils	For full-term and premature infants with no special nutritional requirements	Available fortified with iron, 1.8 mg/100 cal, nucleotides, 72 mg/L Also available in 22 and 24 cal/oz with iron
Good Start Supreme (Nestlé) and Good Start Supreme DHA & ARA	Hydrolyzed whey	Lactose, maltodextrin	Palm olein, soy, safflower, coconut oils	For full-term infants	Lower osmolality; lower protein, calcium, sodium, vitamin E; may be less expensive than other brand-name formulas; contains DHA and ARA†
Similac Neosure Advance (with iron) (Ross)	Nonfat cow's milk; whey/casein ratio—50:50	Corn syrup and lactose	MCT oils	Preterm infants, 22 cal/oz	Protein, 2.6 g/100 cal Phosphorus, 62 mg/100 cal Calcium, 105 mg/100 cal; contains DHA and ARA†
Enfamil AR Lipil (Mead Johnson)	Nonfat milk; demineralized whey	Lactose, rice starch, maltodextrin	Palm olein, soy, coconut, HOSun oils	Mild gastroesophageal reflux	Iron fortified; contains DHA and ARA†

Major formula companies such as Ross and Mead Johnson have a variety of formulas containing 22, 24, and 30 cal/oz, with high- or low-iron concentrations intended for use in preterm infants. In addition, major retail companies manufacture their own brands of full-term infant formulas that comply with the Food and Drug Administration guidelines for infant formula composition. This list is not an exhaustive list of all infant and child formula.

HOSun, High-oleic sunflower; *MCT*, medium-chain triglyceride.

*All formulas provide 20 kcal/oz except as noted in product information from the formula manufacturers. For the most current information, consult product labels or package enclosures.

†DHA and ARA are important in development of brain and eyes.

Normal and Special Infant and Child Formulas—cont'd

Formula (Manufacturer)	Protein Source	Carbohydrate Source	Fat Sources	Indications for Use	Comments (Nutritional Considerations)
Commercial Infant Formulas—cont'd					
Enfamil Lipil with Iron (Mead Johnson)	Whey, nonfat cow's milk	Lactose	Palm olein, soy, coconut, HOSun, *Mortierella alpina,* and *Crypthecodinum cohnii* oils	For full-term infants	Iron fortified; contains DHA and ARA† Available fortified with iron, 12 mg/L Also available in 22 and 24 cal/oz
Similac Advance and Similac Advance 2 (Ross)	Whey protein concentrate	Lactose	High oleic safflower, soy, coconut oils	For full-term infants	Contains DHA and ARA†; iron fortified Advance 2 is for children 9-24 months old
Enfamil Prosobee Lipil (Mead Johnson)	Soy protein isolate	Corn syrup solids	Palm, soy, coconut, HOSun oils	With milk protein allergy, lactose intolerance, lactase deficiency, galactosemia	Hypoallergenic, zero band antigen; lactose and sucrose free; contains DHA and ARA†
Enfamil Next Step Prosobee Lipil (Mead Johnson)	Soy Protein	Corn syrup solids	Palm, coconut, sunflower oils	For children 9-24 months	Contains DHA and ARA†
Enfamil EnfaCare Lipil (Mead Johnson)	Nonfat cow's milk; whey/casein ratio—60:40	Lactose and corn syrup solids (powder); maltodextrin and corn syrup solids (liquid)	MCT, coconut, soy, high-oleic vegetable oils	Preterm infants, 22 cal/oz	Contains DHA and ARA†; iron fortified
Similac Special Care Advance 20 and 24 (Ross)	Nonfat cow's milk and whey concentrate	Corn syrup solids and lactose	Soy, coconut, MCT oils	Preterm infants, 20 and 24 cal/oz	Contains DHA and ARA†; iron fortified; available in low-iron form
Enfamil Premature Lipil (Mead Johnson)	Nonfat cow's milk; whey/casein ratio—60:40	Corn syrup, lactose	MCT, soy, and high-oleic vegetable oils	Preterm infants, 20 and 24 cal/oz	Contains DHA and ARA†; low iron and iron fortified
Similac Isomil (Ross)	Soy protein isolate	Corn syrup, sucrose	Soy, coconut oils	With milk protein allergy, lactose intolerance, lactase deficiency, galactosemia	Hypoallergenic; lactose-free
Similac Isomil Advance and Isomil 2 Advance (Ross)	Soy protein isolate, L-methionine	Corn syrup, sucrose	Soy, oleic, coconut oils	For full-term infants; infants with gas, fussiness; spitting up; non–milk-based formula	Contains DHA, ARA†; lactose-free Advance 2 is for children 9-24 months old

Continued

Normal and Special Infant and Child Formulas—cont'd

Formula (Manufacturer)	Protein Source	Carbohydrate Source	Fat Sources	Indications for Use	Comments (Nutritional Considerations)
Commercial Infant Formulas—cont'd					
Similac Isomil DF (Ross)	Soy protein isolate	Corn syrup and sucrose	Soy, coconut oils	For use with antibiotic-induced diarrhea in infants >6 months and toddlers	Lessens amount and duration of watery stools; contains fiber; lactose-free
Enfamil Lacto-Free Lipil (Mead Johnson)	Milk protein isolate	Corn syrup solids	Palm olein, soy, HOSun oils	With lactose intolerance, lactase deficiency, galactosemia	Lactose-free; contains DHA and ARA†
Similac Lactose Free Advance (Ross)	Milk isolate	Sucrose, glucose oligomers	Soy, coconut oils	With lactose malabsorption	Iron fortified; contains DHA and ARA†
For Infants and Toddlers with Malabsorption Syndromes, Milk Allergy (Hydrolysate Formulas)					
RCF (Ross Carbohydrate Free) (Ross)	Soy protein isolate		Soy, coconut oils	With carbohydrate intolerance	Carbohydrate added according to amount infant will tolerate
Portagen (Mead Johnson)	Sodium caseinate	Corn syrup solids, sucrose, lactose	MCT (coconut source), corn oil	For impaired fat absorption secondary to pancreatic insufficiency, bile acid deficiency, intestinal resection, lymphatic anomalies	Nutritionally complete
Nutramigen Lipil (Mead Johnson)	Casein hydrolysate, L-amino acids‡	Corn syrup solids, modified corn starch	Corn, soy oils	For infants and children sensitive to food proteins; use in galactosemic patients	Nutritionally complete; hypoallergenic formula; lactose- and sucrose-free; contains DHA and ARA†
Pregestimil Lipil (Mead Johnson)	Casein hydrolysate, L-amino acids‡	Corn syrup solids, modified corn starch, dextrose	MCT, soy, HOSun oils	Disaccharidase deficiencies, malabsorption syndromes, cystic fibrosis, intestinal resection	Nutritionally complete; easily digestible protein, carbohydrate, and fat; lactose- and sucrose-free; contains DHA and ARA†
Similac Alimentum Advance (Ross)	Casein hydrolysate, L-amino acids‡	Sucrose, modified tapioca starch	Safflower, MCT, oleic soy oils	For colicky infants with protein sensitivity or infants with protein or fat maldigestion (cystic fibrosis)	Nutritionally complete; contains DHA and ARA†; iron fortified; lactose free; hypoallergenic formula

†DHA and ARA are important in development of brain and eyes.

‡L-Amino acids include L-cystine, L-tyrosine, and L-tryptophan, which are reduced in hydrolyzed, charcoal-treated casein.

Normal and Special Infant and Child Formulas—cont'd

Formula (Manufacturer)	Protein Source	Carbohydrate Source	Fat Sources	Indications for Use	Comments (Nutritional Considerations)
Specialty Formulas					
Neocate§	Free amino acids	Corn syrup solids	MCT, safflower oils	For infants sensitive to cow's milk, soy, and hydrolyzed protein formulas	Nutritionally complete; lactose-free; high osmolality; low-fat
Similac PM 60/40 (Ross)	Whey protein concentrate, sodium caseinate (60:40 ratio)	Lactose	Coconut, corn oils	For newborns predisposed to hypocalcemia and infants with impaired renal, digestive, and cardiovascular functions	Low calcium, potassium, and phosphorus; relatively low solute load; Na = 7 mEq/L; available in powder only
Diet Modifiers					
Polycose (Ross)		Glucose polymers (corn syrup solids)		Used to increase calorie intake, as in failure-to-thrive infants	Carbohydrate only; a powdered or liquid calorie supplement; powder: 23 kcal/tbsp
MCT Oil‖	Contains no protein	Contains no carbohydrate	90% MCT (coconut source)	Supplement in fat malabsorption conditions	Fat only: 8.3 kcal/g; 115 kcal/tbsp May be suitable for gluten-free diet
Similac Natural Care Advance (Ross)	Nonfat cow's milk; whey protein concentrate	Hydrolyzed cornstarch, lactose	MCT, coconut, soy oils	For low-birth-weight infants; fed mixed with human milk or fed alternately with human milk; improves vitamin and mineral content of human milk	Protein—2.7 g/100 cal; osmolality—300 mOsm/kg water, 24 cal/oz; low iron; liquid not intended as sole source of nutrients
Similac Human Milk Fortifier (Ross)	Whey protein, nonfat dry milk	Corn syrup solids	MCT oil	For breast milk fortification in preterm infants	Fortification in excess of one package per 25 ml human milk is not recommended
Enfamil Human Milk Fortifier (Mead Johnson)	Whey protein concentrate, casein	Corn syrup solids, lactose	Trace	For low-birth-weight infants; fed mixed with human milk; increases protein, calories, calcium, phosphorus, and other nutrients	Used only as human milk fortifier, not as separate formula Has added iron to reduce need for iron supplementation

§Scientific Hospital Supplies, Gaithersburg, Md.
‖Novartis Medical Nutrition, Fremont, Mich.

Continued

Normal and Special Infant and Child Formulas—cont'd

Formula (Manufacturer)	Protein Source	Carbohydrate Source	Fat Sources	Indications for Use	Comments (Nutritional Considerations)
For Infants and Children with Phenylketonuria¶					
Phenyl-free 1 (Mead Johnson)	Casein hydrolysate, L-amino acids‡	Corn syrup solids, modified tapioca starch	Corn oil	For infants and children	111 mg phenylalanine per quart of formula (20 cal/oz); must be supplemented with other foods to provide minimal phenylalanine
Phenyl-free 2 (Mead Johnson)	L-Amino acids‡	Sucrose, corn syrup solids, modified tapioca starch	Corn, coconut oils	For children over 1 year of age	Phenylalanine-free; permits increased supplementation with normal foods; lactose-free
Phenyl-free 2 HP (Mead Johnson)	L-Amino acids‡	Corn syrup, sugar, modified corn starch	Soy	For women with maternal PKU and older children who require fewer calories than Phenyl-free 2	Lactose-free; gluten-free
Phenex-1 (Ross)	L-Amino acids‡	Hydrolyzed cornstarch	Soy, coconut, palm oils	For infants	Phenylalanine-free; fortified with L-tyrosine, L-glutamine, L-carnitine, taurine; contains vitamins, minerals, trace elements
Phenex-2 (Ross)	L-Amino acids‡	Hydrolyzed cornstarch	Soy, coconut, palm oils	For children and adults	Phenylalanine-free; fortified with L-tyrosine, L-glutamine, L-carnitine, taurine; contains vitamins, minerals, trace elements
Pro-Phree (Ross)	None	Hydrolyzed cornstarch	Soy, coconut, palm oils	For infants and toddlers requiring reduced protein intake	Must be supplemented with protein; has vitamins, minerals, trace elements; L-carnitine and taurine

¶Ross Laboratories and Mead Johnson manufacture several specialty formulas for metabolic disorders for infants and children. For a comprehensive list of metabolic disease formulas the reader should contact either Ross Laboratories or Mead Johnson.

Guidelines for Feeding During the First Year

BIRTH TO 6 MONTHS (BREAST- OR BOTTLE-FEEDING)

Breast-Feeding

Most desirable complete diet for first half-year*

May require supplements of fluoride (0.25 mg) after 6 months of age

May require iron by 4 to 6 months of age

Requires supplements of vitamin D (200 International units/day) beginning during the first 2 months

Formula

Iron-fortified commercial formula is a complete food for the first half-year.*

Requires fluoride supplements (0.25 mg) after 6 months of age when the concentration of fluoride in the drinking water is below 0.3 parts per million (ppm)

Evaporated milk formula requires supplements of vitamin C, iron, and fluoride (in accordance with the fluoride content of the local water supply) after child is 6 months of age.

SIX TO 12 MONTHS (SOLID FOODS)

May begin to add solids by 4 to 6 months of age

First foods are strained, pureed, or finely mashed.

Finger foods such as teething crackers, raw fruit, or vegetables can be introduced by 6 to 7 months.

Chopped table food or commercially prepared junior foods can be started by 9 to 12 months.

With the exception of cereal, the order of introducing foods is variable; a recommended sequence is weekly introduction of other foods, beginning with vegetables, then fruits, and then meat.

As the quantity of solids increases, the amount of formula should be limited to approximately 900 ml (30 ounces) daily and fruit juice to less than 120 ml (4 ounces) daily.

Method of Introduction

Introduce solids when infant is hungry.

Begin spoon-feeding by pushing food to back of tongue because of infant's natural tendency to thrust tongue forward.

Use small spoon with straight handle; begin with 1 or 2 teaspoons of food; gradually increase to 2 to 3 tablespoons per feeding.

Introduce one food at a time, usually at intervals of 4 to 7 days, to identify food allergies.

As the amount of solid food increases, decrease the quantity of milk to prevent overfeeding.

Never introduce foods by mixing them with the formula in the bottle.

Cereal

Introduce commercially prepared, iron-fortified infant cereals, and give daily until 18 months of age.

Rice cereal usually introduced first because of its low allergenic potential

Can discontinue supplemental iron once iron-fortified cereal is given

Fruits and Vegetables

Applesauce, bananas, and pears are usually well tolerated.

Avoid fruits and vegetables marketed in cans that are not specifically designed for infants because of variable and sometimes high lead content and addition of salt, sugar, and/or preservatives.

Offer fruit juice only from a cup, not a bottle, to reduce the development of "nursing caries." Limit fruit juice to no more than 4 to 6 oz daily.

Meat, Fish, and Poultry

Avoid fatty meats.

Prepare meats by baking, broiling, steaming, or poaching.

Include organ meats such as liver, which has a high iron, vitamin A, and vitamin B complex content.

If soup is given, be sure all ingredients are familiar to child's diet.

Avoid commercial meat and vegetable combinations because protein is low.

Eggs and Cheese

Serve egg yolk hard boiled and mashed, soft cooked, or poached.

Introduce egg white in small quantities (1 teaspoon) after the first year of age to detect an allergy.

Use cheese as a substitute for meat and as a finger food.

---

*Breast-feeding or commercial formula-feeding is recommended up to 12 months of age. After 1 year, whole cow's milk can be given.

This section may be photocopied and distributed to families.

Source: Wilson D, Hockenberry MJ: *Wong's clinical manual of pediatric nursing,* ed 7. Copyright © 2008, Mosby, St Louis.

Developmental Milestones Associated with Feeding

Age (Months)	Development
Birth	Has sucking, rooting, and swallowing reflexes
	Feels hunger and indicates desire for food by crying; expresses satiety by falling asleep
1	Has strong extrusion reflex
3-4	Extrusion reflex fading
	Begins to develop hand-eye coordination
4-5	Can approximate lips to the rim of a cup
5-6	Can use fingers to feed self a cracker
6-7	Chews and bites
	May hold own bottle but may not drink from it (prefers for it to be held)
7-9	Refuses food by keeping lips closed; has taste preferences
	Holds a spoon and plays with it during feeding
	May drink from a straw
	Drinks from a cup with assistance
9-12	Picks up small morsels of food (finger foods) and feeds self
	Holds own bottle and drinks from it
	Drinks from a household cup without assistance but spills some
	Uses a spoon with much spilling
12-18	Drools less
	Drinks well from a household cup but may drop it when finished
	Holds cup with both hands
	Begins to use a spoon but turns it before reaching mouth
24	Can use a straw
	Chews food with mouth closed and shifts food in mouth
	Distinguishes between finger and spoon foods
	Holds small glass in one hand; replaces glass without dropping
	Uses spoon correctly but with some spilling
36	Spills small amount from spoon
	Begins to use fork; holds it in fist
	Uses adult pattern of chewing, which involves rotary action of jaw
48	Rarely spills when using spoon
	Serves self finger foods
	Eats with fork; held with fingers
54	Uses fork in preference to spoon
72	Spreads with knife
84	Cuts tender food with knife

Immunizations

Licensed Vaccines and Toxoids Available in the United States and Recommended Routes of Administration

Vaccine[a]	Route
Adenovirus[b]	Oral
Anthrax[b]	Subcutaneous
Bacillus of Calmette and Guérin (BCG)	Intradermal or subcutaneous
Cholera	Subcutaneous, intramuscular, or intradermal[c]
Diphtheria-tetanus–acellular pertussis (DTaP)	Intramuscular
Diphtheria-tetanus-pertussis (DTP)	Intramuscular
DTaP-Hib conjugate[d]	Intramuscular
Haemophilus influenzae type b conjugate (Hib)[d]	Intramuscular
Hepatitis A	Intramuscular
Hepatitis B	Intramuscular[e]
Hib conjugate–hepatitis B	Intramuscular
Human papillomavirus (recombinant)	Intramuscular
Influenza	Intramuscular
Japanese encephalitis	Subcutaneous
Measles	Subcutaneous
Measles-mumps-rubella (MMR)	Subcutaneous
Measles-mumps-rubella 1 varicella (MMRV)	Subcutaneous
Measles-rubella	Subcutaneous
Meningococcal	Intramuscular (MCV4); subcutaneous (MPSV4)
Mumps	Subcutaneous
Pertussis	Intramuscular
Pneumococcal (polysaccharide; PPV)	Intramuscular or subcutaneous
Pneumococcal (polysaccharide-protein conjugate; PCV)	Intramuscular
Poliovirus vaccine, inactivated (IPV)	Subcutaneous
Rabies	Intramuscular or intradermal[f]
Rotavirus	Oral
Rubella	Subcutaneous
Tetanus	Intramuscular
Tetanus-diphtheria (Td or DT)	Intramuscular
Tetanus and diphtheria toxoids and acellular pertussis (Tdap)	Intramuscular
Typhoid (parenteral)	Subcutaneous[g]
Typhoid (Ty21a)	Oral
Varicella	Subcutaneous
Yellow fever	Subcutaneous

Modified from American Academy of Pediatrics: Active and passive immunization. In Pickering LK, editor: *2006 Red book: report of the Committee on Infectious Diseases*, ed 27, Elk Grove Village, Ill, 2006, The Academy.

[a]Additional vaccines that are licensed but not available to the general public include oral poliovirus and smallpox vaccinia. For a list of currently licensed vaccines, see Food and Drug Administration website: *http://www.fda.gov/cber/vaccine/licvacc.htm.*

[b]Available only to U.S. Armed Forces.

[c]Intradermal dose is lower than subcutaneous dose.

[d]May be administered in combination products or as reconstituted products with DTP or DTaP if approved by the Food and Drug Administration for the child's age and if administration of other vaccine is justified.

[e]Not administered in dorsogluteal muscle (buttock) because of possible reduced immunologic response.

[f]Intradermal dose of rabies vaccine, human diploid cell (HDCV), is lower than intramuscular dose and is used only for preexposure vaccination. Rabies vaccine, adsorbed (RVA), should not be used intradermally. Another rabies vaccine, PCEC (purified chicken embryo cell culture), RabAvert, may be given by intramuscular route only for preexposure or postexposure prophylaxis in persons who are sensitive to the other rabies vaccines.

[g]Booster doses may be administered intradermally unless vaccine that is acetone killed and dried is used.

Product Brand Names and Manufacturers and Distributors for Principal Childhood Vaccine Types

Product	Brand Name (Manufacturer, Distributor)
DTaP: Diphtheria and tetanus toxoids and acellular pertussis vaccine	Infanrix (SBB, distributed by SB) Tripedia (SP) Daptacel (SP)
Tdap: Tetanus, reduced diphtheria, acellular pertussis adsorbed (booster)	Boostrix (booster for ages 10-18 yr) (GlaxoKlineSmith) Adacel (booster for ages 11 to 64) (SP)
DTaP-Hib: Diphtheria and tetanus toxoids and acellular pertussis and *Haemophilus influenzae* type b vaccine	TriHIBit* (ActHIB Hib reconstituted with Tripedia DTaP) (SP) Pediarix (DTaP, HepB, IPV) (SBB)
DTwP: Diphtheria and tetanus toxoids and whole-cell pertussis vaccine	No trade name (SP)
HepA: Hepatitis A vaccine	Havrix (SBB, distributed by SB) Vaqta (MRK) Twinrix (HepA and HepB—ages 18 and above) (SBB)
HepB: Hepatitis B vaccine	Engerix-B (SBB, distributed by SB) Recombivax HB (MRK)
Hib: *H. influenzae* type b conjugate vaccine	
HbOC: Oligosaccharides conjugated to diphtheria CRM_{197} toxin protein	HibTITER (WLV)
PRP-OMP: Polyribosylribitol phosphate polysaccharide conjugated to a meningococcal outer membrane protein	PedvaxHIB (MRK)
PRP-T: Polyribosylribitol phosphate polysaccharide conjugated to tetanus toxoid	ActHIB (SP)
Hib-HepB: *H. influenzae* type b and hepatitis B vaccine	Comvax (Hib component = PRP-OMP) (MRK)
Human papillomavirus (types 6,11,16,18), recombinant	Gardasil (MRK)
IPV: Trivalent inactivated polio vaccine (killed Salk type)	IPOL (SP)
MMR: Measles, mumps, rubella vaccine	M-M-R II (MRK)
Measles-mumps-rubella+varicella (MMRV)	ProQuad (MRK)
PCV: Pneumococcal conjugate vaccine	Prevnar (WLV)
PPV: Pneumococcal polysaccharide vaccine	Pneumovax (MRK)
TIV (influenza): Trivalent inactivated influenza vaccine—(SP)	Fluvirin (Chiron) Fluzone (SP)
MCV4 (meningococcal conjugate): Quadrivalent, groups A, C, Y, and W-135	Menactra (SP)
MPSV4 (meningococcal polysaccharide): Groups A, C, Y, and W-135	Menomune (SP)
Influenza—live-attenuated (LAIV)	FluMist (Medimmune)
Varicella live vaccine	Varivax (MRK)
Rotavirus	RotaTeq (MRK)

Modified from American Academy of Pediatrics: Combination vaccines for childhood immunization: recommendations of the Advisory Committee on Immunization Practices (ACIP), the American Academy of Pediatrics (AAP), and the American Academy of Family Physicians (AAFP), *Pediatrics* 103(5):1072, 1999; and American Academy of Pediatrics, Committee on Infectious Diseases, Pickering L, editor: *2006 Red book: report of the Committee on Infectious Diseases,* ed 27, Elk Grove Village, Ill, 2006, The Academy.

MRK, Merck & Co.; *NAV,* North American Vaccine; *SB,* SmithKline Beecham Pharmaceuticals; *SBB,* SmithKline Beecham Biologicals; *SP,* Sanofi Pasteur; *WLV,* Wyeth-Lederle vaccines.

*TriHIBit is licensed only for the fourth dose, recommended at ages 12-15 mo in the vaccination series.

ATRAUMATIC CARE

Immunizations

To Minimize Local Reactions from Vaccines

Select a needle of adequate length (2.5 cm [1 inch] in infants) to deposit the antigen deep in the muscle mass.

Needle length is an important factor and must be considered for each individual child; fewer reactions to immunizations are observed when the vaccine is given deep into the muscle rather than into subcutaneous tissue; contrary to previous belief, deep intramuscular tissue has a better blood supply and fewer pain receptors than adipose tissue, thus providing an optimum site for immunizations with fewer side effects.

Inject into the vastus lateralis or ventrogluteal muscle; the deltoid may be used in children 18 months of age or older or in infants receiving hepatitis B vaccine.

Use an air bubble to clear the needle after injecting the vaccine (theoretically beneficial but unproved).

To Minimize Pain

Apply the topical anesthetic EMLA to the injection site and cover with an occlusive dressing for at least 1 hour.*

Apply the topical anesthetic LMX4 (4% lidocaine; formerly Ela-Max) to the injection site 30 minutes before the injection; there is no evidence that an occlusive dressing is required except to prevent ingestion or accidental application to the eyes in infants.

Apply a vapocoolant spray (e.g., ethyl chloride or FluoriMethane) directly to the skin or to a cotton ball that is placed on the skin for 15 seconds immediately before the injection (Reis and Holubkov, 1997).

It is recommended that a concentrated oral sucrose solution (24%; 1 to 2 ml), and nonnutritive sucking (pacifier), be administered orally 2 minutes before the injection, during the injection, and up to 3 minutes after the procedure to decrease neonatal pain with immunizations.

In preschool children, use distraction, such as telling the child to "take a deep breath and blow and blow and blow until I tell you to stop."

NOTE: Changing the needle on the syringe after drawing up the vaccine and before injecting it has not been shown to decrease local reactions. In children 4 to 6 years of age, the administration of sequential injections or simultaneous injections of vaccines did not alter their perceptions of distress, but parents preferred the simultaneous method (Horn and McCarthy, 1999).

References

Reis EC, Holubkov R: Vapocoolant spray is equally effective as EMLA cream in reducing immunization pain in school-aged children, *Pediatrics* 100(6):1025, 1997; Halperin BA, Halperin SA, McGrath P, and others: Use of lidocaine-prilocaine patch to decrease intramuscular injection pain does not adversely affect the antibody response to diphtheria–tetanus–acellular pertussis–inactivated poliovirus–*Haemophilus influenzae* type b conjugate and hepatitis B vaccines in infants from birth to 6 months of age, *Pediatr Infect Dis* 21(5):399-405, 2002; and Horn MI, McCarthy AM: Children's responses to sequential versus simultaneous immunization injections, *J Pediatr Health Care* 13(1):18-23, 1999.

*The use of the EMLA patch before administration of diphtheria-tetanus–acellular pertussis–inactivated poliovirus–*Haemophilus influenzae* type b (DTaP-IPV-Hib) and hepatitis B vaccines did not decrease antibody titers in immunized infants and was effective in reducing pain in 6-month-old children (Halperin, Halperin, McGrath, and others, 2002). The patch, however, is no longer available.

COMMUNITY FOCUS

Combination Vaccines

Combination vaccines are vaccines that have been combined into one solution or medium so the child receives fewer needle punctures at a given time. A number of combination vaccines licensed for use in the United States are listed in the box on p. 210. The use of combination vaccines provides equivalent immunogenicity; however, it is important that these vaccines be given to the appropriate-age child. For example, the DTaP/Hib combination vaccine (TriHIBit) should not be used for the first three doses at 2, 4, or 6 months but may be used as a booster after any Hib conjugate vaccine in children aged 12 months or older. There is no advantage in administering monovalent vaccines to infants and children when combination vaccines are just as effective.

COMMUNITY FOCUS

Improving Immunization Among Children and Adolescents

Strategies that may increase immunization compliance include giving parents vaccine information at the time of the newborn's discharge and at well-child visits, mailing reminder cards, making immunization services readily available, removing barriers to vaccination (e.g., long waiting times, appointment-only systems), and taking every opportunity to immunize children when they enter a health care facility (e.g., emergency departments, ambulatory clinics, private offices, hospitals).

Despite improving vaccination rates among infants and young children, adolescents are often incompletely immunized. An immunization update is an important part of adolescent preventive care, especially at 11 to 12 years of age. With the exception of pregnant teenagers, all adolescents should receive a second dose of the measles, mumps, and rubella (MMR) vaccine unless they have documentation of two MMR vaccinations after the first 12 months of life. All adolescents who have not previously completed the three-dose series of the hepatitis B vaccine should initiate or complete the series at age 11 to 12 years.

Adolescents ages 11 to 12 years and no older than 16 years should receive a dose of the tetanus and diphtheria toxoids and acellular pertussis (Tdap) vaccine if they have received the primary series of vaccinations and if no dose has been received during the previous 5 years. Unvaccinated adolescents who lack a reliable history of chickenpox should receive the varicella virus vaccine at ages 11 to 12 years.

The first dose (in a series of three) of human papillomavirus vaccine (Gardasil) is now recommended for females who are 11 to 12 years of age; the complete series of vaccinations may be completed within 6 months of the first dose. Adolescent females who have not been vaccinated should consider this vaccine, which is designed to prevent human papillomavirus, a cause of cervical cancer.

Hepatitis A vaccine should be given to all adolescents who have not yet been vaccinated for hepatitis A, especially those who are traveling to or living in countries where the hepatitis A virus is endemic or communities with high rates of hepatitis A, those who have chronic liver disease, those who are intravenous drug users, and adolescent men who have sex with other men. Adolescents who have chronic disorders or underlying medical conditions that place them at high risk for complications associated with the disease, such as influenza, should receive the appropriate vaccines. The meningococcal vaccine (MCV4) is now recommended for all older children (ages 11 and older) and adolescents who have not previously received the polysaccharide meningococcal vaccine (MPSV4) before or when entering college, especially if planning to live in a college dormitory.

Recommended Immunization Schedule for Persons Aged 0 to 6 Years—United States, 2007

DEPARTMENT OF HEALTH AND HUMAN SERVICES • CENTERS FOR DISEASE CONTROL AND PREVENTION

Recommended Immunization Schedule for Persons Aged 0–6 Years—UNITED STATES • 2007

Vaccine ▼ Age ▶	Birth	1 month	2 months	4 months	6 months	12 months	15 months	18 months	19–23 months	2–3 years	4–6 years
Hepatitis B[1]	HepB	HepB		*see footnote 1*	HepB				HepB Series		
Rotavirus[2]			Rota	Rota	Rota						
Diphtheria, Tetanus, Pertussis[3]			DTaP	DTaP	DTaP		DTaP				DTaP
Haemophilus influenzae type b[4]			Hib	Hib	*Hib*[4]	Hib		Hib			
Pneumococcal[5]			PCV	PCV	PCV	PCV				PCV PPV	
Inactivated Poliovirus			IPV	IPV	IPV						IPV
Influenza[6]					Influenza (Yearly)						
Measles, Mumps, Rubella[7]						MMR					MMR
Varicella[8]						Varicella					Varicella
Hepatitis A[9]						HepA (2 doses)				HepA Series	
Meningococcal[10]										MPSV4	

Range of recommended ages

Catch-up immunization

Certain high-risk groups

This schedule indicates the recommended ages for routine administration of currently licensed childhood vaccines, as of December 1, 2006, for children aged 0–6 years. Additional information is available at http://www.cdc.gov/nip/recs/child-schedule.htm. Any dose not administered at the recommended age should be administered at any subsequent visit, when indicated and feasible. Additional vaccines may be licensed and recommended during the year. Licensed combination vaccines may be used whenever any components of the combination are indicated and other components of the vaccine are not contraindicated and if approved by the Food and Drug Administration for that dose of the series. Providers should consult the respective Advisory Committee on Immunization Practices statement for detailed recommendations. Clinically significant adverse events that follow immunization should be reported to the Vaccine Adverse Event Reporting System (VAERS). Guidance about how to obtain and complete a VAERS form is available at **http://www.vaers, hhs.gov** or by telephone, **800-822-7967**.

1. Hepatitis B vaccine (HepB). *(Minimum age: birth)*

At birth:

- Administer monovalent HepB to all newborns before hospital discharge.
- If mother is hepatitis surface antigen (HBsAg)-positive, administer HepB and 0.5 mL of hepatitis B immune globulin (HBIG) within 12 hours of birth.
- If mother's HBsAg status is unknown, administer HepB within 12 hours of birth. Determine the HBsAg status as soon as possible and if HBsAg-positive, administer HBIG (no later than age 1 week).
- If mother is HBsAg-negative, the birth dose can only be delayed with physician's order and mother's negative HBsAg laboratory report documented in the infant's medical record.

After the birth dose:

- The HepB series should be completed with either monovalent HepB or a combination vaccine containing HepB. The second dose should be administered at age 1–2 months. The final dose should be administered at age ≥24 weeks. Infants born to HBsAg-positive mothers should be tested for HBsAg and antibody to HBsAg after completion of ≥3 doses of a licensed HepB series, at age 9–18 months (generally at the next well-child visit).

4-month dose:

- It is permissible to administer 4 doses of HepB when combination vaccines are administered after the birth dose. If monovalent HepB is used for doses after the birth dose, a dose at age 4 months is not needed.

2. Rotavirus vaccine (Rota). *(Minimum age: 6 weeks)*

- Administer the first dose at age 6–12 weeks. Do not start the series later than age 12 weeks.
- Administer the final dose in the series by age 32 weeks. Do not administer a dose later than age 32 weeks.
- Data on safety and efficacy outside of these age ranges are insufficient.

3. Diphtheria and tetanus toxoids and acellular pertussis vaccine (DTaP). *(Minimum age: 6 weeks)*

- The fourth dose of DTaP may be administered as early as age 12 months, provided 6 months have elapsed since the third dose.
- Administer the final dose in the series at age 4–6 years.

4. *Haemophilus influenzae* type b conjugate vaccine (Hib). *(Minimum age: 6 weeks)*

- If PRP-OMP (PedvaxHIB® or ComVax® [Merck]) is administered at ages 2 and 4 months, a dose at age 6 months is not required.
- TriHiBit® (DTaP/Hib) combination products should not be used for primary immunization but can be used as boosters following any Hib vaccine in children aged ≥12 months.

5. Pneumococcal vaccine. *(Minimum age: 6 weeks for pneumococcal conjugate vaccine [PCV]; 2 years for pneumococcal polysaccharide vaccine [PPV])*

- Administer PCV at ages 24–59 months in certain high-risk groups. Administer PPV to children aged ≥2 years in certain high-risk groups. See *MMWR* 2000;49(No. RR-9):1–35.

6. Influenza vaccine. *(Minimum age: 6 months for trivalent inactivated influenza vaccine [TIV]; 5 years for live, attenuated influenza vaccine [LAIV])*

- All children aged 6–59 months and close contacts of all children aged 0–59 months are recommended to receive influenza vaccine.
- Influenza vaccine is recommended annually for children aged ≥59 months with certain risk factors, health-care workers, and other persons (including household members) in close contact with persons in groups at high risk. See *MMWR* 2006;55(No. RR-10):1–41.
- For healthy persons aged 5–49 years, LAIV may be used as an alternative to TIV.
- Children receiving TIV should receive 0.25 mL if aged 6–35 months or 0.5 mL if aged ≥3 years.
- Children aged <9 years who are receiving influenza vaccine for the first time should receive 2 doses (separated by ≥4 weeks for TIV and ≥6 weeks for LAIV).

7. Measles, mumps, and rubella vaccine (MMR). *(Minimum age: 12 months)*

- Administer the second dose of MMR at age 4–6 years. MMR may be administered before age 4–6 years, provided ≥4 weeks have elapsed since the first dose and both doses are administered at age ≥12 months.

8. Varicella vaccine. *(Minimum age: 12 months)*

- Administer the second dose of varicella vaccine at age 4–6 years. Varicella vaccine may be administered before age 4–6 years, provided that ≥3 months have elapsed since the first dose and both doses are administered at age ≥12 months. If second dose was administered ≥28 days following the first dose, the second dose does not need to be repeated.

9. Hepatitis A vaccine (HepA). *(Minimum age: 12 months)*

- HepA is recommended for all children aged 1 year (i.e., aged 12–23 months). The 2 doses in the series should be administered at least 6 months apart.
- Children not fully vaccinated by age 2 years can be vaccinated at subsequent visits.
- HepA is recommended for certain other groups of children, including in areas where vaccination programs target older children. See *MMWR* 2006;55(No. RR-7):1–23.

10. Meningococcal polysaccharide vaccine (MPSV4). *(Minimum age: 2 years)*

- Administer MPSV4 to children aged 2–10 years with terminal complement deficiencies or anatomic or functional asplenia and certain other high-risk groups. See *MMWR* 2005;54(No. RR-7):1–21.

The Recommended Immunization Schedules for Persons Aged 0–18 Years are approved by the Advisory Committee on Immunization Practices (http://www.cdc.gov/nip/acip), the American Academy of Pediatrics (http://www.aap.org), and the American Academy of Family Physicians (http://www.aafp.org).

SAFER • HEALTHIER • PEOPLE™

(From Centers for Disease Control and Prevention: Recommended immunization schedules for persons aged 0-18 years—United States, 2007, *Morbid Mortal Week Rep* 55[51&52], Q1-Q4, 2007.)

Recommended Immunization Schedule for Persons Aged 7 to 18 Years–United States, 2007

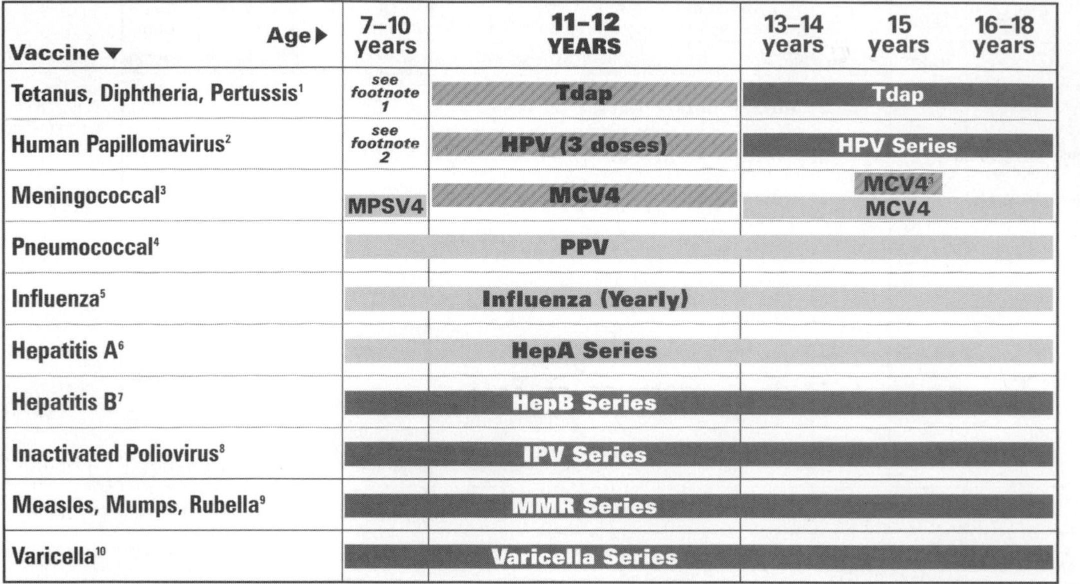

Department of Health and Human Services • Centers for Disease Control and Prevention

Recommended Immunization Schedule for Persons Aged 7–18 Years—UNITED STATES • 2007

Vaccine ▼ / Age ▶	7–10 years	11–12 YEARS	13–14 years	15 years	16–18 years
Tetanus, Diphtheria, Pertussis[1]	see footnote 1	Tdap	Tdap		
Human Papillomavirus[2]	see footnote 2	HPV (3 doses)	HPV Series		
Meningococcal[3]	MPSV4	MCV4		MCV4[3]	
			MCV4		
Pneumococcal[4]	PPV				
Influenza[5]	Influenza (Yearly)				
Hepatitis A[6]	HepA Series				
Hepatitis B[7]	HepB Series				
Inactivated Poliovirus[8]	IPV Series				
Measles, Mumps, Rubella[9]	MMR Series				
Varicella[10]	Varicella Series				

Range of recommended ages

Catch-up immunization

Certain high-risk groups

This schedule indicates the recommended ages for routine administration of currently licensed childhood vaccines, as of December 1, 2006, for children aged 7–18 years. Additional information is available at **http://www.cdc.gov/nip/recs/child-schedule.htm.** Any dose not administered at the recommended age should be administered at any subsequent visit, when indicated and feasible. Additional vaccines may be licensed and recommended during the year. Licensed combination vaccines may be used whenever any components of the combination are indicated and other components of the vaccine are not contraindicated and if approved by the Food and Drug Administration for that dose of the series. Providers should consult the respective Advisory Committee on Immunization Practices statement for detailed recommendations. Clinically significant adverse events that follow immunization should be reported to the Vaccine Adverse Event Reporting System (VAERS). Guidance about how to obtain and complete a VAERS form is available at **http://www.vaers.hhs.gov** or by telephone, **800-822-7967**.

1. Tetanus and diphtheria toxoids and acellular pertussis vaccine (Tdap). *(Minimum age: 10 years for BOOSTRIX® and 11 years for ADACEL™)*
- Administer at age 11–12 years for those who have completed the recommended childhood DTP/DTaP vaccination series and have not received a tetanus and diphtheria toxoids vaccine (Td) booster dose.
- Adolescents aged 13–18 years who missed the 11–12 year Td/Tdap booster dose should also receive a single dose of Tdap if they have completed the recommended childhood DTP/DTaP vaccination series.

2. Human papillomavirus vaccine (HPV). *(Minimum age: 9 years)*
- Administer the first dose of the HPV vaccine series to females at age 11–12 years.
- Administer the second dose 2 months after the first dose and the third dose 6 months after the first dose.
- Administer the HPV vaccine series to females at age 13–18 years if not previously vaccinated.

3. Meningococcal vaccine. *(Minimum age: 11 years for meningococcal conjugate vaccine [MCV4]; 2 years for meningococcal polysaccharide vaccine [MPSV4])*
- Administer MCV4 at age 11–12 years and to previously unvaccinated adolescents at high school entry (at approximately age 15 years).
- Administer MCV4 to previously unvaccinated college freshmen living in dormitories; MPSV4 is an acceptable alternative.
- Vaccination against invasive meningococcal disease is recommended for children and adolescents aged ≥2 years with terminal complement deficiencies or anatomic or functional asplenia and certain other high-risk groups. See *MMWR* 2005;54(No. RR-7):1–21. Use MPSV4 for children aged 2–10 years and MCV4 or MPSV4 for older children.

4. Pneumococcal polysaccharide vaccine (PPV). *(Minimum age: 2 years)*
- Administer for certain high-risk groups. See *MMWR* 1997;46(No. RR-8):1–24, and *MMWR* 2000;49(No. RR-9):1–35.

5. Influenza vaccine. *(Minimum age: 6 months for trivalent inactivated influenza vaccine [TIV]; 5 years for live, attenuated influenza vaccine [LAIV])*
- Influenza vaccine is recommended annually for persons with certain risk factors, health-care workers, and other persons (including household members) in close contact with persons in groups at high risk. See *MMWR* 2006;55 (No. RR-10):1–41.
- For healthy persons aged 5–49 years, LAIV may be used as an alternative to TIV.
- Children aged <9 years who are receiving influenza vaccine for the first time should receive 2 doses (separated by ≥4 weeks for TIV and ≥6 weeks for LAIV).

6. Hepatitis A vaccine (HepA). *(Minimum age: 12 months)*
- The 2 doses in the series should be administered at least 6 months apart.
- HepA is recommended for certain other groups of children, including in areas where vaccination programs target older children. See *MMWR* 2006;55 (No. RR-7):1–23.

7. Hepatitis B vaccine (HepB). *(Minimum age: birth)*
- Administer the 3-dose series to those who were not previously vaccinated.
- A 2-dose series of Recombivax HB® is licensed for children aged 11–15 years.

8. Inactivated poliovirus vaccine (IPV). *(Minimum age: 6 weeks)*
- For children who received an all-IPV or all-oral poliovirus (OPV) series, a fourth dose is not necessary if the third dose was administered at age ≥4 years.
- If both OPV and IPV were administered as part of a series, a total of 4 doses should be administered, regardless of the child's current age.

9. Measles, mumps, and rubella vaccine (MMR). *(Minimum age: 12 months)*
- If not previously vaccinated, administer 2 doses of MMR during any visit, with ≥4 weeks between the doses.

10. Varicella vaccine. *(Minimum age: 12 months)*
- Administer 2 doses of varicella vaccine to persons without evidence of immunity.
- Administer 2 doses of varicella vaccine to persons aged <13 years at least 3 months apart. Do not repeat the second dose, if administered ≥28 days after the first dose.
- Administer 2 doses of varicella vaccine to persons aged ≥13 years at least 4 weeks apart.

The Recommended Immunization Schedules for Persons Aged 0–18 Years are approved by the Advisory Committee on Immunization Practices (http://www.cdc.gov/nip/acip), the American Academy of Pediatrics (http://www.aap.org), and the American Academy of Family Physicians (http://www.aafp.org).

SAFER • HEALTHIER • PEOPLE™

(From Centers for Disease Control and Prevention: Recommended immunization schedules for persons aged 0-18 years—United States, 2007, *Morbid Mortal Week Rep* 55[51&52], Q1-Q4, 2007.)

Catch-Up Immunization Schedule for Persons Aged 4 Months to 18 Years Who Start Late or Who Are More Than 1 Month Behind

Catch-up Immunization Schedule for Persons Aged 4 Months–18 Years Who Start Late or Who Are More Than 1 Month Behind

UNITED STATES • 2007

The table below provides catch-up schedules and minimum intervals between doses for children whose vaccinations have been delayed. A vaccine series does not need to be restarted, regardless of the time that has elapsed between doses. Use the section appropriate for the child's age.

Vaccine	Minimum Age for Dose 1	Minimum Interval Between Doses			
		Dose 1 to Dose 2	Dose 2 to Dose 3	Dose 3 to Dose 4	Dose 4 to Dose 5
CATCH-UP SCHEDULE FOR PERSONS AGED 4 MONTHS–6 YEARS					
Hepatitis B[1]	Birth	**4 weeks**	**8 weeks** (and 16 weeks after first dose)		
Rotavirus[2]	6 wks	**4 weeks**	**4 weeks**		
Diphtheria, Tetanus, Pertussis[3]	6 wks	**4 weeks**	**4 weeks**	**6 months**	**6 months**[3]
Haemophilus influenzae type b[4]	6 wks	**4 weeks** if first dose administered at age <12 months **8 weeks (as final dose)** if first dose administered at age 12-14 months **No further doses needed** if first dose administered at age ≥15 months	**4 weeks**[4] if current age <12 months **8 weeks (as final dose)**[4] if current age ≥12 months and second dose administered at age <15 months **No further doses needed** if previous dose administered at age ≥15 months	**8 weeks (as final dose)** This dose only necessary for children aged 12 months–5 years who received 3 doses before age 12 months	
Pneumococcal[5]	6 wks	**4 weeks** if first dose administered at age <12 months and current age <24 months **8 weeks (as final dose)** if first dose administered at age ≥12 months or current age 24–59 months **No further doses needed** for healthy children if first dose administered at age ≥24 months	**4 weeks** if current age <12 months **8 weeks (as final dose)** if current age ≥12 months **No further doses needed** for healthy children if previous dose administered at age ≥24 months	**8 weeks (as final dose)** This dose only necessary for children aged 12 months–5 years who received 3 doses before age 12 months	
Inactivated Poliovirus[6]	6 wks	**4 weeks**	**4 weeks**	**4 weeks**[6]	
Measles, Mumps, Rubella[7]	12 mos	**4 weeks**			
Varicella[8]	12 mos	**3 months**			
Hepatitis A[9]	12 mos	**6 months**			
CATCH-UP SCHEDULE FOR PERSONS AGED 7–18 YEARS					
Tetanus, Diphtheria/ Tetanus, Diphtheria, Pertussis[10]	7 yrs[10]	**4 weeks**	**8 weeks** if first dose administered at age <12 months **6 months** if first dose administered at age ≥12 months	**6 months** if first dose administered at age <12 months	
Human Papillomavirus[11]	9 yrs	**4 weeks**	**12 weeks**		
Hepatitis A[9]	12 mos	**6 months**			
Hepatitis B[1]	Birth	**4 weeks**	**8 weeks** (and 16 weeks after first dose)		
Inactivated Poliovirus[6]	6 wks	**4 weeks**	**4 weeks**	**4 weeks**[6]	
Measles, Mumps, Rubella[7]	12 mos	**4 weeks**			
Varicella[8]	12 mos	**4 weeks** if first dose administered at age ≥13 years **3 months** if first dose administered at age <13 years			

1. **Hepatitis B vaccine (HepB).** *(Minimum age: birth)*
   - Administer the 3-dose series to those who were not previously vaccinated.
   - A 2-dose series of Recombivax HB® is licensed for children aged 11–15 years.
2. **Rotavirus vaccine (Rota).** *(Minimum age: 6 weeks)*
   - Do not start the series later than age 12 weeks.
   - Administer the final dose in the series by age 32 weeks. Do not administer a dose later than age 32 weeks.
   - Data on safety and efficacy outside of these age ranges are insufficient.
3. **Diphtheria and tetanus toxoids and acellular pertussis vaccine (DTaP).** *(Minimum age: 6 weeks)*
   - The fifth dose is not necessary if the fourth dose was administered at age ≥4 years.
   - DTaP is not indicated for persons aged ≥7 years.
4. ***Haemophilus influenzae* type b conjugate vaccine (Hib).** *(Minimum age: 6 weeks)*
   - Vaccine is not generally recommended for children aged ≥5 years.
   - If current age <12 months and the first 2 doses were PRP-OMP (PedvaxHIB® or ComVax® [Merck]), the third (and final) dose should be administered at age 12–15 months and at least 8 weeks after the second dose.
   - If first dose was administered at age 7–11 months, administer 2 doses separated by 4 weeks plus a booster at age 12–15 months.
5. **Pneumococcal conjugate vaccine (PCV).** *(Minimum age: 6 weeks)*
   - Vaccine is not generally recommended for children aged ≥5 years.
6. **Inactivated poliovirus vaccine (IPV).** *(Minimum age: 6 weeks)*
   - For children who received an all-IPV or all-oral poliovirus (OPV) series, a fourth dose is not necessary if third dose was administered at age ≥4 years.
   - If both OPV and IPV were administered as part of a series, a total of 4 doses should be administered, regardless of the child's current age.
7. **Measles, mumps, and rubella vaccine (MMR).** *(Minimum age: 12 months)*
   - The second dose of MMR is recommended routinely at age 4–6 years but may be administered earlier if desired.
   - If not previously vaccinated, administer 2 doses of MMR during any visit with ≥4 weeks between the doses.
8. **Varicella vaccine.** *(Minimum age: 12 months)*
   - The second dose of varicella vaccine is recommended routinely at age 4–6 years but may be administered earlier if desired.
   - Do not repeat the second dose in persons aged <13 years if administered ≥28 days after the first dose.
9. **Hepatitis A vaccine (HepA).** *(Minimum age: 12 months)*
   - HepA is recommended for certain groups of children, including in areas where vaccination programs target older children. See *MMWR* 2006;55(No. RR-7):1–23.
10. **Tetanus and diphtheria toxoids vaccine (Td) and tetanus and diphtheria toxoids and acellular pertussis vaccine (Tdap).** *(Minimum ages: 7 years for Td, 10 years for BOOSTRIX®, and 11 years for ADACEL™)*
    - Tdap should be substituted for a single dose of Td in the primary catch-up series or as a booster if age appropriate; use Td for other doses.
    - A 5-year interval from the last Td dose is encouraged when Tdap is used as a booster dose. A booster (fourth) dose is needed if any of the previous doses were administered at age <12 months. Refer to ACIP recommendations for further information. See *MMWR* 2006;55(No. RR-3).
11. **Human papillomavirus vaccine (HPV).** *(Minimum age: 9 years)*
    - Administer the HPV vaccine series to females at age 13–18 years if not previously vaccinated.

Information about reporting reactions after immunization is available online at **http://www.vaers.hhs.gov** or by telephone via the 24-hour national toll-free information line 800-822-7967. Suspected cases of vaccine-preventable diseases should be reported to the state or local health department. Additional information, including precautions and contraindications for immunization, is available from the National Center for Immunization and Respiratory Diseases at **http://www.cdc.gov/nip/default.htm** or telephone, **800-CDC-INFO (800-232-4636)**.

DEPARTMENT OF HEALTH AND HUMAN SERVICES • CENTERS FOR DISEASE CONTROL AND PREVENTION • SAFER • HEALTHIER • PEOPLE

(From Centers for Disease Control and Prevention: Recommended immunization schedules for persons aged 0-18 years—United States, 2007, *Morbid Mortal Week Rep* 55[51&52], Q1-Q4, 2007.)

Routine Immunization Schedule for Infants and Children–Canada, 2005

Age at Vaccination	DTaP[1]	IPV	Hib[2]	MMR	Td[3] or DTap[4]	HepB[5] (Three Doses)	V	PC	MC
Birth									
2 mo	X	X	X					X[6]	X[9]
4 mo	X	X	X			Infancy		X	X
6 mo	X	(X)[8]	X			or		X	X
12 mo				X		preadolescence	X[9]	X	
18 mo	X	X	X	(X)[10] or		(9-13 yr)			or
4-6 yr	X	X		(X)[10]					
14-16 yr					X[4]				X[7]

Schedule for Children <7 Years of Age Not Immunized in Early Infancy

Timing	DTaP[1]	IPV	Hib	MMR	Td[3] or DTap[4]	HepB[5] (Three Doses)	V	P	M
First visit	X	X	X[11]	X[12]		X	X[9]	X[6]	X[7]
2 mo later	X	X	X	(X)[10]		X		(X)	(X)
2 mo later	X	(X)[8]						(X)	
6-12 mo later	X	X	(X)[11]			X			
4-6 yr of age[13]	X	X							
14-16 yr of age					X				

Schedule for Children ≥7 Years of Age Not Immunized in Early Infancy

Timing	DTaP[4]	IPV	MMR	HepB[5] (Three Doses)	V	M
First visit	X	X	X	X	X	X[7]
2 mo later	X	X	X[10]	X	(X)[9]	
6-12 mo later	X	X		X		
10 yr later	X					

From *Canadian immunization guide,* ed 6, 2002 (updated March 2005), Health Canada. Reproduced with permission of the Minister of Health, Public Health Agency of Canada, Canada, 2006.

dTap, Tetanus and diphtheria toxoid, acellular pertussis, adolescent/adult type with reduced diphtheria and pertussis components; *DTaP,* diphtheria, tetanus, pertussis (acellular) vaccine; *HepB,* hepatitis B vaccine; *Hib, Haemophilus influenzae* type b conjugate vaccine; *IPV,* inactivated poliovirus vaccine; *M,* meningococcal vaccine; *MC,* meningococcal C conjugate vaccine; *MMR,* measles, mumps, and rubella vaccine; *P,* pneumococcal vaccine; *PC,* pneumococcal conjugate vaccine; *Td,* tetanus and diphtheria toxoid, adult type with reduced diphtheria toxoid; *V,* varicella.

[1]DTaP (diphtheria, tetanus, acellular or component pertussis) vaccine is the preferred vaccine for all doses in the vaccination series, including completion of the series in children who have received more than one dose of DPT (whole cell) vaccine.

[2]Hib schedule shown is for PRP-T or HbOC vaccine. If PRP-OMP is used, give at 2, 4, and 12 months of age.

[3]Td (tetanus and diphtheria toxoid), a combined adsorbed "adult type" preparation for use in people >7 years of age, contains less diphtheria toxoid than preparations given to younger children and is less likely to cause reactions in older people.

[4]dTap adult formulation with reduced diphtheria toxoid and pertussis component.

[5]Hepatitis B vaccine can be routinely given to infants or preadolescents, depending on the provincial or territorial policy; three doses at 0, 1, and 6 months are preferred. The second dose should be administered at least 1 month after the first dose, and the third at least 2 months after the second dose. A two-dose schedule for adolescents is also possible.

[6]Recommended schedule, number of doses, and subsequent use of 23-valent polysaccharide pneumococcal vaccine depend on the age of the child when vaccination is begun.

[7]Recommended schedule and number of doses of meningococcal vaccine depend on the age of the child.

[8]This dose is not needed routinely but can be included for convenience.

[9]Children ages 12 months to 12 years should receive one dose of varicella vaccine. Individuals >13 years of age should receive two doses at least 28 days apart.

[10]A second dose of MMR is recommended at least 1 month after the first dose for the purpose of better measles protection. For convenience, options include giving it with the next scheduled vaccination at 18 months of age or with school entry (4 to 6 years) vaccinations (depending on the provincial or territorial policy), or at any intervening age that is practicable. The need for a second dose of mumps and rubella vaccine is not established, but it may be of benefit (given for convenience as MMR). The second dose of MMR should be given at the same visit as DTaP IPV (+Hib) to ensure high uptake rates.

[11]Recommended schedule and number of doses depend on the product used and age of the child when vaccination is begun. Not required past age 5.

[12]Delay until subsequent visit if child is <12 months of age.

[13]Omit these doses if the previous doses of DTaP and polio were given after the fourth birthday.

Recommended Doses of Hepatitis B Vaccines,* 2006

	Vaccine†	
	Recombivax HB‡ Dose, mcg (ml)	**Engerix-B§ Dose, mcg (ml)**
Infants of HBsAg-negative mothers, children, and adolescents younger than 20 years of age	5 (0.5)	10 (0.5)
Infants of HBsAg-positive mothers (HBIG [0.5 ml] also is recommended)	5 (0.5)	10 (0.5)
Adults 20 years of age or older	10 (1)	20 (1)
Patients undergoing dialysis and other immunosuppressed adults	40 (1)‖	40 (2)¶

From American Academy of Pediatrics, Committee on Infectious Disease, Pickering LK, editor: *2006 Red book: report of the Committee on Infectious Diseases,* ed 27, Elk Grove Village, Ill, 2006, The Academy.

**HBsAg*, Hepatitis B surface antigen; *HBIG*, hepatitis B immune globulin.

†Vaccines should be stored at 2° to 8° C (36° to 46° F). Freezing destroys effectiveness. Both vaccines are administered in a three- or four-dose schedule; four doses may be administered if a birth dose is given and a combination vaccine is used to complete the series. Only single-antigen hepatitis B vaccine can be used for the birth dose. Single-antigen or combination vaccine containing hepatitis B vaccine may be used to complete the series.

‡Available from Merck and Company, West Point, Pa. A combination of hepatitis B (Recombivax, 5 mcg) and *Haemophilus influenzae b* (PRP-OMP) vaccine is licensed for use at 2, 4, and 12 to 15 months of age (Comvax). A two-dose schedule, administered at 0 months and 4 to 6 months later, is available for adolescents 11 to 15 years of age using the adult dose of Recombivax HB (10 mcg). A combination of hepatitis B (Recombivax, 5 mcg) and *Haemophilus influenzae* type b (PRP-OMP) vaccine is recommended for use at 2, 4, and 12 to 15 months of age (Comvax); this vaccine cannot be administered at birth, before 6 weeks of age, or after 71 months of age.

§Available from GlaxoSmithKline Biologicals, Rixensart, Belgium. The U.S. Food and Drug Administration has approved this vaccine for use in an optional four-dose schedule at 0, 1, 2, and 12 months. A combination of diphtheria and tetanus toxoids and acellular pertussis (DTaP), inactivated poliovirus (IPV), and hepatitis B (Engerix-B, 10 mcg) is recommended for use at 2, 4, and 6 months of age (Pediarix); this vaccine cannot be administered at birth, before 6 weeks of age, or at or above 7 years of age.

‖Special formulation for dialysis patients.

¶Two 1-ml doses given in one site in a four-dose schedule at 0, 1, 2, and 6 months of age.

Guide to Tetanus Prophylaxis in Routine Wound Management, 2006

	Clean, Minor Wounds		All Other Wounds*	
History of Adsorbed Tetanus Toxoid (Doses)	**Td or Tdap†**	**TIG**	**Td or Tdap†**	**TIG‡**
Unknown or <3	Yes	No	Yes	Yes
≥3§	No‖	No	No¶	No

Data from American Academy of Pediatrics, Committee on Infectious Diseases, Pickering L, editor: *2006 Red book: report of the Committee on Infectious Diseases,* ed 27, Elk Grove Village, Ill, 2006, The Academy.

Td, Tetanus, diphtheria; *Tdap*, booster tetanus toxoid, reduced diphtheria toxoid, and acellular pertussis; *TIG*, tetanus immune globulin.

*Such as, but not limited to, wounds contaminated with dirt, feces, soil, and saliva, puncture wounds, avulsions, and wounds resulting from missiles, crushing, burns, and frostbite.

†Tdap is preferred to Td for adolescents who never have received Tdap. Td is preferred to tetanus toxoid (TT) for adolescents who received Tdap previously or when Tdap is not available.

§If only three doses of *fluid* toxoid have been received, then a fourth dose of toxoid, preferably an adsorbed toxoid, should be given.

‖Yes, if ≥10 years since last dose.

¶Yes, if ≥5 years since last dose. (More frequent boosters are not needed and can accentuate side effects.)

‡Immune Globulin Intravenous should be used when TIG is not available.

Possible Side Effects of Recommended Childhood Immunizations and Nursing Responsibilities

Immunization	Reaction	Nursing Responsibilities
Hepatitis B virus	Well tolerated, few side effects	Explain to parents reason for this immunization. Consider that cost for three injections may be a factor.
Diphtheria	Fever usually within 24-48 hours Soreness, redness, and swelling at injection site Behavioral changes: drowsiness, fretfulness, anorexia, prolonged or unusual crying	Nursing responsibilities for DTP/DTaP apply to immunizations for diphtheria, tetanus, and pertussis. Instruction for DTP/DTaP: advise parents of possible side effects.
Tetanus	Same as for diphtheria but may include urticaria and malaise All may have delayed onset and last several days Lump at injection site may last for weeks, even months, but gradually disappears	Acetaminophen is recommend for prophylactic use at time of DTP/DTaP or Tdap immunization and every 4-6 hours for a total of three doses. Advise parents to notify practitioner *immediately* of any unusual side effects, such as those listed under pertussis on p. 220.
Pertussis	Same as for tetanus but may include loss of consciousness, convulsions, persistent inconsolable crying episodes, generalized or focal neurologic signs, fever (temperature at or above 40.5° C [105° F]), systemic allergic reaction	Before administering next dose of DTP/DTaP, or Tdap inquire about reactions, especially those listed on p. 220.
Haemophilus influenzae type b	Mild local reactions (erythema, pain) at injection site Low-grade fever	Advise parents of possible mild side effects.
Poliovirus (IPV)	No serious adverse effects have been associated with the currently available product Rare reactions possible Trace amounts of neomycin, streptomycin, and polymyxin B may be present in IPV (American Academy of Pediatrics, 2006)	Advise parents of safety of IPV (i.e., no vaccine-associated polio paralysis with inactivated virus).
Measles	Anorexia, malaise, rash, and fever may occur 7-10 days after immunization Rarely (estimated risk 1:1 million doses) encephalitis may occur.	Advise parents of more common side effects and recommend use of antipyretics (acetaminophen) for fever. If a persistent fever with other obvious signs of illness occurs, have parents notify physician immediately.
Mumps	Essentially no side effects other than a brief, mild fever	See general comment to parents.*

American Academy of Pediatrics, Committee on Infectious Diseases, Pickering L, editor: *2006 Red book: report of the Committee on Infectious Diseases,* ed 27, Elk Grove Village, Ill, 2006, The Academy.

DTaP, Diphtheria-tetanus–acellular pertussis; *DTP,* diphtheria-tetanus-pertussis; *MMR,* measles-mumps- rubella vaccine; *Tdap,* tetanus toxoid, reduced diphtheria toxoid, and acellular pertussis (booster); *TIV,* trivalent inactivated influenza vaccine.

*General comment to parents regarding each immunization: benefit of being protected by immunization is believed to greatly outweigh risk from the disease.

Possible Side Effects of Recommended Childhood Immunizations and Nursing Responsibilities–cont'd

Immunization	Reaction	Nursing Responsibilities
Rubella	Fever, lymphadenopathy, or mild rash that lasts 1 or 2 days within a few days after immunization Arthralgia, arthritis, or paresthesia of the hands and fingers may occur approximately 2 weeks after vaccination; more common in older children and adults.	Advise parents of side effects, especially of time delay before joint swelling and pain; assure them that these symptoms will disappear.
Varicella	Pain, tenderness, or redness at the injection site Mild, vaccine-associated maculopapular or varicelliform rash at the vaccine site or elsewhere	Advise parents of possible side effects. If necessary, recommend use of acetaminophen for pain.
Hepatitis A	No severe reactions have been reported. Local erythema may occur in some cases.	Explain to parents and teens rationale for immunization. Encourage parents in high-risk areas to immunize children, especially teens and preteens.
Pneumococcal (PCV and PPV)	Fever, fussiness, decreased appetite, drowsiness, local erythema, interrupted sleep, diarrhea, vomiting, and hives	Explain to parents benefits and rationale for vaccination in children younger than 2 years and older than 2 years if in high-risk category.
Meningococcal	MCV4—See p. 222 for contraindications. Pain at injection site, fever, headache, fatigue, malaise, chills, anorexia, vomiting, diarrhea, rash MPSV4—Pain and redness at injection site, transient fever, urticaria, wheezing, and rash (extremely rare)	Explain to parents benefits and rationale for immunization, especially in adolescents and in small children at higher risk for meningococcal disease.
Influenza	TIV (trivalent inactivated vaccine)—Fever and local reactions: fever possible in children <24 mo, local reactions occur primarily in children >13 yr Live-attenuated influenza vaccine (LAIV)—Fever, rhinitis, nasal congestion NOTE: Children with severe anaphylactic reaction to chicken or egg protein should not receive the inactivated influenza vaccine.	Explain to parents and adolescents rationale for vaccine; explain that the vaccine will *not* give the child a mild case of influenza.
Human papillomavirus	Localized pain, swelling and erythema, fever Syncope in adolescents†	Explain to parents and adolescent benefit and rationale for immunization and necessity of completing vaccination series
Rotavirus	Diarrhea, vomiting, runny nose and sore throat, ear infection, wheezing and coughing	Explain to parents rationale for immunization.

†Centers for Disease Control and Prevention: Quadrivalent human papillomavirus vaccine, Recommendation of the Advisory Committee on Immunization Practices (ACIP), *Morbid Mortal Wkly Rep* 56(10):1-24, 2007.

2 - HEALTH PROMOTION

Contraindications and Precautions to Vaccinations[a]

True Contraindications	Precautions[b]	Not Contraindications (Vaccines May Be Administered)
General for All Vaccines (DTaP, Td, Tdap, IPV, MMR, Hib, Hepatitis B, Varicella, Pneumococcal, Hepatitis A, Influenza, Meningococcal, Rotavirus, Human Papillomavirus)		
Anaphylactic reaction to a vaccine contraindicates further doses of that vaccine Anaphylactic reaction to vaccine component is a contraindication to use of vaccines containing that substance	Latex allergy Moderate or severe illnesses with or without fever	Mild to moderate local reaction (soreness, redness, swelling) after a dose of injectable antigen Mild acute illness with or without low-grade fever Current antimicrobial therapy Convalescent phase of illnesses Preterm birth (same dosage and indications as for normal, full-term infants) Recent exposure to infectious disease History of penicillin or other nonspecific allergies or family history of such allergies Pregnancy or mother of household contact Unimmunized household contact Immunodeficient household contact Breastfeeding or lactating mother
Diphtheria, Tetanus, and Pertussis or Acellular Pertussis Vaccine (DTP or DTaP)		
Encephalopathy within 7 days of administration of previous dose of DTaP/DTP	Fever of ≥40.5° C (105° F) within 48 hr after vaccination with prior dose of DTaP Collapse or shocklike state (hypotonic-hyporesponsive episode) within 48 hr of receiving prior dose of DTaP Seizures within 3 days of receiving prior dose of DTaP[c] Persistent, inconsolable crying lasting ≥3 hr within 48 hr of receiving prior dose of DTaP Guillain-Barré syndrome (GBS) within 6 weeks after dose[d]	Temperature of <40.5° C (105° F) after previous dose of DTaP Family history of seizures[c] Family history of sudden infant death syndrome Family history of adverse event after DTaP administration

Modified from American Academy of Pediatrics, Committee on Infectious Diseases, Pickering L, editor: *2006 Red book: report of the Committee on Infectious Diseases,* ed 27, Elk Grove Village, Ill, 2006, The Academy.

[a]This information is based on the recommendations of the Advisory Committee on Immunization Practices (ACIP) and those of the Committee on Infectious Diseases (Red Book Committee) of the American Academy of Pediatrics (AAP). Sometimes these recommendations vary from those contained in manufacturer's package inserts. For more detailed information, consult published recommendations of ACIP and AAP and manufacturers' package inserts.

[b]Events or conditions listed as precautions, although not contraindications, should be carefully reviewed. Benefits and risks of administering a specific vaccine to an individual under the circumstances should be considered. If risks are believed to outweigh benefits, vaccination should be withheld; if benefits are believed to outweigh risks (e.g., during an outbreak or foreign travel), vaccination should be administered. Whether and when to administer DTaP to children with proven or suspected underlying neurologic disorders should be decided on individual basis. It is prudent on theoretic grounds to avoid vaccinating pregnant women.

[c]Acetaminophen given before administering DTaP and thereafter every 4 hr for 24 hr should be considered for children with personal history or family history of convulsions in siblings or parents.

[d]A decision to administer additional doses of DTaP should be made on the consideration of the benefit of further immunization versus the risk of recurrence of GBS.

Contraindications and Precautions to Vaccinations—cont'd

True Contraindications	Precautions[b]	Not Contraindications (Vaccines May Be Administered)
Diphtheria, Tetanus (DT, Td)		
Severe allergic reaction after a previous dose or to a vaccine component	GBS $\leq$6 weeks after previous dose of tetanus toxoid–containing vaccine Moderate or severe acute illness with or without fever	Same as DTaP or DTP
Inactivated Poliovirus Vaccine (IPV)		
Anaphylactic reaction to neomycin or streptomycin	Pregnancy	Breast-feeding Diarrhea
Measles, Mumps, Rubella Vaccine (MMR)		
Pregnancy Known altered immunodeficiency (hematologic and solid tumors, congenital immunodeficiency, and long-term immunosuppressive therapy) Anaphylactic reaction to neomycin or gelatin Known altered immunodeficiency (hematologic and solid tumors, congenital immunodeficiency, severe HIV infection, and long-term immunosuppressive therapy)	Recent immunoglobulin administration (within 3-11 months) Immunoglobulin products and MMR should not be given simultaneously; if unavoidable, give at different sites and revaccinate or test for seroconversion in 3 months; if immunoglobulin is given first, MMR should not be given for at least 3-6 months, depending on dose; if MMR is given first, immunoglobulin should not be given for 2 weeks Thrombocytopenia or thrombocytopenia purpura Tuberculosis or positive TST[e]	Simultaneous tuberculosis skin testing[f] Breast-feeding Pregnancy of mother of recipient Immunodeficient family member or household contact Infection with HIV Nonanaphylactic reactions to eggs or neomycin
***Haemophilus influenzae* Type B Vaccine (Hib)**		
None identified other than those listed in General for All Vaccines	None identified	History of Hib disease
Hepatitis B Virus Vaccine		
Severe allergic reaction after a previous dose or to a vaccine component.	Preterm birth[g]	Pregnancy

HIV, Human immunodeficiency virus; *TST,* tuberculin skin test.

[e]A theoretic basis exists for concern that measles vaccine might exacerbate tuberculosis. Before administering MMR to persons with untreated active TB, initiating antituberculosis therapy is warranted.

[f]Measles vaccination may temporarily suppress tuberculin reactivity. MMR vaccine may be given after or on the same day as tuberculin skin testing. If MMR has been given recently, delay TB skin test until 4 to 6 weeks after administration of MMR.

[g]Birth weight less than 2000 grams and unknown or HBsAg-positive mother is not a contraindication for vaccination.

Continued

Contraindications and Precautions to Vaccinations—cont'd

True Contraindications	Precautions[b]	Not Contraindications (Vaccines May Be Administered)
Varicella Vaccine		
Severe allergic reaction after a previous dose or to a vaccine component (e.g., neomycin or gelatin) Infection with HIV Known altered immunodeficiency (hematologic and solid tumors, congenital immunodeficiency, and long-term immunosuppressive therapy) Pregnancy	Recent Immune Globulin administration (see *Measles* in AAP 2006 reference) Family history of immunodeficiency	Breast-feeding Consider MMR for mildly symptomatic HIV-infected children (see AAP 2006 reference)
Pneumococcal Vaccine (PCV)		
Severe allergic reaction after a previous dose or to a vaccine component	Moderate or severe acute illness with or without fever A child who has received pneumococcal polysaccharide vaccine (PPV) previously should wait at least 2 months before receiving PCV.	Minor illnesses with or without fever Mild upper respiratory tract infection Allergic rhinitis
Influenza Vaccine (Inactivated/Live-Attenuated)[h]		
Severe allergic reaction after a previous dose or to a vaccine component including eggs Egg hypersensitivity LAIV should not be administered to persons taking salicylates, with known or suspected immune deficiency, with a history of GBS, or who have a reactive airway disease or other chronic disorder considered high risk for severe influenza.	GBS within 6 weeks after previous influenza immunization	Pregnancy
Rotavirus Vaccine		
Severe allergic reaction after a previous dose or to a vaccine component Infants born to HIV-positive mother Known or suspected weakened immune system caused by radiation, drugs, or conditions such as leukemia, blood disorders, cancer	Altered immunocompetence Moderate to severe acute gastroenteritis Moderate to severe febrile illness Chronic gastrointestinal diseases Intussusception	Pregnancy Previous history of rotavirus infection; history of intussusception; temperature ≥100.5° F (38.1° C); close contact with immunocompromised person(s); blood transfusion or immunoglobulins within previous 42 days

[b]Events or conditions listed as precautions, although not contraindications, should be carefully reviewed. Benefits and risks of administering a specific vaccine to an individual under the circumstances should be considered. If risks are believed to outweigh benefits, vaccination should be withheld; if benefits are believed to outweigh risks (e.g., during an outbreak or foreign travel), vaccination should be administered. Whether and when to administer DTaP to children with proven or suspected underlying neurologic disorders should be decided on individual basis. It is prudent on theoretic grounds to avoid vaccinating pregnant women.

[h]See James JM, Zeiger RS, Lester MR, and others: Safe administration of influenza vaccine to patients with egg allergies, *J Pediatr* 133:624-628, 1998.

Contraindications and Precautions to Vaccinations—cont'd

True Contraindications	Precautions[b]	Not Contraindications (Vaccines May Be Administered)
Meningococcal Vaccine		
MCV4/MPSV4: Allergy to vaccine components, including diphtheria toxoid and possible reaction to latex; history of GBS		Pregnancy
Tetanus (Booster Toxoid), Reduced Diphtheria Toxoid, Acellular Pertussis Adsorbed (Tdap)		
Serious reaction to any vaccine component History of encephalopathy (e.g., coma, prolonged seizures) within 7 days of administration of a pertussis vaccine that is not attributable to another identifiable cause.	GBS ≤6 weeks after previous dose of a tetanus toxoid vaccine Progressive neurologic disorder, uncontrolled epilepsy, or progressive encephalopathy until the condition has stabilized	Temperature ≥105° F (40.5° C) within 48 hours after DTP/DTaP immunization not attributable to another cause Collapse or shocklike state within 48 hours after DTP/DTaP immunization Persistent crying lasting 3 hours or longer, occurring within 48 hours after DTP/DTaP immunization Convulsions with or without fever, occurring within 3 days after DTaP/DTP immunization History of entire limb swelling reaction after pediatric DTaP/DTP or Td immunization that was not an Arthus hypersensitivity reaction Stable neurologic disorder, including well-controlled seizures, history of seizure disorder, and cerebral palsy Brachial neuritis Latex allergy other than anaphylactic allergies (e.g., history of contact to latex gloves)[i] Immunosuppression, including persons with HIV Antibiotic use Intercurrent minor illness
Human Papillomavirus Vaccine		
Pregnancy; hypersensitivity to yeast or any vaccine component		Immunosuppressed female; minor acute illness; lactation

[i]The tip and rubber plunger of the Boostrix needleless syringe contain latex and should not be used to administer vaccine to adolescents with a history of severe allergy to latex; the single dose vials of Boostrix and Adacel preparations do not contain latex.

2 - HEALTH PROMOTION

Keeping Current on Vaccine Recommendations

It is much easier to keep current if you know where to look for the official recommendations of the American Academy of Pediatrics (AAP) and the Centers for Disease Control and Prevention's (CDC) Advisory Committee on Immunization Practices (ACIP). The primary sources are publications and the Internet. You can also contact each organization to request information:

American Academy of Pediatrics
141 Northwest Point Blvd.
PO Box 747
Elk Grove Village, IL 60009
(888) 227-1770
Fax: (847) 228-1281
Website: *http://www.aap.org*

Centers for Disease Control and Prevention
1600 Clifton Rd. NE
Atlanta, GA 30333
(404) 639-3311
Information hotline: (800) 232-2522 or (800) 232-7468
International travel hotline: (877) 394-8747
Spanish hotline: (800) 232-0233
Website: *http://www.cdc.gov;* National Immunization Program at CDC: *http://www.cdc.gov/nip*

The AAP's Report of the Committee on Infectious Diseases, known as the *Red Book*, is an authoritative source of information on vaccines and other important pediatric infectious diseases. However, it sometimes lacks an in-depth review and reference list of controversial issues. The recommendations in the *Red Book* first appear in the journal *Pediatrics* and/or the *AAP News*. Typically, the most recent immunization schedule appears in the January issue of the journal.

The CDC now offers a valuable resource tool for parents and clinicians online. The tool will print out an individualized vaccination schedule with dates associated with each vaccination based on the child's date of birth. Clinicians can use this tool for children under 5 years of age to serve as a reminder for parents. Nurses should note that the personalized tool is based on the current immunizations schedule and may need to be adjusted with the yearly updates from the AAP and ACIP. The tool is available at *http://www2a.cdc.gov/nip/kidstuff/newscheduler_le/*.

A publication of the CDC, *Morbidity and Mortality Weekly Report* (MMWR), contains comprehensive reviews of the literature and important background data regarding vaccine efficacy and side effects. To receive an electronic copy, send an e-mail message to *listserv@listserv.cdc.gov.* The body content should read: subscribe mmwr-toc. Electronic copy also is available from the CDC's website at *http://www.cdc.gov* or from the CDC's file transfer protocol server at *http://ftp.cdc.gov.* To subscribe for a paper copy, contact:

Superintendent of Documents
U.S. Government Printing Office
Washington, DC 20402
(202) 512-1800

Immunization Gateway: Your Vaccine Fact-Finder at *http://www.immunofacts.com* provides direct links to all of the best vaccine resources on the Internet.

The **Immunization Action Coalition** at *http://www.immunize.org* offers substantial immunization information for healthcare workers. This informative website provides a variety of immunization publications in various languages for public education including blank immunization schedules and information about various diseases for which there are vaccines.

Vaccine information statements (VISs) are available by calling your state or local health department. They can also be downloaded from the Immunization Action Coalition's website at *http://www.immunize.org/vis* or the CDC's website at *http://www.cdc.gov/nip/publications/vis.* Another resource to keep up to date on the vaccines that are licensed and commercially available is the Food and Drug Administration's Center for Biologic and Research *(http://www.fda.gov/cber/index.html).*

Safety and Injury Prevention

Child Safety Home Checklist

SAFETY: FIRE, ELECTRICAL, BURNS

- ☐ Guards in front of or around any heating appliance, fireplace, or furnace (including floor furnace)*
- ☐ Electrical wires hidden or out of reach*
- ☐ No frayed or broken wires; no overloaded sockets
- ☐ Plastic guards or caps over electrical outlets or furniture in front of outlets*
- ☐ Hanging tablecloths out of reach, away from open fires*
- ☐ Smoke and carbon monoxide detectors tested and operating properly
- ☐ Matches and other lighters (such as butane) stored out of child's reach*
- ☐ Large, deep ashtrays throughout house (if used)
- ☐ Small stoves, heaters, and other hot objects (cigarettes, candles, coffee pots, slow cookers) placed where they cannot be tipped over or reached by children
- ☐ Hot water heater set at 49° C (120° F) or lower
- ☐ Pot handles turned toward back of stove or toward center of table
- ☐ No loose clothing worn near stove
- ☐ No cooking or eating hot foods or liquids with child standing nearby or sitting in lap
- ☐ All small appliances, such as iron, turned off, disconnected, and placed out of reach when not in use
- ☐ Cool, not hot, mist vaporizer used
- ☐ Fire extinguisher available on each floor and checked periodically
- ☐ Electrical fuse box and gas shutoff accessible
- ☐ Family escape plan in case of a fire practiced periodically; fire escape ladder available on upper-level floors
- ☐ Telephone number of fire or rescue squad and address of home with nearest cross street posted near phone

SAFETY: SUFFOCATION AND ASPIRATION

- ☐ Small objects stored out of reach*
- ☐ Toys inspected for small, removable parts or long strings*
- ☐ Hanging crib toys and mobiles placed out of reach
- ☐ Plastic bags stored away from young child's reach, large plastic garment bags discarded after tying in knots*
- ☐ Mattress or pillow should not be covered with plastic or in such a way that is accessible to child*
- ☐ Crib designed according to federal regulations (crib slats less than 2⅜ inches [6 cm] apart) with snug-fitting mattress*†
- ☐ Crib positioned away from other furniture or windows*
- ☐ Portable playpen gates up at all times while in use*
- ☐ Accordion-style gates not used*
- ☐ Bathroom doors kept closed and toilet seats down or toilet lid fasteners used*
- ☐ Faucets turned off firmly*
- ☐ Pool fenced with locked gate
- ☐ Proper safety equipment at poolside
- ☐ Electric garage door openers stored safely and garage door adjusted to rise when door strikes object
- ☐ Doors of ovens, trunks, dishwashers, refrigerators, and front-loading clothes washers and dryers kept closed*
- ☐ Unused appliances such as refrigerators securely closed with lock or doors removed*
- ☐ Food served in small, noncylindric pieces*
- ☐ Toy chests without lids or with lids that securely lock in open position*
- ☐ Buckets and wading pools kept empty when not in use*
- ☐ Clothesline above head level
- ☐ At least one member of household trained in basic life support (CPR) including first aid for choking‡

SAFETY: POISONING

- ☐ Toxic substances, including batteries, placed on a high shelf, preferably in a locked cabinet
- ☐ Toxic plants hung or placed out of reach*
- ☐ Excess quantities of cleaning fluid, paints, pesticides, drugs, and other toxic substances not stored in home
- ☐ Used containers of poisonous substances discarded where child cannot obtain access
- ☐ Telephone number of local poison control center and address of home with nearest cross street posted near phone
- ☐ Medicines clearly labeled in childproof containers and stored out of reach
- ☐ Household cleaners, disinfectants, and insecticides kept in their original containers, separate from food and out of reach
- ☐ Smoking only allowed in areas away from children

---

*Safety measures are specific for homes with young children. All safety measures should be implemented in homes where children reside and in homes they visit frequently, such as those of grandparents or babysitters.

†Federal regulations are available from U.S. Consumer Product Safety Commission, (800) 638-CPSC; *http://www.cpsc.gov.*

‡For patient and family education instructions for infant cardiopulmonary resuscitation and infant and child choking see pp. 581 and 582.

This section may be photocopied and distributed to families.

SAFETY: FALLS

☐ Nonskid mats, strips, or surfaces in tubs and showers
☐ Exits, halls, and passageways in rooms kept clear of toys, furniture, boxes, and other items that could be obstructive
☐ Stairs and halls well lit, with switches at both top and bottom
☐ Sturdy handrails for all steps and stairways
☐ Nothing stored on stairways
☐ Treads, risers, and carpeting in good repair
☐ Glass doors and walls marked with decals
☐ Safety glass used in doors, windows, and walls
☐ Gates on top and bottom of staircases and elevated areas, such as porch or fire escape*
☐ Guardrails on upstairs windows with locks that limit height of window opening and access to areas such as fire escape*
☐ Crib side rails raised to full height; mattress lowered as child grows*
☐ Restraints used in high chairs, walkers, or other baby furniture; preferably walkers not used*
☐ Scatter rugs secured in place or used with nonskid backing
☐ Walks, patios, and driveways in good repair

SAFETY: BODILY INJURY

☐ Knives, power tools, and unloaded firearms stored safely or placed in locked cabinet
☐ Garden tools returned to storage racks after use
☐ Pets properly restrained and immunized for rabies
☐ Swings, slides, and other outdoor play equipment kept in safe condition
☐ Yard free of broken glass, nail-studded boards, other litter
☐ Cement birdbaths placed where young child cannot tip them over*

Injury Prevention During Infancy

Major Developmental Accomplishments	Injury Prevention
Age: Birth to 4 Months	
Involuntary reflexes, such as the crawling reflex, may propel infant forward or backward, and the startle reflex may cause the body to jerk. May roll over Has increasing eye-hand coordination and voluntary grasp reflex NOTE: Infants are prone to injury as a result of increasing curiosity about their environment, developing and uncoordinated mobilization skills, increasing skill in handling objects, desire to place objects in mouth or on face, and inability to protect self from potential dangers such as falls from heights (no cognitive basis for cause-effect reasoning).	***Aspiration*** Not as great a danger in this age-group but should begin practicing safeguards early (see Age: 4-7 Months) Never shake baby powder directly on infant; place powder in hand and then on infant's skin; store container closed and out of infant's reach. Hold infant for feeding; do not prop bottle. Know emergency procedures for choking.* Use pacifier with one-piece construction and loop handle. ***Suffocation and Drowning*** Keep all plastic bags stored out of infant's reach; discard large plastic garment bags after tying in a knot. Do not cover mattress with plastic. Use a firm mattress and loose blankets; no pillows. Make sure crib design follows federal regulations—crib slats less than 2⅜ (6 cm) apart—and mattress fits snugly. Position crib away from other furniture, windows, and radiators. Do not tie pacifier on a string around infant's neck. Remove bibs at bedtime. Never leave infant alone in bath. Do not leave infant under 12 months alone on adult or youth mattress. ***Falls*** Always raise crib rails. Never leave infant unguarded on a raised surface. When in doubt as to where to place child, use the floor. Restrain child in infant seat and never leave child unattended while the seat is resting on a raised surface. Avoid using a high chair until child can sit well with support. ***Poisoning*** Not as great a danger in this age-group but should begin practicing safeguards early (see Age: 4 to 7 Months).

*For patient and family education instructions for care of the choking infant, see p. 581; for use of child safety seats, see p. 237.

Injury Prevention During Infancy—cont'd

Major Developmental Accomplishments	Injury Prevention
Age: Birth to 4 Months—cont'd	
	Burns Install smoke detectors in home. Use caution when warming formula in microwave oven; always check temperature of liquid before feeding. Check temperature of bath water. Do not pour hot liquids when infant is close by, such as sitting on lap. Beware of cigarette ashes that may fall on infant. Do not leave infant in the sun for more than a few minutes; keep exposed skin covered. Use sunscreen. Wash flame-retardant clothes according to label directions. Use cool-mist vaporizers. Do not leave child in parked car. Check surface heat of restraint before placing child in car seat. ***Motor Vehicles*** Transport infant in federally approved, rear-facing car seat,* preferably in back seat. Do not place infant on the seat or in lap. Do not place child in a carriage or stroller behind a parked car. Do not place infant or child in front passenger seat with an air bag (unless it can be deactivated). ***Bodily Damage*** Avoid sharp, jagged objects. Keep diaper pins closed and away from infant.
Age: 4 to 7 Months	
Rolls over Sits momentarily Grasps and manipulates small objects Resecures a dropped object Has well-developed eye-hand coordination Can focus on and locate very small objects Mouthing is very prominent (places objects in mouth) Can push up on hands and knees Crawls backward	***Aspiration*** Keep buttons, beads, syringe caps, and other small objects out of infant's reach. Keep floor free of any small objects. Do not feed infant hard candy, nuts, food with pits or seeds, or whole or cylindric pieces of hot dog. Exercise caution when giving teething biscuits because large chunks may be broken off and aspirated. Do not feed while infant is lying down. Inspect toys for removable parts. Keep baby powder, if used, out of reach. Avoid storing large quantities of cleaning fluid, paints, pesticides, and other toxic substances in home. Discard used containers of poisonous substances. Do not store toxic substances in food containers. Discard used button-sized batteries; store new batteries in safe area. ***Suffocation*** Keep all latex balloons out of reach. Remove all crib toys that are strung across crib or playpen when child begins to push up on hands or knees. ***Falls*** Restrain in a high chair. Keep crib rails raised to full height. ***Poisoning*** Make sure that paint on walls, furniture, windowsills, and toys does not contain lead. Place toxic substances on a high shelf or in locked cabinet. Hang plants or place them out of reach. Know telephone number of local poison control center (usually listed in front of telephone directory), and post near phone.

Continued

Injury Prevention During Infancy—cont'd

Major Developmental Accomplishments	Injury Prevention
Age: 4 to 7 Months—cont'd	
	Burns Place hot objects (e.g., cigarettes, candles, incense) on high surface. Limit exposure to sun; apply sunscreen. ***Motor Vehicles*** See Age: Birth to 4 months. ***Bodily Damage*** Give toys that are smooth and rounded, preferably made of wood or plastic; avoid long, pointed objects as toys. Avoid toys that are excessively loud. Keep sharp objects out of infant's reach.
Age: 8 to 12 Months	
Crawls and creeps Stands, holding on to furniture Stands alone Cruises around furniture Walks Climbs Pulls on objects Throws objects Is able to pick up small objects; has pincer grasp Explores by putting objects in mouth Dislikes being restrained Explores away from parent Has increasing understanding of simple words and phrases	***Aspiration*** Keep lint and small objects off floor, off furniture, and out of reach of children. Take care in feeding solid table food to ensure that very small pieces are given. Do not use beanbag toys or allow child to play with dried beans. (See also under Age: 4 to 7 months.) ***Suffocation and Drowning*** Keep doors of ovens, dishwashers, refrigerators, coolers, and front-loading clothes washers and dryers closed at all times. If storing an unused appliance, such as a refrigerator, remove the door. Supervise contact with inflated balloons; immediately discard popped balloons and keep uninflated balloons out of reach. Fence swimming pools; keep gate locked. Always supervise when near any source of water, such as cleaning buckets, drainage areas, and toilets. Keep bathroom doors closed. Eliminate unnecessary pools of water. Keep one hand on child at all times when child is in tub. ***Falls*** Avoid mobile (wheeled) walkers, especially near stairs, decks, or porches with drop-off surface.† Fence stairways at top and bottom if child has access to either end. Dress infant in safe shoes and clothing (e.g., soles that do not "catch" on floor, tied shoelaces, pant legs that do not touch floor). Ensure that furniture is sturdy enough for child to pull self to standing position and cruise. ***Poisoning*** Do not describe medications as a candy. Do not administer medications unless prescribed by a practitioner. Put away medications and poisons immediately after use; replace child-protector caps properly. ***Burns*** Place guards in front of or around any heating appliances, fireplaces, or furnace. Keep electrical wires hidden or out of reach. Place plastic guards over electrical outlets; place furniture in front of outlets. Keep hanging tablecloths out of reach (child may pull down hot liquids or heavy or sharp objects).

†Because there is a considerable risk of major and minor injuries and even death from the use of walkers, and because there is no clear benefit from their use, the AAP recommends a ban on the manufacture and sale of mobile infant walkers in the United States. The particular risk of walkers in households with stairs is falls. (American Academy of Pediatrics, Committee on Injury and Poison Prevention: Injuries associated with infant walkers, *Pediatrics* 95[5]:778-780, 1995.)

Injury Prevention During Early Childhood (1 to 5 Years of Age)

Developmental Abilities Related to Risk of Injury	Injury Prevention
Walks, runs, and climbs Able to open doors and gates Can ride tricycle Can throw ball and other objects	***Motor Vehicles*** Use federally approved car restraint. Supervise child while playing outside. Do not allow child to play on curb or behind a parked car. Do not permit child to play in piles of leaves, snow, or large cardboard container in trafficked areas. Supervise tricycle riding. Lock fences and doors if children not directly supervised. Teach child to obey pedestrian safety rules: • Obey traffic regulations; walk only in crosswalks and when traffic signal indicates it is safe to cross. • Stand back a step from curb until it is time to cross. • Look left, right, and left again, and check for turning cars before crossing street. • Use sidewalks; when there is no sidewalk, walk on left, facing traffic. • At night, wear clothing in light colors and with fluorescent material attached.
Able to explore if left unsupervised Has great curiosity Helpless in water, unaware of its danger; depth of water has no significance	***Drowning*** Supervise closely when near any source of water, including buckets. Keep bathroom door and lid on toilet closed. Have fence around swimming pool; lock gate. Teach swimming and water safety (not a substitute for protection).
Able to reach heights by climbing, stretching, standing on toes, and using objects as a ladder Pulls objects Explores any holes or openings Can open drawers and closets Unaware of potential sources of heat or fire Plays with mechanical objects Turn pot handles toward back of stove.	***Burns*** Place electric appliances, such as coffee maker, frying pan, and popcorn popper, toward back of counter. Place guardrails in front of radiators, fireplaces, or other heating elements. Store matches and cigarette lighters in locked or inaccessible area; discard carefully. Place burning candles, incense, hot foods, ashes, embers, and cigarettes out of reach. Do not let tablecloth hang within child's reach. Do not let electrical cord from iron or other appliance hang within child's reach. Cover electrical outlets with protective devices. Keep electrical wires hidden or out of reach. Do not allow child to play with electrical appliances, wires, or lighters. Stress danger of open flames; explain what "hot" means. Always check bath water temperature; set hot water heater at 48.9° C (120° F) or lower; do not allow children to play with faucets. Apply a sunscreen with sun protection factor (SPF) 15 or higher when child is exposed to sunlight (Community Focus box, Reducing Sun Exposure)
Explores by putting objects in mouth Can open drawers, closets, and most containers Climbs Cannot read warning labels Does not know safe dose or amount	***Poisoning*** Place all potentially toxic agents (including plants) in a locked cabinet or out of reach. Replace medications and poisons immediately; replace child-resistant caps properly. Do not refer to medications as candy. Do not store large supplies of toxic agents. Promptly discard empty poison containers; never reuse to store a food item. Teach child not to play in trash containers. Never remove labels from containers of toxic substances. Know number and location of nearest poison control center (usually listed in front of telephone directory), and post near phone.

Continued

Injury Prevention During Early Childhood (1 to 5 Years of Age)—cont'd

Developmental Abilities Related to Risk of Injury	Injury Prevention
Able to open doors and some windows Goes up and down stairs Depth perception unrefined Gait is unsteady (toddler) Climbs on objects Unaware of potential danger from objects, situations	***Falls*** Keep screen in window, nail securely, and use guardrail. Place gates at top and bottom of stairs. Keep doors locked or use child-resistant doorknob covers at entry to stairs, high porch, or other elevated area, such as laundry chute. Remove unsecured or scatter rugs. Apply nonskid mats in bathtubs or showers. Keep crib rails fully raised and mattress at lowest level. Place carpeting under crib and in bathroom. Keep large toys and bumper pads out of crib or playpen (child can use these as "stairs" to climb out); move to youth bed when child is able to crawl out of crib. Avoid using walkers with wheels, especially near stairs. Dress in safe clothing (e.g., soles that do not "catch" on floor, tied shoelaces, pant legs that do not touch floor). Keep child restrained in vehicles; never leave unattended in shopping cart or stroller. Supervise at playgrounds; select play areas with soft ground cover and safe equipment (Community Focus box, Playground Safety).
Puts things in mouth May swallow hard or inedible pieces of food Explores places and things (natural curiosity)	***Choking and Suffocation*** Avoid large, round chunks of meat, such as whole hot dogs (slice lengthwise, then into short pieces). Avoid fruit with pits, fish with bones, dried beans, hard candy, chewing gum, nuts, popcorn, grapes, and marshmallows. Choose large, sturdy toys without sharp edges or small, removable parts. Discard old refrigerators, ovens, and other appliances; if storing old appliance, remove doors. Keep automatic garage door transmitter in inaccessible place. Select toy boxes or chests without heavy, hinged lids. Keep window blind cords out of child's reach. Remove drawstrings from clothing.
Still clumsy in many skills Easily distracted from tasks Unaware of potential danger from situations and strangers or other people	***Bodily Damage*** Avoid giving sharp or pointed objects (e.g., knives, scissors, toothpicks), especially when walking or running. Do not allow lollipops or similar objects in mouth when walking or running. Teach safety precautions (e.g., to carry fork or scissors with pointed ends away from face). Store all dangerous tools, garden equipment, and firearms in locked cabinets. Be alert to danger from animals, including household pets. Use safety glass and decals on large glassed areas, such as sliding glass doors. Teach personal safety: • Teach name, address, and phone number and to ask for help from appropriate people (cashier, security guard, police officer) if lost; have identification on child (e.g., sewn in clothes or inside shoe). • Avoid letting child wear personalized clothing in public places. • Teach child to never go with a stranger. • Teach child to tell parents if anyone makes child feel uncomfortable in any way. • Always listen to child's concerns regarding behavior of others. • Teach child to say "no" when confronted with uncomfortable situations.

COMMUNITY FOCUS

Reducing Sun Exposure

Remember that tanning indicates sun injury, and the risk of skin cancer begins in childhood.

Keep infants and children out of the sun as much as possible.

Use carriage with hood when taking infants outdoors.

Use stroller with canopy for older infants.

Schedule activities to avoid child's sun exposure between 10 AM and 4 PM whenever possible.

Take increased precautions when living or vacationing in the mountains or the tropics.

Protect child with clothing (e.g., sun hat, long-sleeved shirt, long pants) when outdoors; avoid sandals (wear closed shoes).

Avoid sheer clothing or bathing suits that allow the sun's rays to penetrate the fabric.

Use sunscreen with sun protection factor (SPF) of at least 15.

Apply sunscreen liberally to exposed areas:

- Use a waterproof sunscreen if possible.
- Apply a small amount of sunscreen on the child's back as a test; if the child develops a rash contact the pediatrician.
- Apply a broad-spectrum sunscreen to protect against UVA and UVB rays.
- Apply 30 minutes before every exposure.
- Apply on cloudy as well as sunny days.
- Apply even when child plays in shade (sun reflects from sand, snow, cement, and water).
- Reapply liberally every 2 to 3 hours and after child goes in the water or sweats heavily.
- Use sunscreen for protection, not for prolonged sun exposure.

Check with child's practitioner regarding any medications that child is taking that may cause photosensitivity, and observe for any evidence of side effects (rash, redness, swelling).

Use UV-blocking sunglasses when possible to protect child's eyes.

Examine skin regularly for signs of any change in pigmented nevi (rapid growth, crusting, ulceration, bleeding, change in pigmentation, development of inflamed satellite lesions, loss of normal skin lines) or subjective symptoms (tenderness, pain, itching).

If child has sunburn with blistering, pain, or fever, contact the pediatrician.

Encourage child to avoid lamps or tanning parlors, and explain hazards of same.

Set a good example by following these guidelines.

Modified from American Academy of Pediatrics: *Protecting your child from the sun*, Elk Grove Village, Ill, The Academy, retrieved March 22, 2007, from *http://www.aap.org/family/protectsun.htm.*

COMMUNITY FOCUS

Playground Safety

Be certain that playground equipment has no sharp edges, corners, or projections.

Make sure that concrete footings are not exposed.

Examine area to make sure that there is a safe, resilient surface under equipment (e.g., sand, wood chips, composite material) to reduce the impact from a fall.

Be certain that the size of the equipment matches child.

Make sure there are no holes or other places where fingers, arms, legs, and necks could get caught.

Slides should not have an incline of more than 30 degrees and should have evenly spaced rungs for climbing and protective tunnels.

S-hooks on swings must be closed.

Check for litter, broken glass, exposed wires, electrical outlets, and animal excreta.

COMMUNITY FOCUS

Recreational Water Illness

Since the 1980s there has been an increase in the number of childhood illnesses and deaths related to swallowing, breathing, or having contact with contaminated water in wading or swimming pools, spas, ponds, streams, rivers and lakes. Common illnesses may include gastrointestinal and respiratory tract illness and neurologic, skin, eye, and wound infections. To avoid such illnesses the following are recommended for children and adults:

- Avoid swimming when ill or having diarrhea.
- Do not swallow recreational pool water.
- Avoid swimming in untreated, stagnant pools of water.
- Observe child closely for water swallowing in recreational water.
- Wash hands after each diaper change.
- Change diapers in restroom, not by recreational water.
- Wash child's perianal area with soap and water before entering recreational water.
- Wash hands with soap and water after using restroom (keep a supply of hand disinfectant moist towelettes on hand for such uses).

Modified from American Academy of Pediatrics, Committee on Infectious Diseases, Pickering L, editor: *2006 Red book: report of the Committee on Infectious Diseases,* ed 27, Elk Grove Village, Ill, 2006, The Academy.

Injury Prevention During School-Age Years

Developmental Abilities Related to Risk of Injury	Injury Prevention
Is increasingly involved in activities away from home Is excited by speed and motion Is easily distracted by environment Can be reasoned with	***Motor Vehicles*** Educate child regarding proper use of seat belts while riding in a vehicle. Maintain discipline while in a vehicle (e.g., children must keep arms inside, must not lean against doors, must not interfere with driver). Remind parents and children that no one should ride in the bed of a pickup truck. Emphasize safe pedestrian behavior. Insist on wearing safety apparel (e.g., a helmet) when applicable, such as when riding a bicycle, motorcycle, moped, or all-terrain vehicle (Figure 2-2) (Community Focus boxes, Bicycle Safety and Safe Use of All-Terrain Vehicles).
Is apt to overdo; has poorly defined awareness of own limitations/boundaries May work hard to perfect a skill Has cautious, but not fearful, gross motor actions Likes swimming	***Drowning*** Teach child to swim. Teach basic rules of water safety. Select safe and supervised places to swim. Check sufficient water depth for diving. Teach child to swim with a companion. Make sure child wears an approved flotation device in water or while boating. Advocate for legislation requiring fencing around pools. Learn cardiopulmonary resuscitation (CPR).
Has increasing independence Is adventuresome Enjoys trying new things	***Burns*** Make sure smoke detectors are in home. Set hot-water heater temperature at 48.9° C (120° F) to avoid scald burns. Instruct child in behavior involving contact with potential burn hazards (e.g., gasoline, matches, bonfires or barbecues, lighter fluid, firecrackers, cigarette lighters, cooking utensils, chemistry sets) and to avoid climbing or flying kites around high-tension wires. Instruct child in proper behavior in the event of fire (e.g., fire drills at home and school). Teach child safe cooking methods (use low heat; avoid frying; be careful of steam burns, scalds, or exploding food, especially from microwaving). Apply a sunscreen with SPF 15 or higher when child is exposed to sunlight.
Adheres to group rules May be easily influenced by peers Has strong allegiance to friends	***Poisoning*** Educate child regarding hazards of taking nonpresciption and prescription drugs and chemicals, including aspirin and alcohol. Teach child to say "no" if offered illegal or dangerous drugs or alcohol. Keep potentially dangerous products in properly labeled receptacles—preferably locked and out of reach.

Injury Prevention During School-Age Years—cont'd

Developmental Abilities Related to Risk of Injury	Injury Prevention
Has increased physical skills Needs strenuous physical activity Is interested in acquiring new skills and in perfecting attained skills Is daring and adventurous, especially with peers Frequently plays in hazardous places Confidence often exceeds physical capacity. Desires group loyalty and has strong need for friends' approval Attempts hazardous feats Accompanies friends to potentially hazardous facilities Is likely to overdo Growth in height exceeds muscular growth and coordination.	***Bodily Damage*** Help provide facilities for supervised activities. Encourage playing in safe places. Keep firearms safely locked up except during adult supervision. Teach proper care of, use of, and respect for devices with potential danger (e.g., power tools, firecrackers). Teach children animal safety (Community Focus box, Animal Safety). Stress eye, ear, and mouth protection when using potentially hazardous objects or devices or when engaged in potentially hazardous sports (e.g., baseball). Teach safety regarding use of corrective devices (glasses); if child wears contact lenses, monitor duration of wear to prevent corneal damage. Stress careful selection, use, and maintenance of sports and recreation equipment such as skateboards and in-line skates (Community Focus box, Skateboard and In-line Skate Safety). Emphasize proper conditioning, safe practices, and use of safety equipment for sports or recreational activities. Caution against engaging in hazardous sports, such as those involving trampolines. Use safety glass and decals on large glassed areas, such as sliding glass doors. Use window guards to prevent falls. Teach name, address, and phone number and how to ask for help from appropriate people (cashier, security guard, police officer) if lost; have identification on child (sewn in clothes, inside shoe). Teach stranger safety: • Do not let child wear personalized clothing in public places. • Caution child to never go with a stranger. • Have child tell parents if anyone makes child feel uncomfortable in any way. • Always listen to child's concerns regarding behavior of others. • Teach child to say "no" when confronted with uncomfortable situations.

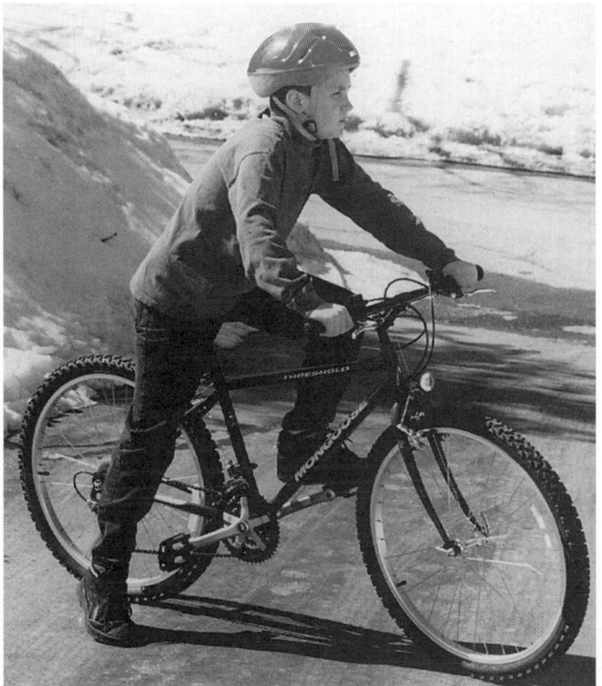

FIGURE **2-2** Proper bicycle helmet fit. A helmet should sit on top of the head in a level position and not rock back and forth or from side to side. If the child cannot see the edge of the brim at the extreme upper range of vision, the helmet is probably out of place. Adjust the chin straps so that when buckled they hold the helmet firmly in place. Try to remove the helmet without undoing the chin strap. If the helmet comes off or shifts over the eyes, readjust and try again. If no adjustment seems to work, this helmet is not a good fit; try another. Make sure child *always* fastens the strap when wearing the helmet.

COMMUNITY FOCUS

Bicycle Safety

Always wear properly fitted bicycle helmet that is U.S. Consumer Product Safety Commission (CPSC) or Snell Memorial Foundation approved (see Figure 2-2); older helmets designated *only* as American National Standards Institute (ANSI) approved no longer meet safety standards.
Replace damaged helmet.
Avoid riding on the handlebar or crossbar.
Ride bicycles with traffic and away from parked cars.
Ride single file.
Walk bicycles through busy intersections using crosswalks only.
Give hand signals well in advance of turning or stopping.
Keep as close to the curb as practical.
Watch for drainage grates, potholes, soft shoulders, and loose dirt or gravel.
Keep both hands on handlebars, except when signaling.
Never ride with more than one person on a bicycle (such as on handlebars or back bumper).
Do not carry packages that interfere with vision or control; do not drag objects behind bike.
Watch for and yield to pedestrians.
Watch for cars backing up or pulling out of driveways; be especially careful at intersections.
Look left, right, then left again before turning into traffic or onto a roadway.
Never hitch a ride by grabbing on to a truck or other vehicle.
Learn rules of the road, and show respect for traffic officers.
Obey all local ordinances.
Wear shoes that fit securely while riding.
Wear light colors at night, and attach fluorescent material to clothing and bicycle.
Be certain the bicycle is the correct size for the rider.
Equip bicycle with proper lights and reflectors.
Have the bicycle inspected to ensure good mechanical condition.
Children passengers must wear appropriate-size helmets and ride in specially designed protective seats. Passengers should be at least 1 year old.

From American Academy of Pediatrics, Committee on Injury and Poison Prevention: Bicycle helmets, *Pediatrics* 108(4):1030-1032, 2001.

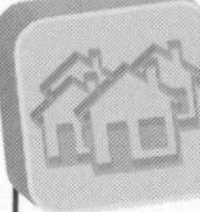

COMMUNITY FOCUS

Safe Use of All-Terrain Vehicles (ATVs)

Adolescents and children under the age of 16 years should not operate an off-road vehicle.
Vehicles should be sturdy and stable; high-quality construction is essential.
Riders should receive instruction from a mature, experienced cyclist or a certified instructor.
Riding should be supervised and allowed only after the rider has demonstrated competence in handling the machine on familiar terrain (preferably licensing is required).
Riders should wear approved helmets designed for motorcycle use (not bicycle), eye protection, and protective reflective clothing (e.g., trousers, boots, gloves).
Parents should prohibit street or paved road use of off-road vehicles.
Riding should be restricted to familiar terrain.
Nighttime riding should not be allowed.
Vehicle should not carry more than one person.
Riders should avoid riding after alcohol consumption.
Parents and other adults should set an example for ATV safety and riding.

Modified from American Academy of Pediatrics, Committee on Injury and Poison Prevention: All-terrain vehicle injury prevention: two-, three-, and four-wheeled unlicensed motorized vehicles, *Pediatrics* 105:1352-1354, 2000. (Statement reaffirmed January 1, 2007.)

COMMUNITY FOCUS

Animal Safety

Never leave a baby or small child alone with a dog.

Teach children to avoid all strange animals, especially wild, sick, or injured ones, who may be carriers of rabies. (Use the same techniques employed in teaching children not to talk to strangers.)

Teach children to avoid aggressive, dangerous, and nervous animals in their neighborhood.

Vaccinate your own dog against rabies.

Be alert to own dog's behavior; avoid child contact if dog appears uncomfortable or is demonstrating aggressive behavior.

Never permit children to break up an animal fight, even when their own pet is involved. Adults must use a rake, broom, or garden hose to separate fighting animals.

Teach children the danger of mistreating or teasing pets (i.e., that animals will bite if mauled, annoyed, or frightened).

Spay or neuter your pets. (Spaying or neutering reduces aggression, not protectiveness.)

Avoid direct eye contact with a threatening dog; remain motionless until the threatening dog leaves the area.

Teach children to never put their face close to an animal. Teach children not to disturb an animal that is eating, sleeping, or caring for its young.

Never approach a strange dog that is confined or restrained; do not keep animals confined with short ropes or chains. (This can make them aggressive or vicious, especially when teased.)

Teach children to not run, ride a bicycle, or skate in front of a dog (it will startle the dog and often encourages chasing the child); teach children the importance of avoiding bike routes where dogs are known to chase vehicles.

Do not allow an inexperienced child or adult to feed a dog. (If the person pulls back when the animal moves to take the food, this can frighten the animal.)

If a dog has not seen you approach, speak to the animal to make it aware of your presence and avoid startling the animal.

Allow a dog to see and sniff a child before allowing the child to pet the animal.

Do not permit a child to lead a large dog.

Train or socialize a dog for appropriate behavior; avoid aggressive play with pets.

Do not adopt pets for children until children demonstrate their maturity and ability to handle and care for pets.

From Humane Society of the United States (HSUS): *Preventing and avoiding dog bites,* Washington, DC, 1998, HSUS; and American Academy of Pediatrics, *A lesson in dog safety can help prevent bites,* retrieved June 12, 2006, from *http://www.aap.org/advocacy/releases/dogbitetips.htm.*

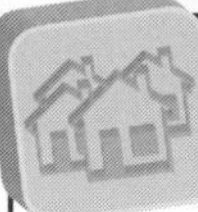

COMMUNITY FOCUS

Skateboard and In-Line Skate Safety

Children younger than 5 years of age should not use skateboards or in-line skates. They are not developmentally prepared to protect themselves from injury. Inexperienced children are encouraged to skate on indoor rinks and to avoid tricks.

Children who ride skateboards or in-line skates should wear helmets and protective equipment (wrist guards, knee pads, and elbow pads) to prevent injury.

The helmet should be certified by one of the following: CPSC, ANSI, or ASTM.

Skaters performing tricks are encouraged to wear heavy-duty protective gear.

Skateboards and in-line skates should never be used near traffic and should be prohibited on streets and highways. Activities that bring motor vehicles and skateboards together (e.g., catching a ride, truck-surfing, or skitching) are especially dangerous.

Some types of use, such as riding homemade ramps on hard surfaces, can be particularly hazardous.

Modified from American Academy of Pediatrics, Committee on Injury and Poison Prevention and Committee on Sports Medicine and Fitness: In-line skating injuries in children and adolescents, *Pediatrics* 101(4):720-722, 1998. (Statement reaffirmed, *Pediatrics* 117(5):1846-1847, 2006.)

Injury Prevention During Adolescence

Development Abilities Related to Risk of Injury	Injury Prevention
Need for independence and freedom Testing independence Age permitted to drive a motor vehicle (varies) Inclination for risk taking Feeling of indestructibility Need for discharging energy, often at expense of logical thinking and other control mechanisms Strong need for peer approval May attempt hazardous feats Peak incidence for practice and participation in sports Access to more complex tools, objects, and locations Can assume responsibility for own actions (Community Focus box)	***Motor and Nonmotor Vehicles*** ***Pedestrian***—Emphasize and encourage safe pedestrian behavior. At night, walk with a friend, not alone. If someone is following you, go to nearest place with people. Do not walk in secluded areas; take well-traveled walkways. ***Passenger***—Promote appropriate behavior while riding in a motor vehicle. ***Driver***—Provide competent driver education; encourage judicious use of vehicle, discourage drag racing, playing chicken; maintain vehicle in proper condition (brakes, tires, etc.). Teach and promote safety and maintenance of motorcycles; promote and encourage wearing of safety apparel, such as a helmet and long trousers. Reinforce teaching about the dangers of drugs, including alcohol, when operating a motor vehicle. ***Drowning*** Teach nonswimmers to swim. Teach basic rules of water safety: Judicious selection of place to swim. Sufficient water depth for diving. Swimming with companion. ***Burns*** Reinforce proper behavior involving contact with burn hazards (gasoline, electric wires, fires). Advise regarding excessive exposure to natural or artificial (ultraviolet) light, such as tanning. Discourage smoking. Encourage use of sunscreen. ***Poisoning*** Educate in hazards of nonprescription, prescription, and recreational drug use, including alcohol. ***Falls*** Teach and encourage general safety measures in all activities. ***Bodily Damage*** Promote proper instruction in sports and safe use of sports equipment. Instruct in safe use of and respect for firearms and other devices with potential danger (e.g., power tools, fireworks). Provide and encourage use of protective equipment when using potentially hazardous devices. Promote access to and/or provision of safe facilities for sports and recreation. Be alert for signs of depression (potential suicide). Discourage use and/or availability of hazardous sports equipment (e.g., trampoline, surfboards). Instruct regarding proper use of corrective devices, such as glasses, contact lenses, and hearing aids. Encourage judicious application of safety principles and prevention.

COMMUNITY FOCUS

Steps for Condom Use*

1. Be careful when opening the package; handle the condom gently, and check for breaks or holes in the condom.
2. Squeeze a dab of water-based contraceptive jelly or cream with nonoxynol-9 into the tip of the condom.
3. Put on the condom as soon as erection occurs and before any vaginal, anal, or oral contact with the penis.
4. Unroll the condom on the erect penis, leaving about ½ inch of space at the tip of the condom.
5. Apply some of the contraceptive cream or jelly around the vagina or anus before entry.
6. Hold the rim of the condom in place when withdrawing the penis.
7. Take the condom off when away from the partner's genitalia.
8. Throw the used condom away. *Never reuse a condom.*
9. Never use an oil-based spermicide or lubricant on a latex condom, as it will damage the condom.

Modified from *Entering adulthood: preventing sexually transmitted diseases*, Santa Cruz, Calif, 1989, Network Publications.
*For additional information on AIDS/HIV, contact CDC National Prevention Information Network (NPIN), PO Box 6003, Rockville, MD 20849, (800) 458-5231; AIDS Info, (800) 448-0440, hearing impaired (888) 480-3739; and CDC index on HIV: *http://www.cdc.gov/hiv.*

Guidelines for Automobile Safety Seats

This important information is provided because motor vehicle crashes cause significant numbers of deaths and injuries in infants and young children. These deaths and injuries are mostly preventable. All states now have laws that require children to be properly secured in motor vehicles. For more information about your laws, contact your state highway safety office.

Remember that the most dangerous place for an infant or child to ride is in the arms or on the lap of another person.

Nurses have a responsibility for educating parents regarding the importance of car restraints and their proper use. Several types of restraints are available: infant-only devices, convertible models for both infants and toddlers, booster seats, built-in forward facing seats, shoulder-lap safety belts, and devices for children with special needs. Some vehicles have manufacturer-installed seats that convert to child car restraints.

The *infant-only restraint* is a semireclined seat (45 to 50 degrees) that faces the rear of the car (Figure 2-3). A rear-facing car seat provides the best protection for the disproportionately heavy head and weak neck of an infant. This position minimizes the stress on the neck by spreading the forces of a frontal crash over the entire back, neck, and head; the spine is supported by the back of the car seat. If the seat were faced forward, the head would whip forward because of the force of the crash, creating enormous stress on the neck. The restraint is anchored to the vehicle with the vehicle's seat belt or LATCH (lower anchors and tethers for children) system, and the restraint has a harness system for securing the infant. The five-point harness system provides the most effective support for infant restraint; the three-point harness system secures only the upper body. Many infant seats have a plastic base that can be left in the car; the seat latches or clicks into the base so that the base does not have to be installed each time the car seat is removed.

The *convertible restraint* is suitable for infants in the rear-facing position (Figure 2-4) and for toddlers in the forward-facing position (Figure 2-5). The transition point for switching to the forward-facing position is defined by the manufacturer but is generally at a body weight of 9 kg (20 pounds) and 1 year of age. If the child weighs 20 pounds or more but is not 1 year old, the rear-facing position is still recommended. It is recommended, for added protection, that infants ride in the rear-facing position until they reach the highest height and weight recommended by the seat manufacturer. Convertible safety seats should be used until the child weighs at least 40 pounds (18 kg) regardless of age and as long as the child fits properly into the seat. The restraint consists of a molded hard plastic with energy-absorbing padding and a special harness system designed to hold the child firmly in the seat and distribute the forces to body areas that can withstand the impact.

Convertible restraints use different types of harness systems: a *five-point harness* that consists of a strap over each shoulder, one on each side of the pelvis, and one between the legs (all five come together at a common buckle), as well as a *padded overhead shield* that uses shoulder straps attached to a shield that is held in place by a crotch strap. With both the infant and toddler restraints, it is important that extra blankets, head cushions,

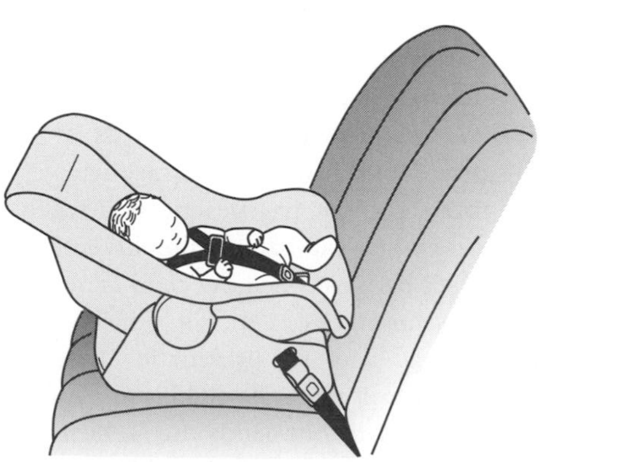

FIGURE **2-3** Rear-facing, infant-only safety seat.

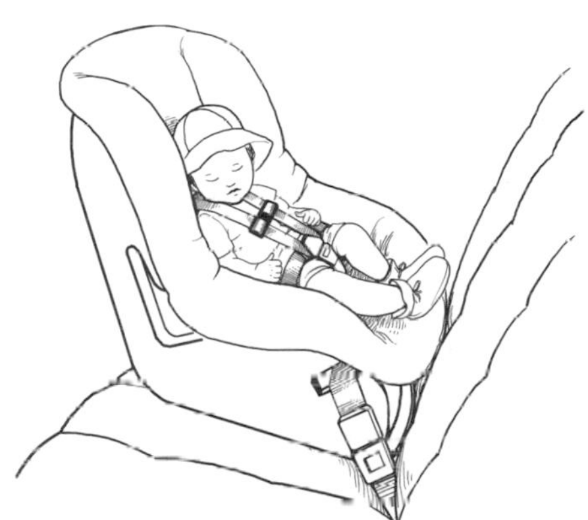

FIGURE **2-4** Convertible seat in rear-facing position for use with infants.

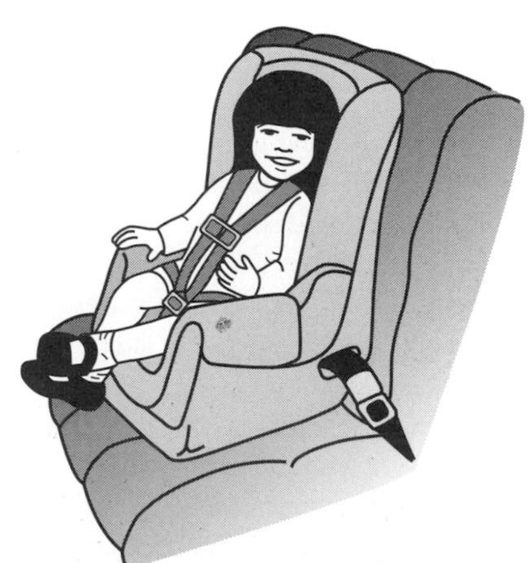

FIGURE **2-5** Convertible seat in forward-facing position for toddlers.

or padding that did not come as original equipment not be added because these "add-ons" create spaces of air between the child and the restraint and decrease support for the back, head, and neck. Cars with free-sliding latch plates on the lap or shoulder belt require the use of a metal locking clip to keep the belt in a tight-holding position. The locking clip is threaded onto the belt above the latch plate (Figure 2-6).

Booster seats are not restraint systems like the convertible devices because they depend on the vehicle belts to hold the child and booster seat in place. Three booster models have been approved by the National Highway Traffic Safety Administration (NHTSA): the high-back belt-positioning seat, which provides head and neck support for the child riding in a vehicle seat without a head rest; the no-back belt-positioning seat, which should be used only if the vehicle seat has a head rest; and a combination seat, which converts from a forward-facing toddler seat to a booster seat. This last model is equipped with a harness for use in toddlers; the harness may be removed and a shoulder-lap belt used when the child outgrows the harness. Booster seats are used for children who are less than 145 cm (4¾ feet) tall and who weigh more than 18 kg (40 pounds), typically those between 4 and 8 years of age. A booster seat should be used until the child is able to sit against the back of the seat with feet hanging down and legs bent at the knees. The belt-positioning booster model raises a child higher in the seat, moving the shoulder part of the belt off the neck and the lap portion of the belt off the abdomen onto the pelvis (Figure 2-7).

Children with special needs may require a restraint system that secures them appropriately in the event of a crash. Examples of such devices include car bed restraints for infants who cannot tolerate a semireclining position and specially adapted molded-plastic chairs for children who have spica casts (Britax Hippo by SnugSeat, [800] 336 7684). The E-Z-On vest is a special safety harness for larger children with poor trunk control. Additional safety restraints and a listing of distributors are available at the SafetyBeltSafe U.S.A. website *(http://www.carseat.org)*, or call (800) 745-SAFE (Spanish: [800] 747-SANO).

Children should use specially designed car restraints until they weigh at least 60 pounds (27 kg) or are 8 years old. Children who outgrow the convertible restraint may still be able to ride safely in a booster seat until the midpoint of the head is higher than the vehicle seat back. If a car safety seat is not available, the lap belt provides more protection than no restraint (except for infants, for whom there is no safe alternative to approved restraint devices). Shoulder-only automatic belts are designed to protect adults. Children should use the manual shoulder belts in the rear seat. Air bags do not take the place of child safety seats or seat belts and can be lethal to young children.

The LATCH universal child safety seat system was implemented as a requirement starting in 2002 for all new automobiles and child safety seats. This system provides a uniform anchorage consisting of two lower anchorages and one upper anchorage in the rear seat of the vehicle. When used appropriately the top anchor (tether) strap prevents the child from pitching forward in a crash. If the tether strap is not used, up to 90% of the restraint's protection is lost. Instructions for proper installation of the tether strap and permanent bracket are included with the car restraint. New child safety seats will have a hook, buckle, strap, or other connector that attaches to the anchorage (Figure 2-8). Seat belts will no longer be used to anchor child safety seats to newer vehicles. The first phase requires all new cars to have an upper anchorage. After fall 2002, all new cars were required to have the entire LATCH system.*

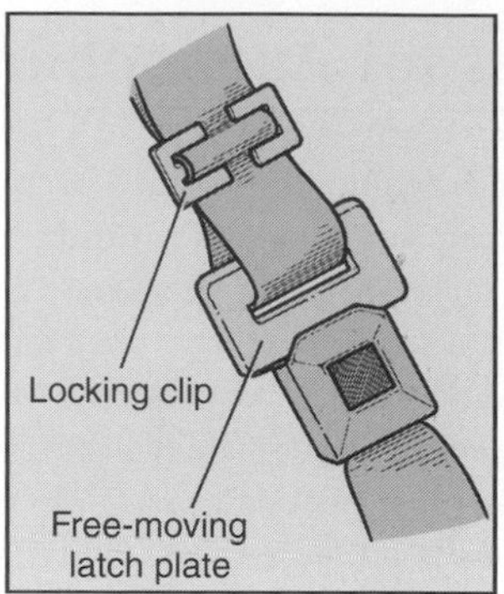

FIGURE **2-6** Locking clip used with free-sliding lap/shoulder belt to keep the belt in a tight holding position.

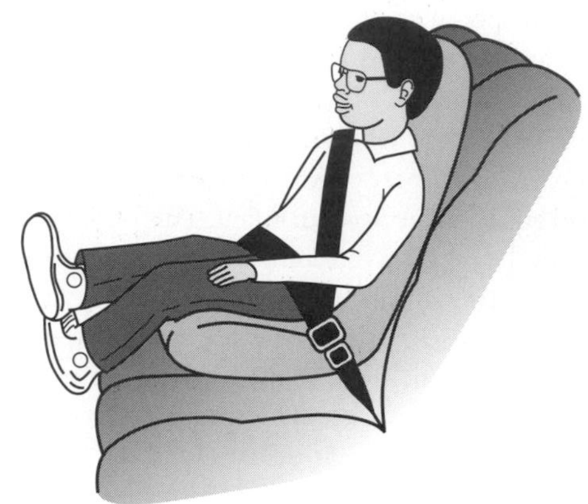

FIGURE **2-7** Automobile booster seat. Note placement of shoulder strap (away from neck and face).

The safest area of the car for children of any age is the middle of the back seat. Children should not ride in the front seat of any activated air bag–equipped car, except in emergencies, and then the vehicle seat must be as far back as possible. Many newer model cars are equipped with a "smart" air bag system that allows air bag deactivation when a child is riding in the passenger seat. Parents should remember to turn the air bag switch back on once the child is no longer in the front seat. Also, many newer model vehicles are equipped with side-impact air bags for protection; these air bags are reported to be safe as long as the child is in a proper restraint system. The NHTSA recommends that vehicle owners with

*U.S. Department of Transportation, National Highway Traffic Safety Administration, 400 Seventh St SW, Washington, DC 20590; (800) 424-9393; *http://www.nhtsa.dot.gov.*

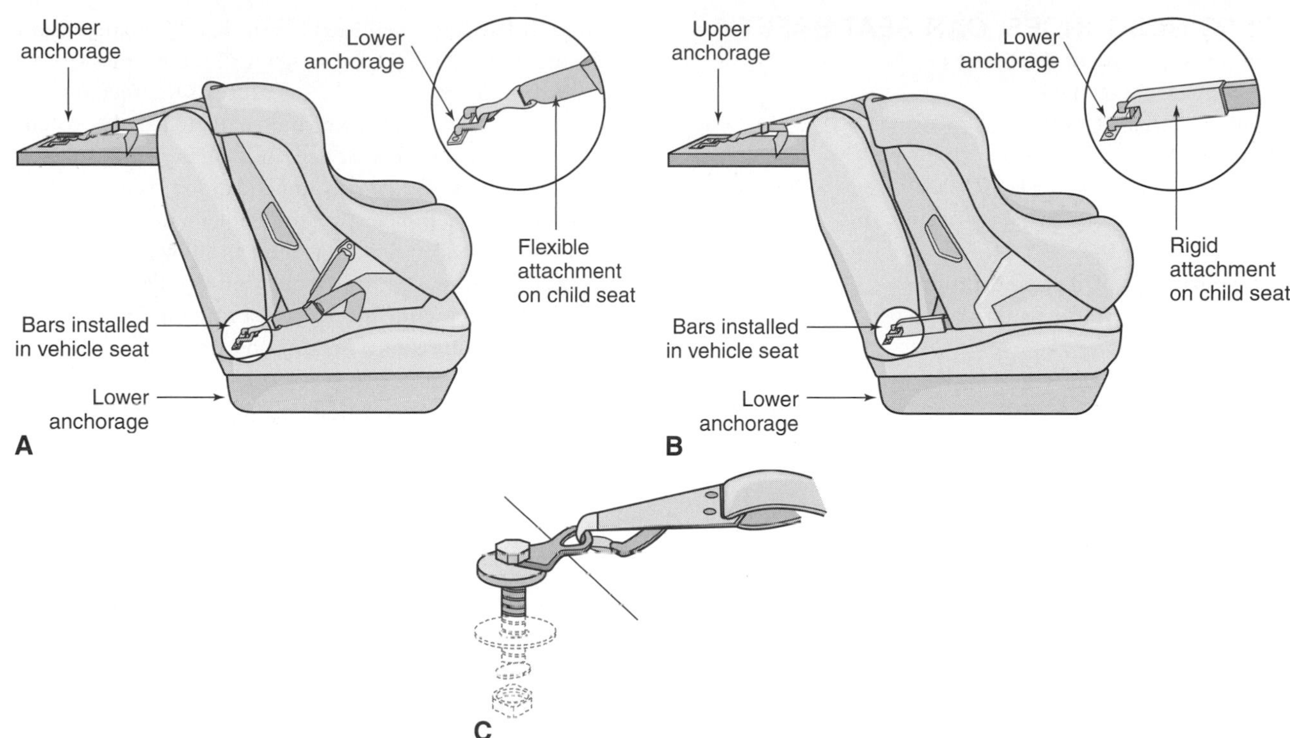

FIGURE **2-8** Lower anchors and tethers for children (LATCH). **A**, Flexible two-point attachment with top tether. **B**, Rigid two-point attachment with top tether. **C**, Top tether. (Courtesy U.S. Department of Transportation, National Highway Traffic Safety Administration.)

side-impact air bags check the manufacturer's recommendations for child safety. The NHTSA (2005) recommends that children not lean on chest-only or head-chest combination side air bags. Because of a large number of adverse events involving serious injuries and even some child fatalities with air bags, some manufacturers designed and installed air bags designed to minimize injury to adults and children at deployment yet still protect the passenger. Because diverse types of air bags continue to be in use, parents are cautioned to continue placing all children younger than 13 years old in the back seat with the proper child restraint system.

SAFETY ALERT

Safety belts should be worn low on the hips, snug, and not on the abdominal area. Children should be taught to sit up straight to allow for proper fit. The shoulder belt is used *only* if it does not cross the child's neck or face.

For any restraint to be effective, it must be used consistently and properly. Examples of misuse include misrouting of the vehicle seat belt through the restraint, failing to use the vehicle seat belt through the restraint, failing to use a tether strap, failing to use the restraint's harness system, and incorrectly positioning the child, especially facing infants forward instead of rearward. To address these issues, nurses must stress correct use of car restraints and rules that ensure compliance and can emphasize to parents that children riding in car safety seats are generally better behaved than children left unrestrained (Community Focus box).

Despite widespread education and publicity regarding seat belt safety restraint and the danger of front seat air bags for children, surveys indicate that children are still placed in potentially lethal situations of either improper seat restraint or no restraint.

COMMUNITY FOCUS

Using Car Safety Restraints

Read manufacturer's directions, and follow them exactly.

Anchor safety seat securely to car's seat, and apply harness snugly to child.

Do not start car until everyone is properly restrained.

Always use the restraint, even for short trips.

If child begins to climb out or undo harness, firmly say, "no." It may be necessary to stop the car to reinforce the expected behavior. Use rewards, such as stars or stickers, to encourage cooperative behavior.

Encourage child to help attach buckles, straps, and shields.

Decrease boredom on long trips. Keep special toys in car for quiet play; talk to child; point out objects, and teach child about them. Stop periodically. If child wishes to sleep, make sure child stays in restraint.

Insist that others who transport children also follow these safety rules.

PARENT RESOURCES, CAR SEAT SAFETY

American Academy of Pediatrics
141 Northwest Point Blvd.
Elk Grove Village, IL 60007
(847) 434-4000
Website: *http://www.aap.org; http://www.aap.org/family/carseatguide.htm*

U.S. Department of Transportation
National Highway Traffic Safety Administration
400 Seventh St., SW
Washington, DC 20590
(888) 327-4236
Website: *http://www.nhtsa.dot.gov*

SafeKids Worldwide
Website: *http://www.safekids.org*
Contact your local SafeKids chapter, which sponsors Seat Belt Fit clinics to ensure that seat belt restraint systems being used are adequate protection. For children with special needs, the following is an available resource for car restraint information:

Automotive Safety Program
Riley Hospital for Children
75 West Dr., Room 004
Indianapolis, IN 46202
(317) 274-2977; (800) 543-6227
Website: *http://www.preventinjury.org*

NEONATAL CAR SEAT EVALUATION: THE PRETERM AND NEAR TERM INFANT

The AAP (1996, 1999)* recommended that infants born before 37 weeks' gestation be evaluated for apnea, bradycardia, or oxygen desaturation episodes before hospital discharge. It has been well established that all infants at lower weights, in particular those weighing 2500 g or less, require certain modifications for existing car seats to prevent slouching sideways or forward, which essentially has the potential for causing airway obstruction and subsequent oxygen desaturation. The AAP recommendations suggested that facilities develop policies for the implementation of a program of evaluation; however, there are few evidence-based practice recommendations published to date delineating specific requirements for such a program. Based on the available literature some suggestions are provided for guidance in providing a car seat evaluation of infants born before 37 weeks of gestation.

- Use the parents' car seat for the evaluation.
- Perform the evaluation 1 to 7 days before the infant's anticipated discharge.
- Secure infant in car seat per guidelines using blanket rolls on side.
- Set pulse oximeter low alarm at 88% (arbitrary).
- Set heart rate low alarm limit at 80 and apnea alarm at 20 seconds (cardiorespiratory monitor).
- Leave the infant undisturbed in car seat for 60 minutes *or* for the time period parents state it takes to arrive at their home.
- Document infant's tolerance to car seat evaluation.
- An episode of desaturation, bradycardia, or apnea (20 seconds or more) constitutes a failure, and evaluation by the practitioner must occur before discharge.
- Repeat the test after 24 hours once modifications are made to the car seat, car bed, or infant's position in either restraint system.
- It is recommended that a certified car seat technician place the infant in the car seat (or bed) if a failure occurs.(see NHTSA website above for car seat inspection station)
- The technician will demonstrate appropriate positioning of the infant in the restraint device to the parents and have the parents do a return demonstration.
- Document the interventions, the infant's tolerance, and the parents' return demonstration.

---

*Modified from American Academy of Pediatrics: Safe transportation of premature and low birth weight infants, *Pediatrics* 97(5):758-760, 1996; American Academy of Pediatrics: Transporting children with special health care needs, *Pediatrics* 104(4):988-992, 1999.

Parental Guidance

Guidance During Infancy

FIRST 6 MONTHS

Teach car safety with use of federally approved car seat, facing rearward, in the middle of the back seat—not in a seat with an air bag.

Understand each parent's adjustment to newborn, especially mother's postpartal emotional needs.

Teach care of infant; assist parents to understand infant's individual needs and temperament and that the infant expresses wants through crying.

Reassure parents that infant cannot be spoiled by too much attention during the first 4 to 6 months.

Encourage parents to establish a schedule that meets needs of child and themselves.

Help parents understand infant's need for stimulation in environment.

Support parents' pleasure in seeing child's growing friendliness and social responses, especially smiling.

Plan anticipatory guidance for safety, including placing infant on back to sleep.

Stress need for immunizations.

Prepare for introduction of solid foods.

Encourage parent to take infant and child CPR class.

SECOND 6 MONTHS

Prepare parents for child's stranger anxiety.

Encourage parents to allow child to cling to them and avoid long separation from either parent.

Guide parents concerning discipline because of infant's increasing mobility.

Encourage use of negative voice and eye contact rather than physical punishment as a means of discipline.

Encourage showing most attention when infant is behaving well, rather than when infant is crying.

Teach injury prevention because of child's advancing motor skills and curiosity.

Encourage parents to leave child with suitable caregiver to allow themselves some free time.

Discuss readiness for weaning.

Explore parents' feelings regarding infant's sleep patterns.

Provide anticipatory guidance for safety.

Guidance During Toddler Years

AGES 12 TO 18 MONTHS

Prepare parents for expected behavioral changes of toddler, especially negativism and ritualism.

Assess present feeding habits, and encourage gradual weaning from bottle to cup and increased intake of solid foods.

Stress expected feeding changes of physiologic anorexia, presence of food fads and strong taste preferences, need for scheduled routine at mealtimes, inability to sit through an entire meal, and lack of table manners.

Assess sleep patterns at night, particularly habit of a bedtime bottle, which is a major cause of dental caries, and procrastination behaviors that delay hour of sleep.

Prepare parents for potential dangers of the home, particularly motor vehicle, poisoning, and falling injuries; give appropriate suggestions for childproofing the home.

Discuss need for firm but gentle discipline and ways in which to deal with negativism and temper tantrums; stress positive benefits of appropriate discipline.

Emphasize importance for both child and parents of brief, periodic separations.

Discuss new toys that use developing gross and fine motor, language, cognitive, and social skills.

Emphasize need for dental supervision, types of basic dental hygiene at home, and food habits that predispose children to caries; stress importance of supplemental fluoride (if adequate amounts are not in potable water source).

Discuss options for safe day care (in home or outside of home) as required by parents' work status.

Provide anticipatory guidance for safety.

AGES 18 TO 24 MONTHS

Stress importance of peer companionship in play.

Explore need for preparation for additional sibling; stress importance of preparing child for new experiences.

Discuss present discipline methods, their effectiveness, and parents' feelings about child's negativism; stress that negativism is important aspect of developing self-assertion and independence and is not a sign of spoiling.

Discuss signs of readiness for toilet training; emphasize importance of waiting for physical and psychologic readiness.

Discuss development of fears, such as of darkness or loud noises, and of habits, such as security blanket or thumb sucking; stress normalcy of these transient behaviors.

Prepare parents for signs of regression in time of stress.

Assess child's ability to separate easily from parents for brief periods under familiar circumstances.

Allow parents opportunity to express their feelings of weariness, frustration, and exasperation; be aware that it is often difficult to love toddlers at times when they are not asleep!

Point out some of the expected changes of the next year, such as longer attention span, somewhat less negativism, and increased concern for pleasing others.

Provide anticipatory guidance for safety.

AGES 24-36 MONTHS

Discuss importance of imitation and domestic mimicry and need to include child in activities.

Discuss approaches toward toilet training, particularly realistic expectations and attitude toward toileting accidents.

Stress uniqueness of toddlers' thought processes, especially regarding their use of language, poor understanding of time, causal relationships in terms of proximity of events, and inability to see events from another's perspective.

Stress that discipline must still be quite structured and concrete and that relying solely on verbal reasoning and explanations leads to confusion, misunderstanding, and even injuries.

Discuss investigation of preschool or daycare center toward completion of second year.

Provide anticipatory guidance for safety.

Guidance During Preschool Years

AGE 3 YEARS

Prepare parents for child's increasing interest in widening relationships.

Discuss and encourage enrollment in preschool.

Emphasize importance of setting limits.

Prepare parents to expect exaggerated tension-reduction behaviors, such as need for security blanket.

Encourage parents to offer choices when child vacillates.

Prepare parents to expect marked changes at 3½ years, when child becomes less coordinated, becomes insecure, and exhibits emotional extremes.

Prepare parents for normal dysfluency in speech, and advise them to avoid focusing on the pattern.

Prepare parents to expect extra demands on their attention as a reflection of child's emotional insecurity and fear of loss of love.

Discuss with parents that equilibrium of 3-year-old will change to the aggressive, out-of-bounds behavior of 4-year-old.

Inform parents to anticipate a more stable appetite with wider food selections.

Stress need for protection and education of child to prevent injury.

AGE 4 YEARS

Prepare parents for more aggressive behavior, including motor activity and offensive language.

Prepare parents to expect resistance to their authority.

Explore parental feelings regarding child's behavior.

Suggest some type of respite for primary caregivers, such as placing child in preschool for part of the day.

Prepare parents for child's increasing sexual curiosity.

Emphasize importance of realistic limit setting on behavior and appropriate discipline techniques.

Prepare parents for highly imaginative 4-year-old who indulges in tall tales (to be differentiated from lies) and who has imaginary playmates.

Prepare parents to expect nightmares or an increase in nightmares, and suggest they make sure child is fully awakened from a frightening dream.

Provide reassurance that a period of calm begins at 5 years of age.

AGE 5 YEARS

Inform parents to expect tranquil period at 5 years.

Help parents to prepare child for entrance into school environment.

Make sure immunizations are up-to-date before child enters school.

Suggest that unemployed mothers or fathers consider own activities when child begins school.

Suggest swimming lessons for child.

Guidance During School-Age Years

AGE 6 YEARS

Prepare parents to expect child's strong food preferences and frequent refusals of specific food items.

Inform parents to expect increasing appetite in child.

Prepare parents for emotionality as child experiences erratic mood changes.

Help parents anticipate continued susceptibility to illness.

Teach injury prevention and safety, especially bicycle safety.

Encourage parents to respect child's need for privacy and to provide a separate bedroom for child, if possible.

Prepare parents for child's increasing interests outside the home.

Help parents understand the importance of encouraging child's interactions with peers.

Encourage balanced diet and exercise for prevention of obesity, diabetes, and other preventable cardiovascular disorders.

AGES 7 TO 10 YEARS

Prepare parents to expect improvement in child's health and fewer illnesses, but inform them that allergies may increase or become apparent.
Prepare parents to expect an increase in minor injuries.
Emphasize caution in selecting and maintaining sports equipment, and reemphasize safety.
Prepare parents to expect increased involvement with peers and interest in activities outside the home.
Emphasize the need to encourage independence while maintaining limit setting and discipline.
Prepare mothers to expect more demands when child is 8 years of age.
Prepare fathers to expect increasing admiration at 10 years of age; encourage father-child activities.
Prepare parents for prepubescent changes in girls.
Discuss safety aspects of online usage and monitor child's involvement in same (see Internet Safety, p. 244)

AGES 11 TO 12 YEARS

Help parents prepare child for body changes of pubescence.
Prepare parents to expect a growth spurt in girls.
Make certain child's sex education is adequate with accurate information.
Prepare parents to expect energetic but stormy behavior at 11, to become more even tempered at 12.
Encourage parents to support child's desire to grow up but to allow regressive behavior when needed.
Prepare parents to expect an increase in exploratory sexual activity such as masturbation.
Instruct parents that the amount of rest child needs may increase.
Help parents educate child regarding experimentation with potentially harmful activities.
Encourage keeping immunizations up to date.

HEALTH GUIDANCE

Help parents understand the importance of regular health and dental care for child.
Encourage parents to teach and model sound health practices, including diet, rest, activity, and exercise.
Stress the need to encourage children to engage in appropriate physical activities.
Emphasize providing a safe physical and emotional environment.
Encourage parents to teach and model safety practices.

COMMUNITY FOCUS

Collaboration Between School Nurses and Teachers

Have complete health records for all students.
Give all teachers a list of students who have health problems.
Designate in teacher grade books those students who have health problems so that substitute teachers can recognize these students and intervene appropriately if problems occur.
If possible, provide adaptive physical education classes for students who cannot attend the regular classes.
Have metered dose inhalers available to all students with asthma for their emergency use in physical education and other classes.
Supervise selection of teams for physical education so that one team is not stacked with all the best players.
Give students an opportunity to redo a skill or activity in physical education if they have not performed well because every child has good and bad days.
Avoid questioning a child's ability in front of other students.
Provide privacy for height and weight checks and vision and hearing screening.

Suggestions submitted by Linda L. Smith, health and physical education teacher.

COMMUNITY FOCUS

Violence in Schools

In recent years, reports of abuse and violence by some children have raised concern for early identification of these individuals. In particular, concern has focused on sudden acts of fatal violence in schools.* In assessing both adults and children, look for a history of animal abuse, torment, or torture. Look also for childhood or adolescent acts of violence toward other children and, possibly, adults. A history of destructiveness to property, such as fire setting, is also significant.

Cruelty to animals and cruelty to humans should be viewed as a continuum of abuse. These acts are not harmless ventings of emotions in healthy individuals; they are warning signs that these individuals need professional intervention. Abusing animals does not dissipate violent emotions; rather, the abuse may fuel them.

*An excellent resource is Dwyer K, Osher D, Warger C: *Early warning, timely response: a guide to safe schools,* Washington, DC, 1998, U.S. Department of Education. Available from U.S. Department of Education, Special Education and Rehabilitative Services, Room 3131, Mary E. Switzer Building, Washington, DC 20202-2524; (877) 433-7827 or (202) 205-9043; telecommunication devices for the deaf (TDD): (202) 205-5465 or Federal Information Relay Service (FIRS): (800) 877-8339; e-mail David_Summers@ed.gov; *http://www.ed.gov/offices/OSERS/OSEP/earlywrn.html.* American Academy of Pediatrics (AAP) policy addresses violence in children with *The role of the pediatrician in youth violence prevention in clinical practice and at the community level.* Available from AAP, Division of Publications, 141 Northwest Point Blvd, PO Box 747, Elk Grove Village, IL 60009-0747; (800) 433-9016; fax (847) 228-1281; *http://www.aap.org.*

Internet Safety*

The Internet and electronic media, including cellular phones, are an ever-present factor in the lives of children, adolescents, and adults. Although direct injury may not occur through the Internet, there is increasing concern about predators who may use such a medium to attract, meet, and harm children and adolescents. Several parent rules may be helpful in providing Internet safety for the child and family:

- Become familiar with the Internet services the child or adolescent uses. Find out what kinds of services the Internet provider provides for home use and methods to block objectionable or offensive material. If blocking services are available, it is recommended that these be used, especially if children are on the Internet frequently. Such blockers often do not prevent scholarly research.
- Become familiar with materials available to Internet users (even if you never avail yourself of such material).
- Discuss with the adolescent or child the types of services he or she accesses and what types of communication or chat rooms the child or adolescent frequents.
- Discuss the benefits and potential hazards of Internet chat rooms according to the child's developmental age.
- Place the computer in a public area of the home.
- Understand and encourage discussion of the fact that not all material printed on the Internet is true.
- Never allow child to meet in person with someone with whom they have chatted on the Internet unless you are present.
- Discourage child or adolescent from providing anyone on the Internet (other than a close known personal friend) with personal information such as entire name, school name, address, telephone or cell phone number, personal photo, or credit card number. This applies to *anyone,* including a representative of the Internet service provider (ISP)—in such cases, a parent should communicate with the company's representative.
- Encourage child to not respond to messages or bulletin boards that include offensive, suggestive, obscene, or threatening information or anything that makes the child or adolescent uncomfortable.
- Help adolescent understand that persons on the Internet may misrepresent themselves for the purpose of committing a crime.
- If pornography, harassing messages, or threats are transmitted to your computer by another person, contact the local authorities and your service provider.
- Discuss Internet safety rules with all household members, including young children.
- Be reasonable in setting rules for computer use, and monitor computer use in the home.
- Monitor time spent on the computer and the time of day when most computer access is popular. Excessive computer activities may suggest a potential problem, especially if child or adolescent does not engage in other social activities with peers.
- Know the type of games children and adolescents are involved in via the Internet; some may not be harmless and may contain adult material.
- The best advice from consumer and government agencies is to apply a filter to block objectionable materials to which you prefer your child not have access. Some ISPs provide a filtering service for subscribers; contact them for service and prices. Examples of Internet filters available to the public (at a price) include Yahoo, MSN, KidsNet, SafeEyes, SafeBrowse, Cyberpatrol, and Cybersitter. Be aware that different filters may only filter as much as 80% of all objectionable materials, whereas others may block research material with objectionable words, phrases, or themes. Consumer Report has ratings of such services at *http://www.consumerreports.org.* Parents may also wish to read through the publication A parent's guide to Internet safety, available at *http://www.fbi.gov/publications.htm.*

Guidance During Adolescence

ENCOURAGE PARENTS TO:

Accept adolescent as a unique individual.

Recognize the influence of peer group.

Respect adolescent's ideas, likes and dislikes, and wishes.

Be involved with school functions and attend adolescent's performances, whether they be sporting events or a school play.

Be involved in adolescents' choice of Internet chat rooms, e-mail, Web "surfing," and cellular phone communication options (see Internet Safety, above)

Listen and try to be open to adolescent's views, even when they differ from parental views.

Avoid criticism about no-win topics.

Provide opportunities for choosing options and to accept the natural consequences of these choices.

*…ection may be photocopied and distributed to families.

Allow young person to learn by doing, even when choices and methods differ from those of adults.
Provide adolescent with clear, reasonable limits.
Clarify home rules and the consequences for breaking them.
Let society's rules and the consequences teach responsibility outside the home.
Allow increasing independence within limitations of safety and well-being.
Be available, but avoid pressing teen too far.
Respect adolescent's privacy.
Try to share adolescent's feelings of joy or sorrow. Respond to feelings as well as to words.
Be available to answer questions, give information, and provide companionship.
Try to make communication clear.
Avoid comparisons with siblings.
Assist adolescent in setting appropriate career goals and in preparing for adult role.
Welcome adolescent's friends into the home, and treat them with respect.
Provide unconditional love.
Be willing to apologize when mistaken.
Prepare adolescent for and guide him or her in relationships with peers that will carry over into adulthood.

BE AWARE THAT ADOLESCENTS:

Are subject to turbulent, unpredictable behavior.
Are struggling for independence.
Are extremely sensitive to feelings and behaviors that affect them.
May receive a different message than what was sent.
Consider friends extremely important.
Have a strong need to belong.

Play

Functions of Play

SENSORIMOTOR DEVELOPMENT

Improves fine and gross motor skills and coordination
Enhances development of all the senses
Encourages exploration of the physical nature of the world
Provides for release of surplus energy
Encourages and enhances communication

INTELLECTUAL DEVELOPMENT

Provides multiple sources of learning:

- Exploration and manipulation of shapes, sizes, textures, and colors
- Experience with numbers, spatial relationships, and abstract concepts
- Opportunity to practice and expand language skills

Provides opportunity to rehearse past experiences to assimilate them into new perceptions and relationships
Helps children to comprehend the world in which they live and to distinguish between fantasy and reality

SOCIALIZATION AND MORAL DEVELOPMENT

Teaches adult roles, including gender role behavior
Provides opportunities for testing relationships
Develops social skills
Encourages interaction and development of positive attitudes toward others
Reinforces approved patterns of behavior and moral standards

CREATIVITY

Provides an expressive outlet for creative ideas and interests
Allows for fantasy and imagination
Enhances development of special talents and interests

SELF-AWARENESS

Facilitates the development of self-identity
Encourages regulation of own behavior
Allows for testing of own abilities (self-mastery)
Provides for comparison of own abilities with those of others
Allows opportunities to learn how own behavior affects others

THERAPEUTIC VALUE

Provides for release from tension and stress
Allows expression of emotions and release of unacceptable impulses in a socially acceptable fashion
Encourages experimentation and testing of fearful situations in a safe manner
Facilitates nonverbal and indirect verbal communication of needs, fears, and desires
Meets own ongoing developmental needs

CULTURAL VALUE

Allows expression of cultural values and beliefs

General Trends During Childhood

Age	Social Character of Play	Content of Play	Most Prevalent Type of Play	Characteristics of Spontaneous Activity	Purpose of Dramatic Play	Development of Ethical Sense
Infant	Solitary	Social-affective	Sensorimotor	Sense-pleasure	Self-identity	
Toddler	Parallel	Imitative	Body movement	Intuitive judgment	Learning gender role	Beginning of moral values
Preschool	Associative	Imaginative	Fantasy Informal games	Concept formation Reasonably constant ideas	Imitating social life Learning social roles	Developing concern for playmates Learning to share and cooperate
School-age	Cooperative	Competitive games and contests Fantasy	Physical activity Group activities Formal games Play acting	Testing concrete situations and problem solving Adding fresh information	Vicarious mastery	Peer loyalty Playing by the rules Hero worship
Adolescent	Cooperative	Competitive games and contests Daydreaming	Social interaction	Abstract problem solving	Presenting ideas	Causes and projects

Guidelines for Toy Safety*

SELECTION

Select toys that suit the skills, abilities, and interests of children.

Select toys that are safe for the specific child; look for a label that indicates the intended age-group. Toys that are safe for one age-group may not be safe for another.

- For infants, toddlers, and all children who still mouth objects, avoid toys with small parts that may pose a fatal choking hazard or aspiration hazard. Toys in this category are usually labeled as "not recommended for children under 3 years."
- For infants, avoid toys with strings or cords that are 6 inches or longer because they may cause strangulation.
- For all children under 8 years old, avoid electric toys with heating elements.
- For children under 5 years old, avoid arrows or darts.

Check for safety labels, such as "flame retardant" or "flame resistant."

Select toys durable enough to survive rough play; look for sturdy construction, such as tightly secured eyes and nose on stuffed animals, or any small parts.

Select toys light enough that they will not cause harm if one falls on a child.

Look for toys with smooth, rounded edges. Avoid toys with sharp edges that can cut or that have sharp points. Points on the inside of the toy can puncture if the toy is broken.

Avoid toys with any shooting or throwing objects that can injure eyes.

- This includes toys with which other missiles, such as sticks or pebbles, might be used as substitutes for the intended projectiles.
- Arrows and darts used by children should have soft tips such as rubber suction cups and should be manufactured from resilient materials; make certain the tips are securely attached.

Make certain that materials in toys are nontoxic.

Avoid toys that make loud noises that might be damaging to a child's hearing.

- Even some squeaking toys are too loud when held close to the ear.
- If selecting caps for cap guns, look for the label required by federal law to be on boxes or packages of caps, which states: "Warning—Do not fire closer than 1 foot to the ear. Do not use indoors."

---

*Another helpful resource is *Toy safety: guidelines for parents* from American Academy of Pediatrics, Division of Publications, 141 Northwest Point Blvd., Elk Grove Village, IL 60007-1098; (800) 433-9016.

If selecting a toy gun, be certain that the barrel or the entire gun is brightly colored to avoid being mistaken for a real gun.
Check toy instructions for clarity. They should be clear to an adult and, when appropriate, to the child.

SUPERVISION

Maintain a safe play environment:
- Remove and discard plastic wrappings on toys immediately; they could suffocate a child.
- Remove large toys, bumper pads, and boxes from playpens; an adventuresome child can use such items as a means of climbing or falling out.

Set ground rules for play.
Supervise young children closely during play.
Teach children how to use toys properly and safely.
Instruct older children to keep their toys away from younger brothers, sisters, and friends.
Keep children who are playing with riding toys away from stairs, hills, traffic, and swimming pools.
Establish and enforce rules regarding protective gear:
- Insist that children wear helmets when using bicycles, skateboards, or in-line skates.
- Insist that children wear gloves and wrist, elbow, and knee pads when using skateboards or in-line skates.
- Ensure that protective sports equipment is worn for softball, baseball, football, soccer, hockey, and other contact sports.

Instruct children on electrical safety:
- Teach children the proper way to unplug an electric toy—pull on the plug, not the cord.
- Teach children to beware of electrical appliances and even electrically operated playthings; often children are unfamiliar with the hazards of electricity in association with water.

Teach children the safe use of items that under certain circumstances can cause injury—scissors, knives, needles, heating elements, loops, long strings, and cords.

MAINTENANCE

Regularly inspect old and new toys for breakage, loose parts, and other potential hazards.
- Look for jagged or sharp edges or broken parts that might constitute a choking hazard.
- Check movable parts to make certain they are attached securely to the toys; sometimes pieces that are safe when attached to the toy become a danger when detached.
- Examine outdoor toys for rust and weak or sharp parts that could be a danger to children.
- Check electrical cords and plugs for cracked or fraying parts.

Maintain toys in good repair, without possible hazards such as sharp edges, splinters, weak seams, or rust.
- Make repairs immediately, or discard the toy out of reach of children.
- Sand sharp or splintered surfaces on wooden toys so they are smooth.
- Use only paint labeled "nontoxic" to repaint toys, toy boxes, or children's furniture.

STORAGE

Provide a safe place for children to store toys:
- Select a toy chest or toy box that is ventilated, free of self-locking devices that could trap a child inside. Make sure it has a lid designed not to pinch a child's fingers or fall on a child's head.
- To avoid entrapment and suffocation, containers other than toy chests used for storage purposes should be fitted with spring-loaded support devices if they have a hinged lid.

Teach children to store toys safely in order to prevent accidental injury from stepping, tripping, or falling on them.
Playthings meant for older children and adults should be safely stowed away on high shelves, in locked closets, or in other areas unavailable to young children.

Play During Infancy

Age (Months)	Visual Stimulation	Auditory Stimulation	Tactile Stimulation	Kinetic Stimulation
Suggested Activities				
Birth-1	Hang bright, shiny object within 20-25 cm (8-10 inches) of infant's face and in midline. Hang mobiles with black-and-white designs.	Talk to infant; sing in soft voice. Play music box, radio, television. Have ticking clock or metronome nearby.	Hold, caress, cuddle. Keep infant warm. Infant may like to be swaddled.	Rock infant; place in cradle. Use stroller or carrier for walks.
2-3	Provide bright objects. Make room bright with pictures or mirrors. Take infant to various rooms while doing chores. Place in infant seat for vertical view of environment.	Talk to infant. Include in family gatherings. Expose to various environmental noises other than those of home. Use rattles, wind chimes.	Caress infant while bathing, at diaper change. Comb hair with a soft brush.	Use infant swing. Take in car for rides. Exercise body by moving extremities in swimming motion. Use cradle gym.
4-6	Place infant in front of safety (unbreakable) mirror. Give brightly colored toys to hold (small enough to grasp).	Talk to infant; repeat sounds infant makes. Laugh when infant laughs. Call infant by name. Crinkle different papers by infant's ear. Place rattle or bell in hand.	Give infant soft squeeze toys of various textures. Allow to splash in bath. Place nude on soft, furry rug and move extremities.	Use swing or stroller. Bounce infant in lap while holding in standing position. Support infant in sitting position; let infant lean forward to balance self. Place infant on floor to crawl, roll over, sit.
6-9	Give infant large toys with bright colors, movable parts, and noise makers. Place unbreakable mirror where infant can see self. Play peek-a-boo, especially hiding face in a towel. Make funny faces to encourage imitation.	Call infant by name. Repeat simple words, such as "dada," "mama," "bye-bye." Speak clearly. Name parts of body, people, and foods. Tell infant what you are doing. Use "no" only when necessary. Give simple commands. Show how to clap hands, bang a drum.	Let infant play with fabrics of various textures. Have bowl with foods of different sizes and textures to feel. Let infant catch running water. Encourage "swimming" in large bathtub or shallow pool. Give wad of sticky tape to manipulate.	Hold upright to bear weight and bounce. Pick up, say "up." Put down, say "down." Place toys out of reach, encourage infant to get them. Play pat-a-cake.
9-12	Show infant large pictures in books. Take infant to places where there are animals, many people, different objects (shopping center). Play ball by rolling it to child, demonstrate throwing it back. Demonstrate building a two-block tower.	Read infant simple nursery rhymes. Point to body parts and name each one. Imitate sounds of animals.	Give infant finger foods of different textures. Let infant mess up and squash food. Let infant feel cold (ice cube) or warm (bath water); say what temperature each is. Let infant feel a breeze (fan blowing).	Give large push-pull toys. Place furniture in a circle to encourage cruising on floor. Turn in different positions.

This section may be photocopied and distributed to families.

Play During Infancy—cont'd

Age (Months)	Visual Stimulation	Auditory Stimulation	Tactile Stimulation	Kinetic Stimulation
Suggested Toys				
Birth-6	Nursery mobiles Unbreakable mirrors See-through crib bumpers Contrasting colored sheets	Music boxes Musical mobiles Crib dangle bells Small-handled clear rattle	Stuffed animals Soft clothes Soft or furry quilt Soft mobiles	Rocking crib or cradle Weighted or suction toy Infant swing
6-12	Various colored blocks Nested boxes or cups Books with rhymes and bright pictures Strings of big beads Simple take-apart toys Large ball Cup and spoon Large puzzles Jack-in-the-box	Rattles of different sizes, shapes, tones, and bright colors Squeaky animals and dolls Recordings of light, rhythmic music	Soft, different-textured animals and dolls Sponge toys, floating toys Squeeze toys Teething toys Books with textures and objects, such as fur and zippers	Activity box for crib Push-pull toys Wind-up swing

Play During Toddlerhood

Physical Development	Social Development	Mental Development and Creativity
Suggested Activities		
Provide spaces that encourage physical activity. Provide sandbox, swing, and other scaled-down playground equipment.	Provide replicas of adult tools and equipment for imitative play. Permit child to help with adult tasks. Encourage imitative play. Provide toys and activities that allow for expression of feelings. Allow child to play with some actual items used in the adult world; for example, let child help wash dishes or play with pots and pans and other utensils (check for safety).	Provide opportunities for water play. Encourage building, drawing, and coloring. Provide various textures in objects for play. Provide large boxes and other safe containers for imaginative play. Read stories appropriate to age. Monitor TV viewing.
Suggested Toys		
Push-pull toys Rocking horse, stick horse Riding toy Balls (large) Blocks (unpainted) Pounding board Low gym and slide Pail and shovel Containers Play-Doh	Record player or tape recorder Purse Housekeeping toys (broom, dishes) Toy telephone Dishes, stove, table and chairs Mirror Puppets, dolls, stuffed animals (check for safety [e.g., no button eyes])	Wooden puzzles Cloth picture books Paper, finger paint, thick crayons Blocks Large beads to string Wooden shoe for lacing Appropriate TV programs, videos, music CDs

Play During Preschool Years

Physical Development	Social Development	Mental Development and Creativity
Suggested Activities		
Provide spaces for the child to run, jump, and climb. Teach child to swim. Teach simple sports and activities.	Encourage interactions with neighborhood children. Intervene when children become destructive. Enroll child in preschool.	Encourage creative efforts with raw materials. Read stories. Monitor TV viewing. Attend theater and other cultural events appropriate to child's age. Take short excursions to park, seashore, museums, zoo.
Suggested Toys		
Medium-height slide Adjustable swing Vehicles to ride Tricycle Wading pool Wheelbarrow Sled Wagon Roller skates, speed graded to skill	Child-sized playhouse Dolls, stuffed toys Dishes, table Ironing board and iron Cash register, toy typewriter, computer Trucks, cars, trains, airplanes Play clothes for dress-up Doll carriage, bed, high chair Doctor and nurse kits Toy nails, hammer, saw Grooming aids, play makeup, or shaving kits	Books Jigsaw puzzles Musical toys (xylophone, piano, drum, horns) Picture games Blunt scissors, paper, glue Newsprint, crayons, poster paint, large brushes, easel, finger paint Flannel board and pieces of felt in colors and shapes Records, tapes Dry erase board Sidewalk chalk (different colors) Wooden and plastic construction sets Magnifying glass, magnets

Unit 3

Evidence-Based Pediatric Nursing Interventions

Terri Brown

Preparing Children for Procedures Based on Developmental Characteristics

INFANCY: DEVELOPING A SENSE OF TRUST AND SENSORIMOTOR THOUGHT

Attachment to Parent

Involve parent in procedure if desired.*

Keep parent in infant's line of vision.

If parent is unable to be with infant, place familiar object with infant (e.g., stuffed toy).

Stranger Anxiety

Have usual caregivers perform or assist with procedure.*

Make advances slowly and in nonthreatening manner.

Limit number of strangers entering room during procedure.*

Sensorimotor Phase of Learning

Use sensory soothing measures during procedure (e.g., stroking skin, talking softly, giving pacifier).

Use analgesics (e.g., topical anesthetic, intravenous opioid) to control discomfort.*

Cuddle and hug infant after stressful procedure; encourage family to comfort infant.

Increased Muscle Control

Expect older infants to resist.

Restrain adequately.

Keep harmful objects out of reach.

Memory for Past Experiences

Realize that older infants may associate objects, places, or persons with prior painful experiences and will cry and resist at the sight of them.

Keep frightening objects out of view.*

Perform painful procedures in a separate room (not in crib or bed).*

Use nonintrusive procedures whenever possible (e.g., axillary temperature, oral medication).*

Imitation of Gestures

Model desired behavior (e.g., opening mouth).

TODDLER: DEVELOPING A SENSE OF AUTONOMY AND SENSORIMOTOR TO PREOPERATIONAL THOUGHT

Use same approaches as for infant in addition to the following.

Egocentric Thought

Explain procedure in relation to what child will see, hear, taste, smell, and feel.

Emphasize those aspects of procedure that require cooperation (e.g., lying still).

Tell child it is acceptable to cry, yell, or use other means to express discomfort verbally.

Negative Behavior

Expect treatments to be resisted; child may try to run away.

Use firm, direct approach.

Ignore temper tantrums.

Use distraction techniques (e.g., singing a song with child).

Restrain adequately.

Animism

Keep frightening objects out of view. (Young children believe objects have lifelike qualities and can harm them.)

Limited Language Skills

Communicate using behaviors.

Use a few simple terms familiar to child.

Give one direction at a time (e.g., "Lie down," then "Hold my hand").

Use small replicas of equipment; allow child to handle equipment.

Use play; demonstrate on doll but avoid child's favorite doll, because child may think doll is really feeling the procedure.

Prepare parents separately to avoid child's misinterpreting words.

Limited Concept of Time

Prepare child shortly or immediately before procedure.

Keep teaching sessions short (about 5 to 10 minutes).

Have preparations completed before involving child in procedure.

Have extra equipment nearby (e.g., alcohol swabs, new needle, adhesive bandages) to avoid delays.*

Tell child when procedure is completed.

Striving for Independence

Allow choices when they exist but realize that child may still be resistant and negative.

Allow child to participate in care and to help whenever possible (e.g., drink medicine from a cup, hold a dressing).

PRESCHOOLER: DEVELOPING A SENSE OF INITIATIVE AND PREOPERATIONAL THOUGHT

Egocentric

Explain procedure in simple terms and in relation to how it affects child (as with toddler, stress sensory aspects).

Demonstrate use of equipment.

*Applies to any age.

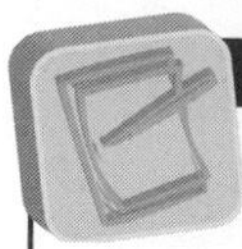

GUIDELINES

Selecting Nonthreatening Words or Phrases

Words and Phrases to Avoid	Suggested Substitutions
Shot, bee sting, stick	Medicine under the skin
Organ	Special place in body
Test	See how [specify body part] is working
Incision	Special opening
Edema	Puffiness, swelling
Stretcher, gurney	Rolling bed
Stool	Child's usual term
Dye	Special medicine
Pain	Hurt, discomfort, "owie," "boo-boo"
Deaden	Numb, make sleepy
Cut, fix	Make better
Take (as in "take your temperature or blood pressure")	See how warm you are; check your pressure; hug your arm
Put to sleep, anesthesia	Special sleep
Catheter	Tube, straw
Monitor	TV screen
Electrodes	Stickers, ticklers
Specimen	Sample
Start an IV	Slip a tube in the blue line

Allow child to play with miniature or actual equipment.

Encourage playing out experience on a doll both before and after procedure to clarify misconceptions.

Use neutral words to describe the procedure (Guidelines box).

Increased Language Skills

Use verbal explanation but avoid overestimating child's comprehension of words.

Encourage child to verbalize ideas and feelings.

Concept of Time and Frustration Tolerance Still Limited

Implement same approaches as for toddler but may plan longer teaching session (10 to 15 minutes); may divide information into more than one session.

Illness and Hospitalization May Be Viewed as Punishment

Clarify why each procedure is performed; a child will find it difficult to understand how medicine can taste bad and make him or her feel better at the same time.

Ask for child's thoughts regarding why a procedure is performed.

State directly that procedures are never a form of punishment.

Animism

Keep equipment out of sight, except when shown to or used on child.

Fears of Bodily Harm, Intrusion, and Castration

Point out on drawing, doll, or child where procedure will be performed.

Emphasize that no other body part will be involved.

Use nonintrusive procedures whenever possible (e.g., axillary temperatures, oral medication).

Apply an adhesive bandage over puncture site.

Encourage parental presence.

Realize that procedures involving genitalia produce anxiety.

Allow child to wear underpants with gown.

Explain unfamiliar situations, especially noises or lights.

Striving for Initiative

Involve child in care whenever possible (e.g., to hold equipment, remove dressing).

Give choices when they exist, but avoid excessive delays.

Praise child for helping and for attempting to cooperate; never shame child for lack of cooperation.

SCHOOL-AGE CHILD: DEVELOPING A SENSE OF INDUSTRY AND CONCRETE THOUGHT

Increased Language Skills; Interest in Acquiring Knowledge

Explain procedures using correct scientific or medical terminology.

Explain reason for procedure using simple diagrams of anatomy and physiology.

Explain function and operation of equipment in concrete terms.

Allow child to manipulate equipment; use doll or another person as model to practice using equipment whenever possible (doll play may be considered childish by older school-age child).

Allow time before and after procedure for questions and discussion.

Improved Concept of Time

Plan for longer teaching sessions (about 20 minutes).

Prepare before procedure.

Increased Self-Control

Gain child's cooperation.

Tell child what is expected.

Suggest ways of maintaining control (e.g., deep breathing, relaxation, counting).

Striving for Industry

Allow responsibility for simple tasks (e.g., collecting specimens).

Include in decision making (e.g., what time of day to perform procedure, the preferred site).

Encourage active participation (e.g., removing dressings, handling equipment, opening packages).

Developing Relationships with Peers

May prepare two or more children for same procedure or encourage one peer to help prepare another.

Provide privacy from peers during procedure to maintain self-esteem.

ADOLESCENT: DEVELOPING A SENSE OF IDENTITY AND ABSTRACT THOUGHT

Increasingly Capable of Abstract Thought and Reasoning

Supplement explanations with reasons why procedure is necessary or beneficial.

Explain long-term consequences of procedures.

Realize that adolescent may fear death, disability, or other potential risks.

Encourage questioning regarding fears, options, and alternatives.

Conscious of Appearance

Provide privacy.

Discuss how procedure may affect appearance (e.g., scar) and what can be done to minimize it.

Emphasize any physical benefits of procedure.

Concerned More with Present Than with Future

Realize that immediate effects of procedure are more significant than future benefits.

Striving for Independence

Involve in decision making and planning (e.g., choice of time and place; individuals present during procedure, such as parents; what clothing to wear).

Impose as few restrictions as possible.

Suggest methods of maintaining control.

Accept regression to more childish methods of coping.

Realize that adolescent may have difficulty in accepting new authority figures and may resist complying with procedures.

Developing Peer Relationships and Group Identity

Same as for school-age child but assumes even greater significance.

Allow adolescents to talk with other adolescents who have had the same procedure.

Play During Hospitalization

Functions of Play in the Hospital

Facilitates mastery over an unfamiliar situation

Provides opportunity for decision making and control

Helps to lessen stress of separation

Provides opportunity to learn about parts of body, their functions, and own disease or disability

Corrects misconceptions about the use and purpose of medical equipment and procedures

Helps children have an age-appropriate understanding of illness and treatment

Aids in assessment and diagnosis

Meets ongoing developmental needs

Provides for continuation of development

Speeds recovery and rehabilitation

Provides diversion and brings about relaxation

Helps the child feel more secure in a strange environment

Provides a means to release tension and express feelings

Encourages interaction and development of positive attitudes toward others

Provides an expressive outlet for creative ideas and interests

Provides a means for accomplishing therapeutic goals

THERAPEUTIC PLAY ACTIVITIES FOR HOSPITALIZED CHILDREN

Fluid Intake

Make snow cones or freezer pops using child's favorite juice.

Cut gelatin into fun shapes.

Make game of taking sip when turning page of book or during games such as Simon Says.

Use small medicine cups; decorate the cups.

Color water with food coloring or powdered drink mix.

Have a tea party; pour at small table.

Let child fill a syringe and squirt it into mouth or use it to fill small, decorated cups.

Cut straw in half, and place in small container (much easier for child to suck liquid).

Decorate straw; place small sticker on straw.

Use a "crazy" straw.

Make a progress poster; give rewards for drinking a predetermined quantity.

Play "fluid checkers" using medicine cups with different colors of juice; every time someone gets 'jumped' they must drink some juice.

Deep Breathing

Blow bubbles with bubble blower.

Blow bubbles with straw (no soap).

Blow on pinwheel, feathers, whistle, harmonica, balloons, toy horns, or party noisemakers.

Practice on band instruments.

Have blowing contest using balloons, boats, cotton balls, feathers, marbles, Ping-Pong balls, pieces of paper; blow such objects over a tabletop goal line, over water,

through an obstacle course, up in the air, against an opponent, or up and down a string.
Move paper or cloth from one container to another using suction from a straw.
Use blow bottles with colored water to transfer water from one side to the other (bubble painting).
Dramatize scenes, such as "I'll huff and puff and blow your house down" from the "Three Little Pigs."
Do straw-blowing painting.
Take a deep breath and "blow out the candles" on a birthday cake.
Use a little paint brush to paint nails with water, then blow nails dry.

Range of Motion and Use of Extremities

Throw beanbags at fixed or movable target; toss wadded paper into a wastebasket.
Touch or kick Mylar balloons held or hung in different positions (if child is in traction, hang balloon from trapeze). Latex balloons and latex gloves inflated into balloons pose a choking hazard and also present the risk of an allergic reaction.
Play tickle toes; have child wiggle them on request.
Play games such as Twister or Simon Says.
Play pretend and guess games (e.g., imitate a bird, butterfly, horse).
Have tricycle or wheelchair races in safe area.
Play kick or throw ball with soft foam ball in safe area.
Position bed so that child must turn to view television or doorway.
Have child climb wall with fingers like a spider.
Pretend to teach aerobic dancing or exercise; encourage parents to participate.
Encourage swimming if feasible.
Play video games or pinball (fine motor movement).
Play hide and seek game; hide toy somewhere in bed (or room, if ambulatory), and have child find it using specified hand or foot.
Provide clay to mold with fingers.
Have child paint or draw on large sheets of paper placed on floor or wall.
Encourage combing own hair; play beauty shop with "customer" in different positions.

Soaks

Play with small toys or objects (cups, syringes, soap dishes) in water.
Wash dolls or toys.
Pick up marbles or pennies* from bottom of bath container.
Make designs with coins on bottom of container.
Pretend a boat is a submarine by keeping it immersed.
During soaks, read to child, sing with child, or play game such as cards, checkers, or other board game (if both hands are immersed, move the board pieces for the child).
Sitz bath: Give child something to listen to (music, stories) or look at (Viewmaster, book).

Tension Release Activities

Muscle relaxation exercises
Distraction by telling stories or singing
Breathing through party blower or pinwheel
Blowing or watching bubbles
Counting
Looking at pop-up books
Squeezing Nerf or stress ball
Playing handheld games
Giving detailed explanation of procedure
Soothing touches or hugs
Deep breathing
Building tower blocks and knocking them over to allow acceptable, safe outlet for aggression
Playing with Play-Doh
Punching holes in bottom of plastic cup, filling with water, and letting it rain on child

Injections

Let child handle syringe (without needle), vial, and alcohol swab and pretend to give an injection to doll or stuffed animal.
Use syringes to decorate cookies with frosting, squirt paint, or target shoot into a container.
Draw a "magic circle" on area before injection; draw smiling face in circle after injection (but avoid drawing on puncture site).
Allow child to have a collection of syringes (without needles); make wild creative objects with syringes.
If child is receiving multiple injections or venipunctures, make a progress poster; give rewards for predetermined number of injections.
Have child count to 10 or 15 during injection or "blow the hurt away."

Ambulation

Give child something to push:
- Toddler, push-pull toy
- School-age child, wagon or a doll in a stroller or wheelchair
- Adolescent, decorated intravenous (IV) stand

Have a parade; make hats, drum, and so on.
Encourage foot pointing.
Have a treasure hunt or interdepartmental field trip.

Immobilization or Isolation

Flashlight play—use flashlights to create designs on wall or ceiling.
Use isolation pen pals or phone pals to provide social experience for confined children.
Play "traction" basketball or volleyball with soft ball.
Unit scrapbook—view photographs of people and places on unit.
Make bed into a pirate ship or airplane with decorations.
Move patient's bed frequently, especially to playroom, hallway, or outside.

*Small objects such as marbles or coins are unsafe for young children because of possible aspiration.

Informed Consent to Treat Child

Health Insurance Portability and Accountability Act (HIPAA)

The first-ever federal privacy standards to protect patients' medical records and other health information provided to health plans, doctors, hospitals, and other health care providers took effect on April 14, 2003. Developed by the Department of Health and Human Services (HHS), these new standards provide patients with access to their medical records and more control over how their personal health information is used and disclosed. For further information see the website *http://www.hhs.gov/ocr/hipaa.*

Consent Considerations

Children are considered minors (usually until 18 years of age), and, except under special circumstances, the parent or the person designated as legal guardian for the child is required to give informed consent before medical treatment is implemented or any procedure is performed on the child. Separate permission is also required for the following:

- Major surgery
- Minor surgery—for example, cutdown, biopsy, dental extraction
- Diagnostic tests with an element of risk—for example, bronchoscopy, needle biopsy, angiography
- Medical treatments with an element of risk—for example, blood transfusion, thoracentesis or paracentesis, radiation therapy, and shock therapies
- Other hospital situations that require written parental permission include the following:
  - Taking photographs for medical, educational, or other public use
  - Removal of the child from the hospital against medical advice
  - Postmortem examinations, except when ordered by the medical examiner in cases of unexplained deaths, such as sudden infant death, violent death, or suspected suicide
  - Release of medical information
- Exceptions to the previously mentioned regulations include the following:
  - Informed consent of persons in loco parentis (in place of the parent)—Permission granted by the person responsible for the child during parents' absence
  - Oral informed consent—Telephone consent or oral consent from a parent who is unable to sign (have witness to verbal consent)
  - Mature or emancipated minor—A person who is legally underage but who is recognized as having the legal capacity of an adult, such as an unmarried pregnant minor, a minor who is married, or a minor who lives apart from the parents and is self-supporting (varies by state)
  - Situations in which children need prompt medical or surgical treatment and a parent is not readily available to give consent
  - Parental negligence—When children need protection from their parents, such as when parents neglect or impose improper punishment on a child or refuse needed treatment; or when parents' refusal is a direct violation of the law
  - Suspicion of sexual or physical abuse

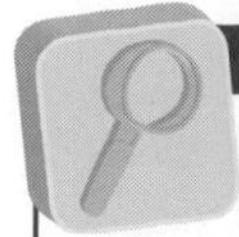

EVIDENCE-BASED PRACTICE

Informed Consent and Assent in Children

Janet DeJean

Ask the Question

Question

At what age should children be able to participate in the informed consent or assent process?

Objective

To determine when it is appropriate to involve the pediatric patient in medical decisions

Background

Medical decisions in the past primarily were the sole responsibility of physicians. With the evolution of family-centered care, parents have become more informed and involved in health care decisions for their children. Parents or legal guardians are responsible for the informed consent for the treatment of their minor child. As times have changed, so has the practice of including children in the decision-making process. Assent, a child's agreement to participate, should include information to help a child to understand his or her condition and the tests and treatments he or she will experience. Health care providers need to assess the patient's understanding and response and avoid any undue pressure to participate. Patient agreement should be expressed.

Search for Evidence

Search Strategies

Search selection criteria included English language publications within the past 10 years and research-based articles on informed consent and assent in children receiving medical treatment.

Databases Used

Cochrane Collaboration, Joanna Briggs Institute, PubMed, MD Consult

Critically Analyze the Evidence

There are numerous opinions on when and how a child should be involved in the medical decision-making process. The determining factor is the child's developmental readiness and the medical procedure involved.

The American Academy of Pediatrics' (1995) position is that patients should participate in decision making commensurate with their development. No specific minimum age for a child is identified.

The Children's Oncology Group (2005) states that in clinical research trials for cancer treatment, a child needs to be at least 9 years of age before he or she would have the ability to understand research-related information.

Two research studies evaluated the understanding of assent. Each recommended a different age of understanding.

- Ondrusek, Abramovitch, Pencharz, and others (1998) found that in subjects younger than 9 years, understanding of most aspects of a clinical nutrition study involving a nontherapeutic blood sample was poor to nonexistent.
- Tait, Voepel-Lewis, and Malviya (2003) found children ages 11 years and older had significantly greater understanding of the study protocol, benefits, and freedom to withdraw from a clinical anesthesia or surgical study.

Wendler (2006) suggests that children are capable of assent when they become able to understand the research in question at approximately 14 years of age. Assent is not required when the prospect of direct benefit of treatment is available only within the context of research. Sustained dissent should be respected in all cases.

Two research studies were found examining institutional review board (IRB) practices of determining when assent should be attained. All of the IRBs in these two studies support obtaining assent for children before clinical trials.

- Kimberly, Hoehn, Feudtner, and others (2006) compared 55 different IRBs across the United States. The majority of the IRBs (83%) included methods for documenting assent, whereas only 45% identified specific age ranges for obtaining assent. The ages ranged from 7 to 18 years.
- Whittle, Shah, Wilfond, and others (2004) interviewed 188 chairpersons of IRBs nationwide. Half the IRBs had a method they required investigators to follow in determining which children are capable of assent, most commonly an age cutoff.

Apply the Evidence: Nursing Implications

- Children should be assessed for understanding and ability to participate in the assent process.
- The age for assent ranged from 7 to 14 years in numerous published articles on obtaining assent in children.
- The complex nature of some research studies and interventions may preclude children younger than 7, 9, 11, or 14 years of age from complete understanding.
- Assent should not be sought when the prospect of direct treatment benefit is available only within the context of research.
- Sustained dissent should be respected.
- Consent should be obtained at the age of 18 years.

References

American Academy of Pediatrics Committee on Bioethics: Informed consent, parental permission, and assent in pediatric practice, *Pediatrics* 95(2):314-317, 1995.

Children's Oncology Group: *Guidelines for involving children in decision-making about research participation,* 2005, Children's Oncology Group.

Kimberly M, Hoehn K, Feudtner C, and others: Variation in standards of research compensation and child assent practices: a comparison of 69 institutional review board–approved informed permission and assent forms for three multicenter pediatric clinical trials, *Pediatrics* 117:1706-1711, 2006.

Ondrusek N, Abramovitch R, Pencharz P, and others: Empirical examination of the ability of children to consent to clinical research, *J Med Ethics* 24(3):158-165, 1998.

Tait A, Voepel-Lewis T, Malviya S: Do they understand, part II. Assent of children participating in clinical anesthesia and surgery research, *Anesthesiology* 98(3):609-614, 2003.

Wendler D: Assent in paediatric research: theoretical and practical considerations, *J Med Ethics* 32(4):229-234, 2006.

Whittle A, Shah S, Wilfond B, and others: Institutional review board practices regarding assent in pediatric research, *Pediatrics* 113(6):1747-1752, 2004.

General Hygiene and Care

Skin Care

General Guidelines

Cleanse skin with gentle soap (e.g., Dove) or cleanser (e.g., Cetaphil). Rinse well with plain, warm water.

Provide daily cleansing of eyes, oral area, diaper or perineal area, and any areas of skin breakdown.

Apply moisturizing agents after cleansing to retain moisture and rehydrate skin.

Use minimum tape and adhesives. On very sensitive skin, use a protective, pectin-based or hydrocolloid skin barrier between skin and tape and adhesives.

Use adhesive remover (if skin is not fragile) or water when removing tape or adhesives.

Place pectin-based or hydrocolloid skin barriers directly over excoriated skin. Leave barrier undisturbed until it begins to peel off. With wet, oozing excoriations, place a small amount of stoma powder (as used in ostomy care) on site, remove excess powder, and apply skin barrier. Hold barrier in place for several minutes to allow barrier to soften and mold to skin surface. See Table 3-1 for common wound care products.

Alternate electrode placement sites and thoroughly assess skin underneath electrodes at least every 24 hours.

Be certain fingers or toes are visible whenever extremity is used for IV or arterial line.

Reduce friction by keeping skin dry (may apply absorbent powder such as cornstarch) and using soft, smooth bed linen and clothes.

Use a draw sheet to move a child in bed or onto a gurney to reduce friction and shearing injuries; do not drag the child from under the arms.

Keep skin free of excess moisture (e.g., urine or fecal incontinence, wound drainage, excessive perspiration).

Do not massage reddened, bony prominences because this can cause deep tissue damage; provide pressure relief to these areas instead.

Routinely assess the child's nutritional status. A child who is on nothing by mouth (NPO) status for several days and who is receiving only IV fluids is nutritionally at risk. This can also affect the skin's ability to maintain its integrity. Hyperalimentation should be considered for these children at risk.

Identify children who are at risk for skin breakdown before it occurs. Employ measures such as *pressure-reducing devices* (reduce pressure more than would usually occur on a regular hospital bed or chair) or *pressure-relieving devices* (maintain pressure below that which would cause capillary closing) to prevent breakdown.

Pressure Reduction and Relief Devices

Description	Advantages	Disadvantages	Examples*
Overlay†			
Foam: Varying density; 2- to 4-inch convoluted and nonconvoluted	Primarily pressure reduction, although in children may have pressure relief advantages; can be cut to fit cribs	Can be soiled by incontinent patient; inability to reduce skin moisture because of lack of airflow	Aerofoam, BioGard, DuraPedic, GeoMatt, Ultra Form Pediatric (does not include ordinary convoluted foam mattresses)
Gel or water filled: Pressure reduction; water or gel conforms to patient's contours	One-time charge; low cost for water; gels are expensive Relieves pressure and shear; nonpowered, easy cleaning	Mattress is a dense collection of viscous fluid cells; there have been reports that the mattress is cold to the touch; patients may have to spare vital calories to warm the mattress Heavy	Aqua-Pedics (water and gel), Tender Gel and Water, Theracare (water and gel), RIK mattress
Alternating-pressure mattress: An overlay with rows of air cells and pump; pump cycles air to provide inflation and deflation over pressure points	Intent is to relieve pressure points to create pressure gradients that enhance blood flow	Studies show inconsistent results; some have reported very low deflation interface pressures, but only the deflation pressures were used for analysis; tissue interface pressures during inflation are consistently higher and must be incorporated into the statistical analysis; clinical trials indicate higher pressure ulcer incidence rates when compared with other products	AeroPulse, AlphaBed, AlphaCare, BetaBed, Bio Flote, Dyna-CARE, Lapidus, PCA Systems, Pillo-Pump, Tenderair
Static air: Designed with interlocking air cells that provide dry flotation; inflated with a blower	Mattress overlays that are designed with multiple chambers, allowing air exchange between the compartments	Pressure reduction depends on adequate air volume and periodic reinflation	DermaGard, K-Soft, Koala-Kair, Roho, Sof-Care, Tenderair
Low–air-loss specialty overlay: Multiple airflow cushions that cover the entire bed; pressures can be set and controlled by a blower	Surface materials are constructed to reduce friction and shear and to eliminate moisture; pressure relief; can be used for prevention and/or treatment of ulcers	Surface mattress and pump are a rental item; not available for cribs	Acucair, Bio Therapy, CLINICARE, CRS 4000, RibCor Therapeutic Mattress Pad, TheraPulse, Select Firstep, Dynapulse

Modified from Hagelgans NA: Pediatric skin care issues for the home care nurse, *Pediatr Nurs* 19(5):499-507, 1993.
Material revised by Ivy Razmus, MSN, RN.
*This list is a representative sampling of products and is not intended to be all-inclusive. No endorsement of any product is intended. Within each category, products must be individually evaluated on their efficacy as comfort, pressure-reducing, or pressure-relieving devices. All products within a category do not necessarily perform equally.
†A device that is made to fit over a regular hospital mattress.

Pressure Reduction and Relief Devices—cont'd

Description	Advantages	Disadvantages	Examples*
Specialty Beds‡			
Low–air-loss beds: Bed surface consists of inflated air cushions; each section is adjusted for optimum pressure relief for patient's body size; some models have built-in scales	Provides pressure relief in any position; treatment for stages III and IV pressure ulcers; available in pediatric crib sizes	Bed is more bulky than a hospital bed, and some homes may not be able to accommodate its size; reimbursement is questionable	Air Plus, Flexicair, KinAir III Mediscus For cribs: Pedcare, PNEU-CARE/PEDI, Clinitron, TheraPulse, KCI's PediDyne, BariKare, with FirstStep, Select Heavy Duty
Low–air-loss mattress replacements	Provides pressure relief in any position; fits on hospital frame	Requires mattress storage	Flexicair Eclipse SilkAir—home use
Air-fluidized beds: Air is blown through beads to "float" patient	Provides pressure relief for oncology patients and for treatment of full-thickness pressure ulcers, postoperative flaps, burns; lighter-weight home care units available	Can be difficult to transfer patient	Clinitron At Home, Clinitron Elexis, Clinitron Fluid Air, Skytron, Elite, Clinitron Uplift Fluid Air
Kinetic therapy: Therapy surfaces that provide continuous gentle side-to-side rotation of 40 degrees or more on each side; table-based or cushion-based	Has been demonstrated to improve mucous transport, redistribute pulmonary blood flow, and mobilize pulmonary interstitial fluid; has been used for trauma victims and unstable spinal cord injuries (should use table-based; once stabilized, may use cushion-based)	Used only in acute care settings	Cushion-based: With air loss: BioDyne II, EfficaCC, Pulmonex, Triadyne, Pro-Turn, Synergy, Pneu-Care Plus, Pediadyne Table-based: Without air loss: RotoRest, Delta, Keane Mobility bed
Continuous lateral rotation beds (CLRT): Less than 40 degrees side-to-side rotation	Helps reposition unstable spinal cord injury patient; promotes comfort and shifts pressure points		BariAir, Q2Plus, Effica Pulmonex

‡High-tech beds used in place of the standard hospital bed. These are normally used on a rental basis and are intended for short-term use. They usually provide pressure relief and eliminate shear, friction, and maceration.

TABLE 3-1 Common Wound Care Products

Type of Product*	Indication	Function	Frequency of Dressing Change	Comments
Transparent film (e.g., Tegaderm)	Skin tears, intravenous access and tube sites, partial thickness wounds, primary and secondary dressing	Provides moist wound healing, impermeable to fluid and bacteria, promotes autolytic debridement No absorption	Daily Up to 7 days over intravenous sites	Seals wound from contaminants
Hydrocolloid (e.g., DuoDerm)	Pressure ulcers, partial- and full-thickness wounds, skin tears, tape anchor	Occlusive Impermeable to bacteria and contaminants Promotes autolytic debridement Minimal absorption	Up to 7 days	Do not place over infected or heavily draining wounds
Alginates, hydrofibers—calcium, collagen and silver (e.g., Aquacel, Fibrocal)	Moderate to large drainage, partial- and full-thickness wounds, dehiscence, infected areas, bleeding areas	Absorptive	Daily, but depends on amount of drainage Silver impregnated 3-7 days	Excellent for packing tunneling and undermining Trauma-free removal
Barrier dressings (e.g., Stomahesive wafer, Coloplast wafer)	Protect periwound, tube or tape anchor	Protect skin from drainage or adhesive stripping	Up to once weekly	Excellent around G tube sites, apply around wounds or on skin to attach tape
Barrier cream or ointment (e.g., Sensicare, Criticaid, Laniseptic)	Perineal and diaper areas	Protects skin from moisture	With each diaper change	Some impregnated with antifungals Choose those formulated to stick to moist lesions
Foam (e.g., Lyofoam, Mepilex, Allevyn, Polymem)	Moderate to heavy drainage, partial- and full-thickness wounds	More absorptive than gauze	Depends on drainage, up to 7 days	Excellent around leaking tubes and tracheostomy sites Available with fenestration Comfortable Nonadherent, trauma-free removal

*This table does not endorse any product. It is intended to provide the practitioner an "at a glance" reference for products used successfully in pediatric patients.

TABLE 3-1 **Common Wound Care Products—cont'd**

Type of Product*	Indication	Function	Frequency of Dressing Change	Comments
Silver (e.g., Silvasorb dressing and gel, Arglaes powder)	Infected or colonized full- and partial-thickness wounds	Depends on dressing type Available in foam, hydrocolloid, hydrofiber, alginate, and powder	Depends on dressing type, usually 3 to 7 days	Consider in wounds recalcitrant to previous treatments Controls odor
Wound gel (e.g., Curosal)	Dry, partial- and full-thickness wounds, burns	Adds moisture, promotes epithelization, fills up dead space	Once or twice daily Do not allow to dry out	Easy to use
Hydrogel dressing (e.g., Carragauze, Carradress)	Burns, partial- and full-thickness wounds, painful wounds	Adds moisture, aids autolytic debridement, minimal to moderate absorption	Daily	Nonadherent; trauma- and pain-free removal
Beclapermin gel (e.g., Regranex)	Diabetic, neuropathic, and granular ulcers	Promotes granulation	Daily	Contraindicated in infected and necrotic wounds Refrigerate Expensive
Enzymatic debrider (e.g., Accuzyme)	Necrotic wounds in patients who are not surgical candidates	Selectively dissolves necrotic tissue	Once or twice daily	Cross-hatch eschar with a scalpel for enzyme penetration Cover with moist NS gauze to activate Avoid use with silver or mercury
Gauze	All wound types	Minor absorption, mild debridement	3-4 times per day	Dries out Poor absorbancy Can macerate periwound Requires increased labor costs and supplies secondary to dressing change frequency

EVIDENCE-BASED PRACTICE

Wound Care

Shannon Stone McCord

Ask the Question

Questions

In children, what interventions prevent wounds?

In children, what cleansers should be used once wounds are present?

In children, what is known about wound debridement?

In children, what dressings are more effective in reducing healing time and pain?

Objective

To apply evidence-based wound care principles when providing wound care to children

Background

Provision of wound care to children is based on adult wound care principles derived from research studies on adults and wound care products. Although many of these principles apply in pediatrics, the patient's developmental age, size, and age must be taken into consideration.

Search for Evidence

Search Strategies

Search selection criteria included English language publications and research-based articles on wound care in the neonatal and pediatric population.

Databases Used

National Guideline Clearinghouse (AHRQ), Cochrane Collaboration, PubMed, Medscape

Critically Analyze the Evidence

Eliminate the Cause

The first step to wound healing is to eliminate the cause of the wound. Multiple interventions can prevent epidermal injury (Agency for Health Care Policy and Research [AHCPR], 1992; Wooten and Hawkins, 2005; McCord, McElvain, Sachdeva, and others, 2004; McLane, Bookout, McCain, and others, 2003; Santiago, 2003):

- Eliminate pressure secondary to medical devices such as tracheostomy tubes, wheelchairs, braces, and gastrostomy tubes.
- Reduce friction with proper positioning in bed.
- Turn the patient every 1 to 2 hours.
- Decrease the risk of infection by providing skin conditioning.
- Apply appropriate infection-control practices.

Wound Cleansing

Numerous studies have demonstrated that normal saline (NS) is the least damaging cleanser to cells, because it has a neutral pH. Other antiseptics such as povidone-iodine, hydrogen peroxide, Dakin's solution, and alcohol should not be used in open wounds, particularly at full strength, because they are toxic to white cells and fibroblasts and can impair wound healing. Study suggestions (Krasner, Rodeheaver, and Sibbald, 2001; Baranoski and Ayello, 2004; Lineweaver, Howard, Soucy, and others, 1985; Lund, Kuller, Lane, and others, 1999; Bryant, 2002; Bennett, Rosenblum, Perlov, and others, 2001; Fernandez, Griffiths, and Ussia, 2002; Moore and Cowman, 2005; Association of Women's Health, Obstetric and Neonatal Nurses, 2001) also include the following:

- Cleanse all wounds with NS or a saline-based wound cleanser with surfactant.
- Cleansing with drinkable tap water may be as effective as cleansing with sterile water or sterile saline.
- For intact periwound skin, soap and water may be used.

Debridement

According to studies (AHCPR, 1992; Baranoski and Ayello, 2004; Bryant, 2002; Krasner, Rodeheaver, and Sibbald, 2001; Heggars, 2003), debridement of necrotic tissue decreases the bacterial load within the wound, controls and prevents wound infection, and promotes healing. Debridement restores circulation and allows adequate oxygen delivery to the wound. Necrotic tissue stimulates an inflammatory process in the wound bed and interrupts the chemical and biologic process necessary for recruiting microphages and fibroblasts that deposit collagen, which is necessary for new cell growth. The nurse should debride wounds of necrotic tissue based on the wound type and depth and patient condition. Methods of debridement include mechanical ("wet to dry"), hydrotherapy, pulsed lavage, sharp or surgical, enzymatic, and autolytic. An exception is that stable, dry eschar to heels or ulcers to feet and toes where there is poor blood supply should not be debrided.

Dressings

The studies that were consulted (Winter, 1963; Ovington, 2001; Mertz, 1985; Berger, 2000; Valencia, 2001; Vermeulen, Ubbink, Goossens, and others, 2004; Dickson and Bodnaryk, 2006; Lund, Osborne, Kuller, and others, 2001; Nemeth, Eaglstein, Taylor, and others, 1991; Lawrence, Lilly, and Kidson, 1992) found that moist wound healing is two or three times faster than when wounds are left open to air. Moisture-retentive dressings such as transparent and hydrocolloid dressings accelerate wound healing, protect the wound, decrease bacterial wound contamination and infection, and reduce scarring. Comparatively, wet-to-dry dressings are associated with increases in labor costs, dressing change frequency, wound healing time, infection rates, pain, disruption of newly formed healthy tissue, and dispersal of bacteria on removal.

Dressing type and dressing change frequency should be based on the wound type and location, phase of wound healing, and amount of exudate. Many of the newer dressings allow for reduced dressing changes because they absorb more drainage and promote a moist wound healing environment. In addition, wound gels provide moisture to a wound bed while eliminating dead space. If a wound is infected or bacterial colonization is suspected, antibacterial ointments are indicated to reduce the bacterial bioburden and promote moist wound healing.

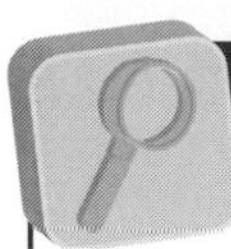

EVIDENCE-BASED PRACTICE

Wound Care—cont'd

Packing wounds with absorptive materials reduces wound exudate and abscess development and prevents skin maceration. There is insufficient evidence to suggest whether one dressing or topical product is more effective at healing a wound than another. There is evidence to suggest that wet-to-dry gauze dressings are more painful to patients on removal (Vermeulen, Ubbink, Goossens, and others, 2004).

Premature and newborn infants are prone to epidermal stripping and skin tears secondary to an immature epidermal-dermal bond. Avoid tape when possible. Secure dressings with a stretchy overwrap or use Montgomery straps. Frame wounds with a barrier dressing and adhere tape to the barrier. Apply non–alcohol-based skin preparation barriers under tape and dressings (AWHONN, 2001).

Apply the Evidence: Nursing Implications

- Identify and eliminate causes of wounds.
- Cleanse wounds with NS or a wound cleanser. Avoid placing chemical solutions and disinfectants in wounds.
- Cleanse intact skin with mild, neutral pH–balanced cleansers.
- Debride wounds of necrotic, devitalized tissue (exception: do not debride stable, dry eschar on feet and heels and on patients at risk for poor wound healing because of diabetes, immunocompromise, ischemia, poor circulation, or poor nutrition).
- Apply dressings that provide a moist wound environment.
- Pack wounds to eliminate dead space, absorb exudate, and prevent abscess formation.
- Dressing change frequency should be based on wound type and location, amount of pain and exudate, and the need for wound assessment. Most wounds require a daily dressing change.
- Protect the periwound skin with a barrier dressing or protective wipe to prevent epidermal injury.
- Avoid tape and secure dressings with stretchy wraps.

References

Agency for Health Care Policy and Research, U.S. Department of Health and Human Services: *Pressure ulcers in adults: prediction and prevention.* Clinical Practice Guideline No. 3, 1992, The Department.

Association of Women's Health, Obstetric and Neonatal Nurses: *Evidence-based clinical practice guideline: neonatal skin care,* Washington, DC, 2001, The Association.

Baranoski S, Ayello E: *Wound care essentials: practice principles,* Philadelphia, 2004, Lippincott Williams & Wilkins.

Bennett L, Rosenblum R, Perlov C, and others: In vivo comparison of topical agents on wound repair, *Plast Reconstr Surg* 108(3):675-687, 2001.

Berger R: A newly formulated triple antibiotic ointment minimizes scarring, *Cutis* 65:401-404, 2000.

Bryant R: *Acute and chronic wounds: nursing management,* ed 2, St Louis, 2002, Mosby.

Dickson D, Bodnaryk K: Neonatal intravenous extravasation injuries: evaluation of a wound care protocol, *Neonatal Netw* 25(1):13-19, 2006.

Fernandez R, Griffiths R, Ussia C. Water for wound cleansing. In *The Cochrane Database of Systematic Reviews 2002,* Issue 4. Article No. CD003861. DOI: 10.1002/14651858.CD003861.

Heggars J: Assessing and controlling wound infection, *Clin Plast Surg* 30:25-35, 2003.

Krasner D, Rodeheaver G, Sibbald G: *Chronic wound care: a clinical source book for healthcare professionals,* ed 3, Wayne, Penn, 2001, Health Management Publications.

Lawrence J, Lilly H, Kidson A: Wound dressings and airborne dispersal of bacteria, *Lancet* 339:807, 1992.

Lineweaver W, Howard R, Soucy D, and others: Topical antimicrobial toxicity, *Arch Surg* 120(3):267, 1985.

Lund C, Kuller J, Lane A, and others: Neonatal skin care: the scientific basis for practice, *Neonatal Netw* 18(4):241-254, 1999.

Lund C, Osborne J, Kuller J, and others: Neonatal skin care: clinical outcomes of the AWHONN/NANN evidence-based clinical practice guideline, Association of Women's Health, Obstetric and Neonatal Nurses and the National Association of Neonatal Nurses, *J Obstet Gynecol Neonatal Nurs* 30(1):41-51, 2001.

McCord S, McElvain V, Sachdeva R, and others: Risk factors associated with pressure ulcers in the pediatric intensive care unit, *J Wound Ostomy Continence Nurs* 31(4):179-183, 2004.

McLane K, Bookout K, McCain J, and others: The 2003 national pediatric pressure ulcer and skin breakdown prevalence survey: a multisite study, *J Wound Ostomy Continence Nurs* 1(4):168-177, 2004.

Mertz P: Occlusive wound dressings to prevent bacterial invasion and wound infection, *J Am Acad Dermatol* 12:662-668, 1985.

Moore ZEH, Cowman S: Wound cleansing for pressure ulcers. In *The Cochrane Database of Systematic Reviews 2005,* Issue 4. Article No. CD004983. DOI: 10.1002/14651858.CD004983.pub2.

Nemeth A, Eaglstein W, Taylor J, and others: Faster healing and less pain in skin biopsy sites treated with an occlusive dressing, *Arch Dermatol* 127(110):1679-1683, 1991.

Ovington L: Hanging wet to dry dressings out to dry, *Home Health Care Nurse* 19(8):477-484, 2001.

Santiago I: A sore spot in pediatrics: risk factors for pressure ulcers, *Pediatr Nurs* 29(4):278-282, 2003.

Valencia I: New developments in wound care for infants and children, *Pediatr Ann* 30(4):211-218, 2001.

Vermeulen H, Ubbink D, Goossens A, and others: Dressings and topical agents for surgical wounds healing by secondary intention. In *The Cochrane Database of Systematic Reviews 2004,* Issue 1. Article No. CD003554. DOI: 10.1002/14651858.CD003554.pub2.

Winter G: Effect of air drying and dressings on the surface area of a wound, *Nature* 197:91-92, 1963.

Wooten M, Hawkins K: *WOCN position statement: clean versus sterile: management of chronic wounds,* 2005, Wound, Ostomy and Continence Nurses Society.

ADHESIVES

Decrease use as much as possible.

Use transparent adhesive dressings to secure IV lines, catheters, and central lines.

Consider use of hydrogel electrodes.

Consider pectin barriers (Hollihesive,* DuoDerm†) beneath adhesives to protect skin.

Secure pulse oximeter probe or electrodes with elasticized dressing material (carefully avoid restricting blood flow).

Do not use adhesive remover, solvents, and bonding agents.

Adhesive removal can be facilitated using water, mineral oil, petrolatum, or alcohol-based foam hand cleanser.

Remove adhesives or skin barriers slowly, supporting the skin underneath with one hand and gently peeling away the product from the skin with the other hand. (CAUTION: Scissors are not to be used for tape or dressing removal because of hazard of cutting skin or amputating tiny digits.)

TREATING SKIN BREAKDOWN

Irrigate wound every 4 to 8 hours with warm normal saline (NS) using a 30-ml or larger syringe and 20-gauge Teflon catheter.

Culture wound and treat if signs of infection are present (excessive redness, swelling, pain on touch, heat, resistance to healing).

Use transparent adhesive dressing for uninfected wounds.

Use hydrocolloid for deep, uninfected wounds (leave in place for 5 to 7 days); warm barrier in hand for several minutes to soften before applying to skin.

Apply hydrogel with or without antibacterial or antifungal ointments (as ordered) for infected wounds (may need to moisten before removal).

Avoid use of antiseptic solutions for wound cleansing (used for intact skin only).

TREATING DIAPER DERMATITIS

Maintain clean, dry skin; use absorbent diapers, and change often.

If mild irritation occurs, use petrolatum barrier.

For developing dermatitis, apply a generous quantity of zinc-oxide barrier.

For severe dermatitis, identify cause and treat (frequent stooling from spina bifida, severe opiate withdrawal, malabsorption syndrome).

Treat *Candida albicans* with antifungal ointment or cream.

Avoid powders and antibiotic ointments.

NEONATAL GUIDELINES

General Skin Care

Assessment

Assess skin every day or once a shift for redness, dryness, flaking, scaling, rashes, lesions, excoriation, or breakdown.

Evaluate and report abnormal skin findings, and analyze for possible causation.

Intervene according to interpretation of findings or physician order.

Bathing

Initial Bath

- Assess for stable temperature a minimum of 2 to 4 hours before first bath.
- Use cleansing agents with neutral pH and minimal dyes or perfume, in water.
- Do not completely remove vernix.
- Bathe preterm infant <32 weeks in sterile water alone.

Routine

- Decrease frequency of baths to every second or third day by daily cleansing of eye, oral, and diaper areas and pressure points.
- Use cleanser or soaps no more than two or three times a week.
- Avoid rubbing skin during bathing or drying.
- Immerse stable infants fully (except head) in an appropriate-sized tub.
- Use swaddled immersion bathing technique: slow unwrapping after gently lowering into water for sensitive, but stable, infants needing assistance with motor system reactivity.

Emollients

Follow hospital protocol or consider the following:

- Apply petroleum-based ointment without preservative sparingly to body (avoid face, head) every 6 to 12 hours during the first 2 to 4 weeks for infants <32 weeks (except when neonate is in radiant heat source).
- Apply emollient as needed to infants >32 weeks for dry, flaking skin.

Antiseptic Agents

Apply before invasive procedures.

Apply chlorhexidine gluconate (CHG) two times, air dry for 30 seconds; remove completely with sterile water or sterile saline solution after procedure.

Avoid use of alcohol.

Transepidermal Water Loss

Minimize transepidermal water loss (TEWL) and heat loss in small premature infants over 30 weeks by:

- Measuring ambient humidity during first weeks of life
- Considering an increase in humidity to >70% by using one or more of the following options or hospital guidelines:
  - Transparent dressings
  - Emollient application every 6 to 8 hours or according to hospital protocol
  - Servocontrolled humidifying incubator

---

*Hollister, Libertyville, Il.

†Convatec/Bristol-Myers Squibb Co, Princeton, NJ.

Skin Breakdown Prevention

Decrease pressure from externally applied forces using water, air, or gel mattresses, sheepskin, or cotton bedding.

Provide adequate nutrition, including protein, fat, and zinc.

Apply transparent adhesive dressings to protect arms, elbows, and knees from friction injury.

Use tracheostomy and gastrostomy dressings for drainage and relief of pressure from tracheostomy or gastrostomy tube (Hydrasorb* or Lyofoam†).

Use emollient in the diaper area (groin, thighs) to reduce urine irritation.

Other Skin Care Concerns

Use of Substances on Skin

Evaluate all substances that come in contact with infant's skin.

Before using any topical agent, analyze components of preparation and:

- Use sparingly and only when necessary.
- Confine use to smallest possible area.
- Whenever possible and appropriate, wash off with water.
- Monitor infant carefully for signs of toxicity and systemic effects.

Use of Thermal Devices

Avoid heat lamps because of increased potential for burns. If needed, measure actual temperature of exposed skin every 15 minutes.

When using heating pads:

- Change infant's position every 15 minutes initially, then every 1 to 2 hours.
- Preset temperature of heating pads <40° C (<104° F).

When using preheated transcutaneous electrodes:

- Avoid use on infants <1000 g.
- Set at lowest possible temperature (<44° C [<111.2° F]), and secure with plastic wrap.
- Use pulse oximetry rather than transcutaneous monitoring whenever possible.

When prewarming heels before phlebotomy, avoid temperatures >40° C.

Warm ambient humidity, direct away from infant; use aerosolized sterile water and maintain ambient temperature so as not to exceed 40° C.

Bathing

Never leave infant or small child unattended in a bathtub.

Hold infant who is unable to sit alone.

Support infant's head securely with one hand or grasp the infant's farther arm firmly and rest the head comfortably on your wrist.

Closely supervise the infant or child who is able to sit without assistance.

Place a pad in the bottom of the tub to prevent slipping and loss of balance.

Offer older children the option of a shower, if available.

Use judgment regarding the amount of supervision older children require.

Children with mental and/or physical limitations such as severe anemia or leg deformities and suicidal or psychotic children (who may commit bodily harm) require close supervision.

Clean the ears, between skinfolds, the neck, the back, and the genital area carefully.

Retract the foreskin of uncircumcised boys gently once it is mobile (usually older than 3 years of age), clean the exposed surfaces, and replace the foreskin. Never forcefully retract the foreskin.

Provide more extensive assistance with bathing and other aspects of hygienic care to children who are debilitated: Encourage them to perform as much as they are capable of without overtaxing their energies.

Expect increasing involvement with improved strength and endurance.

Modified from Kuller JM: Skin breakdown: risk factors, prevention, and treatment, *NINR* 1(1):33-42, 2001; Johnson FE, Maikler VE: Nurses' adoption of the AWHONN/NANN Neonatal Skin Care Project, *NINR* 1(1):59-67, 2001; Lund CH, Kuller J, Lott JW: Neonatal skin care: clinical outcomes of the AWHONN/NANN evidence-based clinical practice guideline, *J Obstet Gynecol Neonatal Nurs* 30(1):41-51, 2001; Taquino LT: Promoting wound healing in the neonatal setting: process versus protocol, *J Perinatal Neonatal Nurs* 14(1):108-118, 2000; Lund C, Lane A, Raines DA: Neonatal skin care: the scientific basis for practice, *J Obstet Gynecol Neonatal Nurs* 28(3):241-254, 1999; Malloy MB, Perez-Woods R: Neonatal skin care: prevention of skin breakdown, *Pediatr Nurs* 17(1):41-48, 1991.

*Kendall Co., Mansfield, MA.

†Convatec/Bristol-Myers Squibb Co, Princeton, NJ.

Hair Care

Brush and comb hair or help children with hair care at least once daily. Avoid using most standard combs for African-American children because they can cause hair breakage and discomfort.

Style hair for comfort and in a manner pleasing to the child and parents.

Do not cut hair without parental permission, although clipping hair to provide access to scalp vein for needle insertion is permissible.

Shampoo hair in the tub or shower, or transport the child by gurney to an accessible sink or washbasin. If the child is unable to be transported, shampoo in the bed with adequate protection and/or with specially adapted equipment or positioning.

Wash hair of the newborn every 2 to 3 days as part of the bath.

Wash hair and scalp as needed in later infancy and childhood.

Teenagers may need more frequent hair care and shampoos.

Use commercial dry shampoo products on a short-term basis.

Skin Closure (Suture or Staple) Removal Procedure

Determine that sutures have been in place an adequate length of time. This length of time varies depending on area of the body sutured. Some guidelines are 3 days for the eyelids; 3 to 4 days for the neck; 5 days for the face and scalp; 7 days for the trunk and upper extremities; and 8 to 10 days for the lower extremities.

Position patient to allow access to stitches without putting undue tension on incision.

Assess wound for any signs of infection (redness, swelling, heat, drainage) or of wound not healing (dehiscence).

Clean wound with NS or antiseptic. Hydrogen peroxide may be used to remove any scabs over stitches.

Remove stitches (technique varies based on type of stitch).

SIMPLE INTERRUPTED SUTURES

Simple interrupted sutures are the most widely used type of stitch; each stitch is placed and tied individually.

Use forceps to firmly grasp knot and pull taught to expose underside of knot. Insert scissors underneath stitch to side of knot. Clip stitch with scissors while continuing to pull on knot with forceps. Gently pull knot with forceps to remove stitch completely. To minimize infection, stitch should be cut as close to skin as possible so that external parts of stitch do not pass through wound. Repeat process for additional sutures.

SIMPLE CONTINUOUS SUTURES

Simple continuous sutures consist of a series of stitches; only the first and last stitches are tied.

Use forceps to firmly grasp knot and pull taught to expose underside of knot. Insert scissors underneath stitch to side of knot. Clip stitch with scissors. To minimize infection, stitch should be cut as close to skin as possible so that external parts of stitch do not pass through wound. Move down to the next suture in line, keeping on the same side of wound. Clip this stitch with scissors. Gently pull stitch with forceps to remove. Continue this process of cutting and removing stitches, working down the same side of wound.

STAPLES

Insert lower jaw of staple extractor underneath first staple. Push jaws of staple remover together. Once jaws are firmly closed, pull extractor toward you to remove staple. Continue this process, removing every other staple, then remove the remainder.

Assess for possible complications. If incision begins to separate, leave remainder of stitches in place and use skin closure strips (Steri-Strips) to secure opening area of wound. Notify physician.

Use dressing as needed if wound is draining.

Procedures Related to Maintaining Safety

Ensure that environmental safety measures are in operation, such as the following:
- Nonsmoking policy
- Good illumination
- Floors clear of fluid or objects that might contribute to falls
- Nonskid surfaces in showers and tubs
- Electrical equipment maintained in good working order, used only by personnel familiar with its use, and not in contact with moisture or near tubs
- Beds of ambulatory patients locked in place and at a height that allows easy access to the floor
- Proper care and disposal of small, breakable items, such as thermometers and bottles
- A well-organized fire plan known to all staff members
- All windows secure
- Electrical outlets covered to prevent burns

Be sure the child is wearing a proper identification band.

Check bath water carefully before placing the child in the bath.

Use furniture that is scaled to the child's proportions and sturdy and well balanced to prevent tipping over.

Securely strap infants and small children into infant seats, feeding chairs, and strollers.

Do not leave infants, young children, and youngsters who are agitated or cognitively impaired unattended on treatment tables, on scales, or in treatment areas.

Keep portholes in incubators securely fastened when not attending the infant.

Prevent child's access to tubs, laundry bags or chutes, elevators, medication rooms, and medication and cleaning carts.

Keep crib sides up and fastened securely.
- Leave crib sides up regardless of child's ability to get out, and even when the crib is unoccupied, to remove the temptation for the child to climb in.
- Never turn away from an infant or small child in a crib that has the sides down without maintaining contact with the child's back or abdomen to prevent rolling, crawling, or jumping from the open crib.

Place the child who may climb over the side of the crib in a specially constructed crib with a cover or one that has a safety net placed over the top.
- Tie net to the frame in such a manner that there is ready access to the child in case of emergency.
- Never tie nets to the movable crib sides or use knots that do not permit quick release.

Do not tie balloons or other objects with long ties or strings to cribs because they can pose an entanglement hazard.

Do not place cribs within reach of heating units, appliances, dangling cords, outlets, or other objects that can be reached by curious hands.

Pillows should not be placed in cribs with children chronologically or developmentally less than 12 months old except to therapeutically position a patient per medical orders.

Assess the safety of toys brought to the hospital for children, and determine whether they are appropriate to the child's age and condition.

Inspect toys to make certain they are allergy-free, washable, and unbreakable and that they have no small, removable parts that can be aspirated or swallowed.

All objects within reach of children younger than 3 years should pass the choke tube test. A toilet paper roll is a handy guide. If a toy or object fits into the cylinder (items less than $1\frac{1}{4}$ inches across or balls smaller than $1\frac{3}{4}$ inches), it is a potential choking danger to the child.

Set limits for the child's safety.

Make sure children understand where they are permitted to go and what they are permitted to do in the hospital.

Enforce the limitations consistently, and repeat them as frequently as necessary to make certain that they are understood.

Transporting

Carry infants and small children for short distances within the unit:
- In the horizontal position, hold or carry small infants with the back supported and the thighs grasped firmly by the carrying arm.
- In the football hold, support the infant on the nurse's arm with the head supported by the hand and the body held securely between the body and elbow.
- In the upright position, hold the infant with the buttocks on the nurse's forearm and the front of the body resting against the chest. Support the infant's head and shoulders with the other arm to allow for any sudden movement by the infant.

For more extended trips, use a suitable conveyance:
- Determine the method of transporting children by considering their age, condition, and destination.
- Use appropriate safety belts and/or raised sides to secure child.
- Transport infants in their incubators, cribs, strollers, wheeled feeding chairs, and tables or in wagons with raised sides.

Use wheelchairs or gurneys with side rails for older children.

Ambulation may be appropriate for children who are not on cardiac or pulse oximetry monitors.

Preventing Falls

Multiple interventions are needed to minimize pediatric patients' risk of falling. Once individual children are identified as at risk for falling, visual identification and communication of the risk among all health care providers is essential. Reduce the risk of falling through patient, family, and staff education.

Identify hospitalized children at risk for falling. Perform a fall risk assessment on patients on admission and throughout hospitalization to identify patients at high risk for falls. Risk factors for hospitalized children include:

- Medication effects: postanesthesia or sedation; analgesics or narcotics, especially in those who have never had narcotics in the past and in whom effects are unknown
- Altered mental status: secondary to seizures, brain tumors, or medications
- Altered or limited mobility: skill at ambulation secondary to developmental abilities, disease process, tubes, drains, casts, splints, or other appliances; new to ambulating with assistive devices such as walkers or crutches
- Postoperative children: risk of hypotension or syncope secondary to large blood loss, a heart condition, or extended bedrest
- History of falls
- Infants or toddlers in cribs with side rails down or on the daybed with family members

Visually identify patients at risk with one or more of the following:

- Post signs on the door and at the bedside.
- Apply a special colored armband labeled "Fall Precautions."
- Label the chart with a sticker.
- Document information on the chart.

Alter the environment:

- Keep bed in lowest position, breaks locked, and side rails up.
- Place call bell within reach.
- Ensure that all necessary and desired items are within reach (e.g., water, glasses, tissues, snacks).
- Offer toileting on a regular basis, especially if patient is on diuretics or laxatives.
- Keep lights on at all times, including dim lights while sleeping.
- Lock wheelchairs before transferring patients.
- Ensure that patient has appropriate size gown and nonskid footwear. Do not allow gowns or ties to drag on the floor when ambulating.
- Keep floor clean and free of clutter. Post "wet floor" sign if floor was recently mopped or is wet.
- Encourage patient to sit on the side of the bed to get bearings before standing, especially if patient has been on extended bedrest.
- Ensure that patient has glasses on if he or she normally wears them.

Educate patients and family members:

- Patients (as age appropriate):
  - Assist with ambulation even though the child may have ambulated well before hospitalization.
  - Patients who have been lying in bed will need to get up slowly, sitting on the side of the bed before standing.
- Family members:
  - Call the nursing staff for assistance, and do not allow patients to get up independently.
  - Keep the side rails of the crib or bed up whenever patient is in the crib or bed.
  - Do not to leave infants on the daybed; put them in the crib with the side rails up.
  - When all family members need to leave the bedside, notify the nursing staff before leaving and ensure that the patient is in the bed or crib with side rails up and call bell within reach (if appropriate).

Restraining Methods and Therapeutic Hugging

The Joint Commission (2001) defines restraint as "any method, physical or mechanical, which restricts a person's movement, physical activity, or normal access to his or her body." Before initiating restraints, the nurse completes a comprehensive assessment of the patient to determine whether the need for a restraint outweighs the risk of not using one. Restraints can result in loss of dignity, violation of patient rights, psychological harm, physical harm, and even death. Alternative methods should first be considered and documented in the patient's record. The nurse is responsible for selecting the least restrictive type of restraint. Using less restrictive restraints is often possible by gaining the cooperation of the child and parents.

The two types of restraints used with children are classified as medical-surgical and behavioral restraints. When a standard or protocol states that immobilization is required 100% of the time as a part of the procedure or postprocedural care process, the restraint device is considered a part of routine care. For example, the postoperative use of elbow restraints after a cleft lip repair, if written in the protocol or standard of care and used in 100% of patients, would not fall under the Joint Commission or Centers for Medicare and Medicaid Services mandates for restraints.

Medical-surgical restraints are used for children with an artificial airway or airway adjunct for delivery of oxygen, indwelling catheters, tubes, drains, lines, pacemaker wires, or suture sites. The medical-surgical restraint is used to ensure that safe care is given to the patient. The potential risks of the restraint are offset by the potential benefit of providing safer care. Criteria have been developed that outline when medical-surgical restraints may be instituted. These situations include:

- Risk for interruption of therapy used to maintain oxygenation or airway patency
- Risk of harm if indwelling catheter, tube, drain, line, pacemaker wire, or sutures are removed, dislodged, or ruptured
- Patient confusion, agitation, unconsciousness, or developmental inability to understand direct requests or instructions

Medical-surgical restraints can be initiated by an individual order or by protocol; the use of the protocol must be authorized by an individual order. Continued use of restraints must be renewed each day. Patients are monitored at least every 2 hours.

Behavioral restraints are limited to situations with a significant risk of patients physically harming themselves or others because of behavioral reasons and when nonphysical interventions are not effective. Before initiating a behavioral restraint, the nurse should assess the patient's mental, behavioral, and physical status to determine the cause for the child's behavior that may be harmful to the patient or others. If behavioral restraints are indicated, a collaborative approach involving the patient, if appropriate, the family, and the health care team should be used. An order must be obtained as soon as possible, but no longer than 1 hour after the initiation of behavioral restraints. Behavioral restraints for children must be reordered every 1 to 2 hours, based on age. A Licensed Independent Practitioner (LIP) must conduct an in-person evaluation within 1 hour and again every 4 hours until restraints are discontinued. Children in behavioral restraints must be *continuously* observed and assessed every 15 minutes. Assessment components include signs of injury associated with applying restraint, nutrition/hydration, circulation and range-of-motion of extremities, vital signs, hygiene and elimination, physical and psychological status and comfort, and readiness for discontinuation of restraint. Use clinical judgment in setting a schedule of when each of these parameters needs to be evaluated because every parameter must be assessed during each 15-minute physical assessment.

Restraints with ties must be secured to the bed or crib frame, not the siderails. Suggestions for increasing safety and comfort while the child is in a restraint include leaving one finger breadth between skin and the device (Figure 3-1); tying knots that allow for quick release; ensuring the restraint does not tighten as the child moves; decreasing wrinkles or bulges in the restraint; placing jacket restraints over an article of clothing; placing limb restraints below waist level, below knee level, or distal to the IV; and tucking in dangling straps (Selekman and Snyder, 1997).

An alternative approach for temporary restraint is therapeutic holding. Therapeutic holding is the use of a secure, comfortable, temporary holding position that provides close physical contact with the parent or caregiver for 30 minutes or less. The use of restraints can often be avoided with adequate preparation of the child; parental or staff supervision of the child; or adequate protection of a vulnerable site, such as an infusion device. The nurse needs to assess the child's development, mental status, potential to hurt others or self, and safety. The nurse should carefully consider alternative measures to using restraints. Some examples of alternative measures include bringing a child to the nurses' station for continuous observation, providing diversional activities such as music, or encouraging the participation of the parents.

Examples of mechanical restraints are presented in Table 3-2.

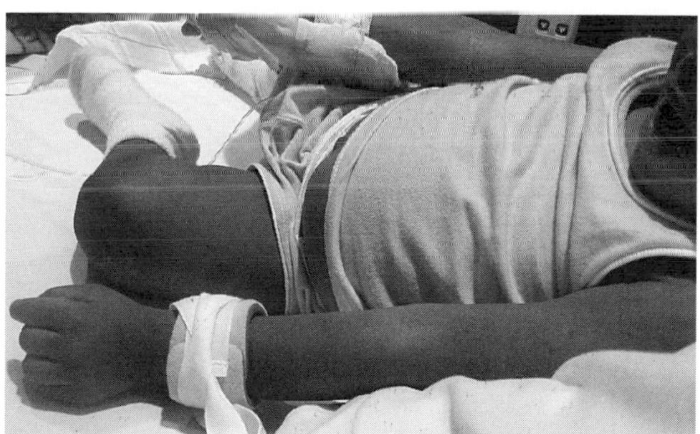

FIGURE **3-1** Wrist restraints.

TABLE 3-2 Types of Mechanical Restraints

Type	Function	Description
Jacket restraint	To prevent child from climbing out of crib or bed	Waist-length, sleeveless jacket with back closure fastened with ties Long ties on bottom of jacket secure child to crib, chair, or bed
Elbow restraint	To prevent child from bending elbow To prevent child from reaching head, face, neck, or chest	Soft, padded commercial restraints Muslin square with vertical pockets to contain tongue depressors that supply vertical rigidity and horizontal flexibility; ties secure the device around the arm Padded large-diameter towel roller Tubular plastic container with top and bottom removed and suitably padded for comfort and safety
Arm and leg restraints	To immobilize one or more extremities: For treatments For procedures To facilitate healing To control child's movements To immobilize extremities To provide temporary restraining device for short procedures	Soft, padded commercial restraints (see Figure 3-1) Place opened sheet or blanket on flat surface with one corner folded to the center Place infant on blanket with shoulders at blanket fold and feet toward opposite corner Place infant's right arm straight against side of body Pull side of blanket on right side firmly across right shoulder and chest Secure beneath left side of body Place left arm straight against side Bring remaining side of blanket across left shoulder and chest Secure beneath body Fold lower corner, bring up to shoulders, and secure ends beneath body Fasten in place with safety pins or tape Modification for chest examination: Left and right corners are brought over arms only to, but not including, chest and secured under body. Bottom corner is secured at waist rather than at shoulders.

Positioning for Procedures

See Atraumatic Care box.

Extremity Venipuncture or Injection

Place child on parent's (or assistant's) lap, with the child facing toward the parent and in the straddle position (Figure 3-2).

For venipuncture, place child's arm on a firm surface such as the treatment table (for support) and on top of a soft cloth or towel.

Have assistant or parent immobilize child's arm for venipuncture.

Have parent hug the child around the back to hold the child's free arm.

Place child on parent's (or assistant's) lap, with the child facing away from the parent (Figure 3-3).

To hold the child's legs still, place them between the parent's legs. This position is appropriate for an injection into the thigh; or, for an injection into the arm, place child in parent's (or assistant's) lap, with the child facing sideward (Figure 3-4).

Place the child's arm closest to the parent under the parent's arm, and wrap toward the back.

Have the parent hold the arm receiving the injection against the child's body.

ATRAUMATIC CARE

Analgesia and Sedation

For painful procedures, the child should receive adequate analgesia or sedation to minimize pain and the need for excessive restraint. For local anesthesia, use buffered lidocaine to reduce stinging sensation or apply LMX, EMLA, or lidocaine iontophoresis. (See Evidence-Based Practice boxes.)

Some painful procedures, such as bone marrow tests, can be performed without restraint using general anesthesia with proper anesthesia monitoring availability (e.g., propofol [Diprivan]).

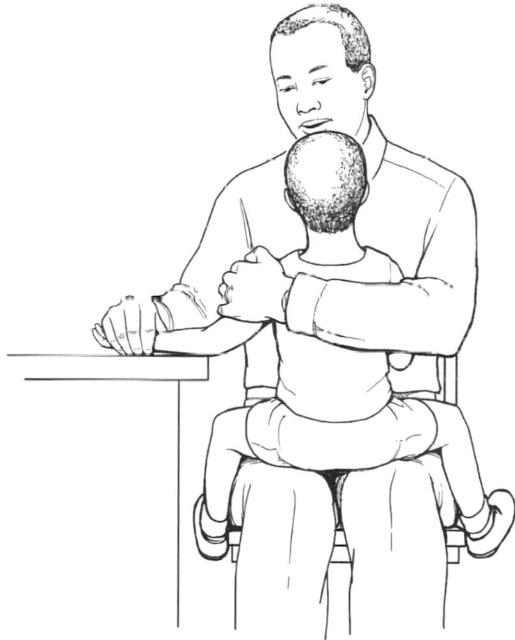

FIGURE **3-2** Chest-to-chest straddle position.

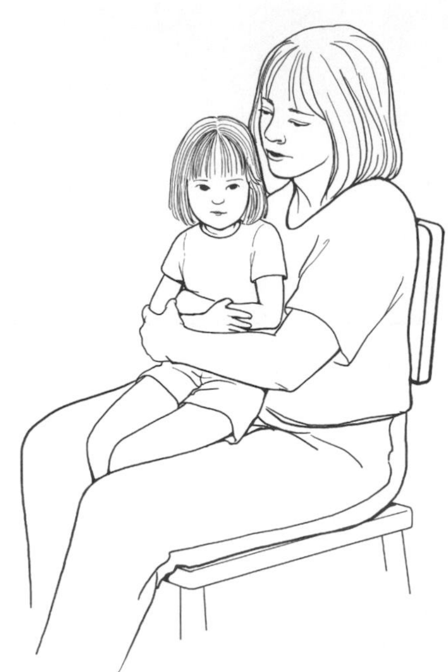

FIGURE **3-3** Chest-to-back sitting position with legs secured.

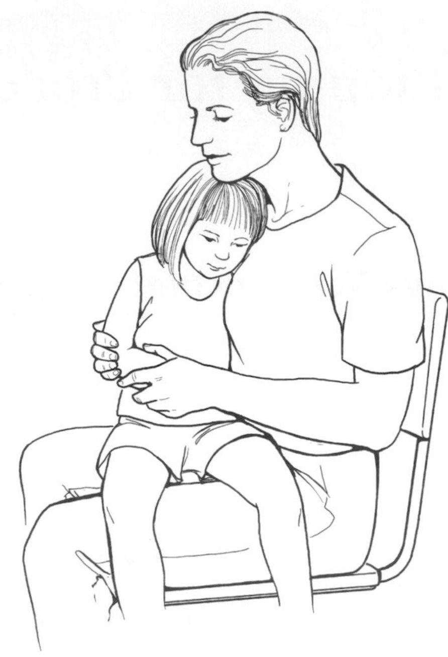

FIGURE **3-4** Side-sitting position.

Femoral Venipuncture

Place infant supine with legs in frog position to provide extensive exposure of the groin.

Restrain legs in frog position with hands while controlling the child's arm and body movements with downward and inward pressure of forearms.

Cover genitalia to protect the operator and the venipuncture site from contamination if the child urinates during the procedure.

Site is not advisable for long-term venous access in mobile child because of risk of infection and trauma to flexion area.

Subdural Puncture (Through Fontanel or Bur Holes)

Place active infant in mummy restraint.

Position supine with head accessible to examiner.

Control head movement with firm hold on each side of the head.

Nose and/or Throat Access

Position supine with face accessible to examiner.

Control head and arms by holding child's extended arms over and close to the head, thus immobilizing both head and arms.

Ear Access

Place child in parent's (or assistant's) lap with the child's body sideways and the ear to be examined away from the parent (Figure 3-5). Place the child's arm closest to the parent under the parent's arm and wrap toward the back.

Have the parent hold the other arm against the child's body and use the free arm to hold the head against the parent's chest.

To hold the child's legs still, place them between the parent's legs.

This can also be performed with the parent standing (Figure 3-6).

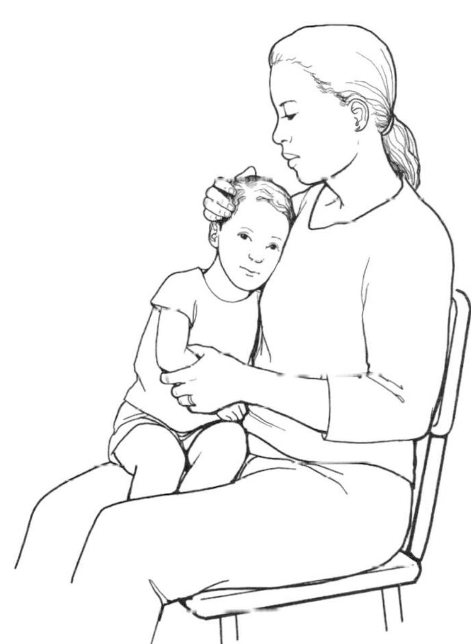

FIGURE **3-5** Side-sitting position with head and legs secured.

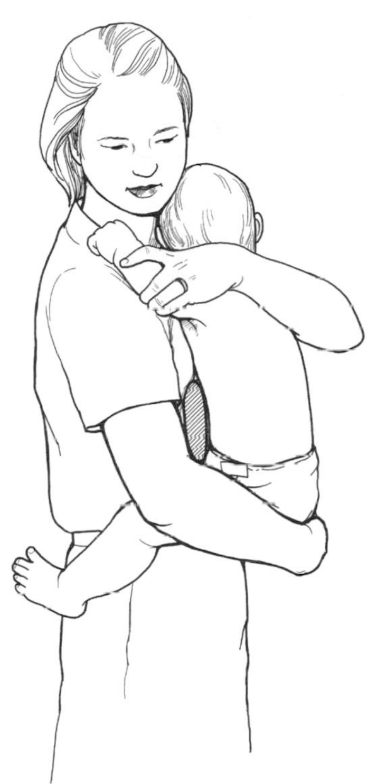

FIGURE **3-6** Chest-to-chest straddle standing position.

Lumbar Puncture

INFANT

Place infant in sitting position with buttocks extended over the edge of the table and head flexed on chest.

In neonates, use side-lying position with modified head extension to decrease respiratory distress during procedure. Pulse oximetry and heart rate monitoring are advisable.

Immobilize arms and legs with nurse's hands.

Observe child for difficulty in breathing.

CHILD

Place child on side with back close to or extended over the edge of examining table, head flexed, and knees drawn up toward the chest.

Reach over the top of the child, and place one arm behind child's neck and the other behind the knees.

Stabilize this position by clasping own hands in front of the child's abdomen.

Take care that excessive pressure does not compromise circulation or breathing and that the nose and mouth are not covered by the restrainer's body.

Bone Marrow Examination

For posterior iliac site:

- Position child prone.
- Place a small pillow or folded towel under the hips to raise them slightly.
- Apply restraint at upper body and lower extremities, preferably with two persons.

For anterior iliac site or tibia:

- Position child supine.
- Apply restraint at upper body and lower extremities, preferably with two persons.

Urinary Catheterization

Have the parent sit in a chair or on an examining table with a back support. Place the child leaning back in the parent's lap with the parent's arms hugging the child's upper body (Figure 3-7).

Place the child's legs in the frog position, with the parent's legs over the child's to stabilize them. In this comfortable position the perineum is exposed for the procedure.

Place the child supine in bed with legs in the frog position. Raise head of bed as much as possible while still allowing good visualization of the perineum. A semiupright position is less stressful to a child.

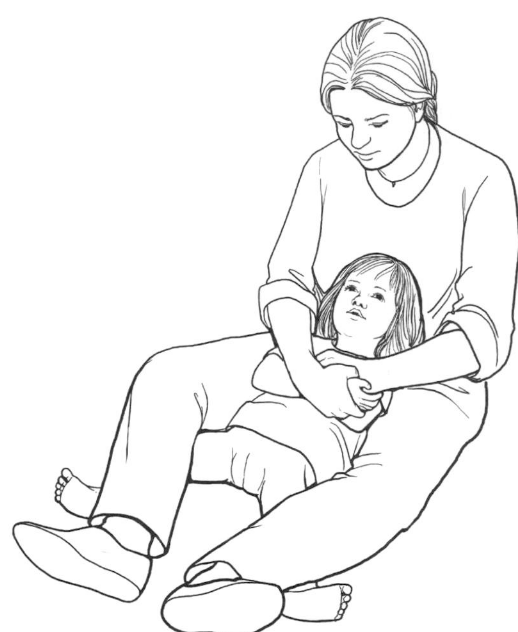

FIGURE **3-7** Semireclining position with legs secured.

Collection of Specimens

Urine

See Safety Alert.

NON–TOILET-TRAINED CHILD*

Use a collection bag; cut a small slit in the diaper and pull the bag through to allow room for urine to collect and to facilitate checking the contents. To obtain small amounts of urine, use a syringe without a needle to aspirate urine directly from the diaper; if diapers with absorbent gelling material that traps urine are used, place a small gauze dressing, some cotton balls, or a urine collection device inside the diaper to collect urine, then aspirate the urine with a syringe.

Check bag frequently, and remove as soon as specimen is available.

Urine collected for culture should be tested within 30 minutes, refrigerated, or placed in a sterile container with a preservative.

TOILET-TRAINED YOUNG CHILD*

Child may not be able to urinate on request.

Child may be more successful if potty chair or bedpan is placed on the toilet.

Use terms familiar to the child, such as "pee pee," "wee wee," or "tinkle."

Enlist parent's assistance.

TOILET-TRAINED OLDER CHILD

Child is cooperative but appreciates explanation of what specimen is for.

Provide privacy and a receptacle, preferably with some means of concealing it, such as a paper bag.

SAFETY ALERT

The American Academy of Pediatrics recommends that urine collected by the bag can be used to determine whether it is necessary to obtain a catheterized urine specimen for culture. For best results, the perineal area should be washed thoroughly before applying the urine collection bag, with prompt removal of the bag as soon as voiding occurs. Leaving the device in situ for more than 1 hour is more likely to yield a contaminated urine specimen

BLADDER CATHETERIZATION

Bladder catheterization is employed for the following reasons:

- Collection of a urine specimen
- Diagnostic testing
- Continuous urinary drainage
- Intravesical instillation of medications or chemotherapeutic agents

Materials Needed

Sterile gloves (Safety Alert)

Catheter (see Safety Alert)

- Select a catheter based on the purpose of the procedure, the age and gender of the child, and any history of prior urologic surgery.
- When collecting a urine specimen or completing a diagnostic test requiring catheterization for a brief period, use:
  - A 4-5 French catheter or 15-inch feeding tube for the infant
  - A 5-8 French catheter or 15-inch feeding tube for the toddler or school-aged child
  - An 8-12 French in-and-out catheter or 8 French, 15-inch feeding tube for the adolescent girl
  - An 8-12 French, straight tipped or coudé-tipped in-and-out catheter for the adolescent boy
- When placing an indwelling catheter, use:
  - A 5 French feeding tube or a 6-8 French Foley catheter with a 3-ml retention balloon for the infant
  - A 6-8 French Foley catheter with a 3-5-ml retention balloon for the toddler or school-aged child
  - An 8-12 French Foley catheter with a 5-ml retention balloon for the adolescent girl

SAFETY ALERT

Nonlatex catheters and sterile gloves should be used for all infants and children with known latex allergy, with latex sensitivity, or on latex precautions (e.g., children with conditions associated with frequent exposure to latex-containing products).

3 - EVIDENCE-BASED PEDIATRIC NURSING INTERVENTIONS

*See Patient and Family Education, p. 506.

- An 8-16 French Foley catheter with a 5-ml retention balloon for the adolescent boy
- Larger French sizes (14 to 16) are reserved for older adolescents with more fully developed prostates. A coudé-tipped catheter is selected for the adolescent boy with a history of urologic surgery.

Catheter tray

- Catheter insertion trays are available that provide a cost-effective alternative to gathering individual supplies for catheterization. These kits may come with or without a catheter, and both should be available for use with children. When a tray is not accessible, the following materials are needed in addition to the catheter: Betadine cleanser with cotton balls, sterile draping, a syringe with 5 ml of sterile water, and sterile, water-soluble lubricating jelly.

Container for urine collection

- When collecting a specimen or completing a diagnostic test, an appropriate urine specimen container and 500-ml basin are used; when inserting an indwelling catheter, a bedside drainage bag is obtained before the procedure. When inserting a Foley catheter, it is preferable to use a preconnected (closed) system containing catheter and bedside drainage bag.

Procedure

1. Assemble necessary equipment.
2. Explain procedure to child and parents.
   - Give a careful and thorough explanation of the procedure, according to the developmental level of the child, before preparation of the perineum. Include an explanation of the purpose of the catheterization, and reassure child that it is not punishment.
   - Reassure parents that catheterization will not harm their child or damage the urethra or hymen.
   - Reassure child that insertion of the catheter will not feel like having a sharp object inserted but will produce a feeling of pressure and desire to urinate.
3. Give instruction on pelvic muscle relaxation whenever possible.
   - Young child is taught to blow (using a pinwheel is helpful) and to press the hips against the bed or procedure table during catheterization in order to relax the pelvic and periurethral muscles.
   - Older child or adolescent is taught to contract and relax the pelvic muscles, and the relaxation procedure is repeated during catheter insertion. If the youngster vigorously contracts the pelvic muscles when the catheter reaches the striated sphincter (proximal urethra in boys and midurethra in girls), catheter insertion is temporarily stopped. The catheter is neither removed nor advanced; instead the child is assisted to press the hips against the bed or examining table and relax the pelvic muscles. The catheter is then gently advanced into the bladder.
4. Place the infant or child in a supine position with the perineum adequately exposed. Girls may bend the knees and abduct the legs in a froglike position; boys should lie with the penis lying above the upper thighs. For a young child, have the parent sit on the bed or examining table with a back support. Place the child leaning back in the parent's lap with the parent's arms hugging the child's upper body. When the child's legs are in the frog position, the parent's legs can be placed over the child's to stabilize them. In this comfortable position the perineum is exposed for the procedure and the child is helped to lie still.
5. Put on a pair of sterile gloves. (See Safety Alert, p. 277.)
6. Place a sterile drape over the perineum of girls, ensuring that the vagina, labia, and urethral meatus remain exposed. Most catheter insertion kits provide a sterile drape with a diamond-shaped hole in the middle to assist with this. For boys the sterile drape is placed over the upper aspect of the thighs.
7. Place 5 ml of sterile lubricating jelly on the sterile drape. During catheterization of an adolescent or child accustomed to the procedure, the catheter may be placed on the sterile drape laid over the perineum. When an anxious child is being catheterized, the catheter should remain on a sterile field that will not be upset should the child move during the procedure.
8. Cleanse the perineum of girls, including the labia, vaginal introitus, and urethral meatus. Use a new cotton ball for each wipe, moving in a front-to-back motion along each side of the labia minora, along the sides of the urinary meatus, and finally straight down over the urethral opening. For boys, the entire glans penis is cleansed, in an outward circular fashion, using one cotton ball for each wipe. The foreskin is retracted in the uncircumcised boy to ensure adequate exposure. If the foreskin cannot be easily retracted, particular care is taken to ensure that the glans penis is adequately cleaned before catheter insertion.
9. Wipe the cleanser from the skin using sterile cotton balls.
10. *Girls:* Spread the labia (if necessary) using one hand in order to clearly visualize the urethral meatus. With the other hand, grasp the catheter and apply a small amount of sterile lubricant from the sterile field onto the tip of the catheter. (It is rarely necessary to spread the labia in infants; instead, locate the urethra, which often appears as a dimple above the hymen.) Gently insert the catheter until urine return is seen. If inserting an indwelling catheter, advance the catheter an additional 1 to 2 inches before attempting to fill the retention balloon.
11. *Boys:* Hold the penile shaft just under the glans to prevent the foreskin from contaminating the area. Grasp the catheter with the other hand, and apply a small amount of sterile lubricant from the sterile field onto the tip of the catheter. Insert the catheter while gently stretching the penis and lifting it to a 90-degree angle to the body. Resistance may occur when the catheter meets the urethral sphincter. Ask the patient to inhale deeply and advance the catheter at that time. Insert the

catheter until urine return occurs; this may take several seconds longer because of the additional lubricant present in the urethra. If inserting an indwelling catheter, advance until urine return is noted and then advance to the bifurcation of the filling port before filling the retention balloon.

12. When catheterizing for specimen collection, allow 15 to 30 ml for urinalysis and urine culture. Drain bladder, and record postvoid urinary volume if collected soon after urination. Cap the specimen, label, and send it to the laboratory.
13. When inserting an indwelling catheter, gently pull catheter back until resistance is met; this ensures that the retention balloon lies just above the bladder neck. Tape tubing to the leg to avoid pulling or use a commercially available catheter securement device. Hang drainage apparatus to bedframe (avoid bed rails to prevent pulling on catheter).

24-HOUR URINE COLLECTION

Begin and end collection with an empty bladder:

- At time collection begins, instruct child to void, and discard specimen.
- Twenty-four hours after that specimen was discarded, instruct child to void for last specimen.

Save all voided urine during the 24 hours in a refrigerated container marked with date, total time, and child's name.

Non–Toilet-Trained Child

Prepare skin with thin coating of skin sealant (unless contraindicated, such as in premature infant or on irritated and/or nonintact skin), and apply a urine collection bag with a collection tube that allows urine to drain into a large receptacle.

If a collection tube is not available, insert a small feeding tube through a puncture hole at the top of the bag; use a syringe without needle to aspirate urine through the feeding tube.

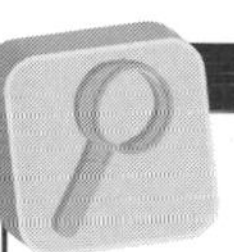

EVIDENCE-BASED PRACTICE

Use of Lidocaine Lubricant for Urethral Catheterization

Marilyn J. Hockenberry

Ask the Question

Question

In children, does a lidocaine lubricant decrease the pain associated with urethral catheterization?

Objective

To evaluate evidence supporting the use of a lidocaine lubricant in decreasing pain in children undergoing urethral catheterization

Background

Urethral catheterization is an invasive procedure for children. Important interventions to minimize the discomfort from this procedure include the expertise of the individual inserting the catheter, choice of an appropriate catheter size and type, and preparation tailored to the child's developmental level. This review further evaluates the use of a lidocaine-based lubricant as an intervention to decrease discomfort associated with this procedure.

Search for Evidence

Search Strategies

Search selection criteria included English language publications within the past 10 years, and research-based and review articles on use of the lidocaine lubricant before urethral catheterization.

Databases Used

Cochrane Collaboration, PubMed, MD Consult, BestBETs, American Academy of Pediatrics

Critically Analyze the Evidence

Smith and Adams (1998) surveyed 46 children's hospitals to determine the existence of standardized practice guidelines for urethral catheter insertion in children. Only 54% of the institutions had a written policy providing guidelines for the procedure, and the hospitals' recommendations lacked consistency.

Grey (1996) published a review of strategies to minimize distress associated with urethral catheterization in children and supported the use of a local anesthetic that contains 2% lidocaine before insertion.

One prospective, double-blind, placebo-controlled trial evaluated the use of lidocaine lubricant for discomfort in 20 children before urethral catheterization. Findings revealed that lidocaine lubricant significantly reduced pain with pediatric urethral catheterization (Gerard, Cooper, Duethman, and others, 2003).

Apply the Evidence: Nursing Implications

- Although only one research study was found to support the use of a topical anesthetic before urethral catheterization, the study found significant reductions in procedural pain. Several publications support its effectiveness in clinical practice.
- A topical anesthetic before urethral catheterization may be helpful, but further evidence is needed.

References

Gerard LL, Cooper CS, Duethman KS, and others: Effectiveness of lidocaine lubricant for discomfort during pediatric urethral catheterization, *J Urol* 170:564-567, 2003.

Grey M: Atraumatic urethral catheterization of children, *Pediatr Nurs* 22(4):306-310, 1996.

Smith AB, Adams LL: Insertion of indwelling urethral catheters in infants and children: a survey of current nursing practice, *Pediatr Nurs* 24(3):229-234, 1998.

Stool

Collect stool without urine contamination, if possible.

NON-TOILET-TRAINED CHILD

Apply a urine collection bag.
Apply diaper over bag.
After bowel movement, use tongue blade to collect stool.
Place specimen in appropriate covered container.

TOILET-TRAINED CHILD

Have child urinate, then flush toilet.
Have child defecate into bedpan or toilet.
To facilitate collecting specimen, place a sheet of plastic wrap over toilet seat, or use a commercial potty hat.
After bowel movement, use tongue blade to collect stool.
Place in appropriate covered container.

Respiratory (Nasal) Secretions

To obtain nasal secretions using a nasal washing:

- Place child supine if maximal restraint needed; upright or semireclining allows the child more control and causes less anxiety.
- Instill 1 to 3 ml sterile NS with a sterile syringe (without needle or with 2 inches of 18- or 20-gauge tubing) into one nostril.
- Aspirate contents with a small, sterile bulb syringe.
- Place in sterile container.

Sputum

Older children and adolescents are able to cough as directed and supply specimens when given proper direction.
Specimens can sometimes be collected from infants and young children who have an endotracheal (ET) tube or tracheostomy by means of tracheal aspiration with a mucous trap or suction apparatus.

Blood

HEEL OR FINGER

Heel lancing has been shown to be more painful than venipuncture; consider venipuncture when the amount of blood from the heel would require much squeezing (e.g., genetic tests).
Puncture should be no deeper than 2 mm.
Obtain necessary equipment, including appropriate specimen container(s).
Explain procedure to child as developmentally appropriate, and provide atraumatic care.
Maintain aseptic technique, and follow Standard Precautions.
To increase blood flow, warm heel by using a commercial heel warmer for 3 minutes before puncture. May hold finger under warm water for a few seconds before puncture.
Prepare area for puncture with antiseptic agent.
Perform puncture on heel or finger in proper location with an automatic lancet device:

- Usual site for heel puncture is outer aspects of heel (Figure 3-8, *A*). Boundaries can be marked by an imaginary line extending posteriorly from a point between the fourth and fifth toes and running parallel to the lateral aspect of the heel and another line extending posteriorly from the middle of the great toe and running parallel to the medial aspect of the heel.
- Usual site for finger puncture is just to the side of the finger pad (see Figure 3-8, *B*), which has more blood vessels and fewer nerve endings. Avoid steadying the finger against a hard surface.

Collect blood sample in appropriate specimen container.
Apply pressure to puncture site with a dry, sterile gauze pad until bleeding stops.
Clean area of prepping agent with water to avoid absorption in neonate.
Praise child for cooperation.
Discard puncture device in puncture-resistant container near site of use.
Document site and amount of blood withdrawn as well as type of test performed.

VEIN

Obtain necessary equipment, including appropriate specimen container(s).
Explain procedure to child as developmentally appropriate, and provide atraumatic care.
Maintain aseptic technique, and use Standard Precautions.
Restrain child only as needed to prevent injury.
Prepare area for puncture with antiseptic agent.
Apply tourniquet; alternative tourniquet for neonate is a rubber band.
Visualize or palpate vein.
Insert needle with bevel up; a slight pop may be felt when entering a child's vein; in small and preterm infants this may not occur.
Withdraw required amount of blood, and place in appropriate container.
Release tourniquet.
Withdraw needle from site, and apply dry, sterile gauze or cotton ball to site with firm pressure until bleeding stops. If antecubital site is used, keep arm extended to reduce bruising.
Clean area of prepping agent with water to decrease absorption in neonate.
Praise child for cooperation.
Discard syringe and needle in puncture-resistant container near site of use.
Document site and amount of blood withdrawn as well as type of test obtained.

ARTERY

Obtain necessary equipment, including appropriate specimen container(s).
Explain procedure to child as developmentally appropriate and provide atraumatic care. Arterial blood samples from punctures are painful and often cause crying and breath holding, which affect the accuracy of blood gas values (decreased PaO_2).
Provide pain intervention with buffered lidocaine, and for infants use sucrose before stick.
Maintain aseptic technique, and use Standard Precautions.
Arterial punctures may be performed using the radial, brachial, or femoral arteries.
Palpate artery for puncture.
Perform *Allen test* to determine adequacy of collateral circulation prior to radial puncture:

- Elevate extremity distal to puncture site, and blanch by squeezing gently (e.g., making a fist); two arteries supplying blood flow to the extremity (radial and ulnar arteries of the wrist) are then occluded.
- Lower extremity, and remove pressure from one artery (ulnar); color return to the blanched extremity in less than 5 seconds indicates adequate collateral circulation.

Prepare area for puncture with antiseptic agent.
Insert needle at a 60- to 90-degree angle.
Withdraw required amount of blood into syringe (or specimen container, as appropriate).
Withdraw needle, and apply pressure to site with a dry, sterile gauze pad for 5 to 10 minutes until bleeding stops. NOTE: Pressure must be applied at the site to prevent a hematoma.
Place specimen in heparinized syringe after removing bubbles from the syringe.
Place specimen on ice.
Clean area of prepping agent with water to decrease absorption in neonate.
Praise child for cooperation.
Discard syringe needle in puncture-resistant container near site of use.
Document site and amount of blood withdrawn as well as type of test performed.

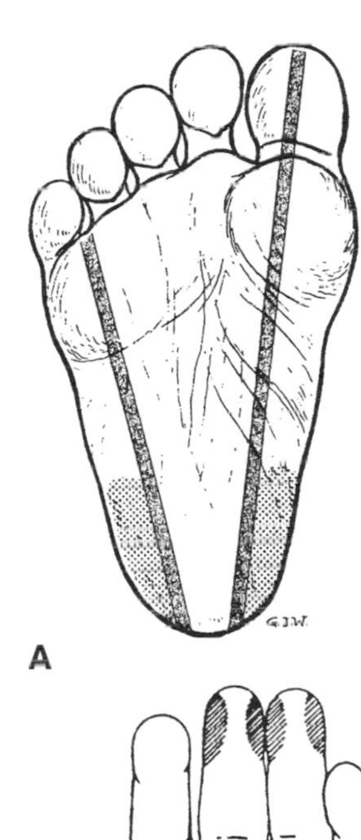

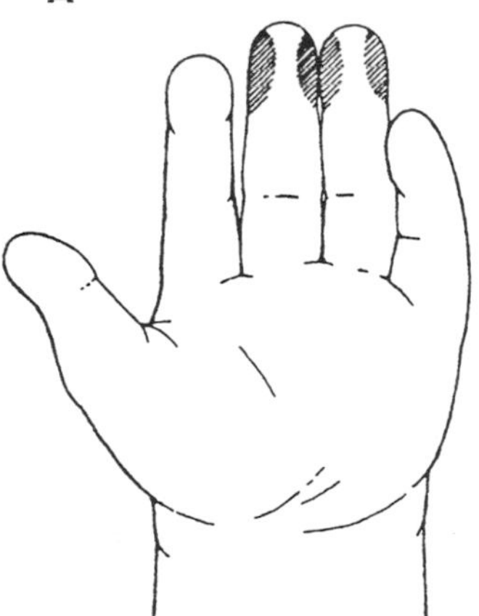

FIGURE **3-8** **A,** Puncture sites *(stippled areas)* on infant's heel. **B,** Puncture sites on fingers. (**B** from Smith DP, Wong DL: *Comprehensive child and family nursing skills,* St Louis, 1991, Mosby.)

Procedures Related to Administration of Medications

General Guidelines

ESTIMATING DRUG DOSAGE

Body surface area as a basis: estimated from height and weight by use of West nomogram (Figure 3-9)

Body surface area related to adult dose:

$$\frac{\text{Body surface area of child}}{\text{Body surface area of adult}} \times \text{Average adult dose} = \text{Estimated child's dose}$$

Body surface area related to average dose per square meter (m^2):

Body surface area of child (m^2) × Dose/m^2 = Estimated child's dose

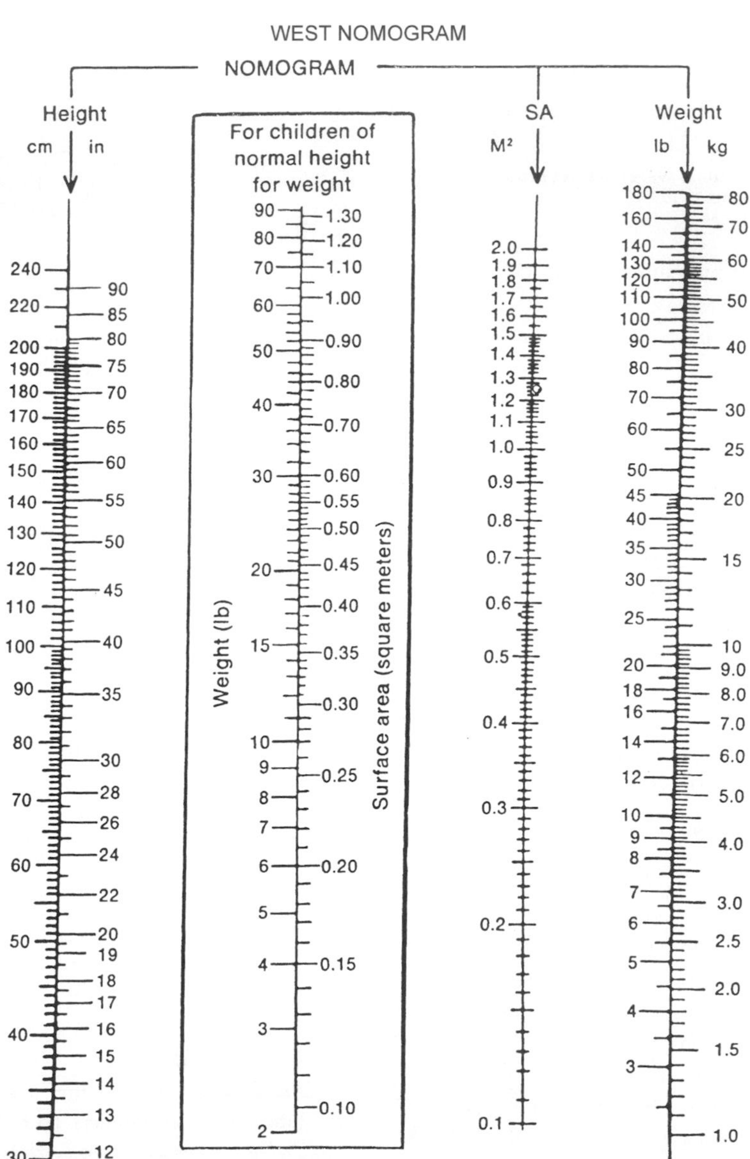

FIGURE **3-9** West nomogram (for estimation of surface areas). The surface area is indicated where a straight line connecting the height and weight intersects the surface area *(SA)* column; or, if the patient is approximately of normal proportion, from the weight alone *(boxed area)*. (Nomogram modified from data of E Boyd by CD West. In Behrman RE, Kliegman RM, Jenson HB, editors: *Nelson textbook of pediatrics,* ed 16, Philadelphia, 2000, Saunders.)

APPROACHES TO PEDIATRIC PATIENTS

Children's reactions to treatments are affected by the following:

- Developmental characteristics, such as physical abilities and cognitive capabilities
- Environmental influences
- Past experiences
- Current relationship with the nurse
- Perception of the present situation

Expect success: use a positive approach.

Provide an explanation appropriate to the child's developmental level.

Allow the child choices whenever they exist.

Be honest with the child.

Involve the child in the treatment in order to gain cooperation.

Allow the child the opportunity to express his or her feelings.

Praise the child for doing his or her best.

Provide distraction for a frightened or uncooperative child.

Spend some time with the child after administering the medication.

Let the child know that he or she is accepted as a person of value. (See also section on preparing children for procedures, p. 253.)

SAFETY PRECAUTIONS

Take a drug allergy history.

Check the following five *R*'s for correctness:

- Right drug
- Right dosage
- Right time
- Right route
- Right child (Always check identification band.)

Double-check drug and dosage with another nurse.

Always double-check the following:

- Digoxin
- Insulin
- Heparin
- Blood
- Chemotherapy
- Cardiotoxic drugs

May also double-check the following:

- Epinephrine
- Opioids (narcotics)
- Sedatives

Be aware of drug-drug or drug-food interactions.

Document all drugs administered.

Monitor child for side effects.

Be prepared for serious side effects (e.g., respiratory depression, anaphylaxis).

Teaching Family to Administer Medication

Family needs to know the following:

- Name of the drug
- Purpose for which the drug is given
- Amount of the drug to be given
- Length of time to be administered (e.g., for IV or inhaled medication)
- Anticipated effects of the drug (therapeutic effects, possible side effects)
- Signs that might indicate an adverse reaction to the drug
- Time(s) to give the drug
- Safe storage of drug (Safety Alert)

Assess the family's level of understanding.

Explain the administration procedure. Instruction needed varies markedly with the intellectual level of the learner and the type and route of medication to be administered.

Demonstrate and have family return the demonstration (if appropriate).

Give written instructions.*

Assist family in scheduling the time for administration around the family routine.

Be certain family knows what to do and whom to contact if any side effects occur.

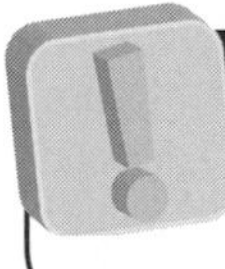

SAFETY ALERT

Dispose of any plastic covers that may be on the ends of syringes. These covers are small enough to be aspirated by young children.†

†Botash SA: Syringe caps: an aspiration hazard, *Pediatrics* 90(1):92-93, 1992.

*See Patient and Family Education related to administering medication beginning on p. 522.

Oral Administration*

1. Follow safety precautions for administration.
2. Select appropriate vehicle, for example, calibrated cup, oral medication syringe, dropper, measuring spoon, or nipple (Safety Alert).
3. Prepare medication:
   - Measure into appropriate vehicle.
   - Crush tablets (except when contraindicated, e.g., time-released or enteric-coated preparations) for children who will have difficulty swallowing; mix with syrup, juice, and so on (Atraumatic Care box).
   - Avoid mixing medications with essential food items, such as milk and formula.
4. Employ safety precautions in identification and administration (Safety Alert).

INFANTS

Hold in semireclining position.

Place oral syringe, measuring spoon, or dropper in mouth well back on the tongue or to the side of the tongue.

Administer slowly to reduce likelihood of choking or aspiration.

Allow infant to suck medication placed in a nipple.

OLDER INFANT OR TODDLER

Offer medication in cup or spoon.

Administer with oral syringe, measuring spoon, or dropper (as with infants).

Use mild or partial restraint with reluctant children.

Do not force actively resistive children because of danger of aspiration; postpone 20 to 30 minutes, and offer medication again.

SAFETY ALERT

Many pediatric medications are given by drops or dropper. A misunderstanding of these terms by parents can result in a potential overdose.† In addition, many droppers that come with medications are marked in tenths of cubic centimeters. If a parent were to use a syringe instead of the dropper, 0.4 cc may be thought to be the same as 4 cc. Educate parents about the correct methods for giving medication, and demonstrate the proper techniques.

†Rudy C: A drop or a dropper: the risk of overdose, *J Pediatr Health Care* 6(1):40, 51-52, 1992.

PRESCHOOL CHILDREN

Use straightforward approach.

For reluctant children, use the following:

- Simple persuasion
- Innovative containers
- Reinforcement, such as stars, stickers, or other tangible rewards for compliance

ATRAUMATIC CARE

Encouraging a Child's Acceptance of Oral Medications

Give the child a flavored ice pop or a small ice cube to suck to numb the tongue before giving the drug.

Mix the drug with a small amount (about 1 teaspoon) of sweet-tasting substance such as honey (except in infants because of the risk of botulism), flavored syrup, jam, fruit puree, sherbet, or ice cream; avoid essential food items, such as formula or milk, because the child may later refuse to eat or drink them.

Give a chaser of water, juice, soft drink, flavored ice pop, or frozen juice bar after the drug.

If nausea is a problem, give a carbonated beverage poured over finely crushed ice before or immediately after the medication.

When medication has an unpleasant taste, have the child pinch the nose and drink the medicine through a straw. (Much of what we taste is associated with smell.)

Flavorings such as apple, banana, and bubble gum can be added at many pharmacies (e.g., FLAVORx) at nominal additional cost. Another alternative is to have the pharmacist prepare the drug in a flavored, chewable troche or lozenge.‡

Infants will suck medicine from a needleless syringe or dropper in small increments (0.25 to 0.5 ml) at a time. Use a nipple or special pacifier with a reservoir for the drug.

‡For information about compounding drugs, contact Technical Staff, Professional Compounding Centers of America (PCCA), 9901 S. Wilcrest Dr., Houston, TX 77099; (800)331-2498; *http://www.pccarx.com.*

SAFETY ALERT

When a dose is ordered that is outside the usual range, or if there is some question regarding the preparation or the route of administration, the nurse always checks with the practitioner before proceeding with the administration, because the nurse is legally liable for any drug administered.

*See Patient and Family Education, p. 523.

Intramuscular Administration*

Obtain necessary equipment.

Explain procedure to child as developmentally appropriate, and provide atraumatic care (Atraumatic Care box).

Use safety precautions in administering medications. (See p. 283.)

Select needle and syringe appropriate to the following:

- Amount of fluid to be administered (syringe size)
- Viscosity of fluid to be administered (needle gauge)
- Amount of tissue to be penetrated (needle length)
- If withdrawing medication from an ampule, use a needle equipped with a filter that removes glass particles; then use a new, nonfilter needle for injection. Replace needle after withdrawing medication from a vial.

Maintain aseptic technique, and follow Standard Precautions.

Provide for sufficient help in restraining the child; children are often uncooperative, and their behavior is usually unpredictable.

Determine the site of injection (see pp. 289-290); make certain muscle is large enough to accommodate volume and type of medication.

- Older children—Select site as with the adult patient; allow child some choice of site, if feasible.
- Following are acceptable sites for infants and small or debilitated children:
  - Vastus lateralis muscle
  - Ventrogluteal muscle

Prepare area for puncture with antiseptic agent and allow to dry completely.

Administer the medication:

- Expose injection area for unobstructed view of landmarks.
- Select a site where the skin is free of irritation and danger of infection; palpate for and avoid sensitive or hardened areas. With multiple injections, rotate sites.
- Place the child in a lying or sitting position; the child is not allowed to stand for the following reasons:
  - Landmarks are more difficult to assess.
  - Restraint is more difficult.
  - The child may faint and fall.
- Grasp the muscle firmly between the thumb and fingers to isolate and stabilize the muscle for deposition of the drug in its deepest part; in obese children spread the skin with the thumb and index finger to displace subcutaneous tissue and grasp the muscle deeply on each side.

ATRAUMATIC CARE

Injections

Select a method to anesthetize the puncture site:

- Apply EMLA on site 2½ hours before intramuscular (IM) injection, or apply LMX on site for a at least 30 minutes before injection.
- Use a vapocoolant spray (e.g., Fluori-Methane or ethyl chloride)* just before injection.
- Use shotblocker before injection at the site.
- For infants use sucrose before injection.

Prepare site with antiseptic and allow to dry completely before skin is penetrated.

Have medication at room temperature.

Use a new, sharp needle with smallest gauge that permits free flow of the medication and safe penetration of muscle.

Decrease perception of pain:

- Distract child with conversation.
- Give child something on which to concentrate (e.g., squeezing a hand or bed rail, pinching own nose, humming, counting, yelling "ouch!").
- Say to child, "If you feel this, tell me to take it out."
- Have child hold a small bandage and place it on puncture site after IM injection is given.

Enlist parents' assistance if they wish to participate and/or assist.

Restrain child *only as needed* to perform procedure safely (See restraining methods and therapeutic hugging, p. 270.)

Insert needle quickly using a dartlike motion.

Avoid tracking any medication through superficial tissues:

- Replace needle after withdrawing medication, or wipe medication from needle with sterile gauze.
- If withdrawing medication from an ampule, use a needle equipped with a filter that removes glass particles; then use a new, nonfilter needle for injection.
- Use the Z track and/or air-bubble technique as indicated.
- Avoid any depression of the plunger during insertion of the needle.

Place a small bandage on puncture site (unless skin is compromised, e.g., in low-birth-weight infant); with young children decorate bandage by drawing a smiling face or other symbol of acceptance.

Hold and cuddle young child, and encourage parents to comfort child; praise older child.

*Abbott K, Fowler-Kerry S: The use of a topical refrigerant anesthetic to reduce injection pain in children, *J Pain Symptom Manage* 10(8):584-590, 1995; Cohen Reis E, Holubkov R: Vapocoolant spray is equally effective as EMLA cream in reducing immunization pain in school-aged children, *Pediatrics* 100(6):E5, 1997.

*See Patient and Family Education related to intramuscular injection (pp. 525-526) and subcutaneous injection (p. 527).

- Insert needle quickly using a dartlike motion.
- Avoid tracking any medication through superficial tissues:
  - Use the Z track and/or air-bubble technique as indicated.
  - Avoid any depression of the plunger during insertion of the needle.
- Aspirate for blood.
  - If blood is found, remove syringe from site, change needle, and reinsert into new location.
  - If no blood is found, inject into a relaxed muscle.
- Inject medication slowly over several seconds.

Remove needle quickly; hold gauze firmly against skin near needle when removing it to avoid pulling on tissue.

Apply firm pressure with dry gauze to the site after injection; massage the site to hasten absorption unless contraindicated (e.g., with iron, dextran).

Clean area of prepping agent with water to decrease absorption of agent in neonate.

Praise child for cooperation.

Discard syringe and needle in puncture-resistant container near site of use.

Record date, time, dose, drug, and site of injection.

Intramuscular Administration: Location, Needle Length, Gauge, and Fluid Administration Amount

	Location of Injection	Needle Length (inches)	Needle Gauge (G)	Suggested Maximum Amount (ml)
Preterm newborn	Anterolateral thigh	5/8	23-25	0.25-0.5*
Term newborn	Anterolateral thigh	5/8	23-25	0.5-1*
Infant (1 month to 12 months)	Anterolateral thigh	5/8-1	22-25	1*
Toddler (13 to 36 months)	Deltoid	5/8-1	22-25	0.5-1*
	Anterolateral thigh or ventrogluteal	5/8-1† 1-1¼‡	22-25	1-2*
Preschool and older children	Deltoid	5/8-1	22-25	0.5-1*
	Anterolateral thigh or ventrogluteal	1-1¼‡	22-25	2-3*
Adolescent	Deltoid	5/8-1 1-1½† 1-1¼§	22-25	1-1.5* 2§
	Anterolateral thigh or ventrogluteal	1-1¼‡ 1-1½†	22-25	2-3* 2-5§

Modified from Becton-Dickinson Media Center: A *guide for managing the pediatric patient: reducing the anxiety and pain of injections*, Franklin Lakes, NJ, 1998, Becton-Dickinson; Centers for Disease Control and Prevention: General recommendations on immunization: recommendations of the Advisory Committee on Immunization Practices (ACIP), *MMWR* 55(RR-15):16-18, 2006; American Academy of Pediatrics; *Red book, 2006 Report of the Committee on Infectious Diseases,* ed 27, Elk Grove Village, IL, 2006, American Academy of Pediatrics, pp 19-21; and Nicoll LH, Hesby A: Intramuscular injection: an integrative research review and guideline for evidence-based practice, *Appl Nurs Res* 16(2):149-162, 2002.

*Evaluate size of muscle mass before administration.

†Centers for Disease Control and Prevention, 2006.

‡American Academy of Pediatrics, 2006.

§Nicoll and Hesby, 2002.

EVIDENCE-BASED PRACTICE

Intramuscular Injections in Infants, Toddlers, and Small Children

David Wilson

Ask the Question

Question

In infants, toddlers, and small children, what are the best site, technique, needle size and gauge, and dosage for intramuscular (IM) injections?

Objective

To evaluate the evidence comparing various practices in IM injection administration in infants, toddlers, and small children

Background

Infants and toddlers receive more immunizations than children of any other age. Although several vaccines are available in conjugate form, infants may receive as many as four or five injections per clinic visit. This age-group also has a smaller muscle mass for injectable medications than any other age-group, thus placing them at risk for more pain and potential side effects from injected medications. Many immunizations require IM administration for maximum effectiveness. It is imperative that nurses administering vaccines and other medications to infants and toddlers use an appropriate site, needle size, and amount of medication for the child's size, in addition to adhering to the five rights of drug administration, to minimize adverse effects. Common complications of IM injection include abscess, fibrosis and muscle contractures, nerve injury, and local and systemic reactions (erythema, pain, limited mobility) (Beecroft and Kongelbeck, 1994).

Search the Evidence

Search Strategies

Literature from 1990 to 2006 was reviewed to obtain clinical research studies related to this issue.

Databases Used

CINAHL, PubMed

Critically Analyze the Evidence

The searches reviewed were mostly small studies. There were no randomized trials, double-blinded trials, or large clinical studies addressing the subject of IM injections in children.

Studies in adults indicate that injection pain can be minimized by deep IM administration, because muscle tissue has fewer nerve endings and medications are absorbed faster than with subcutaneous administration (Zuckerman, 2000). Immunizations such as diphtheria-tetanus–acellular pertussis (DTaP) and hepatitis A and B contain an aluminum adjuvant that, if injected into subcutaneous tissue, increases the incidence of local reactions. Inadvertent injection into subcutaneous tissue may be caused by use of a needle too short to reach IM tissue (Zuckerman, 2000).

One study found that 4-month-old infants experienced fewer local side effects (redness, tenderness, and swelling) when immunizations were administered into the anterior aspect of the thigh with a 25-mm (1-inch) needle as opposed to the shorter 16-mm (⅝-inch) needle (Diggle and Deeks, 2000). A subsequent study by the same group found that infants immunized with (ACT-Hib) and a meningococcal vaccine in separate vastus lateralis injection sites with a 1-inch needle had significantly fewer localized reactions (edema, erythema, hardness, tenderness), than infants immunized with the ⅝-inch needle (Diggle, Deeks, and Pollard, 2006).

Another study comparing needle length and injection method found that a longer needle (25 mm) was preferred for injection when bunching the skin and injecting, whereas a shorter needle (16 mm) was perceived as causing fewer localized reactions when the injection was administered with the skin held taut (Grosswasser, Kahn, Bouche, and others, 1997). However, the study's conclusions fail to address whether needle lengths were applicable to both the deltoid and the vastus lateralis muscles.

Cook and Murtagh (2002) made ultrasound measurements of the subcutaneous and muscle layer thickness in 57 children ages 2, 4, 6, and 18 months. These researchers concluded that a 16-mm needle was sufficient to penetrate the anterolateral thigh muscle if the needle is inserted at a 90-degree angle without pinching the muscle, whereas thigh measurements demonstrated that a 25-mm needle was necessary to penetrate the muscle when a 45-degree injection technique was employed. This study supports the concept of longer needle length to fully deposit the medication into the muscle.

In a study by Davenport (2004), needle length proved to be the most significant variable for local reactions in children after injection with 16-mm and 25-mm needles; the 25-mm needle was associated with fewer localized reactions.

Beecroft and Redick (1990) cited numerous differences of opinion regarding IM injection technique among pediatric nurses, highlighting how little agreement there is with regard to injection site and technique among the evaluated nursing texts .

In a study of diphtheria-tetanus-pertussis (DTP) immunizations administered to infants 7 months of age and younger, only 84.6% of injections were administered at the correct site (anterior thigh); an alarming number were given in the dorsogluteal (5.1%) and deltoid (2.6%) muscles (Daly, Johnston, and Chung, 1992).

Beecroft and Kongelbeck (1994) evaluated pediatric IM injections and concluded that the ventrogluteal site is the site of choice in children of all ages and no reports of complications at this site appeared in the literature. The ventrogluteal site is relatively free of important nerves and vascular structures, the site is easily identified by landmarks, and the subcutaneous tissue is thinner in that area. To date, no reports can be found in the literature to refute the claims made by these researchers.

Nicoll and Hesby (2002) developed a clinical practice guideline for intramuscular injection in children and adults; the guideline recommends the vastus lateralis as the preferred site for IM injection in infants, the vastus lateralis and deltoid as preferred sites for toddlers and children, and ventrogluteal and deltoid sites for adults. The recommended needle sizes for

Continued

EVIDENCE-BASED PRACTICE

Intramuscular Injections in Infants, Toddlers, and Small Children—cont'd

vastus lateralis injections are ⅝-inch to 1-inch (age not specified) and for deltoid injections in children needle sizes ⅝-inch to 1¼-inch are recommended.

The American Academy of Pediatrics (AAP, 2006) and the Centers for Disease Control and Prevention (CDC, 2006) recommend that vaccines containing adjuvants such as aluminum (DTaP, hepatitis A and B, diphtheria-tetanus [DT or Td]) be given deep into the muscle to prevent local reactions. In addition, a 16-mm needle may be adequate for injections in infants less than 1 month old, and a 25-mm (1 inch) needle can be used in infants aged 1 to 12 months . The CDC (2006) recommends that toddlers receive injections with a 25- to 32-mm (1-inch to 1¼-inch) needle in the deltoid if muscle size is adequate; a minimum of a 1-inch long needle is recommended for anterolateral thigh injection in toddlers. Both the AAP (2006) and the CDC (2006) recommend a 22- to 25- gauge needle for all intramuscular childhood immunizations. The deltoid muscle may be used for immunizations in toddlers with adequate muscle mass, older children, and adolescents. Diggle (2003) recommends the deltoid muscle for IM injections in children over 1 year of age. When multiple vaccines are given, two may be given in the thigh (anterior and lateral) because of its larger size. The AAP (2006) recommends that injections in the anterolateral thigh be given at least 2.5 cm (1 inch) apart so that local reactions are less likely to overlap. The dorsogluteal muscle should be avoided in infants and toddlers, and perhaps even in smaller preschoolers with smaller muscle mass, because of the possibility of damaging the sciatic nerve.

No research or supportive data were found regarding the amount of medication to be given at the different sites in infants and toddlers; although a table from one text had suggested amounts, the basis for these recommendations is unknown. In general, 1 ml of medication is recommended for infants younger than 12 months; however, no data can be found to refute or support such a recommendation. Furthermore, small and preterm infants may tolerate only up to 0.5 ml in each muscle to prevent local complications.

In summary, some discrepancy remains in actual clinical practice regarding IM injection sites, amount of drug injected, and needle size in infants and toddlers. Further research is needed to address the following issues:

- What is the appropriate muscle in which an IM injection can be administered with fewest adverse effects in infants and toddlers?
- What is the appropriate needle size based on the infant or toddler's age and weight?
- What is the largest safe amount of medication that can be given to infants and toddlers based on weight and muscle size?

Apply the Evidence: Nursing Implications

- Based on the evidence in the literature, the recommendation is to continue administering IM injections to infants in the anterolateral thigh (up to 12 months old), deltoid (12 months and older), and ventrogluteal site. A 22- to 25-gauge needle may be used for immunizations in infants and children because the vaccines available are not viscous solutions.
- Needle length is an important factor in decreasing local reactions; the length should be adequate to deposit the medication into the muscle for IM injections. Recommendations according to age and muscle size vary slightly.

References

American Academy of Pediatrics, Committee on Infectious Diseases, Pickering L, editor: *2006 Red book: report of the Committee on Infectious Diseases,* ed 27, Elk Grove Village, Ill, 2006, AAP.

Beecroft PC, Kongelbeck SR: How safe are intramuscular injections? *AACN Clin Issues* 5(2):207-215, 1994.

Beecroft PC, Redick SA: Intramuscular injection practices of pediatric nurses: site selection, *Nurse Educ* 15(4):23-28, 1990.

Centers for Disease Control and Prevention: General recommendations on immunization, *MMWR Morb Mortal Wkly Rep* 55(RR-15):14-17, 2006.

Cook IF, Murtagh J: Needle length required for intramuscular vaccination of infants and toddlers: an ultrasonographic study, *Aust Fam Physician* 31(3):295-297, 2002.

Daly JM, Johnston W, Chung Y: Injection sites utilized for DPT immunizations in infants, *J Community Health Nurs* 9(2):87-94, 1992.

Davenport JM: A systematic review to ascertain whether the standard needle is more effective than a longer or wider needle in reducing the incidence of local reaction in children receiving primary immunization, *J Adv Nurs* 46(1):66-77, 2004.

Diggle L: The administration of child vaccines, part 11, Childhood vaccinations, *Pract Nurse* 25(12):63-69, 2003.

Diggle L, Deeks J: Effect of needle length on incidence of local reactions to routine immunisation in infants aged 4 months: randomised controlled trial, *BMJ* 321(7266):931-933, 2000.

Diggle L, Deeks J, Pollard AJ: Effect of needle size on immunogenicity and reactogenicity of vaccines in infants: a randomized controlled trial. *BMJ* 333(7568): 563-564, 2006.

Groswasser J, Kahn A, Bouche B, and others: Needle length and injection technique for efficient intramuscular vaccine delivery in infants and children evaluated through an ultrasonographic determination of subcutaneous and muscle layer thickness, *Pediatrics* 100(3 Pt 1):400-403, 1997.

Nicoll LH, Hesby A: Intramuscular injection: an integrative research review and guideline for evidence-based practice, *Appl Nurs Res* 16(2):149-162, 2002.

Zuckerman J: The importance of injecting vaccines into muscle, *BMJ* 321(7271):1237-1238, 2000.

Intramuscular Injection Sites in Children

Site	Discussion

Vastus Lateralis

GREATER TROCHANTER*
Sciatic nerve
Femoral artery
Site of injection (vastus lateralis)
Rectus femoris
KNEE JOINT*

Location*

Palpate to find greater trochanter and knee joints; divide vertical distance between these two landmarks into thirds; inject into middle one third.

Needle Insertion and Size

Insert needle at 90-degree angle between syringe and upper thigh in infants and in young children.
22-25 gauge, 5/8-1 inch

Advantages

Large, well-developed muscle that can tolerate larger quantities of fluid (0.5 ml [infant] to 2 ml [child])
Easily accessible if child is supine, side lying, or sitting

Disadvantages

Thrombosis of femoral artery from injection in midthigh area (rectus femoris muscle)
Sciatic nerve damage from long needle injected posteriorly and medially into small extremity
More painful than deltoid or gluteal sites

Ventrogluteal

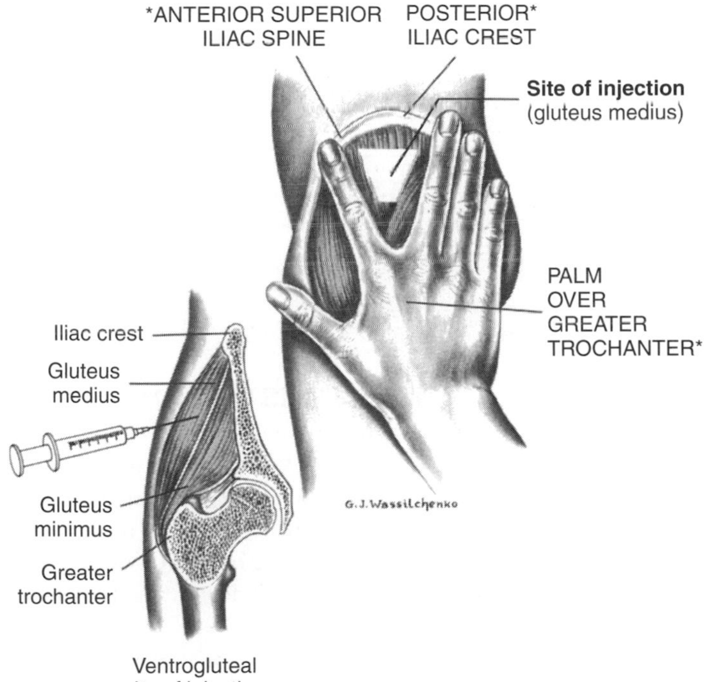

Location*

Palpate to locate greater trochanter, anterior superior iliac tubercle (found by flexing thigh at hip and measuring up to 1-2 cm above crease formed in groin), and posterior iliac crest; place palm of hand over greater trochanter, index finger over anterior superior iliac tubercle, and middle finger along crest of ilium posteriorly as far as possible; inject into center of V formed by fingers.

Needle Insertion and Size

Insert needle perpendicular to site but angled slightly toward greater trochanter.
22-25 gauge, 1/2-1 inch

Advantages

Free of important nerves and vascular structures
Easily identified by prominent bony landmarks
Thinner layer of subcutaneous tissue than in dorsogluteal site, thus less chance of depositing drug subcutaneously rather than intramuscularly
Can accommodate larger quantities of fluid (0.5 ml [infant] to 2 ml [child])
Easily accessible if child is supine, prone, or side lying
Less painful than vastus lateralis

Disadvantages

Health professionals' unfamiliarity with site

*Locations of landmarks are indicated by asterisks on illustrations.

Continued

Intramuscular Injection Sites in Children—cont'd

Site	Discussion
Deltoid	**Location***

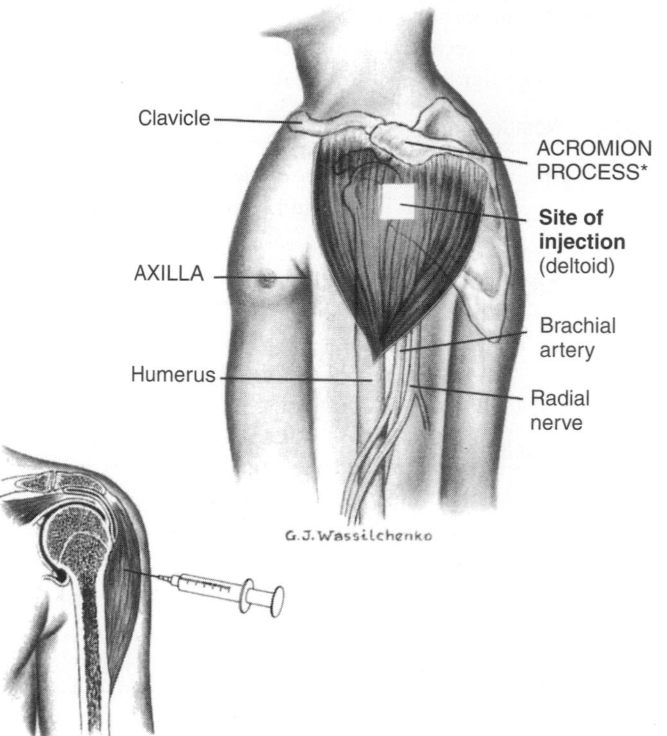

Location*

Locate acromion process; inject only into upper third of muscle that begins about two finger-breadths below acromion but is above axilla.

Needle Insertion and Size

Insert needle perpendicular to site with syringe angled slightly toward elbow.
22-25 gauge, ½-1 inch

Advantages

Faster absorption rates than gluteal sites
Easily accessible with minimum removal of clothing
Less pain and fewer local side effects from vaccines as compared with vastus lateralis

Disadvantages

Small muscle mass; only limited amounts of drug can be injected (0.5-1 ml)
Small margins of safety with possible damage to radial nerve and axillary nerve (not shown, lies under deltoid at head of humerus)

Subcutaneous and Intradermal Administration

Obtain necessary equipment.
Explain procedure to child as developmentally appropriate, and provide atraumatic care. (See Atraumatic Care box on p. 285.)
Maintain aseptic technique, and follow Standard Precautions.
Any site may be used where there are relatively few sensory nerve endings and large blood vessels and bones are relatively deep.
Suggested sites:

- Center third of lateral aspect of upper arm
- Abdomen
- Center third of anterior thigh
- (Avoid the medial side of arm or leg, where skin is more sensitive.)

After injection:

- Clean area of prepping agent with water to decrease absorption of agent in neonate.
- Praise child for cooperation.
- Discard syringe and needle in puncture-resistant container near site of use.
- Record date, time, dose, drug, and site of injection.

NEEDLE SIZE AND INSERTION

Use 26- to 30-gauge needle; change needle before skin puncture if it pierced a rubber stopper on a vial.
Prepare area for puncture with antiseptic agent. Inject small volumes (up to 0.5 ml).

SUBCUTANEOUS ADMINISTRATION

Pinch tissue fold with thumb and index finger.
Using a dartlike motion, insert needle at a 90-degree angle (Figure 3-10). (Some practitioners use a 45-degree angle on children with little subcutaneous tissue or those who are dehydrated. However, the benefit of using the 45-degree angle rather than the 90-degree angle remains controversial.)
Aspirate for blood. (Some practitioners believe it is not necessary to aspirate before injecting subcutaneously; however, this is not universally accepted. Automatic injector devices do not aspirate before injecting.)
Inject medication slowly without tracking through tissues.

*Locations of landmarks are indicated by asterisks on illustrations.

INTRADERMAL ADMINISTRATION

Spread skin site with thumb and index finger if needed for easier penetration.
Insert needle with bevel up and parallel to skin.
Aspirate for blood.
Inject medication slowly.

USE OF INSUFLON FOR SUBCUTANEOUS ADMINISTRATION OF INSULIN

Small indwelling catheter is placed in the subcutaneous tissues.
The average indwelling time is 3 to 5 days.
The catheter is most often inserted in the abdomen, but the buttocks and other areas can also be used. Topical anesthetic cream is recommended before insertion.
Needles 10 mm or shorter should be used for injecting to avoid penetration of the tubing of the catheter.
Using indwelling catheters for up to 4 to 5 days does not affect the absorption of insulin.
The long-term (measured by HbA1c) and short-term glucose control (measured by blood glucose profiles and insulin levels) is not altered.
The dead space of the catheter is about 0.5 unit of U100 so it may be necessary to give 0.5 units extra with the first dose after insertion if the child uses small doses.

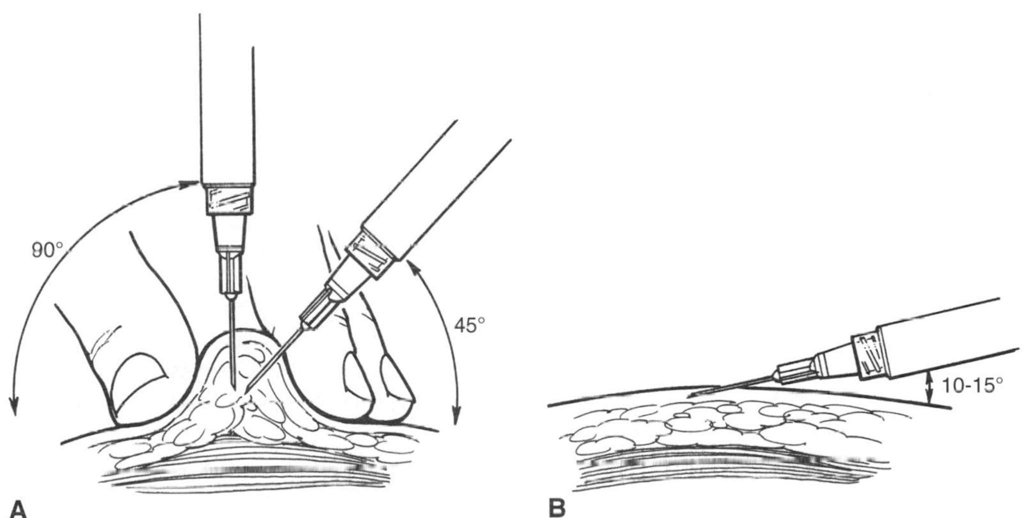

FIGURE **3-10** **A,** Comparison of the angles of insertion for injections. **A,** Subcutaneous (90 degrees or 45 degrees). **B,** Intradermal (10 to 15 degrees).

EVIDENCE-BASED PRACTICE

Medication Safety and Insulin Therapy

Shelly Nalbone

Ask the Question

Question

In children, what practices decrease the number of errors in patients receiving insulin therapy?

Objective

To determine strategies and processes to increase medication safety related to insulin

Background

Medication safety is a concern for health care providers and institutions across the world and receives special attention in almost every health care setting today. In today's fast-paced, technology-based health care arena, medication safety is much more than the "five rights." Medication safety includes not only safe handling, safe storage, and appropriate administration, but also competency of staff who are administering the medication. Despite the heightened awareness, injuries still occur, especially with insulin. According to the Institute for Safe Medication Practices, insulin consistently appears as a top offender, leading to the most harmful and severe adverse events.

Search for Evidence

Search Strategies

Search selection criteria included English language publications within the past 10 years, research-based studies, and pediatric populations.

Continued

EVIDENCE-BASED PRACTICE

Medication Safety and Insulin Therapy—cont'd

Databases Used

National Guideline Clearinghouse (AHRQ), Cochrane Collaboration, PubMed, CINAHL, University of Michigan Evidence-Based Pediatrics, Micromedex, EMBASE, ProQuest, TRIP Database, Medscape, RxMed, STAT!Ref, RxKinetics

Critically Analyze the Evidence

The American Society of Health-System Pharmacists (2006) conducted a review of all relevant literature and evidence-based reviews surrounding insulin therapy focusing on safety and patient outcomes in the hospital setting. Practice recommendations included preprinted order sets or computerized order entry and ongoing and annual training.

A quality improvement project to reduce medication errors and assess a standardized protocol for supplemental sliding scale insulin (SSI) in nonintensive care units was described by Donihi, DeVita, and Korytkowski (2006). Before implementation, more than 20 different types of SSI were used. The number of prescribing errors found on chart review 1 year after implementation was reduced from 10.3 to 1.2 per 100 SSI days. Authors recommend preprinted standardized SSI protocols and intense, ongoing education for direct patient care providers.

Ragone and Lando (2002) evaluated sources of errors and stated that, with the advent of new insulin analogs and premixed insulin combinations, the potential for errors in insulin therapy has increased. Errors have occurred when health care workers have mistaken rapid-acting insulin (Humalog) for glargine at bedtime. Inappropriate use of the proper insulin syringe has also led to errors. Excessive heat, inappropriate labeling of vials after opening, and improper handling of insulin pens can affect the efficacy of insulin. Staff education leads to decreased errors and improved patient outcomes.

Heatlie (2003) found in a qualitative study that long delays existed in the dosing of insulin after blood glucose was obtained. Recommendations included preprinted insulin order forms, increased nursing education surrounding diabetes management, and implementation of a 1-hour time limit from blood glucose specimen to insulin administration.

Davis, Harwood, Midgett, and others (2005) described the safety and efficacy of insulin therapy in intermediate care units. They reviewed staffing patterns, order trends, and past errors. Intense educational offerings were developed and implemented. Three months of data collection revealed 275 correct insulin drip rate calculations out of a possible 276. Audit results indicated that insulin therapy could be safely managed with a 1:5 to 1:6 nurse/patient ratio with proper nursing education.

Cohen, Robinson, and Mandrack (2003) identified methods to increase the safety of medication administration, including preprinted medication orders, the use of "smart pumps" for medication administration, and routine double checking by two licensed nurses when administering high alert medications such as insulin.

Apply the Evidence: Nursing Implications

- Preprinted order sets or computerized order entry for insulin therapy should be used in hospital settings.
- SSI should be a set of standardized protocols for hospitals, and use should be minimized.
- Staff education should be ongoing.
- Direct care provider education should be performed annually and be readily available for just-in-time training.
- Processes should be implemented to include annual education and competency validation for all involved staff.
- Patients receiving insulin therapy should be limited to designated areas of the hospital where staff have received appropriate training and development.
- Well-defined policies should be in place to support appropriate patient placement, safe and effective medication administration, strict insulin management, and judicious documentation.

References

American Society of Health-System Pharmacists: *Professional practice recommendations for safe use of insulin in hospitals,* Bethesda, Md, 2006, Inpatient Care Practitioners.

Cohen H, Robinson E, Mandrack M: Getting to the root of medication errors, *Nursing* 33(9):36-46, 2003.

Davis E, Harwood K, Midgett L, and others: Implementation of a new intravenous insulin method in intermediate-care units in hospitalized patients, *Diabetes Educ* 31(6):818-823, 2005.

Donihi A, DeVita M, Korytkowski M: Use of a standardized protocol to decrease medication errors and adverse events related to sliding scale insulin, *Qual Saf Health Care* 15:89-91, 2006.

Heatlie J: Reducing insulin medication errors: evaluation of a quality improvement initiative, *J Nurs Staff Dev* 19(2):92-98, 2003.

Ragone M, Lando H: Errors of insulin commission? *Clin Diabetes* 20(4):221-222, 2002.

Intravenous Administration*

Obtain necessary equipment.

Explain procedure to child as developmentally appropriate, and provide atraumatic care.

Use pain prevention interventions before procedure.

Maintain aseptic technique, and follow Standard Precautions.

Assess the status of IV infusion to determine that it is functioning properly.

Inspect injection site to make certain the catheter or needle is secure.

Dilute the drug in an amount of solution according to the following:

- Compatibility with infusion fluids or other IV drugs child is receiving
- Size of the child
- Size of the vein being used for infusion
- Length of time over which the drug is to be administered (e.g., 30 minutes, 1 hour, 2 hours)
- Rate at which the drug is to be infused
- Strength of the drug or the degree to which it is toxic to subcutaneous tissues
- Need for fluid restriction

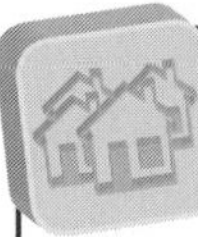

COMMUNITY FOCUS

Preventing Intravenous Site Infections

With the increasing use of intravenous (IV) therapy in the community, preventing infection is essential. The most effective ways to prevent infection of an IV site are to cleanse hands between each patient, wear gloves when inserting an IV catheter, and inspect the insertion site and physical condition of the IV dressing. Proper education of the patient and family regarding signs and symptoms of an infected IV site can help prevent infections from going unnoticed.

Monitor until medication has been infused. Medication is not completely administered until solution in tubing has infused also (amount of solution depends on tubing length).

Praise child for cooperation.

Discard syringe.

Record date, time, dose, drug, and site of injection.

Procedure for Inserting and Taping a Peripheral Intravenous Catheter

Obtain necessary equipment.

Explain procedure to child as developmentally appropriate, and provide atraumatic care.

Verify order, and confirm patient identity.

Follow manufacturer's directions for all devices used.

Wash hands, and observe aseptic technique throughout procedure.

Choose catheter insertion site and an alternative site in case the initial attempt is unsuccessful. A transilluminator can be useful in identifying suitable veins.

Prepare insertion site by applying with friction an antiseptic solution.

Allow solution to dry completely, but do not blow, blot dry, or fan the area.

Don gloves.

Apply tourniquet when site is ready for catheter insertion.

Stretch the skin taut downward below the point of insertion, upward above the site of insertion, or from underneath level with the point of insertion. This technique helps stabilize veins that roll or move away from the catheter as attempts are made to enter the vein.

Inspect catheter, looking for damage (e.g., bent stylet, shavings on the catheter, frayed catheter tip [follow employer's policy for reporting defective devices]).

Insert catheter through the skin, bevel up, at a 30-degree angle, and enter the vein. This direct approach is best for large veins and allows the skin and vein to be entered in one step. The indirect approach for smaller veins enables the catheter to enter the vein from the side perpendicularly. It is sometimes helpful with short veins to start the catheter below the intended site and advance through the superficial layers of skin so that the advancement of the catheter in the vein is a shorter distance. In infants or children with very small veins insert the catheter bevel down, which prevents the needle from puncturing the back wall of the vein and provides an earlier flashback of blood as the vein is entered.

Watch for blood return in the flashback chamber. Some 24-gauge catheters provide visualization of the flashback within the catheter so immediate vein entrance is recognized before the needle punctures the back of the vessel or goes through the other side of the vessel.

Once the flashback is seen, lower the angle between the skin and catheter to 15 degrees. Advance the catheter another $\frac{1}{16}$ to $\frac{1}{8}$ inch to ensure that both the metal stylet and the catheter are inside the vein. Look closely at the IV catheter before inserting it, and note that the stylet tip is slightly longer than the catheter. It is necessary to have both pieces inside the vein before the catheter is advanced. Holding the stylet steady, push the catheter off the stylet and into the vein until the catheter hub is situated against the skin at the insertion site. Activate safety

*Directions for care of intermittent infusion device and central venous catheter are in Patient and Family Education on pp. 531-533.

mechanism if necessary (some safety catheters are passive and activate automatically), remove the stylet, and discard into sharps container. Apply pressure to catheter within the vein to prevent backflow of blood before attachment of tubing.

Collect blood if ordered. Remove the tourniquet. Flush the IV line with NS to check for patency (ease of flushing fluid, lack of resistance while flushing), complaints of pain, or swelling at the site. If line flushes easily, proceed to secure the catheter to the skin.

Connect the T-connector, J-connector, injection cap, or tubing, and reinforce connection with a junction securement device (Luer-Lok, clasping device, threaded device) to prevent accidental disconnection and subsequent air embolism or blood loss.

Place transparent dressing across catheter hub, up to but not including the junction securement device, and surrounding skin.

Further secure the catheter to the skin using tape or adhesive securement devices (e.g., StatLock). Follow manufacturer's directions for adhesive anchors.

Place a ¼ to ½-inch strip of clear tape across the width of the transparent dressing and the catheter hub, but avoid the insertion site. This will serve as an anchor tape strip, and all other tape will be affixed to this strip (tape-on-tape method). This strip will not compromise the transparent dressing properties or interfere with visual inspection of the catheter-skin insertion site.

To stabilize the catheter and junction securement device, attach 1 to 1½ inches of clear tape that is ¼ to ½ inch wide, adhesive side up, to the underneath side of the catheter hub and junction securement device at their connection. Wrap the ends of the tape around the connections, and meet on top to form a V shape (sometimes referred to as a *chevron*); secure the overlapping ends onto the anchor tape strip.

Loop the IV tubing away from the catheter hub and toward the IV fluid source. Secure the looped tubing with a piece of tape on the anchor tape strip. Be certain fingers or toes are visible whenever extremity is used.

Consider use of a commercial protective device (e.g., I.V. House) over the catheter hub and looped tubing. Bending one corner of the tape over and onto itself provides a free tab to lift the tape easily for site visualization.

Documentation of a Peripheral Intravenous Catheter

The entire procedure for inserting and taping a peripheral IV catheter should be documented in the patient's medical record. Important information includes but is not limited to the following.

INTRAVENOUS LINE INSERTION DOCUMENTATION

Normally part of the patient's medical record

The date and time of insertion; name or initials of clinician inserting IV line

Preparation of site, including antiseptic solution used

Manufacturer, gauge, and length of catheter

Site of insertion (e.g., "right ankle," or more specifically "right saphenous vein")

Number of attempts (e.g., "24-gauge, 1-inch Insyte initiated in right saphenous vein in first attempt," or "24-gauge, 1-inch Insyte initiated in right saphenous vein after one unsuccessful attempt to left saphenous vein")

Presence of blood return and name of samples drawn and sent to laboratory if applicable

Activation of junction securement devices (Luer-Lok) and explanation of taping (e.g., "IV catheter secured with transparent dressing and Transpore tape")

Use of armboard

Appearance of site (e.g., site is soft without redness or edema, flushes easily)

Flushing solution, amount used

Connection to IV solution, naming the fluid and amount in the bag

Tolerance of procedure; it is best to describe specific behaviors displayed by the patient or use quotes (e.g., "patient cried during insertion but quieted easily and fell asleep in mom's arms after procedure," or "patient stated, 'That hurt but it feels better now'")

INTRAVENOUS SITE DOCUMENTATION

Can be done on a piece of tape at the site

Date, time, gauge, and length of catheter and initials of nurse initiating

INTRAVENOUS FLUID DOCUMENTATION

Frequently achieved on an IV flow sheet

Date and time of fluid initiation

Type and volume of bag hung (e.g., "500-ml NS")

Type of delivery system used and rate of infusion (e.g., "IV catheter connected to Baxter pump at 25 ml/hr")

Any additives, type and dose, in the primary solution (e.g., "potassium chloride [KCl], 2 mEq/100 ml")

ONGOING INTRAVENOUS SITE ASSESSMENT

Follow hospital's policy but recommended at least every 1 to 2 hours for continuous infusions (can be done in medical record or on the IV flow sheet)

Appearance (e.g., "site is soft without redness or edema" [any protective device needs to be lifted to see the entire site])

Any patient comments regarding IV

DISCONTINUATION OF INTRAVENOUS THERAPY

Can be done in medical record

Reason for discontinuing IV catheter (e.g., "end of therapy," "infiltration," or "accidentally removed")

Integrity of device, including length and condition of catheter

Appearance of site

Dressing applied

Patient tolerance; again direct quotes from patient are best

EVIDENCE-BASED PRACTICE

Use of Transillumination Devices in Obtaining Vascular Access

Jennifer L. Sanders

Ask the Question

Question

In children do transillumination devices decrease the number of attempts needed to obtain vascular access?

Background

Patients, families, and care providers often report difficulty in obtaining vascular access in pediatric patients. In patients such as infants, those with highly pigmented skin, or those who are chronically ill, veins may be difficult to palpate or visualize. This review evaluates studies of the efficacy of using transillumination to increase vein visibility and decrease the number of access attempts.

Objective

To evaluate evidence supporting the use of transillumination devices in obtaining vascular access in pediatric patients.

Search for Evidence

Search Strategies

Search selection criteria included English language publications within the past 30 years, research-based articles on children undergoing venipuncture.

Databases

PubMed, Cochrane Collaboration, MD Consult, BestBETs

Critically Analyze the Evidence

Five articles were found regarding the efficacy of transillumination. All concluded that transillumination aids in decreasing the number of access attempts.

- Forty cases were described in which transillumination was used to decrease the number of peripheral intravenous (PIV) attempts. In these patients, small superficial veins that were not previously visualized or palpated were visualized using the transillumination device. Far fewer attempts were needed, and PIV access of infants and obese children was easier for staff (Kuhns, Martin, Gildersleeve, and others, 1975).
- One article reviewed the safety (related to heat and burns) of transillumination devices. No burns were reported in a sample of 10 neonates, even when the transillumination device was used for up to 20 minutes (Curran, 1980).
- A letter to the editor focused on the method of using two fiberoptic lights as a venous transilluminator. PIV access was usually successful on the first attempt because of the increased visualization of the superficial venous anatomy (Dinner, 1992).
- A sample of 100 infants ages 2 to 36 months was evaluated for PIV access using a simple otoscope for transillumination. In 40 of the 100 infants, a vein was visible using the otoscope for transillumination. In 23 of these children, transillumination was used after a vein could not be visualized or palpated. In 17 others, one previous attempt to gain PIV access had failed. With transillumination, 39 of 40 PIV attempts were successful on the first attempt. One patient required a second attempt (Goren, Laufer, Yativ, and others, 2001).
- A sample of 240 patients was randomized to receive PIV access either with or without transillumination with the Veinlite. Patients were either less than 3 years old and required elective insertion of an IV, or were 3 to 21 years of age with a chronic illness who were previously identified as having difficult access. Those patients in the Veinlite group were significantly more likely to have a successful IV insertion on the first or second attempt (Katsogridakis, Seshadri, Sullivan, and others, 2005).

Apply the Evidence: Nursing Implications

- Transillumination should be used before PIV access to decrease the number of attempts needed to successfully obtain access.
- Education and practice in this technique are needed for success. Since the veins stand out so clearly with transillumination, they appear more superficial than they are.
- An assistant may be needed to hold the device when using the transilluminator to obtain PIV access.
- The heat and temperature of the transilluminator should be monitored to prevent injury to the patient's skin.
- Appropriate equipment should be used to increase the likelihood of visualization of the vasculature.

References

Curran JS: A restraint and transillumination device for neonatal arterial/venipuncture: efficacy and thermal safety, *Pediatrics* 66(1):128-130, 1980.

Dinner M: Transillumination to facilitate venipuncture in children (letter to editor), *Anesthesiol Analg* 74:467-477, 1992.

Goren A, Laufer J, Yativ N, and others: Transillumination of the palm for venipuncture in infants, *Pediatr Emerg Care* 17(2):130-131, 2001.

Katsogridakis Y, Seshadri R, Sullivan C, and others: *Veinlite transillumination in the pediatric emergency department: a therapeutic interventional trial,* retrieved Aug 2005 from *http://www.veinlite.com/public.html.*

Kuhns LR, Martin AJ, Gildersleeve RT, and others: Intense transillumination for infant venipuncture, *Radiology* 116:734-735, 1975.

EVIDENCE-BASED PRACTICE

Peripheral Intravenous Site Care

Joy Hesselgrave

Ask the Question

Question

In children, what site preparation, dressing, and stabilization measures for peripheral intravenous catheters (PIVs) are optimum for preventing complications and extending dwell time?

Objective

To determine optimum PIV site care in children

Background

PIVs are routinely used in pediatrics to deliver intravenous fluids, medications, and blood products. Meticulous care in starting and maintaining the pediatric PIV extends the longevity and prevents complications (infection, infiltration, dislodgment, phlebitis, pain, and anxiety).

Search for Evidence

Search Strategies

Search selection criteria included English language and research-based publications within the past 20 years on PIV site care.

Databases Used

National Guidelines Clearinghouse (AHQR), Cochrane Collaboration, Joanna Briggs Institute, PubMed, TRIP Database Plus, MD Consult, PedsCCM, BestBETs

Critically Analyze the Evidence

Site Preparation

Multiple studies cited as the basis of the Centers for Disease Control and Prevention recommendations by O'Grady, Alexander, Dellinger, and others (2002) indicate that the skin should be disinfected with an appropriate antiseptic before PIV catheter insertion. A 2% chlorhexidine-based preparation is preferred, but tincture of iodine, an iodophor, or 70% alcohol can be used. Allow the antiseptic to air dry before catheter insertion. There is no recommendation at this time for the use of chlorhexidine in infants younger than 2 months old.

The Infusion Nurses Society (2006) recommends cleansing the skin with a preparation that combines alcohol with either chlorhexidine gluconate or povidone-iodine before PIV insertion. For neonates, use only chlorhexidine or povidone-iodine without alcohol and remove with sterile water or NS to prevent absorption (Association of Women's Health, Obstetric and Neonatal Nurses, 2001).

Site Dressing

Multiple studies indicate that either gauze dressings or clear semipermeable dressings are acceptable for PIV sites. Several studies cite clinician preference for the semipermeable dressing because of better visibility of the insertion site and no need to perform dressing changes. Neonatal guidelines recommend a transparent adhesive dressing or clear tape at the PIV site (Callaghan, Copnell, and Johnson, 2002; Tripepi-Bova, Woods, and Loach, 1997; Hoffmann, Wester, Kaiser, and others, 1988).

A prospective randomized trial with 2088 peripheral catheters using four different dressings indicated that the rate of colonization among catheters dressed with transparent semipermeable dressings is comparable to that obtained with gauze dressings and that the dressing may be left on until the catheter is removed (Maki and Ringer, 1987).

Gauze dressings that prevent visualization of the insertion site should be changed every 48 hours. Transparent semipermeable membrane dressings may remain on the site for the duration of the PIV unless they become wet or soiled or the integrity of the dressing is compromised (Infusion Nurses Society, 2006).

Stabilization or Securement Devices

A prospective study of 105 PIV placements compared a control group using traditional transparent dressing (Tegaderm) and tape with a study group that used transparent dressings and a catheter securement device (StatLock) (Wood, 1997). The control group had a 65% complication rate (dislodgments, infiltration, and phlebitis) versus a 20% complication rate in the study group, indicating a 45% reduction in overall PIV therapy complications in the study group.

When comparing tape, StatLock, and Hub-Guard for a 96-hour PIV protocol change, researchers found that PIVs with StatLock produced a statistically significant improved survival rate (52%)

EVIDENCE-BASED PRACTICE

Peripheral Intravenous Site Care—cont'd

compared with tape (8%) or HubGuard (9%) (Smith, 2006). Securement devices may extend the life of a PIV.

Dwell Time

In pediatric patients, PIV catheters may remain in place until a complication occurs or the therapy is complete (O'Grady, Alexander, Dellinger, and others, 2002).

Results of a prospective study of 525 pediatric patients with PIVs determined that the overall risk of PIV catheter complication was extremely low and would not be reduced substantially by routine catheter replacement (Shimandle, Johnson, Baker, and others, 1999).

Apply the Evidence: Nursing Implications

The evidence supports multiple skin cleansing guidelines and leaving PIVs in children until they develop complications or become dislodged. PIV sites may be dressed with either gauze or clear dressings, with the advantage of clear dressings allowing continuous site visualization. Commercial securement or protection devices extend the life of the PIV in the pediatric patient. Other implications include the following:

- Provide topical local anesthetic or oral sucrose for pain prevention as appropriate for age before PIV insertion.
- For children older than 2 months, chlorhexidine is the preferred skin cleanser. For younger infants, nonalcohol-based cleansers are preferred and should be removed with sterile water or sterile NS to prevent absorption.
- Select the vein that is most distal on the extremity and one that allows the child optimum movement (e.g., avoid over the joint). Veins on the scalp may be used in infants. Subsequent PIVs should be proximal to the previous IV site.
- Apply a clear semipermeable dressing or gauze dressing and tape. The semipermeable dressing allows better visualization of the PIV and may remain on the site for the length of therapy as long as integrity is maintained. If a gauze dressing is used, assess it regularly and replace it every 48 hours. Gauze dressings may be preferred for patients who are diaphoretic or in whom blood is oozing from the insertion site.
- If the child is mobile, consider using a securement or protection device (e.g., StatLock, HubGuard, Ray-Marshall Shield, IV House, IV Shield, IV Pro).
- Discontinue PIV if complications occur or when it is no longer needed.

References

Association of Women's Health, Obstetric and Neonatal Nurses: *Neonatal skin care: evidence-based clinical practice guideline,* 2001, retrieved from National Guideline Clearinghouse, *http://www.guideline.gov.*

Callaghan S, Copnell B, Johnson L: Comparison of two methods of peripheral intravenous cannula securement in the pediatric setting, *J Infus Nurs* 25(4):256-264, 2002.

Hoffmann K, Wester S, Kaiser D, and others: Bacterial colonization and phlebitis-associated risk with transparent polyurethane film for peripheral intravenous site dressings, *Am J Infect Control* 16(3):101-106, 1998.

Infusion Nurses Society: *Policies and procedures for infusion nursing,* ed 3, South Norwood, Mass, 2006, The Society.

Maki D, Ringer M: Evaluation of dressing regimens for prevention of infection with peripheral intravenous catheters: gauze, a transparent polyurethane dressing, and an iodophor-transparent dressing, *JAMA* 258(17):2396-2403, 1987.

O'Grady N, Alexander M, Dellinger E, and others: Guidelines for the prevention of intravascular catheter–related infections, *MMWR Morb Mortal Wkly Rep* 51(32), 2002.

Shimandle R, Johnson D, Baker M, and others: Safety of peripheral intravenous catheters in children, *Infect Control Hosp Epidemiol* 20:736-740, 1999.

Smith B: Peripheral intravenous catheter dwell times: a comparison of three securement methods for implementation of a 96-hour scheduled change protocol, *J Infus Nurs* 29(1):14-17, 2006.

Tripepi-Bova K, Woods, K, Loach, M: A comparison of transparent polyurethane and dry gauze dressings for peripheral IV catheter sites rates of phlebitis, infiltration and dislodgement by patients, *Am J Crit Care* 6(5):377-381, 1997.

Wood D: A comparative study of two securement techniques for short peripheral intravenous catheters, *J Intraven Nurs* 20(6):280-285, 1997.

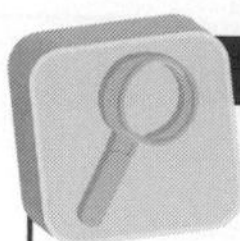

EVIDENCE-BASED PRACTICE

Frequency of Changing Intravenous Administration Sets

Brandi Horvath

Ask the Question

Question

In children, should intravenous (IV) administration sets be changed at 24, 48, 72, or 96 hours to safely prevent patient infection while containing costs?

Objective

To determine the optimum time interval for routine replacement of IV administration sets containing crystalloids or parenteral nutrition when infused using a central or peripheral venous catheter

Background

IV therapy is an important aspect of patient care in a hospital setting. Routine replacement of IV administration sets reduces IV infusion contamination and patient morbidity. Determining the appropriate time interval is integral to optimizing patient outcomes, decreasing risk for bloodstream infection, and decreasing costs.

Search for Evidence

Search Strategies

Search selection criteria included English language publications within past 10 years, and research-based articles on frequency of changing IV administration sets.

Databases Used

National Guideline Clearinghouse (AHRQ), Cochrane Collaboration, Joanna Briggs Institute, PubMed, Infusion Nurses Society, Oncology Nurses Society, MD Consult, BestBETs, TRIP Database Plus, PedsCCM

Critically Analyze the Evidence

A systematic Cochrane review by Gillies, O'Riordan, Wallen, and others (2005) identified the optimum interval for the routine replacement of IV administration sets when infusate or parenteral nutrition solutions are administered. Data results from 13 randomized or quasirandomized controlled trials were pooled to compare different time intervals of administration set changes: every 24 hours versus 48 hours or greater, 48 hours versus at least 72 hours, and 72 hours versus 96 hours. Findings revealed no evidence that changing IV administration sets more often than every 96 hours reduces the incidence of bloodstream infection. There were no differences in results between patients with central and peripheral catheters and those who did or did not receive parenteral nutrition. For IV administration sets including blood or blood products and lipids, the researchers recommending changing the sets every 24 hours.

The Centers for Disease Control and Prevention (O'Grady, Alexander, Dellinger, and others, 2002) recommends changing IV administration sets for crystalloids at no more than 72-hour intervals. Rates of phlebitis were not substantially different for administration sets left in place 96 hours compared with 72 hours. For tubing used to administer blood and blood products or lipid emulsions, replace tubing within 24 hours of starting the infusion.

The Infusion Nurses Society (2006) and Alexander (2006) recommend replacing continuously infusing IV administration sets no more frequently than every 72 hours. Administration sets used intermittently should be changed every 24 hours. Secondary piggyback sets may be changed no more frequently than every 72 hours when attached to a continuously infusing line; once detached from the primary set, they should be changed at 24 hours. Exceptions include sets used with lipids (change at 24 hours if continuous or after each unit if intermittently infused) and blood or blood components (change at the end of 4 hours if continuous or after each intermittent component). All sets should be changed immediately if contamination is suspected.

The Oncology Nursing Society (Camp-Sorreli, 2004) recommends replacing IV administration sets every 96 hours or with catheter change, except for fluids that enhance microbial growth. Tubing used to administer blood, blood products, lipids, or total parenteral nutrition should be replaced 24 hours after initiation of therapy.

Apply the Evidence: Nursing Implications

- Replace IV administration sets every 96 hours.
- Replace tubing used for lipid emulsions, blood, and blood products every 24 hours.
- Replace blood tubing with in-line filters after 2 units or 4 hours, whichever comes first.

References

Alexander M, editor: Infusion nursing standards of practice, *J Infus Nurs* 29(1S):S48-S50, 2006.

Camp-Sorreli D, editor: *Access device guidelines: recommendations for nursing practice and education,* ed 2, Pittsburgh, 2004, Oncology Nursing Society.

Gillies D, O'Riordan L, Wallen M, and others: Optimal timing for intravenous administration set replacement. In *The Cochrane Database of Systematic Reviews 2005,* Issue 4, Article No. CD003588.pub2. DOI: 10.1002/14651858.CD003588.pub2.

Infusion Nurses Society: *Policies and procedures for infusion nursing,* ed 3, South Norwood, Mass, 2006, The Society.

O'Grady N, Alexander M, Dellinger E, and others: Guidelines for the prevention of intravascular catheter-related infections, MMWR *Morb Mortal Wkly Rep* 51(RR-10):1-29, 2002.

Rectal Administration

SUPPOSITORY*

Medications may need to be administered rectally if the oral route is not available Rectal suppositories are usually inserted with the apex (pointed end) first.

RETENTION ENEMA

1. Dilute drug in smallest amount of solution possible.
2. Insert into rectum (Guidelines box). Depending on volume, may use syringe with rubber tubing, enema bottle, or enema bag.
3. Hold or tape buttocks together for 5 to 10 minutes.

GUIDELINES

Administration of Enemas to Children

Age	Amount (ml)	Insertion Distance in Centimeters (inches)
Infant	120-240	2.5 (1)
2-4 years	240-360	5.0 (2)
4-10 years	360-480	7.5 (3)
11 years	480-720	10.0 (4)

Eye, Ear, and Nosc Administration

See Atraumatic Care box.

EYE MEDICATION†

Eye drops are administered in the same manner as to adults. Children, however, require additional preparation (Practice Alert).

ATRAUMATIC CARE

Oral, Eye, Ear, and Nasal Administration

To administer oral, nasal, ear, or optic medication when only one person is available to restrain the child, use the following procedure:

- Place child supine on flat surface (bed, couch, floor).
- Sit facing child so that child's head is between operator's thighs and child's arms are under operator's legs.
- Place lower legs over child's legs to restrain lower body if necessary.
- To administer oral medication, place small pillow under child's head to reduce risk of aspiration.
- To administer nasal medication, place small pillow under child's shoulders to aid flow of liquid through nasal passages.

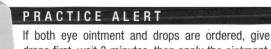

EAR MEDICATION†

Depending on the child's age, the pinna is pulled differently. Such variations are discussed in the Patient and Family Education section.

NOSE DROPS†

Nose drops are administered in the same manner as to adults. Different positions may be used, depending on the child's age.

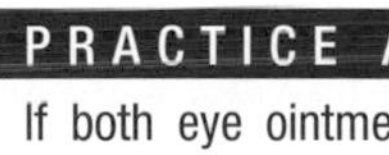

PRACTICE ALERT

If both eye ointment and drops are ordered, give drops first, wait 3 minutes, then apply the ointment. This allows each drug time to work. When possible, administer eye ointments before bedtime or naptime, because the child's vision will be blurred for a while.

3 - EVIDENCE-BASED PEDIATRIC NURSING INTERVENTIONS

*See Patient and Family Education, p. 538.
†See Patient and Family Education, pp. 539 (eye), 540 (ear), and 541 (nose).

Nasogastric, Orogastric, or Gastrotomy Tube Administration

Use elixir or suspension preparations of medication (rather than tablets) whenever possible (Safety Alert).

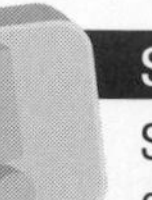

SAFETY ALERT

Sprinkle-type medications should be avoided. However, if there is no other option and the tube is large gauge (18 French or greater), but usually not a Foley catheter, the medication may be given by mixing the sprinkles with a small amount of pureed fruit and thinning with water. The fruit keeps the sprinkles suspended so they do not float to the top. Flush well. This procedure is not recommended for skin-level gastrostomy devices.

Dilute viscous medication or syrup with a small amount of water if possible.

Avoid oily medications because they tend to cling to the sides of the tube.

If administering tablets, crush them to a very fine powder and dissolve drug in a small amount of warm water.

Never crush enteric-coated or sustained-release tablets or capsules.

Do not mix medication with enteral formula unless fluid is restricted. If adding a drug:

- Check with pharmacist for compatibility.
- Shake formula well, and observe for any physical reaction (e.g., separation, precipitation).
- Label formula container with name of medication, dosage, date, and time infusion started.

Have medication at room temperature.

Measure medication in calibrated cup or syringe.

Check for correct placement of nasogastric (NG) or orogastric tube.

Attach syringe (with adaptable tip but without plunger) to tube.

Pour medication into syringe.

Unclamp tube, and allow medication to flow by gravity.

Adjust height of container to achieve desired flow rate (e.g., increase height for faster flow).

As soon as syringe is empty, pour 10 ml of water to flush tubing.

- Amount of water depends on length and gauge of tubing.
- Determine amount before administering any medication by using a syringe to completely fill an unused NG or orogastric tube with water. The amount of flush solution is usually $1\frac{1}{2}$ times this volume.
- With certain drug preparations (e.g., suspensions), more fluid may be needed.

If administering more than one drug at the same time, flush the tube between each medication with clear water.

Clamp tube after flushing, unless tube is left open.

Chemotherapy

Chemotherapy is routinely administered by nurses caring for children with cancer. Table 3-3 provides a summary of the most common agents, their side effects, and toxicities and specific nursing interventions.

TABLE 3-3 Chemotherapeutic Agents Used in the Treatment of Childhood Cancers*

Agent and Administration	Side Effects and Toxicity	Comments and Specific Nursing Considerations
Alkylating Agents		
Mechlorethamine (nitrogen mustard, Mustargen)—IV	N/V† (½-8 hours later) (severe) BMD (2-3 weeks later) Alopecia Local phlebitis	Vesicant‡ May cause phlebitis and discoloration of vein Use within 15 minutes after reconstitution.
Cyclophosphamide (Cytoxan, CTX, Neosar)—PO, IV, IM	N/V (3-4 hours later) (severe at high doses) BMD (10-14 days later) Alopecia Hemorrhagic cystitis Severe immunosuppression Stomatitis (rare) Syndrome of inappropriate antidiuretic hormone (SIADH) with seizures Hyperpigmentation Transverse ridging of nails Infertility Cardiac toxicity	BMD has platelet-sparing effect. Give dose early in day to allow adequate fluids afterward. Mesna is given to prevent hemorrhagic cystitis. Force fluids before administering drug and for 2 days after to prevent chemical cystitis; encourage frequent voiding even during night. Warn parents to report signs of burning on urination or hematuria to practitioner.
Ifosfamide (Ifos, IFF)—IV	Hemorrhagic cystitis BMD (10-14 days later) Alopecia Neurotoxicity—lethargy, disorientation, somnolence, seizures (rare)	Mesna is given to prevent hemorrhagic cystitis. Hydrate as with CTX. Myelosuppression less severe than with CTX.
Melphalan (L-phenylalanine mustard, Alkeran, L-Pam)—PO, IV	N/V (severe) BMD (2-3 weeks later) Diarrhea Alopecia	Potent irritant Give over 30-60 minutes. Administer within 60 minutes of reconstitution.
Procarbazine (Matulane)—PO	N/V (moderate) BMD (3-4 weeks later) Lethargy Dermatitis Myalgia Arthralgia Less commonly: Stomatitis Neuropathy Alopecia Diarrhea Azoospermia Cessation of menses	CNS depressants (phenothiazines, barbiturates) enhance CNS symptoms. Monoamine oxidase (MAO) inhibition sometimes occurs, causing increased norepinephrine; foods containing high levels of tyramine may elevate norepinephrine to toxic levels; foods to avoid are overripe or aged products (e.g., cheese; avocados, bananas; tea, coffee; broad beans, fava beans; red wines; yogurt, chocolate); to avoid drug interactions, all other drugs are avoided unless medically approved.

BMD, Bone marrow depression; *CNS,* central nervous system; ECG, electrocardiogram; *IM,* intramuscular; *IT,* intrathecal; *IV,* intravenous; *N/V,* nausea and vomiting; *PO,* by mouth; *SC,* subcutaneous. For parenteral injections, apply EMLA 60 minutes before IV administration and 2½ hours before IM administration.

*Table includes principal drugs used in the treatment of childhood cancers. Several other conventional and investigational chemotherapeutic agents may be employed in the treatment regimen.

†Nausea and vomiting: Mild = <20% incidence; moderate = 20%-70% incidence; severe = >75% incidence.

‡Vesicants (sclerosing agents) can cause severe cellular damage if even minute amounts of the drug infiltrate surrounding tissue. Only nurses experienced with chemotherapeutic agents should administer vesicants. These drugs must be given through a free-flowing IV line. The infusion is stopped *immediately* if any sign of infiltration (pain, stinging, swelling, redness at needle site) occurs. Interventions for extravasation vary, but each nurse should be aware of the institution's policies and should implement them at once.

Continued

TABLE 3-3 **Chemotherapeutic Agents Used in the Treatment of Childhood Cancers—cont'd**

Agent and Administration	Side Effects and Toxicity	Comments and Specific Nursing Considerations
Alkylating Agents—cont'd		
Dacarbazine (DTIC-Dome)—IV	N/V (especially after first dose) (severe) BMD (7-14 days later) Alopecia Flulike syndrome Burning sensation in vein during infusion (not extravasation)	Vesicant (less sclerosive) Must be given cautiously in patients with renal dysfunction Decrease IV rate or use cold pack along vein to decrease burning.
Cisplatin (Platinol)—IV	Renal toxicity (severe) N/V (1-4 hours later) (severe) BMD (mild, 2-3 weeks later) Ototoxicity Neurotoxicity (similar to that for vincristine) Electrolyte disturbances, especially hypomagnesemia, hypocalcemia, hypokalemia, and hypophosphatemia Anaphylactic reactions may occur.	Renal function (creatinine clearance) must be assessed before drug is given. Must maintain hydration before and during therapy (specific gravity of urine is used to assess hydration.) Mannitol may be given intravenously to promote osmotic diuresis and drug clearance. Monitor intake and output. Monitor for signs of ototoxicity (e.g., ringing in ears) and neurotoxicity; report signs immediately; ensure that routine audiogram is done before treatment for baseline and routinely during treatment. Do not use aluminum needle; reaction with aluminum decreases potency of drug. Monitor for signs of electrolyte loss (e.g., hypomagnesemia—tremors, spasm, muscle weakness, lower extremity cramps, irregular heart-beat, convulsions, delirium). Have emergency drugs at bedside.§
Carboplatin (CBDCA)—IV	BMD (14 days later) N/V (mild) Mild hepatotoxicity Alopecia	Do not use saline dilution. Drug is less nephrotoxic and ototoxic than cisplatin. Do not use aluminum needle.
Thiotepa (triethylene thiophosphoramide, TESPA)—IV, IT, IM, SC, intracavity, intratumor	N/V (mild) BMD (7-14 days later) Headache, dizziness Stomatitis Dermatitis Alopecia	Use 0.22-μm filter when preparing to eliminate haze. Do not use with succinylcholine.
Antimetabolites		
5-Azacytidine (5-AzaC) IV	N/V (moderate) BMD (7-14 days later) Diarrhea	Infuse slowly via IV drip to decrease severity of N/V.

§Emergency drugs include oxygen and parenteral preparations of epinephrine 1:1000, diphenhydramine, or similar antihistamine, aminophylline, corticosteroids, and vasopressors.

TABLE 3-3 Chemotherapeutic Agents Used in the Treatment of Childhood Cancers—cont'd

Agent and Administration	Side Effects and Toxicity	Comments and Specific Nursing Considerations
Antimetabolites—cont'd		
Cytosine arabinoside (Ara-C, Cytosar, cytarabine, arabinosyl cytosine)—IV, IM, SC, IT	Alopecia N/V (mild and severe at high doses) BMD (7-14 days later) ara-C syndrome (fever, conjunctivitis, maculopapular rash) Mucosal ulceration Immunosuppression Hepatitis (usually subclinical)	Crosses blood-brain barrier Use with caution in patients with hepatic dysfunction. Conjunctivitis with high doses Administer steroid eye drops to prevent conjunctivitis.
5-Fluorouracil (5-FU, Adrucil, fluorouracil)—IV	N/V (moderate) Stomatitis BMD (7-14 days later) Alopecia Diarrhea Dermatitis	Infuse slowly via IV. Take on empty stomach.
Mercaptopurine (6-MP, Purinethol)—PO, IV	N/V (mild) Diarrhea Anorexia Stomatitis BMD (4-6 weeks later) Immunosuppression Dermatitis Less commonly may be hepatotoxic	6-MP is an analog of xanthine; therefore allopurinol (Zyloprim) delays its metabolism and increases its potency, necessitating a lower dose (⅓ to ¼) of 6-MP.
Methotrexate (MTX, amethopterin)—PO, IV, IM, IT May be given in conventional doses (mg/m^2) or high doses (g/m^2)	N/V (severe at high doses) Diarrhea Mucosal ulceration (2-5 days later) BMD (10 days later) Immunosuppression Dermatitis Photosensitivity Alopecia (uncommon) Toxic effects include: Hepatitis (fibrosis) Osteoporosis Nephropathy	Side effects and toxicity are dose related. Potency and toxicity increased by reduced renal function, salicylates, sulfonamides, and aminobenzoic acid; avoid use of these substances, such as aspirin. Use sunblock. High-dose therapy Citrovorum factor (folinic acid or leucovorin) decreases cytotoxic action of MTX; used as an antidote for overdose and to enhance normal cell recovery following high-dose therapy; avoid use of vitamins containing folic acid during MTX therapy unless prescribed by physician.
	Pneumonitis (fibrosis) Neurologic toxicity with IT use—Pain at injection site, meningismus (signs of meningitis without actual inflammation, especially fever and headache); potential sequelae—transient or permanent hemiparesis, convulsions, dementia, death	IT therapy Drug *must* be mixed with preservative-free diluent. Report signs of neurotoxicity immediately.

Continued

TABLE 3-3 **Chemotherapeutic Agents Used in the Treatment of Childhood Cancers—cont'd**

Agent and Administration	Side Effects and Toxicity	Comments and Specific Nursing Considerations
Antimetabolites—cont'd		
6-Thioguanine (6-TG, Thioguan)—PO	N/V (mild) BMD (7-14 days later) Stomatitis Rarely: Dermatitis Photosensitivity Liver dysfunction	Side effects are unusual. Take oral dose once daily on an empty stomach.
Plant Alkaloids		
Vincristine (Oncovin)—IV	Neurotoxicity—Paresthesia (numbness); ataxia; weakness; footdrop; hyporeflexia; constipation (adynamic ileus); hoarseness (vocal cord paralysis); ptosis; abdominal, chest, and jaw pain; mental depression Fever N/V (mild) BMD (minimal; 7-14 days later) Alopecia SIADH	Vesicant Report signs of neurotoxicity because may necessitate cessation of drug. Individuals with underlying neurologic problems may be more prone to neurotoxicity. Monitor stool patterns closely; administer stool softener. Excreted primarily by liver into biliary system; administer cautiously to anyone with biliary disease. Maximum dose is 2 mg.
Vinblastine (Velban)— IV	Neurotoxicity (same as for vincristine but less severe) N/V (mild) BMD (especially neutropenia; 7-14 days later) Alopecia	Same as for vincristine
VP-16 (etoposide, VePesid)—IV, PO	N/V (mild to moderate) BMD (7-14 days later) Alopecia Hypotension with rapid infusion Bradycardia Diarrhea (infrequent) Stomatitis (rare) May reactivate erythema of irradiated skin (rare) Allergic reaction with anaphylaxis possible Neurotoxicity	Give slowly via IV drip with child recumbent. Have emergency drugs available at bedside.§
VM-26 (teniposide)—IV	Same as for VP-16	Same as for VP-16

§Emergency drugs include oxygen and parenteral preparations of epinephrine 1:1000, diphenhydramine, or similar antihistamine, aminophylline, corticosteroids, and vasopressors.

TABLE 3-3 Chemotherapeutic Agents Used in the Treatment of Childhood Cancers—cont'd

Agent and Administration	Side Effects and Toxicity	Comments and Specific Nursing Considerations
Antibiotics		
Actinomycin D (dactinomycin, Cosmegen, ACT-D)—IV	N/V (2-5 hours later) (moderate) BMD (especially platelets; 7-14 days later) Immunosuppression Mucosal ulceration Abdominal cramps Diarrhea Anorexia (may last a few weeks) Alopecia Acne Erythema or hyperpigmentation of previously irradiated skin Fever Malaise	Vesicant Enhances cytotoxic effects of radiation therapy but increases toxic effect May cause serious desquamation of irradiated tissue
Doxorubicin (Adriamycin)—IV	N/V (moderate) Stomatitis BMD (7-14 days later) Fever, chills Local phlebitis Alopecia Cumulative-dose toxicity includes: Cardiac abnormalities ECG changes Heart failure	Vesicant (Extravasation may *not* cause pain.) Observe for any changes in heart rate or rhythm and signs of failure. Cumulative dose must not exceed 375 mg/m^2, less with radiation. Warn parents that drug causes urine to turn red (for up to 12 days after administration); this is normal, not hematuria.
Daunorubicin (daunomycin, rubidomycin)—IV	Similar to doxorubicin	Similar to doxorubicin
Bleomycin (Blenoxane)—IV, IM, SC	Allergic reaction—Fever, chills, hypotension, anaphylaxis Fever (nonallergic) N/V (mild) Stomatitis Cumulative dose effects include: Skin—Rash, hyperpigmentation, thickening, ulceration, peeling, nail changes, alopecia Lungs—Pneumonitis with infiltrate that can progress to fatal fibrosis	Should give test dose (SC) before therapeutic dose administered Have emergency drugs at bedside.§ Hypersensitivity occurs with first one to two doses. May give acetaminophen before drug to reduce likelihood of fever Concentration of drug in skin and lungs accounts for toxic effects. Follow pulmonary function tests baseline, before therapy, and after therapy.

Continued

TABLE 3-3 Chemotherapeutic Agents Used in the Treatment of Childhood Cancers—cont'd

Agent and Administration	Side Effects and Toxicity	Comments and Specific Nursing Considerations
Hormones, Corticosteroids		
Prednisone (Meticorten, Deltasone, Paracort)—PO; IM or IV	For short-term use, no acute toxicity Usual side effects are mild; moon face, fluid retention, weight gain, mood changes, increased appetite, gastric effects	Explain expected effects, especially in terms of body image, increased appetite, and personality changes. Monitor weight gain. Recommend moderate salt restriction. Administer with antacid and early in morning (sometimes given every other day to minimize side effects).
Dexamethasone (Decadron)—PO Hydrocortisone (Solu-Cortef)—IV Methylprednisolone (Solu-Medrol)—IV	Irritation, insomnia, susceptibility to infection. Hyperglycemia	May need to disguise bitter taste. (Crush tablet and mix with syrup, jam, ice cream, or other highly flavored substance; use ice to numb tongue before administration; place tablet in gelatin capsule if child can swallow it.) Observe for potential infection sites; usual inflammatory response and fever are absent.
	Long-term effects of long-term steroid administration are mood changes, hirsutism, trunk obesity (buffalo hump), thin extremities, muscle wasting and weakness, osteoporosis, poor wound healing, bruising, potassium loss, gastric bleeding, hypertension, diabetes mellitus, growth retardation, immunosuppression, and avascular necrosis of bone.	Same as for short-term use; in addition, encourage foods high in potassium (bananas, raisins, prunes, coffee, chocolate). Test stools for occult blood. Monitor blood pressure. Test blood for sugar and urine for acetone. Observe for signs of abrupt steroid withdrawal: flulike symptoms, hypotension, hypoglycemia, shock.

TABLE 3-3 **Chemotherapeutic Agents Used in the Treatment of Childhood Cancers—cont'd**

Agent and Administration	Side Effects and Toxicity	Comments and Specific Nursing Considerations
Enzymes		
L-Asparaginase (Elspar)—IV, IM, SQ Erwinia L-Asparaginase PEG-L-Asparaginase (long-acting form)	Allergic reactions (including anaphylactic shock) Fever N/V (mild) Anorexia Weight loss Toxicity Liver dysfunction Hyperglycemia Renal failure Pancreatitis Coagulation abnormalities	Observe patient 1 hour after dose for signs of allergic reaction. Have emergency drugs at bedside.§ Record signs of allergic reaction, such as urticaria, facial edema, hypotension, or abdominal cramps. Check weight daily. Normally, blood urea nitrogen (BUN) and ammonia levels rise as a result of drug; not evidence of liver damage. Check urine for sugar and blood amylase.
Nitrosoureas Carmustine (BCNU)—IV Lomustine (CCNU)—PO	N/V (2-6 hours later) (severe) BMD (3-4 weeks later) Burning pain along IV infusion (usually caused by alcohol diluent) BCNU—Flushing and facial burning on infusion Alopecia	Prevent extravasation; contact with skin causes brown spots. Oral form—Give 4 hours after meals when stomach is empty. Reduce IV burning by diluting drug and infusing slowly via IV drip. Crosses blood-brain barrier
Other Agents		
Hydroxyurea (Hydrea) PO	N/V (mild) Anorexia Less commonly: Diarrhea BMD Mucosal ulceration Alopecia Dermatitis	Must be given cautiously in patients with renal dysfunction

§Emergency drugs include oxygen and parenteral preparations of epinephrine 1:1000, diphenhydramine, or similar antihistamine, aminophylline, corticosteroids, and vasopressors.

Pain Interventions

Pain Assessment

Various pain scales are summarized in Tables 3-4, 3-5, and 3-6.

TABLE 3-4 Summary of Selected Behavioral Pain Assessment Scales for Young Children

Ages of Use	Reliability and Validity	Variables	Scoring Range
Objective Pain Score (OPS) (Hannallah, Broadman, Belman, and others, 1987)			
4 mo–18 yr	Concurrent validity with linear analog pain scale, Spearman's r: 0.721 with scores ≥6 and 0.419 with scores <6 Interrater agreement, coefficient alpha: 0.986 for one rater and 0.983 for the other Concurrent validity with CHEOPS, Pearson correlation coefficient: 0.88 and 0.94	Blood pressure (0-2) Crying (0-2) Moving (0-2) Agitation (0-2) Verbal evaluation/body language (0-2)	0 = no pain; 10 = worst pain
Children's Hospital of Eastern Ontario Pain Scale (CHEOPS) (McGrath, Johnson, Goodman, and others, 1985)			
1-5 yr	Interrater reliability: 90%-99.5% Internal correlation: significant correlations between pairs of items Concurrent validity between CHEOPS and visual analog scale (VAS): 0.91; between individual and total scores of CHEOPS and VAS: 0.50-0.86 Construct validity with preanalgesia and postanalgesia scores: 9.9-6.3	Cry (1-3) Facial (0-2) Child verbal (0-2) Torso (1-2) Touch (1-2) Legs (1-2)	4 = no pain; 13 = worst pain

TABLE 3-4 Summary of Selected Behavioral Pain Assessment Scales for Young Children—cont'd

Ages of Use	Reliability and Validity	Variables	Scoring Range
Nurses Assessment of Pain Inventory (NAPI) (Stevens, 1990)			
Newborn–16 yr	Not tested by original author; later tested by Joyce, Schade, Keck, and others (1994) Interrater agreement: weighted kappa 0.37-0.80 Discriminant validity: statistically significant differences between preanalgesia and postanalgesia scores ($p < .0001$) Reliability: Cronbach alpha: 0.35-0.69	Body movement (0-2) Facial (0-3) Touching (0-2)	0 = no pain; 7 = worst pain
Behavioral Pain Score (BPS) (Robicux, Kumar, Radhakrishnan, and others, 1991)			
3-36 mo	Original article stated, "reliability of the VAS and BPS scores was tested by a k test"; no further testing of reliability or validity mentioned	Facial expression (0-2) Cry (0-3) Movements (0-3)	0 = no pain; 8 = worst pain
Modified Behavioral Pain Scale (MBPS) (Taddio, Nulman, Koren, and others, 1995)			
4-6 mo	Concurrent validity between MBPS and VAS scores: correlation coefficient 0.68 ($p < .001$) and 0.74 ($p < .001$) Construct validity using prevaccination and postvaccination scores with EMLA versus placebo: significantly lower scores with EMLA ($p < .01$) Internal consistency of items: significant correlations between items Interrater agreement ICC: 0.95, $p < .001$ Test-retest reliability: 0.95, $p < .001$	Facial expression (0-3) Cry (0-4) Movements (0, 2, 3)	0 = no pain; 10 = worst pain

Continued

TABLE 3-4 Summary of Selected Behavioral Pain Assessment Scales for Young Children—cont'd

Ages of Use	Reliability and Validity	Variables	Scoring Range
Riley Infant Pain Scale (RIPS) (Schade, Joyce, Gerkensmeyer, and others, 1996)			
<36 mo and for children with cerebral palsy	Interrater agreement using intraclass correlation coefficient: 0.53-0.83, $p < .0001$ Discriminant validity using Mann-Whitney U test with preanalgesia and postanalgesia scores: statistically significant ($p < .001$) Sensitivity: 0.31-0.23 Specificity: 0.86-0.90 Interrater reliability using 2-way cross tabulations and kappa statistics ($r[87] = 0.94$; $p < .001$) and kappa values above 0.50 for each category	0: Neutral face/smiling, calm, sleeping quietly, no cry, consolable, moves easily 1: Frowning/grimace, restless body movements, restless sleep, whimpering, winces with touch 2: Clenched teeth, moderate agitation, sleeps intermittently, difficult to console, cries with touch 3: Full cry expression, thrashing/flailing, sleeping prolonged periods interrupted by jerking or no sleep, screaming/high-pitched cry, inconsolable, screams when touched/moved	0 = no pain; 3 = worst pain
FLACC Postoperative Pain Tool (Merkel, Voepel-Lewis, Shayevitz, and others, 1997)			
2 mo–7 yr	Validity using analysis of variance for repeated measures to compare FLACC scores before and after analgesia; preanalgesia FLACC scores significantly higher than postanalgesia scores at 10, 30, and 60 min ($p < .001$ for each time) Correlation coefficients used to compare FLACC pain scores and OPS pain scores; significant positive correlation between FLACC and OPS scores ($r = 0.80$; $p < .001$); positive correlation also found between FLACC scores and nurses' global ratings of pain ($r[47] = 0.41$; $p < .005$)	Face (0-2) Legs (0-2) Activity (0-2) Cry (0-2) Consolability (0-2)	0 = no pain; 10 = worst pain

TABLE 3-4 Summary of Selected Behavioral Pain Assessment Scales for Young Children—cont'd

Ages of Use	Reliability and Validity	Variables	Scoring Range
FLACC Scale*			
	0	1	2
Face	No particular expression or smile	Occasional grimace or frown, withdrawn, disinterested	Frequent to constant frown, clenched jaw, quivering chin
Legs	Normal position or relaxed	Uneasy, restless, tense	Kicking, or legs drawn up
Activity	Lying quietly, normal position, moves easily	Squirming, shifting back and forth, tense	Arched, rigid, or jerking
Cry	No cry (awake or asleep)	Moans or whimpers, occasional complaint	Crying steadily, screams or sobs, frequent complaints
Consolability	Content, relaxed	Reassured by occasional touching, hugging, or talking to; distractible	Difficult to console or comfort

*From Merkel SI, Voepel-Lewis T, Shayevitz JR, and others: The FLACC: a behavioral scale for scoring postoperative pain in young children, *Pediatr Nurs* 23(3):293-297, 1997. Used with permission of Jannetti Publications, Inc., and the University of Michigan Health System. Can be reproduced for clinical and research use.

TABLE 3-5 Pain Rating Scales for Children

Pain Scale, Description	Instructions	Recommended Age, Comments
FACES Pain Rating Scale*		
Consists of 6 cartoon faces ranging from smiling face for "no pain" to tearful face for "worst pain"	*Original instructions:* Explain to child that each face is for a person who feels happy because there is no pain (hurt) or sad because there is some or a lot of pain. FACE 0 is very happy because there is no hurt. FACE 1 hurts just a little bit. FACE 2 hurts a little more. FACE 3 hurts even more. FACE 4 hurts a whole lot, but FACE 5 hurts as much as you can imagine, although you don't have to be crying to feel this bad. Ask child to choose face that best describes own pain. Record number under chosen face on pain assessment record.	For children as young as 3 yr. Using original instructions without affect words, such as happy or sad, or brief words resulted in same range of pain rating, probably reflecting child's rating of pain intensity. For coding purposes, numbers 0, 2, 4, 6, 8, 10 can be substituted for 0-5 system to accommodate 0-10 system. The FACES provides three scales in one: facial expressions, numbers, and words. Research supports cultural sensitivity of FACES for Caucasian, African-American, Hispanic, Thai, Chinese, and Japanese children.

0	1 or 2	2 or 4	3 or 6	4 or 8	5 or 10
No hurt	Hurts little bit	Hurts little more	Hurts even more	Hurts whole lot	Hurts worst

*Wong-Baker FACES Pain Rating Scale reference manual describing development and research of the scale is available from City of Hope Pain/Palliative Care Resource Center, 1500 East Duarte Road, Duarte, CA 91010, (626) 359-8111, ext. 3829; fax (626) 301-8941; *http://www.elsevierhealth.com/WOW/*. Use of FACES with children is demonstrated in *Whaley and Wong's Pediatric Nursing Video Series*, "Pain Assessment and Management," narrated by Donna Wong, PhD, RN. Available from Mosby, 11830 Westline Industrial Drive, St. Louis, MO 63146; (800) 426-4545; fax (800) 535-9935; *http://www.elsevierhealth.com*.

Continued

TABLE 3-5 Pain Rating Scales for Children—cont'd

Pain Scale, Description	Instructions	Recommended Age, Comments
FACES Pain Rating Scale*—cont'd		
	Brief word instructions: Point to each face using the words to describe the pain intensity. Ask child to choose face that best describes own pain, and record appropriate number.	
Oucher (Beyer, Denyes, and Villarruel, 1992)		
Consists of 6 photographs of Caucasian child's face representing "no hurt" to "biggest hurt you could ever have"; also includes vertical scale with numbers from 0 to 100; scales for African-American and Hispanic children have been developed (Villarruel and Denyes, 1991)	*Numeric scale:* Point to each section of scale to explain variations in pain intensity: "0 means no hurt." "This means little hurts" (pointing to lower part of scale, 1-29). "This means middle hurts" (pointing to middle part of scale, 30-69). "This means big hurts" (pointing to upper part of scale, 70-99). "100 means the biggest hurt you could ever have." Score is actual number stated by child. *Photographic scale:* Point to each photograph and explain variations in pain intensity using following language: 1st picture from the bottom is "no hurt," 2nd is "a little hurt," 3rd is "a little more hurt," 4th is "even more hurt than that," 5th is "pretty much or a lot of hurt," and 6th is "biggest hurt you could ever have." Score pictures from 0 to 5, with bottom picture scored as 0. *General:* Practice using Oucher by recalling and rating previous pain experiences (e.g., falling off bike). Child points to number or photograph that describes pain intensity associated with experience. Obtain current pain score from child by asking, "How much hurt do you have right now?"	Children 3-13 yr Use numeric scale if child can count to 100 by ones and identify the larger of any 2 numbers, or by tens (Jordan-Marsh, Yoder, Hall, and others, 1994). Determine whether child has cognitive ability to use photographic scale; child should be able to rate 6 geometric shapes from largest to smallest. Determine which ethnic version of Oucher to use. Allow child to select version of Oucher, or use version that most closely matches physical characteristics of child. NOTE: Ethnically similar scale may not be preferred by child when given choice of ethnically neutral cartoon scale (Luffy and Grove, 2003).

*Wong-Baker FACES Pain Rating Scale reference manual describing development and research of the scale is available from City of Hope Pain/Palliative Care Resource Center, 1500 East Duarte Road, Duarte, CA 91010, (626) 359-8111, ext. 3829; fax (626) 301-8941; *http://www.elsevierhealth.com/WOW/.* Use of FACES with children is demonstrated in *Whaley and Wong's Pediatric Nursing Video Series,* "Pain Assessment and Management," narrated by Donna Wong, PhD, RN. Available from Mosby, 11830 Westline Industrial Drive, St. Louis, MO 63146; (800) 426-4545; fax (800) 535-9935; *http://www.elsevierhealth.com.*

TABLE 3-5 Pain Rating Scales for Children—cont'd

Pain Scale, Description	Instructions	Recommended Age, Comments
Poker Chip Tool (Hester, Foster, Jordan-Marsh, and others, 1998)		
Uses 4 red poker chips placed horizontally in front of child	Say to child: "I want to talk with you about the hurt you may be having right now." Align chips horizontally in front of child on bedside table, clipboard, or other firm surface. Tell child, "These are pieces of hurt." Beginning at chip nearest child's left side and ending at one nearest right side, point to chips and say, "This (1st chip) is a little bit of hurt and this (4th chip) is the most hurt you could ever have." For a young child or for any child who may not fully comprehend the instructions, clarify by saying, "That means this (1) is just a little hurt, this (2) is a little more hurt, this (3) is more yet, and this (4) is the most hurt you could ever have." Do not give children an option for 0 hurt. Research with Poker Chip Tool has verified that children without pain will so indicate by responses such as, "I don't have any." Ask child, "How many pieces of hurt do you have right now?" After initial use of Poker Chip Tool, some children internalize the concept "pieces of hurt." If child gives response such as "I have one right now," before you ask or before you lay out poker chips, record number of chips on Pain Flow Sheet. Clarify child's answer by statements such as "Oh, you have a little hurt? Tell me about the hurt."	Children as young as 4 yr Determine whether child has cognitive ability to use numbers by identifying larger of any 2 numbers.
Word-Graphic Rating Scale† (Tesler, Savedra, Holzemer, and others, 1991)		
Uses descriptive words (may vary in other scales) to denote varying intensities of pain	Explain to child, "This is a line with words to describe how much pain you may have. This side of the line means no pain, and over here the line means worst possible pain." (Point with your finger where "no pain" is, and run your finger along the line to "worst possible pain," as you say it.)	Children 4-17 yr

†Instructions for Word-Graphic Rating Scale from Acute Pain Management Guideline Panel: *Acute pain management in infants, children, and adolescents: operative and medical procedures; quick reference guide for clinicians,* ACHPR Pub No 92-0020, Rockville, Md, 1992, Agency for Health Care Research and Quality, US Department of Health and Human Services. Word-Graphic Rating Scale is part of the Adolescent Pediatric Pain Tool and is available from Pediatric Pain Study, University of California, School of Nursing, Department of Family Health Care Nursing, San Francisco, CA 94143-0606; (415) 476-4040.

Continued

TABLE 3-5 Pain Rating Scales for Children—cont'd

Pain Scale, Description	Instructions	Recommended Age, Comments
Word-Graphic Rating Scale† (Tesler, Savedra, Holzemer, and others, 1991)—cont'd		
	"If you have no pain, you would mark like this." (Show example.) "If you have some pain, you would mark somewhere along the line, depending on how much pain you have." (Show example.) "The more pain you have, the closer to worst pain you would mark. The worst pain possible is marked like this." (Show example.) "Show me how much pain you have right now by marking with a straight, up-and-down line anywhere along the line to show how much pain you have right now." With millimeter rule, measure from the "no pain" end to mark and record this measurement as pain score.	
	No pain — Little pain — Medium pain — Large pain — Worst possible pain	
Numeric Scale		
Uses straight line with end points identified as "no pain" and "worst pain" and sometimes "medium pain" in the middle; divisions along line marked in units from 0-10 (high number may vary)	Explain to child that at one end of line is 0, which means that person feels no pain (hurt). At other end is usually 5 or 10, which means the person feels worst pain imaginable. The numbers 1-5 or 1-10 are for very little pain to a whole lot of pain. Ask child to choose number that best describes own pain.	Children as young as 5 yr, as long as they can count and have some concept of numbers and their values in relation to other numbers. Scale may be used horizontally or vertically. Number coding should be same as other scales used in facility.
	No pain — Worst pain: 0 1 2 3 4 5 6 7 8 9 10	

†Instructions for Word-Graphic Rating Scale from Acute Pain Management Guideline Panel: *Acute pain management in infants, children, and adolescents: operative and medical procedures; quick reference guide for clinicians,* ACHPR Pub No 92-0020, Rockville, Md, 1992, Agency for Health Care Research and Quality, US Department of Health and Human Services. Word-Graphic Rating Scale is part of the Adolescent Pediatric Pain Tool and is available from Pediatric Pain Study, University of California, School of Nursing, Department of Family Health Care Nursing, San Francisco, CA 94143-0606; (415) 476-4040.

TABLE 3-5 Pain Rating Scales for Children—cont'd

Pain Scale, Description	Instructions	Recommended Age, Comments
Visual Analog Scale (VAS) (Cline, Herman, Shaw, and others, 1992)		
Defined as vertical or horizontal line that is drawn to certain length, such as 10 cm (4 in), and anchored by items that represent extremes of the subjective phenomenon, such as pain, that is measured	Ask child to place mark on line that best describes amount of own pain. With centimeter ruler, measure from "no pain" end to the mark, and record this measurement as the pain score. No pain ——— Worst pain	Children as young as 4.5 yr, preferably 7 yr Vertical or horizontal scale may be used. Research shows that children ages 3-18 yr least prefer VAS compared with other scales (Luffy and Grove, 2003; Wong and Baker, 1988).
Color Tool (Eland and Banner, 1999)		
Uses markers for child to construct own scale that is used with body outline	Present 8 markers to child in random order. Ask child, "Of these colors, which color is like ____?" (the event identified by child as having hurt the most). Place the marker (represents severe pain) away from other markers. Ask child, "Which color is like a hurt, but not quite as much as ____?" (the event identified by child as having hurt the most). Place this marker with the marker chosen to represent severe pain. Ask child, "Which color is like something that hurts just a little?" Place the marker with the other colors. Ask child, "Which color is like no hurt at all?" Show the 4 marker choices to the child in order from worst to no-hurt color. Ask child to show on body outlines where he or she hurts, using markers chosen. After child has colored hurts, ask if they are current hurts or hurts from the past. Ask if child knows why the area hurts if it is not clear to you why it does.	Children as young as 4 yr, provided they know their colors, are not color blind, and are able to construct the scale if in pain

TABLE 3-6 Summary of Pain Assessment Scales for Infants

Ages of Use	Reliability and Validity	Variables	Scoring Range
Postoperative Pain Score (POPS) (Barrier, Attia, Mayer, and others, 1987)			
1-7 mo	Not tested by original authors Later tested by Joyce, Schade, Keck, and others (1994); high interrater agreement (reliability); discriminant validity ($p < .0001$); reliability with high Cronbach alpha ranging from 0.79-0.88	Sleep (0-2) Flexion fingers/toes (0-2) Facial expression (0-2) Sucking (0-2) Quality of cry (0-2) Tone (0-2) Spontaneous motor activity (0-2) Consolability (0-2) Spontaneous excitability (0-2) Sociability (0-2)	0 = worst pain; 20 = no pain
Neonatal Infant Pain Scale (NIPS) (Lawrence, Alcock, McGrath, and others, 1993)			
Average gestational age 33.5 wk	Interrater reliability: 0.92 and 0.97 Construct validity using analysis of variance between before, during, and after procedure scores: F = 18.97, df = 2.42, $p < .001$ Concurrent validity between NIPS and visual analog scale (VAS) using Pearson correlations: 0.53-0.84 Internal consistency using Cronbach alpha: 0.95, 0.87, and 0.88 for before, during, and after procedure scores	Facial expression (0-1) Arms (0-1) Cry (0-2) Legs (0-1) Breathing patterns (0-1) State of arousal (0-1)	0 = no pain; 7 = worst pain
Pain Assessment Tool (PAT) (Hodgkinson, Bear, Thorn, and others, 1994)			
27 wk gestational age–full term	No reliability or validity discussed by original authors	Posture/tone (1-2) Respirations (1-2) Sleep pattern (0-2) Heart rate (1-2) Expression (1-2) Saturations (0-2) Color (0-2) Blood pressure (0-2) Cry (0-2) Nurse's perception (0-2)	4 = no pain; 20 = worst pain

TABLE 3-6 Summary of Pain Assessment Scales for Infants—cont'd

Ages of Use	Reliability and Validity	Variables	Scoring Range
Pain Rating Scale (PRS) (Joyce, Schade, Keck, and others, 1994)			
1-36 mo	Interrater agreement: $r = 0.65$-0.84, $p < .0001$ Discriminant validity: statistically significant *t*-tests ($p < 0.0001$)	0: Smiling, sleeping, no change when moved/touched 1: Takes small amount orally, restless, moving, cries 2: Not drinking/eating, short periods of cries, distracted with rocking or pacifier 3: Change in behavior, irritable, arms/legs shake/jerk, facial grimace 4: Flailing, high-pitched wailing, parents request pain medication, unable to distract 5: Sleeping prolonged periods interrupted by jerking, continuous crying, rapid and shallow respirations	0 = no pain; 5 = worst pain
CRIES (Krechel and Bildner, 1995)			
32-60 wk of gestational age	Concurrent validity between CRIES and POPS: 0.73 ($p < .0001$, n = 1382); Spearman correlation between subjective report and POPS and CRIES: 0.49 ($p < 0.0001$, n > 1300) Discriminant validity using before and after analgesia scores: Wilcoxon sign rank test: mean decline of 3.0 units ($p < .0001$, n = 74) Interrater reliability using Spearman correlation coefficient: $r = 0.72$ ($p < .0001$, n = 680)	Crying (0-2) Requires increased oxygen (0-2) Increased vital signs (0-2) Expression (0-2) Sleepless (0-2)	0 = no pain; 10 = worst pain

Continued

TABLE 3-6 Summary of Pain Assessment Scales for Infants—cont'd

Ages of Use	Reliability and Validity	Variables	Scoring Range
Premature Infant Pain Profile (PIPP) (Stevens, Johnston, Petryshen, and others, 1996)			
28-40 wk of gestational age	Internal consistency using Cronbach alpha: 0.75-0.59; standardized item alpha for 6 items: 0.71 Construct validity using handling versus painful situations: statistically significant differences (paired $t = 12.24$, two-tailed $p < .0001$, and Mann-Whitney $U = 765.5$, $p < .00001$) and using real versus sham heel stick procedures with infants ages 28-30 wk of gestational age ($t = 2.4$, two-tailed $p < .02$, and Mann-Whitney $U = 132$, $p < .016$) and with full-term boys undergoing circumcision with topical anesthetic versus. placebo ($t = 2.6$, two-tailed $p < .02$, or nonparametric equivalent Mann-Whitney U test, $U = 145.7$, two-tailed $p < .02$)	Gestational age (0-3) Eye squeeze (0-3) Behavioral state (0-3) Nasolabial furrow (0-3) Heart rate (0-3) Oxygen saturation (0-3) Brow bulge (0-3)	0 = no pain; 21 = worst pain
Scale for Use in Newborns (SUN) (Blauer and Gerstmann, 1998)			
0-28 days	No reliability; face validity, content validity, construct validity using extreme groups	Central nervous system state (0-4) Movement (0-4) Breathing (0-4) Tone (0-4) Heart rate (0-4) Face (0-4) Mean blood pressure (0-4)	0 = no pain; 28 = worst pain Average baseline score 10-14 A 2 represents normal or baseline value

TABLE 3-6 Summary of Pain Assessment Scales for Infants—cont'd

Ages of Use	Reliability and Validity	Variables	Scoring Range
Neonatal Pain, Agitation, and Sedation Scale (NPASS) (Puchalski and Hummel, 2002)			
Birth (23 wk of gestational age) and full-term newborns up to 100 days	Interrater reliability using ICC: 0.95 CI for preintervention and post-intervention pain scale; 0.95 CI for preintervention and postintervention sedation scale Internal consistency (Cronbach alpha): Preintervention pain scale, 0.75 and 0.71 raters 1 and 2 Postintervention pain scale, 0.25 and 0.27 raters 1 and 2 Preintervention sedation scale, 0.88 and 0.81 raters 1 and 2 Postintervention sedation scale, 0.86 and 0.89 raters 1 and 2	Cry/irritability (0-2) Behavior/state (0-2) Facial expression (0-2) Extremities/tone (0-2) Vital signs—heart rate, respiratory rate, blood pressure, SaO_2 (0-2)	Pain score: 0 = no pain; 10 = intense pain Sedation score: 0 = no sedation; 10 = deep sedation
CRIES Neonatal Postoperative Pain Scale			
	0	1	2
Crying	No	High pitched	Inconsolable
Requires oxygen for saturation >95%	No	<30%	>30%
Increased vital signs	Heart rate and blood pressure less than or equal to preoperative state	Heart rate and blood pressure increase <20% of preoperative state	Heart rate and blood pressure increase >20% of preoperative state
Expression	None	Grimace	Grimace/grunt
Sleepless	No	Wakes at frequent intervals	Constantly awake

Developmental Characteristics of Children's Responses to Pain

YOUNG INFANT

Generalized body response of rigidity or thrashing, possibly with local reflex withdrawal of stimulated area

Loud crying

Facial expression of pain (brows lowered and drawn together, eyes tightly closed, and mouth open and squarish) (Figure 3-11)

Demonstrates no association between approaching stimulus and subsequent pain

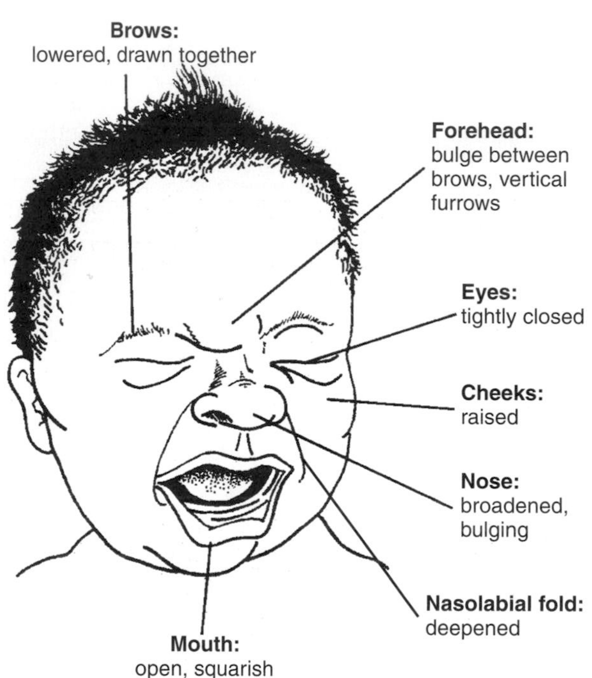

FIGURE **3-11** Facial expression of physical distress is the most consistent behavioral indicator of pain in infants.

OLDER INFANT

Localized body response with deliberate withdrawal of stimulated area

Loud crying

Facial expression of pain or anger (same facial characteristics as pain, but eyes are open)

Physical resistance, especially pushing the stimulus away after it is applied

YOUNG CHILD

Loud crying, screaming

Verbal expressions of "Ow," "Ouch," "It hurts"

Thrashing of arms and legs

Attempts to push stimulus away before it is applied

Uncooperative; needs physical restraint

Requests termination of procedure

Clings to parent, nurse, or other significant person

Requests emotional support, such as hugs or other forms of physical comfort

May become restless and irritable with continuing pain

All of these behaviors may be seen in anticipation of actual painful procedure

SCHOOL-AGE CHILD

May see all behaviors of young child, especially during actual painful procedure but less in anticipatory period

Stalling behavior, such as "Wait a minute" or "I'm not ready"

Muscular rigidity, such as clenched fists, white knuckles, gritted teeth, contracted limbs, body stiffness, closed eyes, wrinkled forehead

ADOLESCENT

Less vocal protest

Less motor activity

More verbal expressions, such as "It hurts" or "You're hurting me"

Increased muscle tension and body control

Data from Craig KD and others: Developmental changes in infant pain expression during immunization injections, *Soc Sci Med* 19(12):1331-1337, 1984; and Katz ER, Kellerman J, Siegel SE: Behavioral distress in children with cancer undergoing medical procedures: developmental considerations, *J Consult Clin Psychol* 48(3):356-365, 1980.

Manifestations of Acute Pain in the Neonate

Physiologic Responses

Vital signs: observe for variations
Increased heart rate
Increased blood pressure
Rapid, shallow respirations
Oxygenation
Decreased transcutaneous O_2 saturation ($tcPO_2$)
Decreased arterial O_2 saturation (SaO_2)
Skin: observe color and character
Pallor or flushing
Diaphoresis
Palmar sweating
Other observations
Increased muscle tone
Dilated pupils
Decreased vagal nerve tone
Increased intracranial pressure

LABORATORY EVIDENCE OF METABOLIC OR ENDOCRINE CHANGES

Hyperglycemia
Lowered pH
Elevated corticosteroids

BEHAVIORAL RESPONSES

Vocalizations: observe quality, timing, and duration
Crying
Whimpering
Groaning
Facial expression: observe characteristics, timing, orientation of eyes and mouth (see Figure 3-11)
Grimaces
Brow furrowed
Chin quivering
Eyes tightly closed
Mouth open and squarish
Body movements and posture: observe type, quality, and amount of movement or lack of movement; relationship to other factors
Limb withdrawal
Thrashing
Rigidity
Flaccidity
Fist clenching
Changes in state: observe sleep, appetite, activity level
Changes in sleep-wake cycles
Changes in feeding behavior
Changes in activity level
Fussiness, irritability
Listlessness

Routes and Methods of Analgesic Drug Administration

ORAL

Preferred because of convenience, cost, and relatively steady blood levels
Higher dosages of oral form of opioids required for equivalent parenteral analgesia
Peak drug effect occurs after 1 to 2 hours for most analgesics
Delay in onset is disadvantage when rapid control of severe pain or of fluctuating pain is desired
See Table 3-7 for several oral nonsteroidal anti-inflammatory drugs used for children

SUBLINGUAL, BUCCAL, AND TRANSMUCOSAL

Tablet or liquid placed between cheek and gum (buccal) or under tongue (sublingual)
Highly desirable because more rapid onset than oral route
Less first-pass effect through liver than oral route, which normally reduces analgesia from oral opioids (unless sublingual or buccal form swallowed, which occurs often in children)
Few drugs commercially available in this form
Many drugs can be compounded into a sublingual troche or lozenge.*
Actiq—Oral transmucosal fentanyl citrate in hard confection base on a plastic holder; indicated only for management of breakthrough cancer pain in patients with malignancies who are already receiving and are tolerant to opioid therapy but can be used for preoperative or preprocedural sedation or analgesia

INTRAVENOUS (BOLUS)

Preferred for rapid control of severe pain
Provides most rapid onset of effect, usually in about 5 minutes
Advantage for acute pain, procedural pain, and breakthrough pain
Needs to be repeated hourly for continuous pain control
Drugs with short half-life (morphine, fentanyl, hydromorphone) are preferred, to avoid toxic accumulation of drug

Data primarily from American Pain Society: *Principles of analgesic use in the treatment of acute pain and chronic cancer pain,* ed 4, Skokie, Ill, 1999, The Society; and McCaffery M, Pasero C: *Pain: a clinical manual,* ed 2, St Louis, 1999, Mosby.

*For further information about compounding drugs in troche or suppository form, contact Professional Compounding Centers of America (PCCA), 9901 South Wilcrest Dr., Houston, TX 77099; (800) 331-2498; *http://www.pccarx.com.*

TABLE 3-7 Nonsteroidal Antiinflammatory Drugs (NSAIDs) Approved for Children*

Drug	Dosage	Comments
Acetaminophen (Tylenol)	10-15 mg/kg/dose every 4-6 hr not to exceed 5 doses in 24 hr or 75 mg/kg/day, orally	Available in numerous preparations Nonprescription Higher dosage range may provide increased analgesia
Choline magnesium trisalicylate (Trilisate)	Children <37 kg (81.5 lb): 50 mg/kg/day divided into 2 doses Children >37 kg (81.5 lb): 2250 mg/day divided into 2 doses	Available in suspension, 500 mg/5 ml Prescription
Ibuprofen (children's Motrin, children's Advil)	Children <6 mo: 5-10 mg/kg/dose every 6-8 hr not to exceed 40 mg/kg/day	Available in numerous preparations Available in suspension, 100 mg/5 ml, and drops, 100 mg/2.5 ml Nonprescription
Naproxen (Naprosyn)	Children >2 yr: 10 mg/kg/day divided into 2 doses	Available in suspension, 125 mg/5 ml, and several different dosages for tablets Prescription
Tolmetin (Tolectin)	Children >2 yr: 20 g/kg/day divided into 3-4 doses	Available in 200-mg, 400-mg, and 600-mg tablets Prescription

Data from Olin BR and others: *Drug facts and comparisons,* St Louis, 2002, Facts and Comparisons.

NOTE: Newer formulations of NSAIDs selectively inhibit one of the enzymes of cyclooxygenase (COX-2, which is responsible for pain transmission) but do not inhibit the other (COX-1). Inhibition of COX-1 decreases prostaglandin production, which is necessary for normal organ function. For example, prostaglandins help maintain gastric mucosal blood flow and barrier protection, regulate blood flow to the liver and kidneys, and facilitate platelet aggregation and clot formation. Theoretically, the COX-2 NSAIDs provide similar analgesic and antiinflammatory benefits with fewer gastric and platelet side effects than the nonselective agents. COX-2 NSAIDs are approved for use in patients older than 18 years of age.

*All NSAIDs in this table (except acetaminophen) have significant antiinflammatory, antipyretic, and analgesic actions. Acetaminophen has a weak antiinflammatory action, and its classification as an NSAID is controversial. Patients respond differently to various NSAIDs; therefore changing from one drug to another may be necessary for maximum benefit. Acetylsalicylic acid (aspirin) is also an NSAID but is not recommended for children because of its possible association with Reye syndrome. The NSAIDs in this table have no known association with Reye syndrome. However, caution should be exercised in prescribing any salicylate-containing drug (e.g., Trilisate) for children with known or suspected viral infection. Side effects of ibuprofen, naproxen, and tolmetin include nausea, vomiting, diarrhea, constipation, gastric ulceration, bleeding nephritis, and fluid retention. Acetaminophen and choline magnesium trisalicylate are well tolerated in the gastrointestinal tract and do not interfere with platelet function. NSAIDs (except acetaminophen) should not be given to patients with allergic reactions to salicylates. All the NSAIDs should be used cautiously in patients with renal impairment.

INTRAVENOUS (CONTINUOUS)

Preferred over bolus and intramuscular injection for maintaining control of pain

Provides steady blood levels

Easy to titrate dosage

SUBCUTANEOUS (CONTINUOUS)

Used when oral and IV routes not available

Provides equivalent blood levels to continuous IV infusion

Suggested initial bolus dose to equal 2-hour IV dose; total 24-hour dose usually requires concentrated opioid solution to minimize infused volume; use smallest gauge needle that accommodates infusion rate

PATIENT-CONTROLLED ANALGESIA

Typically uses programmable infusion pump (IV, epidural, subcutaneous) that permits self-administration of boluses of medication at preset dose and time interval (lockout interval is time between doses)

PCA bolus administration may be combined with initial bolus and continuous (basal or background) infusion of opioid

Optimum lockout interval not known but must be at least as long as time needed for onset of drug; longer lockout requires larger dose

Should effectively control pain during movement or procedures

See Table 3-8 for suggested IV PCA opioid infusion orders

TABLE 3-8 Suggested Intravenous Patient-Controlled Analgesia Opioid Infusion Orders

Drug	Basal Rate (mcg/kg/hr)	Bolus Rate (mcg/kg/dose)	Lockout Period (min)	Maximum Dose/Hour (mg/kg)
Morphine	10-30	10-30	6-10	0.1-0.15
Hydromorphone	3-5	6-10	0.015-0.02	3-5
Fentanyl	0.5-1.00	0.5-1.0	6-10	0.002-0.004

From Yaster M, Krane EJ, Kaplan RF, and others: *Pediatric pain management and sedation handbook,* St Louis, 1997, Mosby.

FAMILY-CONTROLLED ANALGESIA

One family member (usually a parent) or other caregiver is designated child's primary pain manager and has responsibility for pressing PCA button

Guidelines for selecting a primary pain manager for family-controlled analgesia:

- Spends a significant amount of time with the patient
- Is willing to assume responsibility for being primary pain manager
- Is willing to accept and respect patient's reports of pain (if able to provide) as best indicator of how much pain the patient is experiencing; knows how to use and interpret a pain rating scale
- Understands the purpose and goals of patient's pain management plan
- Understands concept of maintaining a steady analgesic blood level
- Recognizes signs of pain and side effects and adverse reactions to opioid

NURSE-CONTROLLED ANALGESIA

Child's primary nurse is designated primary pain manager and is only person who presses PCA button during that nurse's shift

Guidelines for selecting primary pain manager for family-controlled analgesia apply to nurse-controlled analgesia

May be used in addition to a basal rate to treat breakthrough pain with bolus doses; patients are assessed every 30 minutes for the need for a bolus dose

May be used without a basal rate as a means of maintaining analgesia with around-the-clock bolus doses

INTRAMUSCULAR

Not recommended for pain control; not current standard of care

Painful administration (hated by children)

Some drugs (e.g., meperidine) can cause tissue and nerve damage.

Wide fluctuation in absorption of drug from muscle

Faster absorption from deltoid than from gluteal sites

Shorter duration and more expensive than oral drugs

Time-consuming for staff and unnecessary delay for child

INTRANASAL

Available commercially as Stadol NS (butorphanol); approved for those older than 18 years of age; should not be used in patient receiving morphine-like drugs because butorphanol is partial antagonist that will reduce analgesia and may cause withdrawal

INTRADERMAL

Used primarily for skin anesthesia prior to procedures (e.g., before lumbar puncture, bone marrow aspiration, arterial puncture, skin biopsy)

Local anesthetics (e.g., lidocaine) cause stinging, burning sensation

Duration of stinging may depend on type of "caine" used

To avoid stinging sensation associated with lidocaine, buffer the solution by adding 1 part sodium bicarbonate (1 mEq/ml) to 9 to 10 parts 1% or 2% lidocaine with or without epinephrine

NS with preservative and benzyl alcohol also anesthetizes venipuncture sites; use same dose as for buffered lidocaine

TOPICAL/TRANSDERMAL

EMLA and LMX

EMLA (eutectic mixture of local anesthetics [lidocaine and prilocaine]) is available as a cream or anesthetic disk

LMX is available as a nonprescription 4% or 5% lidocaine cream

EMLA and LMX eliminate or reduce pain from most procedures involving skin puncture

Must be placed on intact skin over puncture site and covered by occlusive dressing or applied as anesthetic disk before procedure:

- EMLA requires a minimum of 1 hour
- LMX requires a minimum of 30 minutes

LAT

Lidocaine, adrenaline, and tetracaine; or tetracaine and phenylephrine (tetraphen)

Provides skin anesthesia about 15 minutes after application on nonintact skin

Gel (preferable) or liquid placed on wounds for suturing

Adrenaline must not be used on end arterioles (fingers, toes, tip of nose, penis, earlobes) because of vasoconstriction

Lidocaine Iontophoresis

Uses iontophoresis to transport lidocaine 2% and epinephrine 1:100,000 (Iontocaine) into the skin
A small battery-powered device delivers current via an electrode and speeds the numbing effects of lidocaine
At maximum setting, produces local dermal anesthesia in about 10 minutes to a depth of approximately 10 mm for Numby and 6 mm for LidoSite
May be frightening to young children when they see the device and feel the current
All metal, such as jewelry, is removed from application site to prevent burns
Child should be observed during iontophoresis

Transdermal Fentanyl (Duragesic)

Available as patch for continuous pain control
Safety and efficacy not established in children younger than 12 years of age
Not appropriate for initial relief of acute pain because of long interval to peak effect (12 to 24 hours); for rapid onset of pain relief, an immediate release opioid must be given
Orders for "rescue doses" of an immediate release opioid should be available for breakthrough pain, a flare of severe pain that breaks through the medication being administered at regular intervals for persistent pain
Has duration of up to 72 hours for prolonged pain relief
If respiratory depression occurs, several doses of naloxone may be needed

VAPOCOOLANT

Use of prescription spray coolant, such as Fluori-Methane or ethyl chloride (Pain-Ease); applied to the skin for 10 to 15 seconds immediately before the needle puncture; anesthesia lasts about 15 seconds
Some children dislike the cold; spraying the coolant on a cotton ball and then applying this to the skin may be less uncomfortable
Application of ice to the skin for 30 seconds has been found to be ineffective

RECTAL

Alternative to oral or parenteral routes
Variable absorption rate
Generally disliked by children
Many drugs can be compounded into rectal suppositories*

REGIONAL NERVE BLOCK

Use of long-acting local anesthetic (bupivacaine or ropivacaine) injected into nerves to block pain at site
Provides prolonged analgesia postoperatively, such as after inguinal hernia repair
May be used to provide local anesthesia for surgery, such as dorsal penile nerve block for circumcision or for reduction of fractures

INHALATION

Use of anesthetics, such as nitrous oxide, to produce partial or complete analgesia for painful procedures
Occupational exposure to high levels of nitrous oxide may cause side effects (e.g., headache)

EPIDURAL OR INTRATHECAL

Involves catheter placed into epidural, caudal, or intrathecal space for continuous infusion or single or intermittent administration of opioid with or without a long-acting local anesthetic (e.g., bupivacaine, ropivacaine).
Analgesia primarily from drug's direct effect on opioid receptors in spinal cord.
Respiratory depression is rare but may have slow and delayed onset; can be prevented by checking level of sedation and respiratory rate and depth hourly for initial 24 hours and decreasing dose when excessive sedation is detected.
Nausea, itching, and urinary retention are common dose-related side effects from the epidural opioid.
Mild hypotension, urinary retention, and temporary motor or sensory deficits are common unwanted effects of epidural local anesthetic.
Catheter for urinary retention should be inserted during surgery to decrease trauma to child; if inserted when child is awake, anesthetize urethra with lidocaine.

*For further information about compounding drugs in troche or suppository form, contact Professional Compounding Centers of America (PCCA), 9901 South Wilcrest Dr., Houston, TX 77099; (800) 331-2498; *http://www.pccarx.com.*

Opioid Effects

SIDE EFFECTS OF OPIOIDS

General

Constipation (possibly severe)
Respiratory depression
Sedation
Nausea and vomiting
Agitation, euphoria
Mental clouding
Hallucinations
Orthostatic hypotension
Pruritus
Urticaria
Sweating
Miosis (may be sign of toxicity)
Anaphylaxis (rare)

SIGNS OF TOLERANCE

Decreasing pain relief
Decreasing duration of pain relief

SIGNS OF WITHDRAWAL SYNDROME IN PATIENTS WITH PHYSICAL DEPENDENCE

Initial Signs of Withdrawal

Lacrimation
Rhinorrhea
Yawning
Sweating

Later Signs

Restlessness
Irritability
Tremors
Anorexia
Dilated pupils
Gooseflesh
Nausea and vomiting

See Tables 3-10 to 3-13 (pp. 333-338) for more information on pharmacologic pain management.

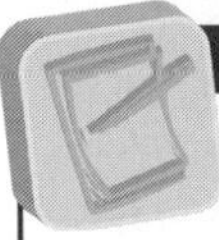

GUIDELINES

Managing Opioid-Induced Respiratory Depression

If Respirations Are Depressed

Assess sedation level
Reduce infusion by 25% when possible
Stimulate patient (shake shoulder gently, call by name, ask to breathe)

If Patient Cannot Be Aroused or Is Apneic

Administer naloxone (Narcan):

- For children weighing less than 40 kg, dilute 0.1 mg naloxone in 10 ml sterile saline to make 10 mcg/ml solution and give 0.5 mcg/kg.
- For children weighing more than 40 kg, dilute 0.4-mg ampule in 10 ml sterile saline and give 0.5 ml.

Administer bolus slow IV push every 2 minutes until effect is obtained.
Closely monitor patient. Naloxone's duration of antagonist action may be shorter than that of opioid, requiring repeated doses of naloxone.

NOTE: Respiratory depression caused by benzodiazepines (e.g., diazepam [Valium] or midazolam [Versed]) can be reversed with flumazenil (Romazicon). Pediatric dosing experience suggests 0.01 mg/kg (0.1 ml/kg); if no (or inadequate) response after 1 to 2 minutes, administer same dose and repeat as needed at 60-second intervals for maximum dose of 1 mg (10 ml).*
*Yaster M, Krane EJ, Kaplan RF, and others: *Pediatric pain management and sedation handbook*, St Louis, 1997, Mosby.

Nonpharmacologic Strategies for Pain Management

GENERAL STRATEGIES

Use nonpharmacologic interventions to supplement, not replace, pharmacologic interventions and use for mild pain and pain that is reasonably well controlled with analgesics. See Table 3-9 for age-appropriate guidelines.

Form a trusting relationship with child and family.

Express concern regarding their reports of pain, and intervene appropriately.

Take an active role in seeking effective pain management strategies.

Use general guidelines to prepare child for procedure.

Prepare child before potentially painful procedures, but avoid "planting" the idea of pain. For example, instead of saying, "This is going to (or may) hurt," say, "Sometimes this feels like pushing, sticking, or pinching, and sometimes it doesn't bother people. Tell me what it feels like to you."

Use "nonpain" descriptors when possible (e.g., "It feels like heat" rather than "It's a burning pain"). This allows for variation in sensory perception, avoids suggesting pain, and gives child control in describing reactions.

Avoid evaluative statements or descriptions (e.g., "This is a terrible procedure" or "It really will hurt a lot").

Stay with child during a painful procedure.

Allow parents to stay with child if child and parent desire; encourage parent to talk softly to child and to remain near child's head.

Involve parents in learning specific nonpharmacologic strategies and in assisting child with their use.

Educate child about the pain, especially when explanation may lessen anxiety (e.g., that pain may occur after surgery and does not indicate something is wrong); reassure that child is not responsible for the pain.

For long-term pain control, give child a doll that represents "the patient" and allow child to do everything to the doll that is done to the child; pain control can be emphasized through the doll by stating, "Dolly feels better after the medicine."

Teach procedures to child and family for later use.

SPECIFIC STRATEGIES

Distraction

Involve parent and child in identifying strong distractors.

Involve child in play; use radio, tape recorder, CD player, or computer game; have child sing or use rhythmic breathing.

Have child take a deep breath and blow it out until told to stop

Have child blow bubbles to "blow the hurt away."

Have child concentrate on yelling or saying "ouch" by focusing on "yelling as loud or soft as you feel it hurt: that way I know what's happening."

Have child look through kaleidoscope (type with glitter suspended in fluid-filled tube) and encourage to concentrate by asking, "Do you see the different designs?"

Use humor, such as watching cartoons, telling jokes or funny stories, or acting silly with child.

Have child read, play games, or visit with friends.

Relaxation

With an infant or young child:

- Hold in a comfortable, well-supported position, such as vertically against the chest and shoulder.
- Rock in a wide, rhythmic arc in a rocking chair or sway back and forth rather than bouncing child.
- Repeat one or two words softly, such as "Mommy's here."

With a slightly older child:

- Ask child to take a deep breath and "go limp as a rag doll" while exhaling slowly; then ask child to yawn (demonstrate if needed).
- Help child assume a comfortable position (e.g., pillow under neck and knees).
- Begin progressive relaxation: starting with the toes, systematically instruct child to let each body part "go limp" or "feel heavy"; if child has difficulty with relaxing, instruct child to tense or tighten each body part then relax it.
- Allow child to keep eyes open, because children may respond better if eyes are open rather than closed during relaxation.

Guided Imagery

Have child identify some highly pleasurable real or imaginary experience.

Have child describe details of the event, including as many senses as possible (e.g., "feel the cool breezes," "see the beautiful colors," "hear the pleasant music").

Have child write down or tape record script.

Encourage child to concentrate only on the pleasurable event during the painful time; enhance the image by recalling specific details through reading the script or playing the tape.

Combine with relaxation and rhythmic breathing.

Positive Self-Talk

Teach child positive statements to say when in pain (e.g., "I will be feeling better soon," "When I go home, I will feel better, and we will eat ice cream").

Thought Stopping

Identify positive facts about the painful event (e.g., "It does not last long").

Identify reassuring information (e.g., "If I think about something else, it does not hurt as much").

Condense positive and reassuring facts into a set of brief statements and have child memorize them (e.g., "Short procedure, good veins, little hurt, nice nurse, go home").

Have child repeat the memorized statements whenever thinking about or experiencing the painful event.

Behavioral Contracting

Informal

May be used with children as young as 4 or 5 years of age.

Use stars, tokens or cartoon character stickers as rewards.

Give uncooperative or procrastinating children (during a procedure) a limited time (measured by a visible timer) to complete the procedure.

Proceed as needed if child is unable to comply.

Reinforce cooperation with a reward if the procedure is accomplished within specified time.

Formal

Use written contract that includes:

- Realistic (seems possible) goal or desired behavior
- Measurable behavior (e.g., agrees not to hit anyone during procedures)
- Contract written, dated, and signed by all persons involved in any of the agreements
- Identified rewards or consequences that are reinforcing
- Goals that can be evaluated
- Commitment and compromise requirements for both parties (e.g., while timer is used, nurse will not nag or prod child to complete procedure)

TABLE 3-9 Nonpharmacologic Pain Interventions by Developmental Age

Developmental Age	Pain Management	Distraction Techniques	Other Considerations
Infant 0-12 months	Call Child Life Specialist Caregiver support Swaddling and positioning Pacifiers	Music Rattles Mobiles Pacifiers	Reacts to caregiver stress or anxiety Sensitive to physical environment
Toddler 1-3 years	Call Child Life Specialist Caregiver support Positioning Incorporate home routines	Music and singing Pacifiers Bubbles Pop-up books Talking, musical toys Comfort items	Reacts to caregiver stress or anxiety Separation anxiety May resist physically
Preschooler 3-5 years	Call Child Life Specialist Caregiver support Positioning Incorporate home routines Simple preparation	Music and singing Bubbles Pop-up books Talking, musical toys Comfort items Counting	Reacts to caregiver stress or anxiety May view pain as punishment May resist physically Allow to watch procedure, if requested
School-age child 5-12 years	Call Child Life Specialist Thorough preparation Caregiver support Positioning Encourage choices	Music TV, video games "I Spy" books Magic wand Bubbles Guided imagery Deep breathing	Younger patients have short attention span May resist physically May blame parents for pain caused May view pain as a punishment Establish rapport to increase cooperation Allow to watch procedure, if requested
Adolescent 12-18 years	Call Child Life Specialist Thorough preparation Allow choices Positioning	Music TV, video games Guided imagery Deep breathing Conversation	May or may not want caregiver presence Allow to watch procedure, if requested May have anxiety related to body image Establish rapport to increase cooperation

Fasting Recommendations Before Sedation and Analgesia*

Ingested Material	Minimum Fasting Period (hr)†
Clear liquids‡	>2
Breast milk	4
Infant formula	6
Nonhuman milk§	6
Light meal‖	6

From American Society of Anesthesiologists: Practice guidelines for preoperative fasting and the use of pharmacologic agents to reduce the risk of pulmonary aspiration: application to healthy patients undergoing elective procedures, *Anesthesiology* 90(3):896-905, 1999; retrieved from *http://www.ASAhq.org/practice/NPO/NPOguide.html.*

*These recommendations apply to healthy patients who are undergoing elective procedures. They are not intended for women in labor. Following the guidelines does not guarantee complete gastric emptying has occurred.

†Fasting periods noted in chart apply to all ages.

‡Examples of clear liquids include water, fruit juices without pulp, carbonated beverages, clear tea, and black coffee.

§Because nonhuman milk is similar to solids in gastric emptying time, the amount ingested must be considered when determining appropriate fasting period.

‖Light meal typically consists of toast and clear liquids. Meals that include fried or fatty foods or meat may prolong gastric emptying time. Both amount and type of foods ingested must be considered when determining appropriate fasting period.

Pain Management During Neonatal Circumcision*

PHARMACOLOGIC INTERVENTIONS

Use of Topical Anesthetic Only

1. One hour before the procedure, administer acetaminophen (e.g., Tylenol, 15 mg/kg) as ordered.
2. Place a thick layer (1 g) of EMLA† or LMX4‡ cream around the penis where the prepuce (foreskin) attaches to the glans. Avoid placing cream on the tip of the penis, where it may come in contact with urethral opening.
3. Cover the penis with a "finger cot" that is cut from a vinyl or latex glove, or a piece of plastic wrap, and secure bottom of covering with tape. Avoid using Tegaderm or large amounts of tape on the skin because removing the adhesive causes pain and can irritate the fragile skin.
4. If the infant urinates during the time anesthetic cream is applied and a significant amount of cream is removed, reapply the cream and covering. The total application of cream should not exceed a surface area of 10 cm^2 (1.25 × 1.25 inches).
5. Remove cream with clean cloth or tissue. Blanching of skin is an expected reaction; erythema and some edema may occur also.
6. Two minutes before starting the procedure, give the infant a 24% sucrose solution. Another dose may be given at the start of the procedure, and a third dose may be given 2 minutes later. Use this solution to coat

*There is sufficient evidence and support for use of a combination of pharmacologic and nonpharmacologic interventions (such as swaddling) to holistically manage neonatal circumcision pain. (Taddio, Pollock, Gilbert-MacLeod, and others, 2000; Anand and International Evidence-Based Group for Neonatal Pain, 2001; Geyer, Ellsbury, Kleiber, and others, 2002; Razmus, Dalton, Wilson, 2004).

†EMLA is approved for use in infants of at least 37 weeks of gestation. Although the package insert warns that patients taking acetaminophen are at greater risk for developing methemoglobinemia, there have been no reported cases of this complication in infants receiving acetaminophen and using EMLA. In fact, there is no evidence that acetaminophen induces methemoglobinemia in humans (Prescott, 1996). The only reported cases of methemoglobinemia from acetaminophen have been in cats and dogs (Hjelle and Grauer, 1986).

‡LMX4 is a 4% lidocaine cream reported to be effective within 30 min of application for venipuncture. There is no need to apply an occlusive dressing over LMX4 cream as recommended for EMLA (Wong, 2003). Use of LMX4 for pain relief of pediatric meatotomy has been reported previously (Smith and Gjellum, 2004.) Despite anecdotal reports of its use in neonatal circumcision, at this time no studies are available regarding the use or effectiveness of LMX4 for neonatal circumcision analgesia.

the pacifier (recoat several times before and during the procedure).

7. After the procedure, apply petrolatum or A&D ointment on a 2×2-inch dressing before diapering infant to prevent the wound from adhering to the dressing or diaper.
8. Administer acetaminophen as ordered 4 hours after the initial dose; give additional doses as needed but not to exceed five doses in 24 hours or a maximum dose of 75 mg/kg/day.

Use of Dorsal Penile Nerve Block or Ring Block

1. One hour before the procedure administer acetaminophen as ordered.
2. One hour before procedure, apply EMLA or LMX4 cream. For the dorsal penile nerve block (DPNB) apply cream to the prepuce as described previously and at the penile base. For the ring block apply cream to the prepuce as described previously and to the shaft of the penis. Use a topical anesthetic in conjunction with the DPNB or ring block to avoid the pain of injecting the anesthetic.
3. Provide a 30-gauge needle to administer the lidocaine.§ For the DPNB, 0.4 ml of lidocaine is infiltrated at the 10:30 and 1:30 o'clock positions in Buck's fascia at the penile base. For the ring block, 0.4 ml of lidocaine is infiltrated subcutaneously on each side of the shaft of the penis below the prepuce.
4. For maximum anesthesia, wait 5 minutes after injection of lidocaine. An alternative anesthetic agent is chloroprocaine, which is as effective as lidocaine after 3 minutes.
5. Approximately 2 minutes before the circumcision, administer concentrated oral sucrose solution as described previously.
6. After the procedure, apply A&D ointment or petrolatum and administer acetaminophen as described previously.

NONPHARMACOLOGIC INTERVENTIONS

In addition to the preceding pharmacologic interventions:

- If Circumstraint board is used, pad with blankets or other thick, soft material such as "lamb's wool." A more comfortable, padded, and physiologic restraint that places the infant semireclining can also decrease distress.||
- Provide the parents, caregiver, or another staff member with the option to hold the infant during the procedure or to be present during the circumcision.
- Swaddle the upper body and legs to provide warmth and containment and to reduce movement.
- If the patient is not swaddled and is unclothed, use a radiant warmer to prevent hypothermia. Shield infant's eyes from overhead lights.
- Prewarm any topical solutions to be used in sterile preparation of the surgical site by placing in a warm blanket or towel.
- Play infant relaxation music before, during, and after procedure; allow parents or other caregiver the option of choosing the music.¶
- After the procedure, remove restraints and swaddle. Immediately have the parent, other caregiver, or nursing staff hold the infant. Continue to have the infant suck on pacifier, or offer feeding.

§In one study the use of buffered lidocaine, which normally reduces stinging sensation of lidocaine, did not provide effective anesthesia for DPNB (Stang, Snellman, Condon, and others, 1997). The study on slow injection of the anesthetics lidocaine and bupivacaine compared 40 versus 80 seconds in patients ages 15 to 53 years (Serour, Mandelberg, Mori, 1998).

||For information on Stang Circ Chair, contact Pedicraft, PO Box 5969, Jacksonville, FL 32247-5969, (800) 223-7649; e-mail: info@pedicraft.com; *http://www.pedicraft.com.*

¶Suggested infant relaxation music: Heartbeat Lullabies by Terry Woodford. Available from Baby-Go-To-Sleep Center, Audio-Therapy Innovations, Inc., PO Box 550, Colorado Springs, CO 80901, (800) 537-7748.

End-of-Life Care Interventions

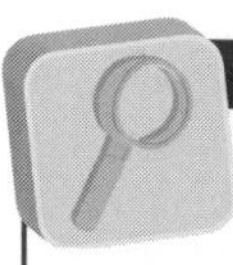

EVIDENCE-BASED PRACTICE

Pediatric Pain and Symptom Management at the End of Life

Angela Ethier

Ask the Question

Question

In children, what is the pain and symptom experience at the end of life?

Background

Infants and children have historically been under treated for pain. Developmental factors add to the complexity of providing care to this patient population. The provision of pediatric palliative care is an emerging specialty. Health care providers have limited training and education in delivering palliative care.

Objective

To evaluate the evidence of infants and children's pain and symptom experience at the end of life

Search for Evidence

Search Strategies

Published studies from 2000 to 2005 using the subject terms *child, palliative care, pain,* and *symptoms* were identified and examined. Retrospective descriptive studies dominated the findings describing infants and children's end-of-life experiences through the use of medical record reviews and provider and parental surveys.

Database Used

PubMed

Critically Analyze the Evidence

Children experienced an average of 11 symptoms during their last week of life (Drake, Frost, and Collins, 2003). Pain, dyspnea, and fatigue were the most frequently documented symptoms, experienced by most children at the end of life (Bradshaw, Hinds, Lensing, and others, 2005; Carter, Howenstein, Gilmer, and others, 2004; Drake and others, 2003; Hongo, Chieko, Okada, and others, 2003). Children and their parents report high distress with pain and symptoms at the end of life. Parents reported pain and suffering as one of the most important factors in deciding to withhold or withdraw their child from life support in the pediatric intensive care unit (Meert, Thurston, and Sarnaik, 2000).

Documentation was scarce related to symptom management. Morphine was the most commonly prescribed pain medication (Drake and others, 2003; Hongo and others, 2003). Parents reported their children as experiencing high levels of pain near the end of life (Contro, Larson, Scofield, and others, 2002). Physicians were more likely than nurses or parents to report that a child's pain and symptoms were well managed at the end of life, and the majority of both provider groups felt the child's physical management was difficult (Andresen, Seecharan, and Toce, 2004; Wolfe, Grier, Klar, and others, 2000).

Barriers to the adequate provision of pediatric palliative care include developmental issues specific to infants and children; symptoms, their causes, how they are related, and effective treatment strategies; lack of education; and reimbursement issues (Harris, 2004). Physicians report reliance on trial and error as they learn to care for children at the end of life and the need for specialty consultations with palliative care service providers (Hilden, Emanuel, Fairclough, and others, 2001).

Apply the Evidence: Nursing Implications

While the philosophy of palliative care encompasses pain and symptom management for infants and children who may not outlive their disease, the provision of that care to ease suffering and provide comfort to those who will die continues to lag. Studies show that children experience significant pain and other distressing symptoms at the end of life that are not well managed. Discrepancies in infant and child pain and suffering continue to exist between providers and parents. Barriers to the provision of pediatric palliative care exist. Improvements are needed in the management of pain and symptoms at the end of life for infants and children.

References

Andresen EM, Seecharan GA, Toce SS: Provider perceptions of child deaths, *Arch Pediatr Adolesc Med* 158:430-435, 2004.

Bradshaw G, Hinds PS, Lensing S, and others: Cancer-related deaths in children and adolescents, *J Palliat Med* 8(1):86-95, 2005.

Carter BS, Howenstein BS, Gilmer MJ, and others: Circumstances surrounding the deaths of hospitalized children: opportunities for pediatric palliative care, *Pediatrics* 114(3):361-366, 2004.

Contro N, Larson J, Scofield S, and others: Family perspectives on the quality of pediatric palliative care, *Arch Pediatr Adolesc Med* 156:1-29, 2002.

Drake R, Frost J, Collins JJ: The symptoms of dying children, *J Pain Symptom Manage* 26(1):594-603, 2003.

Harris B: Palliative care in children with cancer: Which child and when? *J Natl Cancer Inst Monogr* 32:144-149, 2004.

Hilden JM, Emanuel EJ, Fairclough DL, and others: Attitudes and practices among pediatric oncologists regarding end-of-life care: Results of the 1998 American Society of Clinical Oncology Survey, *J Clin Oncol* 19(1):205-212, 2001.

Hongo T, Chieko W, Okada S, and others: Analysis of the circumstances at the end of life in children with cancer: Symptoms, suffering and acceptance, *Pediatr Int* 45:60-64, 2003.

Meert KL, Thurston CS, Sarnaik AP: End-of-life decision-making and satisfaction with care: parental perspectives, *Pediatr Crit Care Med* 1(2):179-185, 2000.

Wolfe J, Grier HE, Klar N, and others: Symptoms and suffering at the end of life in children with cancer, *N Engl J Med* 342(5):326-333, 2000.

Communicating with Families of Dying Children

Listen for an "invitation" to talk about the situation.

"Sometimes I wonder if I am doing the right thing."

"What have other parents done in this situation?"

"Do you know of other children who have survived this?"

"I think the doctor is not telling me everything."

Use open-ended, nonjudgmental questions to explore families' wishes.

"Can you tell me more about how you are feeling?"

"What questions do you (or your child) have that I can have answered for you?"

"What are your concerns (or worries, fears) right now?"

"What is important to you (your child, your family) at this time?"

Common Symptoms Experienced by Dying Children

PAIN

Visceral
Bone
Neuropathic

GASTROINTESTINAL

Anorexia
Nausea and vomiting
Constipation
Diarrhea

GENITOURINARY

Urinary tract infections
Urinary retention

HEMATOLOGIC

Anemia
Bleeding

RESPIRATORY

Cough
Congestion
Shortness of breath
Wheezing

CENTRAL NERVOUS SYSTEM

Fevers and chills
Sleep disturbance
Restlessness or agitation
Seizures

INTEGUMENTARY

Dry skin
Rash or itching
Pressure sores
Edema

EMOTIONAL

Fear
Anxiety
Depression

Physical Signs of Approaching Death

Increased sleeping

Loss of sensation and movement in the lower extremities, progressing toward the upper body

Sensation of heat, although body feels cool

Mottling of skin

Loss of senses:

- Tactile sensation decreases
- Sensitive to light
- Hearing is last sense to fail

Confusion, loss of consciousness, slurred speech

Muscle weakness

Decreased urination, more concentrated urine

Loss of bowel and bladder control

Decreased appetite and thirst

Difficulty swallowing

Change in respiratory pattern:

- Cheyne-Stokes respirations (waxing and waning of depth of breathing with regular periods of apnea)
- "Death rattle" (noisy chest sounds from accumulation of pulmonary and pharyngeal secretions)

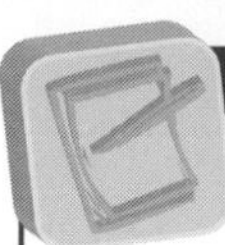

GUIDELINES

Supporting Grieving Families*

General

Stay with the family; sit quietly if they prefer not to talk; cry with them if desired.

Accept the family's grief reactions; avoid judgmental statements (e.g., "You should be feeling better by now").

Avoid offering rationalizations for the child's death (e.g., "You should be glad your child isn't suffering anymore").

Avoid artificial consolation (e.g., "I know how you feel," or "You are still young enough to have another baby").

Deal openly with feelings such as guilt, anger, and loss of self-esteem.

Focus on feelings by using a feeling word in the statement (e.g., "You're still feeling all the pain of losing a child").

Refer the family to an appropriate self-help group or for professional help if needed.

At the Time of Death

Reassure the family that everything possible is being done for the child, if they wish lifesaving interventions.

Do everything possible to ensure the child's comfort, especially relieving pain.

Provide the child and family the opportunity to review special experiences or memories in their lives.

Express personal feelings of loss or frustrations (e.g., "We will miss him so much," or "We tried everything; we feel so sorry that we couldn't save him").

Provide information that the family requests, and be honest.

Respect the emotional needs of family members, such as siblings, who may need brief respites from the dying child.

Make every effort to arrange for family members, especially parents, to be with the child at the moment of death, if they wish to be present.

Allow the family to stay with the dead child for as long as they wish and to rock, hold, or bathe the child.

Provide practical help when possible, such as collecting the child's belongings.

Arrange for spiritual support, such as clergy; pray with the family if no one else can stay with them.

After the Death

Attend the funeral or visitation if there was a special closeness with the family.

Initiate and maintain contact (e.g., sending cards, telephoning, inviting them back to the unit, or making a home visit).

Refer to the dead child by name; discuss shared memories with the family.

Discourage the use of drugs or alcohol as a method of escaping grief.

Encourage all family members to communicate their feelings rather than remaining silent to avoid upsetting another member.

Emphasize that grieving is a painful process that often takes years to resolve.

*"Family" refers to all significant persons involved in the child's life, such as parents, siblings, grandparents, or other close relatives or friends.

3 - EVIDENCE-BASED PEDIATRIC NURSING INTERVENTIONS

Care During the Terminal Phase

PHYSICAL SUPPORT

Provide frequent mouth care to prevent drying, cracking, and bleeding of lips and mucous membranes.

Maintain good hygiene by giving bed baths and using skin lotion as tolerated.

Continue necessary medications to manage symptoms and maintain comfort using IV (if access is easily established) or subcutaneous infusion. Discontinue unnecessary medications and procedures (e.g., vital signs). See Tables 3-7, 3-8, and 3-10 through 3-13 for pain management at the end of life.

See Table 3-14 for common ethical dilemmas in caring for terminally ill children

EMOTIONAL SUPPORT

See Table 3-15.

Encourage family to discuss impending death openly with child and other family members.

Encourage family to continue to speak to child in calm, reassuring voice.

Provide familiar surroundings or objects.

Encourage caregivers to provide one another with periods of respite.

Allow the provision of spiritual and cultural rituals as desired.

Allow family time with child after the death and participation in the preparation of the body if they choose.

TABLE 3-10 Dosage of Selected Opioids for Children

Drug	Appropriate Equianalgesic	Approximate Equianalgesic Parenteral Dose	Recommended Starting Dose (Children <50 kg [110 lb] Body Weight)* Oral	Parenteral
Morphine	30 mg every 3-4 hr	10 mg every 3-4 hr	0.2-0.4 mg/kg every 3-4 hr 0.3-0.6 mg/kg time released every 12 hr	0.1-0.2 mg/kg IM every 3-4 hr 0.02-0.1 mg/kg IV bolus every 2 hr 0.015 mg/kg every 8 min PCA 0.01-0.02 mg/kg/hr IV infusion (neonates) 0.01-0.06 mg/kg/hr IV infusion (child)
Fentanyl (Sublimaze) (oral mucosal form [Actiq])†	Not available	0.1 mg IV	5-15 mcg/kg; maximum dose 400 mcg	0.5-1.5 mcg/kg IV bolus every 30 min 1-2 mcg/hr IV infusion
Codeine‡	200 mg every 3-4 hr	130 mg every 3-4 hr	1 mg/kg every 3-4 hr	Not recommended
Hydromorphone§ (Dilaudid)	7.5 mg every 3-4 hr	1.5 mg every 3-4 hr	0.04-0.1 mg/kg every 3-4 hr	0.02-0.1 mg/kg every 3-4 hr 0.005-0.2 mg/kg IV bolus every 2 hr
Hydrocodone and acetaminophen (Lorcet, Lortab, Vicodin, others)	30 mg every 3-4 hr	Not available	0.2 mg/kg every 3-4 hr	Not available
Levorphanol (Levo-Dromoran)	4 mg every 6-8 hr	2 mg every 6-8 hr	0.04 mg/kg every 6-8 hr	0.02 mg/kg every 6-8 hr
Meperidine (Demerol)‖	300 mg every 2-3 hr	100 mg every 3 hr	Not recommended	0.75 mg/kg every 2-3 hr
Methadone (Dolophine, others)¶	20 mg every 6-8 hr	10 mg every 6-8 hr	0.2 mg/kg every 6-8 hr	0.1 mg/kg every 6-8 hr
Oxycodone (Roxicodone, OxyContin; also in Percocet, Percodan, Tylox, others)	20 mg every 3-4 hr	Not available	2 mg/kg every 3-4 hr#	Not available

Data from Acute Pain Management Guideline Panel: *Acute pain management: operative or medical procedures and trauma: clinical practice guideline,* AHCPR Pub No 92-0032, Rockville, Md, 1992, Agency for Health Care Policy and Research, Public Health Service, US Department of Health and Human Services; Berde C, Ablin A, Glazer J, and others: American Academy of Pediatrics Report of the Subcommittee on Disease-Related Pain in Childhood Cancer, *Pediatrics* 86(5 pt 2):820, 1990.

IM, Intramuscular; *IV,* intravenous; *PCA,* patient-controlled analgesia.

NOTE: Published tables vary in suggested doses that are equianalgesic to morphine. Clinical response is criterion that must be applied for each patient; titration to clinical response is necessary. Because there is not complete cross-tolerance among these drugs, it is usually necessary to use a lower than equianalgesic dose when changing drugs and to retitrate to response.

CAUTION: Recommended doses do not apply to patients with renal or hepatic insufficiency or other conditions affecting drug metabolism and kinetics.

*CAUTION: Doses listed for patients with body weight less than 50 kg (110 lb) cannot be used as initial starting doses in infants less than 6 months of age. For nonventilated infants younger than 6 months, the initial opioid dose should be about ¼ to ⅓ of the dose recommended for older infants and children. For example, morphine could be used at a dose of 0.03 mg/kg instead of the traditional 0.1 mg/kg.

†Actiq is indicated only for management of breakthrough cancer pain in patients with malignancies who are already receiving and are tolerant to opioid therapy, but it can be used for preoperative or preprocedural sedation/analgesia.

‡CAUTION: Codeine doses above 65 mg often are not appropriate because of diminishing incremental analgesia with increasing doses but continually increasing constipation and other side effects. Dosages are from McCaffery M, Pasero C: *Pain: a clinical manual,* ed 2, St Louis, 1999, Mosby.

§For hydromorphone, rectal administration is an alternate route for patients unable to take oral medications, but equianalgesic doses may differ from oral and parenteral doses because of pharmacokinetic differences.

‖Meperidine is not recommended for continuous pain control (i.e., postoperatively) because of risk of normeperidine toxicity.

¶Initial dose is 10%-25% of equianalgesic morphine dose. Parenteral Dolophine is no longer available in the United States.

#CAUTION: Doses of aspirin and acetaminophen in combination with opioid or nonsteroidal antiinflammatory drug preparations must also be adjusted to patient's body weight. Daily dose of acetaminophen should not exceed 75 mg/kg, or 4000 mg.

TABLE 3-11 Co-analgesic Adjuvant Drugs

Category and Drug	Dosage	Indication	Comments
Antidepressants			
Amitriptyline	0.2 to 0.5 mg/kg PO hs Titrate upward by 0.25 mg/kg every 5-7 days as needed Available in 10-mg and 25-mg tablets Usual starting dose is 10-25 mg	Continuous neuropathic pain with burning, aching, dysthesia with insomnia	Provides analgesia by blocking re-uptake of serotonin and norepinephrine, possibly slowing transmission of pain signals Helps with pain related to insomnia and depression (use nortriptyline if patient is oversedated) Analgesic effects seen earlier than antidepressant effects Side effects include dry mouth, constipation, urinary retention
Nortriptyline	0.2 to 1 mg/kg PO AM or bid Titrate up by 0.5 mg q5-7 days Max 25 mg/dose	Neuropathic pain as above without insomnia	
Anticonvulsants			
Gabapentin	5 mg/kg PO at bedtime Increase to bid on day 2, tid on day 3 Max 300 mg/day	Neuropathic pain	Mechanism of action unknown Side effects include sedation, ataxia, nystagmus, dizziness
Carbamazepine	<6 years: 2.5-5 mg/kg PO bid initially Increase weekly prn to optimal response Max 100 mg bid 6 to 12 years: 5 mg/kg PO bid initially Increase weekly prn to optimal dose Usual max: 100 mg/dose bid >12 years: 200 mg PO bid initially Increase weekly prn to optimal response Max: 1.6-2.4 g/24 hr	Sharp, cutting neuropathic pain Peripheral neuropathies Phantom limb pain	Similar analgesic effect as amitriptyline Monitor blood levels for toxicity only Side effects include decreased blood counts, ataxia, and GI irritation
Anxiolytics			
Lorazepam	0.03-0.1 mg/kg q4-6h PO or IV; max 2 mg/dose	Muscle spasm Anxiety	May increase sedation in combination with opioids Can cause depression with prolonged use
Diazepam	0.1-0.3 mg/kg q4-6h PO or IV; max 10 mg/dose		

bid, Twice daily; *GI,* gastrointestinal; *hs,* at bedtime; *IV,* intravenous; *NSAIDs,* nonsteroidal antiinflammatory drugs; *PO,* by mouth; *tid,* three times a day.

TABLE 3-11 Co-analgesic Adjuvant Drugs—cont'd

Category and Drug	Dosage	Indication	Comments
Corticosteroids			
Dexamethasone	Dose dependent on clinical situation; higher bolus doses in cord compression, then lower daily dose Try to wean to NSAIDs if pain allows Cerebral edema: 1-2 mg/kg load then 1-1.5 mg/kg/day divided every 6 hr; max 4 mg/dose Antiinflammatory: 0.08-0.3 mg/kg/day divided every 6-12 hr	Pain from increased intracranial pressure Bony metastasis Spinal or nerve compression	Side effects include edema, GI irritation, increased weight, acne Use gastroprotectants such as H_2 blockers (e.g., ranitidine) or proton pump inhibitors (e.g., omeprazole) for long-term administration of steroids or NSAIDs in end-stage cancer with bony pain
Others			
Clonidine	2-4 mcg/kg PO q4-6h May also use a 100-mcg transdermal patch q7 days for patients > 40 kg	Neuropathic pain Cutting, sharp, electrical, shooting pain Phantom limb pain	Alpha-2 adrenoreceptor agonist modulates ascending pain sensations Routes of administration include oral, transdermal, and spinal Manage withdrawal symptoms Monitor for orthostatic hypertension, decreased heart rate Sedation common
Mexiletine	2-3 mg/kg/dose PO tid May titrate 0.5 mg/kg q2-3 weeks as needed Max 300 mg/dose		Similar to lidocaine, longer acting Stabilizes sodium conduction in nerve cells, reduces neuronal firing Can enhance action of opioids, antidepressants, anticonvulsants Side effects include dizziness, ataxia, nausea, vomiting May measure blood levels for toxicity

TABLE 3-12 Management of Opioid Side Effects

Side Effect	Adjuvant Drugs	Nonpharmacologic Techniques
Constipation	**Senna and docusate sodium** *Tablet:* 2-6 years: Start: ½ tablet once a day; max 1 tablet twice a day 6-12 years: Start 1 tablet once a day; max 2 tablets twice a day >12 years: Start 2 tablets once a day; max 4 tablets twice a day *Liquid:* 1 month–1 year: 1.25-5 ml q hs 1-5 years: 2.5-5 ml q hs 5-15 years: 5-10 ml q hs >15 years: 10-25 ml q hs **Casanthranol and docusate sodium** *Liquid:* 5-15 ml q hs *Capsules:* 1 cap PO q hs **Bisacodyl:** PO or PR 3-12 years: 5 mg/dose/day >12 years 10-15 mg/dose/day **Lactulose** 7.5 ml/day after breakfast Adult: 15-30 ml PO q day **Mineral oil:** 1-2 tsp PO/day **Magnesium citrate** <6 years: 2-4 ml/kg PO once 6-12 years: 100-150 ml PO once >12 years: 150-300 ml PO once **Milk of Magnesia (MOM)** <2 years: 0.5 ml/kg/dose PO once 2-5 years: 5-15 ml PO q day 6-12 years: 15-30 ml PO once >12 years: 30-60 mL PO once	Increase water intake Prune juice, bran cereal, vegetables
Sedation	**Caffeine:** single dose of 1-1.5 mg PO **Dextroamphetamine:** 2.5-5 mg PO in morning and early afternoon **Methylphenidate:** 2.5-5 mg PO in morning and early afternoon Consider opioid switch if sedation is persistent	Caffeinated drinks (e.g., Mountain Dew, cola drinks)
Nausea and vomiting	**Promethazine:** 0.5 mg/kg q4-6h; max 25 mg/dose **Ondansetron:** 0.1-0.15 mg/kg IV or PO q4h; max 8 mg/dose	Imagery, relaxation Deep, slow breathing

bid, Twice daily; *GI,* gastrointestinal; *hs,* at bedtime; *IV,* intravenous; *NSAIDs,* nonsteroidal antiinflammatory drugs; *PO,* by mouth; *tid,* three times a day.

TABLE 3-12 Management of Opioid Side Effects—cont'd

Side Effect	Adjuvant Drugs	Nonpharmacologic Techniques
Nausea and vomiting—cont'd	**Granisetron:** 10-40 mcg/kg q2-4h; max 1 mg/dose **Droperidol:** 0.05-0.06 mg/kg IV q4-6h; can be very sedating	
Pruritus	**Diphenhydramine:** 1 mg/kg IV or PO q4-6h prn; max 25 mg/dose **Hydroxyzine:** 0.6 mg/kg/dose PO q6h; max 50 mg/dose **Naloxone:** 0.5 mcg/kg every 2 minutes until pruritus improves (diluted in a solution of 0.1 mg of naloxone per 10 ml of saline) **Butorphanol:** 0.3-0.5 mg/kg IV (use cautiously in opioid-tolerant children, may cause withdrawal symptoms); max 2 mg/dose because mixed agonist/antagonist	Oatmeal baths, good hygiene Exclude other causes of itching Change opioids
Respiratory depression: Mild to moderate	Hold dose of opioid Reduce subsequent doses by 25%	Arouse gently, give O_2, encourage deep breathing
Respiratory depression: Severe	**Naloxone** *During disease pain management:* 0.5 mcg/kg in 2-minute increments until breathing improves Reduce opioid dose if possible Consider opioid switch *During sedation for procedures:* 5-10 mcg/kg until breathing improves Reduce opioid dose if possible Consider opioid switch	O_2, bag and mask if indicated
Dysphoria, confusion, hallucinations	Evaluate medications, eliminate adjuvant medications with CNS effects as symptoms allow Consider opioid switch if possible **Haloperidol (Haldol):** 0.05-0.15 mg/kg/day divided in two or three doses; max 2-4 mg/day	Rule out other physiologic causes
Urinary retention	Evaluate medications, eliminate adjuvant medications with anticholinergic effects (e.g., antihistamines, tricyclic antidepressants) Occurs with spinal analgesia more frequently than with systemic opioid use **Oxybutynin** 1 year: 1 mg tid 1-2 years: 2 mg tid 2-3 years: 3 mg tid 4-5 years: 4 mg tid >5 years: 5 mg tid	Rule out other physiologic causes In/out or in-dwelling urinary catheter

TABLE 3-13 Selected Analgesics (Equianalgesia)

Drug*	Equal to Oral Morphine (mg)	Equal to Intramuscular/ Intravenous Morphine (mg)
Hydromorphone (Dilaudid), 1 mg	4	1.3
Codeine, 30 mg	4.5	1.5
Meperidine (Demerol), 50 mg	4.8	1.6
Codeine, 30 mg acetaminophen, 300 mg (Tylenol No. 3)	7.2	2.4
Oxycodone, 5 mg acetaminophen, 325 mg (Percocet)	7.2	2.4
Oxycodone, 5 mg aspirin, 325 mg (Percodan)	7.2	2.4
Hydrocodone, 5 mg acetaminophen, 500 mg (Vicodin, Lortab)	9	3
Oxycodone, 5 mg acetaminophen, 500 mg (Tylox)	9	3
Methadone (Dolophine), 10 mg	15	7.5
Acetaminophen (Tylenol), 325 mg	2.7	0.9
Aspirin, 325 mg	2.7	0.9
Acetaminophen (Tylenol Extra Strength), 500 mg	4	1.3
Codeine, 60 mg acetaminophen, 300 mg (Tylenol No. 4)	11.7	3.9
Fentanyl, transdermal patch (Duragesic) (based on 25-mcg/hr patch applied every 3 days = 50 mg oral morphine every 24 hours or divided into six doses = 8.3 mg) or use:	8.3	2.77

Recommended Initial Duragesic Dose Based on Daily Oral Morphine Dose†

Oral 24-Hour Morphine (mg/day)	Duragesic Dose (mg/hr)
45-134	25
135-224	50
225-314	75
315-404	100
405-494	125
495-584	150
585-674	175
675-764	200
765-854	225
855-944	250
945-1034	275
1035-1124	300

Courtesy Betty R. Ferrell, PhD, FAAN, 1999. Used with permission.

NOTE: When converting to oral oxycodone from oral morphine, an appropriate conservative estimate is 15-20 mg of oxycodone per 30 mg of morphine; however, when converting to oral morphine from oral oxycodone, an appropriate conservative estimate is 30 mg of morphine per 30 mg of oxycodone. (McCaffery M, Pasero C: *Pain: a clinical manual,* ed 2, St Louis, 1999, Mosby)

*Oral medication with exception of fentanyl.

†Data from Duragesic package insert, Janssen, Pharmaceutical Products, Titusville, NJ, 2001.

TABLE 3-14 Common Ethical Dilemmas in Caring for Terminally Ill Children

Rationale for Providing to Patient	Rationale for Withholding from Patient
Pain Control	
Comfort is primary goal Improved quality of life Easier dying process if child is pain-free	Side effects of opioids Decreased level of cognition Fear of addiction (unfounded in terminally ill patients)
Chemotherapy or Experimental Therapy	
Prolonged life span Possible increase in quality of life Provides sense that family has done everything they can to save the child	Decreased blood counts, increased risk of infection, bleeding Side effects of treatment may be painful, uncomfortable
Supplemental Nutrition and Hydration (Intravenous, Nasogastric, G-Tube)	
Belief that the child is hungry or thirsty Child cannot or will not eat Fear that child will "starve" to death Primary role of parent to feed and nourish child Parental guilt	Supplemental feedings beyond what child can ingest may actually cause nausea or vomiting Increase in tumor growth (feeding the tumor) Increase in fluid volume may result in congestive heart failure, increased respiratory secretions, and/or pulmonary congestion, which leads to questions of whether or not to implement diuretic Increased urine output leads to increased risk of skin breakdown if child is incontinent Risk of third spacing Death is more comfortable and natural Complaint of thirst is associated with dying process, not level of hydration (Zerwekh, 1997)
Resuscitation	
Family does not want to give up Conflicts with cultural or religious beliefs Denial that child is actually going to die	Allowing nature to take its course Family believes child has suffered enough, does not want aggressive intervention Relieves family of responsibility to stop interventions that might prolong life
Autopsy	
Research to help other children Ability to check genetic link	Religious, cultural belief Family feelings Desecrates body for funeral viewing (an unfounded fear)

Modified from Hockenberry-Eaton MJ: *Essentials of pediatric oncology nursing: a core curriculum,* Glenview, Ill, 1998, Association of Pediatric Oncology Nurses.

TABLE 3-15 Communicating with Dying Children

Approach	Effective Technique
Discuss at the child's level	Gear information to the developmental age of the child, remembering that younger children tend to be concrete thinkers, whereas older children are capable of abstract thought. Begin with the child's experiences: "You've told us how tired you've been lately."
Let the child's questions guide	Begin the conversation with basic information, and let the child's questions direct the conversation.
Provide opportunities for the child to express feelings	Look for clues that child is open to communication. Be accepting of whatever emotion is expressed.
Encourage feedback	Ask the child to summarize what has been heard. This provides the opportunity to clarify misunderstandings.
Use other resources	Books and movies can encourage dialogue. Ask the child to name the people whom he or she can discuss problems with.
Use the child's natural expressive means to stimulate dialogue	Use books, games, art, play, and music to provide a means of expression.

Modified from Doka KJ: *Living with life-threatening illness: a guide for patients, their families, and caregivers,* Lexington, Mass, 1993, Lexington Books.

Strategies for Intervention with Survivors of Sudden Childhood Death

ARRIVAL OF THE FAMILY

Meet the family immediately and escort to a private area.
A health care worker with bereavement training should remain with the family.
Provide information about the extent of illness or injury and treatment efforts (Table 3-16).
If the health care worker must leave the family or if the family requests privacy, return in 15 minutes so the family does not feel forgotten.
Provide tissues and a telephone. Offer coffee, water, and a Bible.

PRONOUNCEMENT OF DEATH

When available, the family's own physician should inform the family of the child's death.
Alternatively, the physician or nurse should introduce himself or herself and establish calm, reassuring eye contact with the parents.
Honest, clear communication that avoids misinterpretation is essential.
Nonverbal communication such as hugging, touching, or remaining with the family in silence may be most empathetic.
Acknowledge the family's guilt, attempt to alleviate it, and deal openly and nonjudgmentally with anger.
Provide information, answer questions, and offer reassurance that everything possible was done for the child.

VIEWING THE BODY

Offer the family the opportunity to see the body; repeat the offer later if they decline.
Before viewing, inform the family of bodily changes they should expect (tubes, injuries, cold skin).
A single staff member should accompany the family but remain inconspicuous.
Offer the opportunity to hold the child.
Allow the family as much time as they need.
Offer parents the opportunity for siblings to view the body.

FORMAL CONCLUDING PROCESS

Discuss and answer questions concerning autopsy and funeral arrangements; obtain signatures on the body release and autopsy forms.
Provide anticipatory guidance regarding symptoms of grief response and their normalcy.
Provide written materials about grief symptoms.
Escort the family to the exit or to their car if necessary.
Provide a follow-up phone call in 24 to 48 hours to answer questions and provide support.
Provide referral for community health nursing visit.
Provide referrals to local support and resource groups (e.g., bereavement groups, bereavement counselors, SIDS groups, Parents of Murdered Children, Mothers Against Drunk Driving).

Modified from Back K: Sudden, unexpected pediatric death: caring for the parents, *Pediatr Nurs* 17(6):571-574, 1991.

TABLE 3-16 Communicating Bad News to Families

Approach	Effective Techniques
Provide a setting conducive to communication	Ensure privacy; use appropriate body language; make eye contact. Have parents choose who will attend.
Determine what the family knows	Ask questions. ("What have you made of all this?" or "What were you told?") Listen to the vocabulary and comprehension of the family. Recognize denial but do not acknowledge it at this stage.
Determine what the family wants to know	Obtain a clear invitation to share information (if this is what the family wants). Use questions such as, "Are you the sort of person who likes to know every detail, or just the basic facts?"
Give information (aligning and educating)	Start at level of family's comprehension and use the same vocabulary. Give information slowly, concisely, and in simple language. Avoid medical jargon. Check regularly to be certain that content is understood.
Respond to family's reactions	Acknowledge all reactions and feelings, particularly using the emphatic response technique (identifying emotion, identifying cause of emotion, and responding appropriately). Expect tears, anger, and other strong emotions.
Close	Briefly summarize major areas discussed. Ask parents if they have other important issues to discuss at this time. Make an appointment for the next meeting.

Modified from Buchman R, Baile W: *How to break bad news to patients with cancer: a practical protocol for clinicians,* Spring Education Book, Alexandria, Va, 1998, American Society of Clinical Oncology.

Procedures Related to Maintaining Fluid Balance or Nutrition

Intravenous Fluid Administration

IV therapy is employed for infants and children for the following reasons:
- Fluid replacement
- Fluid maintenance
- A route for administration of medications or other therapeutic substances (e.g., blood, blood products)

Characteristics of pediatric administration sets may be as follows:
- Small-gauge (23 to 25) needle, flexible over-the-needle catheters (22 to 24 gauge)
- For longer-term administration, consider a midline catheter, peripherally inserted central catheter (PICC), central venous catheter, or implanted port

Sites are as follows:
- Superficial veins of the upper extremities are preferred, then the foot
- Scalp veins (infants)
- A site is chosen that restricts the child's movements as little as possible (e.g., avoid a site over a joint)
- For extremity veins, start with most distal site, especially if irritating or sclerosing agents are to be used

Maintain integrity of IV site.

Maintain strict asepsis, and follow Standard Precautions.

Use small, padded armboard if IV is inserted at a joint or movement restricts flow.

Provide adequate protection of site.

Observe for signs of infiltration, which may include erythema, pain, edema, blanching, streaking on the skin along the vein, and darkened area at the insertion site.

Change IV tubing and solution at regular intervals (no less than 72 hours) according to institution's policy.

Electronic infusion pumps are routinely used with infants and children.

Precautions
- Assess drip rate by assessing amount infused in a given length of time
- Excess buildup of pressure can occur when the:
  - Drip rate is faster than vein can accommodate
  - Catheter is out of vein lumen

ESTIMATES OF DAILY CALORIC EXPENDITURE (UNDER NORMAL CONDITIONS)
Holliday-Segar Method*

	Water			
Body weight	**ml/kg/day**	**ml/kg/hr**	**Electrolytes (mEq/100 ml H_2O)**	
First 10 kg	100	÷ 24 hr/day ≈ 4	Na^+	3
Second 10 kg	50	÷ 24 hr/day ≈ 2	Cl^-	2
Each additional kg	20	÷ 24 hr/day ≈ 1	K^+	2

Example: 8-Year-Old Weighing 25 kg

ml/kg/day			ml/kg/hr		
100 (for first 10 kg) ×	10 kg =	1000 ml/day	4 (for first 10 kg) ×	10 kg =	40 ml/hr
50 (for second 10 kg) ×	10 kg =	500 ml/day	2 (for second 10 kg) ×	10 kg =	20 ml/hr
20 (per additional kg) ×	5 kg =	100 ml/day	1 (per additional kg) ×	5 kg =	5 ml/hr
	25 kg	1600 ml/day		25 kg	65 ml/hr

From Robertson J, Shilkofski N: *The Harriet Lane handbook*, ed 17, St Louis, 2005, Elsevier.
*Not suitable for neonates <14 days old.

Dehydration, diarrhea, and oral rehydration are discussed in Tables 3-17 to 3-20.

TABLE 3-17 Clinical Manifestations of Dehydration

	Isotonic (Loss of Water and Salt)	Hypotonic (Loss of Salt in Excess of Water)	Hypertonic (Loss of Water in Excess of Salt)
Skin			
Color	Gray	Gray	Gray
Temperature	Cold	Cold	Cold or hot
Turgor	Poor	Very poor	Fair
Feel	Dry	Clammy	Thickened, doughy
Mucous membranes	Dry	Slightly moist	Parched
Tearing and salivation	Absent	Absent	Absent
Eyeball	Sunken and soft	Sunken	Sunken
Fontanel	Sunken	Sunken	Sunken
Body temperature	Subnormal or elevated	Subnormal or elevated	Subnormal or elevated
Pulse	Rapid	Very rapid	Moderately rapid
Respirations	Rapid	Rapid	Rapid
Behavior	Irritable to lethargic	Lethargic to comatose; convulsions	Marked lethargy with extreme hyperirritability on stimulation

TABLE 3-18 Intensity of Clinical Signs Associated with Varying Degrees of Isotonic Dehydration in Infants

	Degree of Dehydration		
	Mild	Moderate	Severe
Fluid volume loss	<50 ml/kg	50-90 ml/kg	>100 mg/kg
Skin color	Pale	Gray	Mottled
Skin elasticity	Decreased	Poor	Very poor
Mucous membranes	Dry	Very dry	Parched
Urinary output	Decreased	Oliguria	Marked oliguria and azotemia
Blood pressure	Normal	Normal or lowered	Lowered
Pulse	Normal or increased	Increased	Rapid and thready
Capillary filling time	<2 seconds	2-3 seconds	>3 seconds

TABLE 3-19 Treatment of Acute Diarrhea

Degree of Dehydration	Rehydration Therapy*	Replacement of Stool Losses	Maintenance Therapy
Mild (5%-6%)	ORS, 50 ml/kg within 4 hours	ORS, 10 ml/kg (for infants) or 150-250 ml at a time (for older children) for each diarrheal stool	Breast-feeding, if established, should continue; regular infant formula if tolerated If lactose intolerance suspected, give undiluted lactose-free formula (or half-strength lactose-containing formula for brief period only); infants and children who receive solid food should continue their usual diet
Moderate (7%-9%)	ORS, 100 ml/kg within 4 hours	Same as above	Same as above
Severe (>9%)	IV fluids (Ringer's lactate), 40 ml/kg/hr until pulse and state of consciousness return to normal; then 50-100 ml/kg or ORS	Same as above	Same as above

IV, Intravenous, *ORS,* oral rehydration solution.
*If no signs of dehydration are present, rehydration therapy is not necessary. Proceed with maintenance therapy and replacement of stool losses.

TABLE 3-20 Composition of Some Oral Rehydration Solutions

Formula	Na^+ (mEq/L)	K^+ (mEq/L)	Cl^- (mEq/L)	Base (mEq/L)	Glucose (g/L)
Pedialyte (Ross)*	45	20	35	30 (citrate)	25
Rehydralyte (Ross)	75	20	65	30 (citrate)	25
Infalyte (Mead Johnson)	50	25	45	34 (citrate)	30
WHO (World Health Organization)†	90	20	80	30 (bicarbonate)	20

*Note that there are many generic products available with compositions identical to Pedialyte.
†Must be reconstituted with water.

Blood Product Administration

Nursing administration of blood components and nursing care of the child receiving blood components are discussed in Tables 3-21 and 3-22.

TABLE 3-21 Blood Components and Nursing Administration

Components and Indications	Dose	Nursing Administration
Packed red blood cells (PRBCs) Symptomatic anemia Renal or liver disease Hemolysis Decreased erythropoiesis Thalassemia major Splenic or liver sequestration	Volume packed RBC = weight (kg) × change in hematocrit (Hct) desired	1. Regulate infusion rate using microaggregate filter via infusion pump at 5 ml/kg/hr over 1-2 hours (usual rate). Change the filter after 1-2 units of blood are infused or after 4 hours. 2. Monitor vital signs before transfusion, 15 minutes after initiation, every hour until the end of transfusion.
Whole blood (rarely used) Acute massive blood loss	Volume of whole blood = weight (kg) × change in Hct desired × 2	3. Do not refrigerate blood in the nursing unit. Only the blood bank refrigerator may be used. 4. Ensure that each unit is infused in 4 hours or less. If a longer infusion time is needed, the unit must be divided in the blood bank. 5. Do not infuse solutions other than normal saline in the line with RBCs.
Fresh frozen plasma (FFP) Deficiencies of plasma clotting factors in bleeding patients (e.g., disseminated intravascular coagulopathy [DIC]), liver failure, vitamin K deficiency with bleeding, or replacement of antithrombin III (ATIII), protein C, or protein S	10-15 ml/kg (use within 6-24 hours of thawing)	1. Use microaggregate filter over 1-2 hours every 12-24 hours until hemorrhage stops at a rate of 20 ml/min. 2. Monitor prothrombin time (PT) and partial thromboplastin time (PTT) before and after FFP. 3. Monitor levels of other coagulation factors (e.g., fibrinogen, fibrin split products, D-dimer, ATIII, protein C, and protein S).
Platelets (plt) Active hemorrhage, DIC Thrombocytopenia with bleeding or indicated by clinical status	1 unit/10 kg or 6 units/m^2 intravenously (IV)	1. Regulate infusion rate using 170 μm microaggregate filter at 10 ml/kg/hr, IV push or over 1 hour or as fast as patient can tolerate. 2. Monitor vital signs before transfusion, 15 minutes after initiation, and at the end of infusion. 3. Obtain postplatelet count 1 to 24 hours after infusion.

Continued

TABLE 3-21 Blood Components and Nursing Administration—cont'd

Components and Indications	Dose	Nursing Administration
Granulocytes (rarely used) As an adjunct with other measures in treatment of severe infections in the septic neonate or high-risk patient (e.g., proven bacterial infection in severe neutropenic patient nonresponsive to antibiotic therapy)	10-15 ml/kg IV usually daily × 4 days	1. Monitor vital signs before transfusion, 15 minutes after initiation, and at the end of transfusion. 2. Premedicate 1 hour before transfusion, usually antihistamines, acetaminophen, or steroids. 3. Infuse at slow rate (2-4 hours) using 170 μm blood filter within a 24-hour period. 4. Minimum of 4-6 hours between amphotericin B and granulocyte infusion recommended.
Factor VIII (plasma derived or recombinant) Hemophilia A Acquired factor VIII deficiency	1 unit/kg IV of factor VIII = 2% of factor activity 35-50 units/kg IV of factor VIII every 12-24 hours	1. Use reconstituted factor within 3 hours of mixing. 2. Inject reconstituted factor over 2-5 minutes. 3. Assess for signs of an adverse reaction such as hives, itchy wheals with redness, tightness in chest, wheezing, low blood pressure, or trouble breathing. Notify health care provider immediately if symptoms are present.
Factor IX (plasma derived or recombinant) Hemophilia B	1 unit/kg IV of factor IX = 1% of factor activity 30-50 units/kg IV every 24 hours	
FEIBA (factor eight inhibitor bypass activity) (plasma-derived) Hemophilia A or B with inhibitors (antibodies)	75-100 units/kg IV every 8-24 hours (maximum dose 200 units/kg/day	
Factor VII a (recombinant) Hemophilia A or B with inhibitors	90 mcg/kg IV every 2 hours (35-120 mcg/kg) dosage range	
Cryoprecipitate (CRYO) (rarely used) Control bleeding in patients with DIC Hypofibrinogenemia	4 bags CRYO/10 kg IV	1. Monitor closely: PT/PTT, fibrinogen, fibrinogen split products, D-dimer. 2. Use a filter needle to draw up and administer within 15-30 minutes.

TABLE 3-22 Nursing Care of the Child Receiving Blood Transfusions

Complication	Signs and Symptoms	Precautions and Nursing Responsibilities
Immediate Reactions		
Hemolytic Reactions		
Most severe type, but rare Incompatible blood Incompatibility in multiple transfusions	Chills Shaking Fever Pain at needle site and along venous tract Nausea and vomiting Sensation of tightness in chest Red or black urine Headache Flank pain Progressive signs of shock and/or renal failure Often occur within first 15 minutes	Verify patient identification. Identify donor and recipient blood types and groups before transfusion is begun; verify with another nurse or other practitioner. Transfuse blood slowly for first 15-20 minutes or initial 20% volume of blood; remain with patient. Stop transfusion immediately in event of signs or symptoms, maintain patent intravenous (IV) line, and notify practitioner. Save donor blood to recross-match with patient's blood. Monitor for evidence of shock. Insert urinary catheter, and monitor hourly outputs. Send samples of patient's blood and urine to laboratory for presence of hemoglobin (indicates intravascular hemolysis). Observe for signs of hemorrhage resulting from disseminated intravascular coagulation (DIC). Support medical therapies to reverse shock.
Febrile Reactions		
Most common reaction Leukocyte or platelet antibodies Plasma protein antibodies	Fever Chills Occur within 1-6 hours after transfusion	May give acetaminophen for prophylaxis. Leukocyte-poor RBCs are less likely to cause reaction. Stop transfusion immediately; report to practitioner for evaluation.
Allergic Reactions		
Recipient reacts to allergens in donor's blood.	Urticaria Pruritus Flushing Asthmatic wheezing Laryngeal edema	Give antihistamines for prophylaxis to children with tendency toward allergic reactions. Stop transfusion immediately. Administer epinephrine for wheezing or anaphylactic reaction.
Circulatory Overload		
Too rapid transfusion (even a small quantity) Excessive quantity of blood transfused (even slowly)	Sudden severe headache Precordial pain Tachycardia Dyspnea Rales Cyanosis Dry cough Distended neck veins Hypertension	Transfuse blood slowly. Prevent overload by using PRBCs or administering divided amounts of blood. Use infusion pump to regulate and maintain flow rate. Stop transfusion immediately if signs of overload. Place child upright with feet in dependent position.

Continued

TABLE 3-22 Nursing Care of the Child Receiving Blood Transfusions—cont'd

Complication	Signs and Symptoms	Precautions and Nursing Responsibilities
Immediate Reactions—cont'd		
Air Emboli		
May occur when blood is transfused under pressure	Sudden difficulty in breathing Sharp pain in chest Apprehension	Normalize pressure before container is empty when infusing blood under pressure. Clear tubing of air by aspirating air with syringe at nearest Y-connector if air is observed in tubing; disconnect tubing and allow blood to flow until air has escaped only if a Y-connector is not available.
Hypothermia		
	Chills Low temperature Irregular heart rate Possible cardiac arrest	Use approved mechanical blood warmer or electric warming coil to rapidly warm blood; never use microwave oven. Take temperature if patient complains of chills; if subnormal, stop transfusion.
Electrolyte Disturbances		
Hyperkalemia (in massive transfusions or in patients with renal problems)	Nausea, diarrhea Muscular weakness Flaccid paralysis Paresthesia of extremities Bradycardia Apprehension Cardiac arrest	Use washed RBCs or fresh blood if patient is at risk.
Delayed Reactions		
Transmission of Infection		
	Signs of infection (e.g., jaundice) Toxic reaction: high fever, severe headache or sub-sternal pain, hypotension, intense flushing, vomiting/diarrhea	Blood is tested for antibodies to human immunodeficiency virus (HIV), hepatitis C virus, and hepatitis B core antigen; in addition, blood is tested for hepatitis B surface antigen (HBsAg) and alanine aminotransferase (ALT), and a serology test is performed for syphilis; positive units are destroyed; individuals at risk for carrying certain viruses are deferred from donation. Report any sign of infection and, if occurring during transfusion, stop transfusion immediately, send sample for culture and sensitivity tests, and notify physician.
Alloimmunization		
(Antibody formation) Occurs in patients receiving multiple transfusions	Increased risk of hemolytic, febrile, and allergic reactions	Use limited number of donors. Observe carefully for signs of reactions.
Delayed Hemolytic Reaction		
	Destruction of RBCs and fever 2-10 days after transfusion (anemia, jaundice, dark urine)	Observe for posttransfusion anemia and decreasing benefit from successive transfusions.

EVIDENCE-BASED PRACTICE

Catheter Gauge for Blood Transfusions in Children

Marilyn J. Hockenberry

Ask the Question

Question

In children, what is the smallest gauge catheter that can be used to administer blood products?

Objective

To review the current evidence on catheter size and blood transfusions in children. Concerns exist related to hemolysis caused by small catheter size.

Background

An important consideration when transfusing blood through peripheral catheters is the risk for hemolysis. In young children it is often difficult to place a large catheter size needle into a vein. To ensure that hemolysis does not occur with smaller size catheter gauge needles, an evidence-based search was chosen.

Search for Evidence

Search Strategies

Search selection criteria included English language research-based studies.

Databases Used

PubMed, American Association of Blood Banks, Intravenous Nurses Society, MD Consult

Critically Analyze the Evidence

Six research-based articles were reviewed (1981 to 2004). All studies used an in vitro experimental design to evaluate hemolysis during simulated transfusion of red blood cells (RBCs). Two studies (Levin, Jesurun, Darden, and others, 1986; Herrera and Corless, 1981) used catheters as small as 27 gauge and found no significant hemolysis. Wong, Schreiber, Criss, and others (2004) evaluated the feasibility of RBC transfusion through a small-bore central venous catheter (1.9F = 23-gauge catheter) and found no significant hemolysis. Three additional studies used catheters larger than 23 gauge and also found no hemolysis (Frelich and Ellis, 2001; De la Roche and Gauther, 1993; Wilcox, Barnes, and Mondanlou, 1981).

A search for national published guidelines found that the American Association of Blood Banks (2004, 1999) states that RBCs can be administered safely through 23- to 25-gauge needles.

Apply the Evidence: Nursing Implications

Small-gauge intravenous catheters can be used to safely to administer PRBCs. Considerations should be made for pediatric patients requiring massive transfusions.

References

American Association of Blood Banks: *Primer of blood administration,* Bethesda, Md, 2004, The Association.

American Association of Blood Banks: *Blood transfusion therapy,* Bethesda, Md, 1999, The Association,

De la Roche MR, Gauther L: Rapid transfusion of packed red blood cells: effects of dilution, pressure and catheter size, *Ann Emerg Med* 22(10):1551-1555, 1993.

Frelich R, Ellis MH: The effect of external pressure, catheter gauge, and storage time on hemolysis in RBC transfusion, *Transfusion* 41:799-802, 2001.

Herrera AJ, Corless J: Blood transfusions: effect of speed of infusion and of needle gauge on hemolysis, *J Pediatr* (99)5:757-758, 1981.

Levin GS, Jesurun CA, Darden J, and others: Hemolysis of transfused packed red blood cells, *Perinatol Neonatol* 10:39-42, 1986.

Wilcox GJ, Barnes A, Mondanlou H: Does transfusion using a syringe infusion pump and small-gauge needle cause hemolysis? *Transfusion* 21(6):750-751, 1981.

Wong EC, Schreiber S, Criss VR, and others: Feasibility of red blood cell transfusion through small bore central venous catheters used in neonates, *Pediatr Crit Care Med* (5)1, 2004.

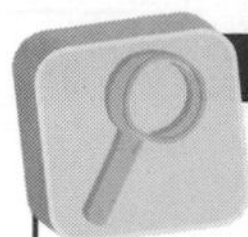

EVIDENCE-BASED PRACTICE

Monitoring Transfused Patients

Marilyn J. Hockenberry

Ask the Question

Question

In children, how long should vital sign monitoring and assessment continue after the completion of blood transfusions?

Objective

To determine when it is safe to discharge a patient after he or she has received a blood product transfusion

Background

A concern during blood transfusion therapy is the risk of an allergic reaction. To develop policies regarding the timing of vial sign monitoring and assessment during blood transfusions in children, an evidence-based practice search was initiated.

Search for Evidence

Search Strategies

Search criteria included English-language publications within the past 16 years, focusing on blood product transfusions and vital sign monitoring in children as well as adults.

Data Bases Used

PubMed, Cochrane Collaboration, UpToDate, MD Consult, CINAHL, OVID, American Association of Blood Banks, Oncology Nursing Society, Intravenous Nurses Society, Association of Pediatric Oncology Nurses

Critically Analyze the Evidence

Incidence of Blood Transfusion Reactions in Children

In a study of 385 pediatric patients who received 7900 blood products (4280 single donor apheresis platelets and 3620 packed red blood cells), the incidence of febrile reactions was less than 1%. Reactions occurred in patients with a history of two or more prior reactions only 3% of the time (Sanders, Maddirala, and Geiger, 2005). One patient required admission to the hospital for febrile neutropenia after developing a fever. No outpatients were admitted specifically to treat a reaction, and no inpatient required transfer to the intensive care unit (ICU) as a result of a transfusion reaction. This researcher also found that premedication with acetaminophen and diphenhydramine was not effective in preventing febrile or allergic reactions. Other researchers have reported a low incidence of transfusion reactions (ranging from 0.03% to 2.2%) when leukoreduced blood products are used (Hebert, Fergusson, Blajchman, and others, 2003; Ezidiegwu, Lauenstein, Rosales, and others, 2004; King, Shirey, Thoman, and others, 2004; Paglino, Pomper, Fisch, and others, 2004; Pruss, Kalus, Radtke, and others, 2004; Yazer, Podlosky, Clarke, and others, 2004; Petz, Swisher, Kleinman, and others, 1996).

Timing of Blood Transfusion Reactions

The most common transfusion reaction, febrile, nonhemolytic transfusion reactions occur within one to six hours after transfusion (Silvergleid, 2004; Petz and others, 1996). In Sanders' study discussed previously (2005), febrile reactions in pediatric patients were rare and no patient receiving a transfusion in the outpatient clinic required hospitalization.

Acute hemolytic transfusion reactions and anaphylactic transfusion reactions often occur within the first 15 minutes of the start of each unit (Silvergleid, 2004; Petz and others, 1996). Patients should be most closely observed during this time period. In hemolytic transfusion reactions, symptoms can occur after a small amount of blood has been transfused and often before the unit is completely transfused (Petz and others, 1996; Kardon, 2005).

Delayed hemolytic transfusion reactions generally occur within 2 to 10 days after transfusion (Petz and others, 1996; Silvergleid, 2004). No immediate side effects are observed.

Assessment Guidelines

The American Association of Blood Banks (AABB, 2005) advises, "...to take and record vital signs before transfusion begins, after the first 15 minutes and every hour until 1 hour after the transfusion has been discontinued" (p.18).

The AABB standard (2004) states, "The patients shall be observed...for an appropriate time thereafter. Specific instructions concerning possible adverse events shall be provided to the patient for a responsible caregiver when direct medical observation or monitoring of the patient will not be available after transfusion." (p.18).

The major transfusion textbook *Clinical Practice of Transfusion Medicine,* ed 3 (Petz and others, 1996), states, "Nursing services typically require that vital signs be checked as often as every 5 minutes during the first 15 minutes and every 15 minutes thereafter" (p. 303). This section of the text goes on to state that because outpatients will not be directly monitored by medical personnel after a transfusion, education of the patient and caregiver about possible signs and symptoms of a delayed transfusion reaction is essential. Specific recommendations for home transfusion therapy are given for monitoring up to 1 hour after the transfusion; however, no specific recommendations are made for the clinic or hospital settings (Petz and others, 1996).

The *Clinical Journal of Oncology Nursing* from the Oncology Nursing Society states that blood transfusion vital signs should be

EVIDENCE-BASED PRACTICE

Monitoring Transfused Patients—cont'd

monitored at the beginning of the transfusion, 15 minutes into a blood product transfusion, and immediately upon transfusion completion (Baldwin, 2002).

The *Core Curriculum* for the Association of Pediatric Oncology Nurses states to monitor the patient for the first 15 minutes and reassess vital signs every hour during the infusion (Kline, Brace O'Neill, Hooke, and others, 2004).

Because severe reactions are most likely to occur within the first 15 minutes of the start of each unit, patients should be most closely observed during this period. Vital signs should be measured and recorded before the start of each unit of blood or blood component, at the end of each transfusion episode. Further observations are at the discretion of each clinical area and need be taken only should the patient become unwell or show signs of a transfusion reaction (Shulman, 2002).

Vital signs should be measured 15 minutes after the start of each unit of blood or blood component and then according to each institution's policy for the remainder of the transfusion (Baldwin, 2002). Transfusion reactions should be considered when assessing a change or deterioration in the patients' condition, particularly in the first 15 minutes after the start of a unit of blood or blood product.

In a recent UpToDate review on general principles of home blood transfusion, the author states, "The patient's vitals signs should be taken prior to the transfusion; every 15 minutes during the first 45 minutes of the transfusion and, if stable, every 30 minutes thereafter; at the conclusion of the transfusion; and 15 or 30 minutes after the transfusion has ended" (Fridey, 1999; Fridley, 2003).

Apply the Evidence: Nursing Implications

- Careful, close assessment during the first 15 minutes of a blood product administration, then every hour while blood product is infusing
- Assessment on completion of each blood product unit and before the initiation of an additional unit
- Assessment at the end of the blood product administration
- Education of parents with children receiving transfusions in the outpatient setting to ensure awareness of possible transfusion reactions
- Routine scheduled vital signs should be resumed in hospitalized patients at the completion of the blood product transfusion

References

American Association of Blood Banks: *Primer of blood administration,* Bethesda, Md, 2005, The Association.

American Association of Blood Banks: *Standards for blood banks and transfusion services,* ed 23, Bethesda, Md, 2004, The Association.

Baldwin PD: Febrile nonhemolytic transfusion reactions, *Clin J Oncol Nurs* 6(3):171-173, 2002.

Ezidiegwu CN, Lauenstein KJ, Rosales LG, and others: Febrile nonhemolytic transfusion reactions. Management by premedication and cost implications in adult patients, *Arch Pathol Lab Med* 128:991-995, 2004.

Fridey JL: *General principles of home blood transfusion,* 2003, retrieved February 7, 2006, from *http:/www.uptodateonline.com/application/topic/topicText.asp?file=transfus/9302&type=A.*

Fridey JL: *The path to safer home transfusion: standardized procedures,* 1999, retrieved February 7, 2006, from *http://www.uptodateonline.com/enterprise.asp?cket1=594267.*

Hebert PC, Fergusson D, Blajchman MA, and others: Clinical outcomes following institution of the Canadian universal leukoreduction program of red blood cell transfusions, *JAMA,* 289:1941-1949, 2003.

Kardon E: *Transfusion reactions. Emergency medicine, hematology and oncology,* 2005, retrieved February 7, 2006, from *http://www.emedicine.com/emerg/topic603.htm.*

King KE, Shirey RS, Thoman SK, and others: Universal leukoreduction decreases the incidence of febrile nonhemolytic transfusion reactions to RBCs, *Transfusion* 44:25-29, 2004.

Kline NE, Brace O'Neill JE, Hooke MC, and others: *Essentials of pediatric oncology nursing: a core curriculum,* Glenview, Ill, 2004, Association of Pediatric Oncology Nurses.

Paglino JC, Pomper GJ, Fisch GS, and others: Reduction of febrile but not allergic reactions to RBCs and platelets after conversion to universal prestorage leukoreduction, *Transfusion* 44(1):16-24, 2004

Petz LD, Swisher SN, Kleinman S, and others, editors: *Clinical practice of transfusion medicine,* New York, 1996, Churchill Livingston.

Pruss A, Kalus U, Radtke H, and others: Universal leukodepletion of blood components results in a significant reduction of febrile nonhemolytic but non-allergic transfusion reactions, *Transfus Apher* 30:41-46, 2004.

Sanders RP, Maddirala SD, Geiger TL: Premedication with acetaminophen or diphenhydramine for transfusion with leucoreduced blood products in children, *Br J Haematol* 130(5):781-787, 2005.

Shulman IA: *Guidance on the length of time a patient must be observed during the start of a transfusion,* e-Network Forum, 2002, California Blood Bank Society, retrieved February 7, 2006, from *http://www.cbbsweb.org/enf/2002/txobservetime.html.*

Silvergleid AJ: *Immunologic blood transfusion reactions,* 2004, retrieved February 7, 2006 from *http:/www.uptodateonline.com/application/topic/topicText.asp?file=transfus/8188&type=A.*

Yazer MH, Podlosky L, Clarke G, and others: The effect of prestorage WBC reduction on the rates of febrile non-hemolytic transfusion reactions to platelet concentrates and RBC, *Transfusion* 44:10-15, 2004.

Peripherally Inserted Central Catheters

Description

Made of Silastic or polyurethane material

Single or double lumen available

Inserted into antecubital fossa and passed through basilic or cephalic vein into superior vena cava (SVC)

Positioning of tip in SVC maximizes hemodilution and reduces likelihood of vessel wall damage, phlebitis, or thrombus formation

Can be placed as a "midline" catheter, also known as a *half-way catheter,* ending near axillary vein (not suitable for total parenteral nutrition [TPN], hyperosmolar solutions, or vesicant chemotherapy)

Benefits

Do not require operating room placement

Can be inserted by specially trained RNs

Can use small insertion needles

Fast placement

Sepsis rates are ≤2%

Care Considerations

Sometimes difficult to thread into SVC

Reports of resistance to removal

Not suitable for rapid fluid replacement because of small lumen size

Five- to 10-ml syringe is used for flushing to prevent catheter wall rupture

Long-Term Central Venous Access Devices

TUNNELED CATHETER (e.g., HICKMAN/ BROVIAC CATHETER)

Description

Silicone, radiopaque, flexible catheter with open ends

One or two Dacron cuffs or Vitacuffs (biosynthetic material impregnated with silver ions) on catheter(s) enhance tissue ingrowth.

May have more than one lumen (Figure 3-12)

Benefits

Reduced risk of bacterial migration after tissue adheres to Dacron cuff or Vitacuff

Easy to use for self-administered infusions

Care Considerations*

Requires daily heparin flushes

Must be clamped or have clamp nearby at all times

Must keep exit site dry

*See Patient and Family Education, p. 533.

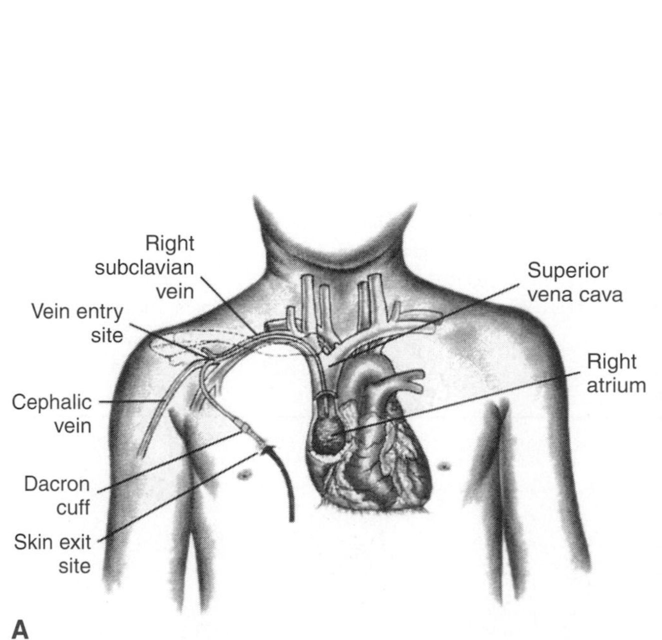

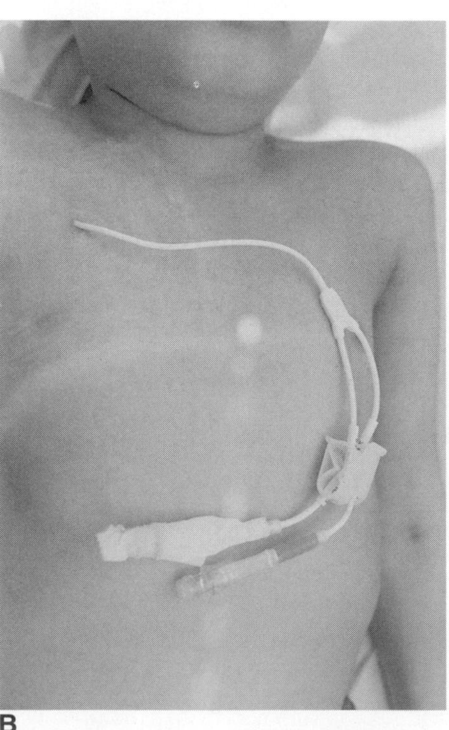

FIGURE **3-12** **A,** Central venous catheter insertion and exit site. **B,** External venous catheter.

Heavy activity restricted until tissue adheres to cuff
Risk of infection still present
Protrudes outside body; susceptible to damage from sharp instruments and may be pulled out; may affect body image
More difficult to repair
Patient and family must learn catheter care

GROSHONG CATHETER

Description

Clear, flexible, silicone, radiopaque catheter with closed tip and two-way valve at proximal end
Dacron cuff or Vitacuff on catheter enhances tissue ingrowth
May have more than one lumen

Benefits

Reduced time and cost for maintenance care; no heparin flushes needed
Reduced catheter damage—No clamping needed because of two-way valve
Increased patient safety because of minimum potential for blood backflow or air embolism
Reduced risk of bacterial migration after tissue adheres to Dacron cuff or Vitacuff
Easily repaired
Easy to use for self-administered infusions

Care Considerations

Requires weekly irrigation with normal saline
Must keep exit site dry
Heavy activity restricted until tissue adheres to cuff
Risk of infection still present
Protrudes outside body; susceptible to damage from sharp instruments and may be pulled out; may affect body image
Patient or family must learn catheter care.

IMPLANTED PORTS (PORT-A-CATH, INFUSAPORT, MEDIPORT, NORPORT, GROSHONG PORT)

Description

Totally implantable metal or plastic device that consists of self-sealing injection port with top or side access with preconnected or attachable silicone catheter that is placed in large blood vessel

Benefits

Reduced risk of infection
Placed completely under the skin; therefore cannot be pulled out or damaged
No maintenance care and reduced cost for family
Heparinized monthly and after each infusion to maintain patency (Groshong port requires only saline)
No limitations on regular physical activity, including swimming
Dressing needed only when port accessed with Huber needle that is not removed
No or only slight change in body appearance (slight bulge on chest)

Care Considerations*

Must pierce skin for access; pain with insertion of needle; can use local anesthetic (EMLA, LMX, or buffered lidocaine) before accessing port (Figure 3-13)
Special noncoring needle (Huber) with straight or angled design must be used to inject into port
Skin preparation needed before injection
Hard to manipulate for self-administered infusions
Catheter may dislodge from port, especially if child plays with port site
Vigorous contact sports generally not allowed

*See Patient and Family Education, p. 537.

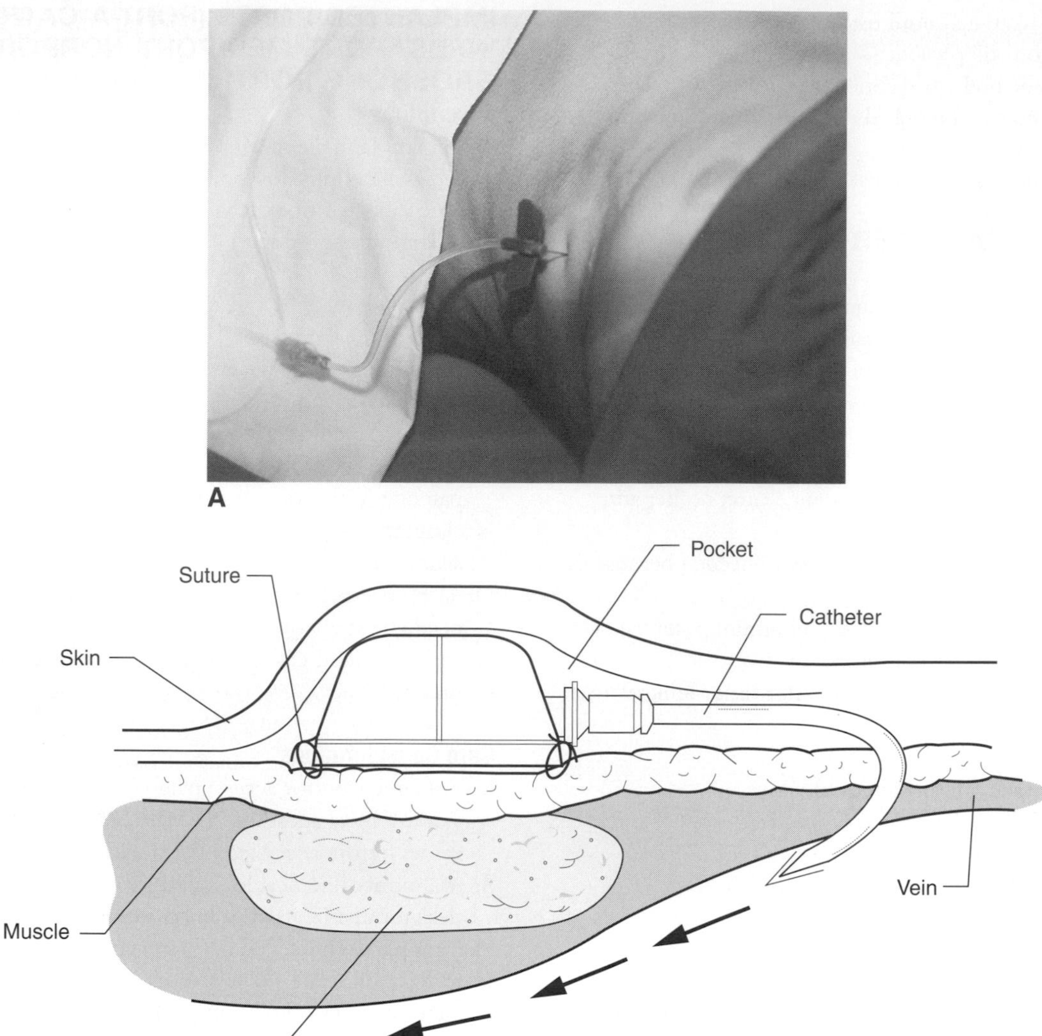

FIGURE **3-13** **A,** Implanted venous access device with Huber placement. **B,** Catheter totally implanted under the skin. The bulge under the skin is the port (Port-a-Cath, Infusaport). To use this system, a special needle is inserted through the skin into the port.

EVIDENCE-BASED PRACTICE

Central Venous Catheter Site Care

Brandi Horvath

Ask the Question

Question

In children with central venous catheters (CVC), is chlorhexidine gluconate a more effective antiseptic solution than povidone-iodine in preventing CVC-related site infections and bacteremia?

Objective

To evaluate the effectiveness of chlorhexidine gluconate versus povidone-iodine as a skin disinfectant for catheter site care

Background

Infection of CVC insertion sites is one of the most common causes of nosocomial bacteremia in children. Historically, povidone-iodine has been used for site care but not without complications. Gram-positive organisms have demonstrated resistance to povidone-iodine, and several studies have documented the irritant and potential toxic effects in neonates.

Search for Evidence

Search Strategies

Search selection criteria included English language publications within the past 10 years and research-based articles on catheter site care and chlorhexidine.

Databases Used

The National Guideline Clearinghouse (AHRQ), Centers for Disease Control and Prevention (CDC), Cochrane Collaboration, Joanna Briggs Institute, PubMed, Infusion Nurses Society, Oncology Nurses Society, MD Consult, BestBETs, TRIP Database Plus

Critically Analyze the Evidence

The CDC (O'Grady, Alexander, Dellinger, and others, 2002) recommends the use of 2% chlorhexidine for disinfecting catheter site before insertion (allow to dry), but tincture of iodine, an iodophor, or 70% alcohol can be used. Iodine needs to remain on the skin for at least 2 minutes or until dry. No recommendations can be made for the use of chlorhexidine in infants younger than 2 months of age. No recommendations can be made regarding the use of topical antibiotic ointments or creams due to the potential to promote fungal infections and antimicrobial resistance. No recommendations are made for the use of impregnated catheters and chlorhexidine sponge dressings to reduce the incidence of infection. Avoid use of sponges in infants less than 7 days old and less than 26 weeks' gestation. Replace the catheter-site dressing when it becomes damp, loosened, or soiled or when inspection of the site is necessary. Replace dressings used on short-term CVC sites every 2 days for gauze dressings and at least every 7 days for transparent dressings, except in those pediatric patients in whom the risk for dislodging the catheter outweighs the benefit of changing the dressing.

The Infusion Nurses Society (2006) recommends the use of alcohol, chlorhexidine gluconate, povidone-iodine, and tincture of iodine. If using povidone-iodine, do not apply alcohol as a second antiseptic. Allow all antiseptics to air dry. Dress vascular access site with sterile gauze and cover with sterile transparent dressings. Gauze dressings should be changed every 48 hours. Semipermeable transparent dressings should be changed at least every seven days, and the interval is dependent on the dressing material, age and condition of the patient, infection rate reported by the organization, environmental conditions, and manufacturer's labeled uses and directions.

The Oncology Nursing Society (Camp-Sorrell, 2004) finds chlorhexidine for preinsertion and postinsertion site catheter care superior to alcohol and povidone-iodine. No recommendations are made for the use of chlorhexidine sponge dressing. Routine application of antibiotic ointment is not recommended because of the risk of fungal infections and antimicrobial resistance. Gauze dressings should be changed every 48 hours. Semipermeable transparent dressings over gauze are treated as gauze dressings and changed every 48 hours. Semi-permeable transparent dressings should be changed every 5 to 7 days or more often, as indicated.

Three evidence-based systematic reviews were found regarding CVC site care.

- In a nursing evidence-based review by Carson (2004), most studies found chlorhexidine to be superior to povidone-iodine for preventing microbial colonization of the CVC insertion site and catheter tip and for decreasing the risk of local site infection. However, there is still conflicting evidence regarding the efficacy of chlorhexidine versus povidone-iodine for preventing CVC-related bacteremia.
- In a metaanalysis of eight studies by Chaiyakunapruk, Veenstra, Lipsky, and Saint (2002), chlorhexidine reduced the risk of catheter-related bloodstream infections by 49% compared with povidone-iodine. In a follow-up review (Chaiyakunapruk, Veenstra, Lipsky, and others, 2003), the use of chlorhexidine rather than povidone-iodine for site care led to a cost savings of $113 for each catheter used.
- In a systematic review focused on bone marrow transplant recipients, chlorhexidine is the recommended antisepsis for prevention of catheter-related infection (Zitella, 2003).

Four randomized controlled trials were found comparing chlorhexidine and povidone-iodine in various populations.

- Chambers, Sanders, Patton, and others (2005) found chlorhexidine sponge dressings (Biopatch) reduced the incidence of exit-site or tunnel infections of central venous catheters in adult neutropenic patients.
- In Garland, Alex, Mueller, and others (2001), 705 neonates and infants in the Biopatch group had a substantial decrease in colonized catheter tips compared with the group that used standard dressings but no difference in rates of catheter related bloodstream infections or bloodstream infections without a source between the two groups. However, Biopatch was associated with localized contact dermatitis in infants of very low birth weight.

Continued

EVIDENCE-BASED PRACTICE

Central Venous Catheter Site Care—cont'd

- In Langgartner, Linde, Lehn, and others (2004), skin disinfection before CVC insertion and daily with dressing changes with propanol-chlorhexidine followed by povidone-iodine was associated with the lowest rate of microbial catheter colonization.
- In a study conducted by Levy, Katz, Solter, and others (2005) in a pediatric cardiovascular intensive care unit, patients with chlorhexidine-impregnated CVC dressing (Biopatch) had a significantly reduced risk of CVC colonization compared with patients with transparent dressing alone. Occurrence of catheter-related bloodstream infection was not different in the two groups.

Apply the Evidence: Nursing Implications

- Two percent chlorhexidine should be used for catheter site antisepsis.
- Two percent chlorhexidine should be used with caution in premature and low-birth-weight infants.
- Chlorhexidine-impregnated sponges (Biopatch) should be used around the catheter site except in low-birth-weight infants in the first 2 weeks of life

References

Camp-Sorrell D, editor: *Access device guidelines: recommendations for nursing practice and education,* ed 2, Pittsburgh, 2004, Oncology Nursing Society.

Carson S: Chlorhexidine versus povidone-iodine for central venous catheter site care in children, *J Pediatr Nurs* 19(1):74-80, 2004.

Chaiyakunapruk N, Veenstra D, Lipsky B, Saint S: Chlorhexidine compared with povidone-iodine solution for vascular catheter-site care: a meta-analysis, *Ann Intern Med* 136:792-801, 2002.

Chaiyakunapruk N, Veenstra D, Lipsky B, and others: Vascular catheter site care: the clinical and economic benefits of chlorhexidine gluconate compared with povidone iodine, *Clin Infect Dis* 37(6):764-771, 2003.

Chambers S, Sanders J, Patton W, and others: Reduction of exit-site infections of tunneled intravascular catheters among neutropenic patients by sustained-release chlorhexidine dressings: results from a prospective randomized controlled trial, *J Hosp Infect* 61:53-61, 2005.

Garland J, Alex C, Mueller C, and others: A randomized trial comparing povidone-iodine to a chlorhexidine-impregnated dressing for prevention of central venous catheter infections in neonates, *Pediatrics* 107(6):1431-1436, 2001.

Infusion Nurses Society: *Policies and procedures for infusion nursing,* ed 3, South Norwood, Mass, 2006, The Society.

Langgartner J, Linde H, Lehn N, and others: Combined skin disinfection with chlorhexidine/propanol and aqueous povidone-iodine reduces bacterial colonisation of central venous catheters, *Intensive Care Med* 30(6):1081-1088, 2004.

Levy I, Katz J, Solter E, and others: Chlorhexidine-impregnated dressing for prevention of colonization of central venous catheters in infants and children: a randomized controlled study, *Pediatr Infect Dis J* 24(8):676-679, 2005.

O'Grady N, Alexander M, Dellinger EP, and others: Guidelines for the prevention of intravascular catheter-related infections, *MMWR Morb Mortal Wkly Rep* 51(RR-10):1-29, 2002.

Zitella L: Central venous catheter site care for blood and marrow transplant recipients, *Clin J Oncol Nurs* 7(3):289-298, 2003.

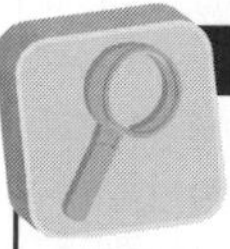

EVIDENCE-BASED PRACTICE

Obtaining Blood Specimens from Central Venous Catheters in Children

Joy Hesselgrave

Ask the Question

Question

In children, do blood specimens obtained from central venous catheters using the discard, reinfusion, or push-pull method yield more accurate samples?

Objective

To evaluate blood specimen accuracy and safety when drawn from central venous catheter by three different methods

Background

Central venous access devices (CVADs) include Port-a-Caths (ports), tunneled central venous catheters, nontunneled central venous catheters, and peripherally inserted central lines (PICCs). Drawing blood specimens from central venous catheters is a routine practice in pediatrics. There are three techniques described in the literature. The discard method involves removing 3 to 10 ml of the first blood aspirate, which may contain saline, heparin, or intravenous fluids, then obtaining the blood specimen. The reinfusion method involves using a stopcock to maintain a closed system and returning the discard specimen after obtaining the blood specimen. In the push-pull method, a 10-ml syringe with 5 ml of saline is attached to the catheter and flushed into the line; 6 ml are withdrawn and pushed back in to the catheter without removing the syringe. This procedure is repeated a total of three or four times. The empty syringe is then removed and a clean syringe or Vacutainer attached to obtain the blood specimen.

3 - EVIDENCE-BASED PEDIATRIC NURSING INTERVENTIONS

EVIDENCE-BASED PRACTICE

Obtaining Blood Specimens from Central Venous Catheters in Children—cont'd

Search for Evidence

Search Strategies

Search selection criteria included English language research-based publications within the past 15 years on pediatric blood specimen collection from central venous access.

Databases Used

National Guideline Clearinghouse (AHRQ), Cochrane Collaboration, Joanna Briggs Institute, PubMed, TRIP database Plus, MD Consult, PedsCCM, BestBETs

Critically Analyze the Evidence

Limited scientific research exists that describes the optimal method for drawing blood samples from CVADs in the pediatric patient.

A convenience sample of paired specimens compared blood drawn from central lines via push-pull method and discard method on 28 pediatric patients 6 months to 12 years of age. Of the 438 pairs of measurements that were compared, 420 or 95.9% were within limits of agreement for hemograms, electrolytes, and glucose. The push-pull method eliminates loss of blood and decreases the amount of times the central line is accessed (Barton, Chase, Latham, and Rayens, 2004).

Forty-two nonneutropenic pediatric patients aged 2 to 20 years were randomly assigned to one of two syringe-handling methods for blood sampling. The discard specimen, routinely reinfused, was collected using the usual clean procedure and an exaggerated unclean alternative procedure. Neither the sterile specimens nor the unclean specimens grew organisms, thus suggesting that the reinfusion of the blood specimen would be safe. This study did not evaluate for clots in the discard specimen (Hinds, Wentz, Hughes, and others, 1991).

Thirty bone marrow transplant units were surveyed to evaluate how blood samples were drawn from CVADs. The average patient age was 5 to 16 years. Seventy-five percent of the units used the discard method, with the volume of discard ranging from 0.5 to 10 ml and an average of 4 to 6 ml. Fourteen percent used the reinfusion method, and 11% used the push-pull or mixing method (Keller, 1994).

The Infusion Nurses Society (2006) recommends that the discard method be used when drawing blood samples from CVADs. The discard volume should be 1.5 to 2 times the fill volume of the CVAD.

Frey (2003) summarizes evidence for the practice of all three blood sampling methods. The discard method is most widely reported, with disadvantages including blood loss, blood exposure risk for clinicians, and the potential to confuse the discard specimen for the blood sample. The reinfusion method does not deplete blood volume but risks blood exposure for clinician and potential to reinfuse a contaminated specimen or clots in the discard volume. The push-pull or mixing method demonstrates accuracy for other than coagulation and drug levels and reduces blood loss and clinician exposure risk.

Apply the Evidence: Nursing Implications

- There is limited pediatric research that clearly supports any particular central line blood sampling method as being superior. All three methods yield accurate results and appear safe. The discard method is the most frequently reported in the literature and benchmarking. However, if there is a concern about blood volume, the push-pull or reinfusion method should be considered.
- If the catheter has multiple lumens, use the distal lumen for laboratory specimen collection.
- Infusions should be stopped and lumens clamped before blood sampling.
- Cleanse the injection cap with antiseptic agent and allow to dry before drawing laboratory specimens.
- Attach a syringe or stopcock depending on specimen method selected, to the injection cap, not directly to the catheter hub. The injection cap at the catheter hub should be removed only if blood cultures are drawn.

References

Barton S, Chase T, Latham B, Rayens M: Comparing two methods to obtain blood specimens from pediatric central venous catheters, *J Pediatr Oncol Nurs* 21(6):320-326, 2004.

Frey M: Drawing blood samples from vascular access devices, *J Infus Nurs* 26(5):285-293, 2003.

Hinds PS, Wentz T, Hughes W, and others: An investigation of the safety of the blood reinfusion step used with tunneled venous access devices in children with cancer, *J Pediatr Oncol Nurs* 8(4):59-64, 1991.

Infusion Nurses Society: *Policies and procedures for infusion nursing,* ed 3, South Norwood, Mass, 2006, The Society.

Keller CA: Methods of drawing blood samples through central venous catheters in pediatric patients undergoing bone marrow transplant: results of a national survey, *Oncol Nurs Forum* 21(5):879-884, 1994

Heparin Flush Catheters

	Intermittent		Dormant	
	Age ≤2 Years or Catheter Gauge ≤24 g	Age >2 Years	Age ≤2 Years or Catheter Gauge ≤24 g	Age >2 Years
Peripheral lines (Heplock)	10 units/ml; 1 ml heparin after medications or every 8 hours	5 ml normal saline after medications or every 8 hours	10 units/ml; 1 ml heparin every 8 hours	5 ml normal saline every 8 hours
External central line (nonimplanted, tunneled, or peripherally inserted central catheter [PICC])	10 units/ml; 3 ml heparin after medications		10 units/ml; 3 ml heparin every day	100 units/ml; 3 ml heparin every day
Totally implanted central line (TIVAS)	10 units/ml; 5 ml heparin after medications		100 units/ml, 5 ml every month; or 10 units/ml, 5 ml every day if accessed	100 units/ml; 5 ml heparin every month or every day if accessed
Midline	10 units/ml; 3 ml heparin in a 5-ml syringe after medications or every 8 hours		10 units/ml; 3 ml heparin in a 5-ml syringe every 8 hours	
Arterial and central venous pressure continuous monitored lines	Heparin, 2 units/ml, in 55-ml syringes run at 1 ml/hr		N/A	
Neonates and Infants				
Peripheral lines (Heplock)	2 units/ml; 2 ml heparin to check for line patency and between medications and/or TPN known to be incompatible		2 units/ml; 2 ml heparin every 8 hours	
Percutaneous central catheter	2 units/ml in 20-ml syringe run at 0.2 ml/hr		N/A	
Surgically placed central venous catheter ≤5 French	2 units/ml; 2 ml heparin to check for line patency and between medications and/or TPN known to be incompatible		2 units/ml; 2 ml heparin every 8 hours	
Surgically placed central venous catheter >5 French	2 units/ml; 3 ml heparin to check for line patency and between meds and/or TPN known to be incompatible		2 units/ml; 3 ml heparin every 8 hours	

Adapted from Texas Children's Hospital, Houston, Texas.
N/A, Not applicable; *TPN*, total parenteral nutrition.

EVIDENCE-BASED PRACTICE

Normal Saline or Heparinized Saline Flush Solution in Pediatric Intravenous Lines

David Wilson

Ask the Question

Question

Is there a significant difference in the longevity of intravenous (IV) intermittent infusion locks in children when normal saline (NS) is used as a flush instead of a heparinized saline (HS) solution?

Background

Intermittent infusion devices (heparin locks) are often used in children who require intermittent infusions of medications such as antibiotics yet do not require continuous fluid infusion. In the past it has been common practice to flush such locks with an HS solution to maintain patency.

Objective

The objective of this study is to determine whether intermittent flush solution of saline is sufficient to maintain patency in children's infusion locks.

Search for Evidence

Search Strategies

Selection criteria included evidence within the past 15 years with the following terms: saline vs heparin intermittent flush, children's heparin lock flush, heparin lock patency, peripheral venous catheter in children

Databases Used

CINAHL, PubMed

Critically Analyze the Evidence

- A systematic Cochrane Review by Shah and Sinha (2002) revealed eight studies (Alpan, Eyal, Springer, and others, 1984; Goldberg, Sankaran, and Givelichian, and others, 1999; Heilskov, Kleiber, Johnson, and others, 1998; Kotter, 1996; Moclair and Bates, 1995; Mudge, Forcier, and Slattery, 1998; Paisley, Stamper, Brown, and others, 1997; Treas and Latinis-Bridges, 1992) that were randomized or quasirandomized trials of HS administration versus NS, placebo, or no treatment in neonates. The authors of the review concluded that the heterogeneity among the studies, variability in methodological quality and clinical details, and variability in reporting outcomes resulted in no strong evidence regarding the effectiveness and safety of heparin to prolong catheter life in neonates.
- No significant statistical difference was found between HS and NS flushes for maintaining catheter patency in children (Hanrahan, Kleiber, and Fagan, 1994; Kotter, 1996; Schultz, Drew, and Hewitt, 2002; Hanrahan, Kleiber, and Berends, 2000; Heilskov, Kleiber, Johnson, and others, 1998).
- Several studies reported increased incidence of pain or erythema with HS flushing of infusion devices (Hanrahan, Kleiber, and Fagan, 1994; Robertson, 1994; Nelson and Graves, 1998; McMullen, Fioravanti, Pollack, and others, 1993).
- Several studies found increased patency and/or longer dwell times with HS solutions versus NS in 24-gauge catheters (Mudge, Forcier, and Slattery, 1998; Danek and Noris, 1992; Beecroft, Bossert, Chung, and others, 1997; Gyr, Burroughs, Smith, and others, 1995; Hanrahan, Kleiber, and Berends, 2000).
- Younger children and lower gestational age in preterm neonates were associated with shorter patency of IV catheters (Paisley, Stamper, Brown, and others, 1997; Robertson, 1994; McMullen, Fioravanti, Pollack, and others, 1993).
- Infusion devices flushed with NS lasted longer than those flushed with HS (Nelson and Graves, 1998; Le Duc, 1997; Goldberg, Sankaran, Givelichian, and others, 1999).
- When measured and reported, length of time between flushing peripheral devices affected dwell time (Crews, Gnann, Rice, and others, 1997; Gyr, Burroughs, Smith, and others, 1995).
- None of the studies cited anticoagulation-associated complications with HS, which is a concern in preterm neonates who are at higher risk for development of clotting problems as a result of heparin (Klenner, Fusch, Rakow, and others, 2003).

Apply the Evidence: Nursing Implications

- Further research is needed with larger samples of children, especially preterm neonates, using small-gauge catheters (24 gauge) and other gauge catheters, flushed with NS and HS as intermittent infusion devices only (no continuous infusions); variables to be considered should include catheter dwell time; medications administered; period between regular flushing and flushing associated with medication administration; pain, erythema, or other localized complications; concentration and amount of heparin solutions used; flush method (positive pressure technique versus no specific technique); reason for IV device removal; and complications associated with either solution.
- NS is a safe alternative to HS flush in infants and children with intermittent IV locks larger than 24 gauge; smaller neonates may benefit from HS flush (longer dwell time), but the evidence is inconclusive for all weight ranges and gestational ages.

References

Alpan G, Eyal F, Springer C, and others: Heparinization of alimentation solutions administered through peripheral veins in premature infants: a controlled study, *Pediatrics* 74(3):375-378, 1984.

Beecroft PC, Bossert E, Chung K, and others: Intravenous lock patency in children: dilute heparin versus saline, *J Pediatr Pharm Practice* 2(4):211-223, 1997.

Crews BE, Gnann KK, Rice MH, and others: Effects of varying intervals between heparin flushes on pediatric catheter longevity, *Pediatr Nurs* 23(1):87-91, 1997.

Danek GD, Noris EM: Pediatric IV catheters: efficacy of saline flush, *Pediatr Nurs* 18(2):111-113, 1992.

Goldberg M, Sankaran R, Givelichian L, and others: Maintaining patency of peripheral intermittent infusion devices with heparinized

Continued

3 - EVIDENCE-BASED PEDIATRIC NURSING INTERVENTIONS

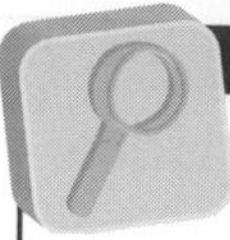

EVIDENCE-BASED PRACTICE

Normal Saline or Heparinized Saline Flush Solution in Pediatric Intravenous Lines—cont'd

saline and saline: a randomized double blind controlled trial in neonatal intensive care and a review of literature, *Neonat Intensive Care* 12(1):18-22, 1999.

Gyr P, Burroughs T, Smith K, and others: Double blind comparison of heparin and saline flush solutions in maintenance of peripheral infusion devices, *Pediatr Nurs* 21(4):383-389, 1995.

Hanrahan KS, Kleiber C, Berends S: Saline for peripheral intravenous locks in neonates: evaluating a change in practice, *Neonat Netw* 19(2):19-24, 2000.

Hanrahan KS, Kleiber C, Fagan C: Evaluation of saline for IV locks in children, *Pediatr Nurs* 20(6):549-552, 1994.

Heilskov J, Kleiber C, Johnson K, and others: A randomized trial of heparin and saline for maintaining intravenous locks in neonates, *J Soc Pediatr Nurs* 3(3):111-116, 1998.

Klenner AF, Fusch C, Rakow A, and others: Benefit and risk of heparin for maintaining peripheral venous catheters in neonates: a placebo-controlled trial, *J Pediatr* 143(6):741-745, 2003.

Kotter RW: Heparin vs. saline for intermittent intravenous device maintenance in neonates, *Neonat Netw* 15(6):43-47, 1996.

Le Duc K: Efficacy of normal saline solution versus heparin solution for maintaining patency of peripheral intravenous catheters in children, *J Emerg Nurs* 23(4):306-309, 1997.

McMullen A, Fioravanti ID, Pollack D, and others: Heparinized saline or normal saline as a flush solution in intermittent intravenous lines in infants and children, *MCN* 18(2):78-85, 1993.

Moclair A, Bates I: The efficacy of heparin in maintaining peripheral infusions in neonates, *Eur J Pediatr* 154(7):567-570, 1995.

Mudge B, Forcier D, Slattery MJ: Patency of 24-gauge peripheral intermittent infusion devices: a comparison of heparin and saline flush solutions, *Pediatr Nurs* 24(2):142-149, 1998.

Nelson TJ, Graves SM: 0.9% Sodium chloride injection with and without heparin for maintaining peripheral indwelling intermittent infusion devices in infants, *Am J Heath Syst Pharm* 55:570-573, 1998.

Paisley MK, Stamper M, Brown T, and others: The use of heparin and normal saline flushes in neonatal intravenous catheters, *J Pediatr Nurs* 23(5):521-527, 1997.

Robertson J: Intermittent intravenous therapy: a comparison of two flushing solutions, *Contemp Nurs* 3(4):174-179, 1994.

Schultz AA, Drew D, Hewitt H: Comparison of normal saline and heparinized saline for patency of IV locks in neonates, *Appl Nurs Res* 15(1):28-34, 2002.

Shah PS, Sinha AK: Heparin for prolonging peripheral intravenous catheter use in neonates, *Cochrane Database Syst Rev 2002* (2):1-26, 2002.

Treas LS, Latinis-Bridges B: Efficacy of heparin in peripheral venous infusion in neonates, *J Obstet Gynecol Neonatal Nurs* 21(3):214-219, 1992.

3 - EVIDENCE-BASED PEDIATRIC NURSING INTERVENTIONS

Tube Feeding

The purpose of tube feeding is to supply gastrointestinal feeding for the child who is unable to take nourishment by mouth because of anomalies of the throat or esophagus, impaired swallowing capacity, severe debilitation, respiratory distress, or unconsciousness.

PROCEDURE: PLACEMENT OF A NASOGASTRIC OR OROGASTRIC TUBE

1. Place the child supine with the head slightly hyperflexed or in a sniffing position (nose pointed toward ceiling). (See Patient and Family Education, p. 549.)
2. Measure the tube for approximate length of insertion, and mark the point with a small piece of tape. Two standard methods of measuring length are as follows:
   - Measuring from nose to earlobe, then to the end of the xiphoid process
   - Measuring from nose to earlobe, then to a point midway between the xiphoid process and umbilicus
3. Lubricate the tube with sterile water or water-soluble lubricant, and insert through one of the nares or the mouth to the predetermined mark. In older infants and children, the tube is passed through the nose and the position alternated between nostrils. An indwelling tube is almost always placed through the nose. Because most young infants are obligatory nose breathers, insertion through the mouth may be used for intermittent gavage feedings because it causes less distress and also helps to stimulate sucking.
   - When using the nose, slip the tube along the base of the nose and direct it straight back toward the occiput.
   - When entering through the mouth, direct the tube toward the back of the throat.
   - If the child is able to swallow on command, synchronize passing the tube with swallowing.
4. Confirm placement by x-ray if available. Document pH and color of aspirate with initial placement and ongoing placement checks (see Evidence-Based Practice box).
5. Stabilize the tube by holding or taping it to the cheek, not to the forehead because of possible damage to the nostril. To assist in maintaining correct placement, measure and record the amount of tubing extending from the nose or mouth to the distal port when the tube is first positioned. Recheck position before each feeding. A hydrocolloid barrier (DuoDerm or Coloplast) may be placed on the cheeks to protect the skin from tape irritation.

PROCEDURE: FEEDING THROUGH THE TUBE

1. Whenever possible, hold the infant or young child during the feeding to associate the comfort of physical contact with the procedure. When this is not possible, place the infant or child supine or slightly toward the right side with head and chest slightly elevated.
   - Use a folded blanket under the head and shoulders for infants and a pillow for small children.
   - Raise the head of the bed for larger children.
   - If possible, allow infant to suck on a pacifier during feeding for association of suck and satiation (feeling satisfied).
2. Warm the formula to room temperature. Do not microwave.
3. For feedings delivered by mechanical pump, pour formula into bag or syringe, and prime tubing. Connect to patient and set desired rate.
4. For gravity feedings via syringe, pour formula into the barrel of the syringe attached to the feeding tube. To start the flow, give a gentle push with the plunger, but then remove the plunger and allow the fluid to flow into the stomach by gravity. To prevent nausea and regurgitation, the rate of flow should not exceed 5 ml every 5 to 10 minutes in preterm and very small infants and 10 ml/min in older infants and children. The rate is determined by the diameter of the tubing and the height of the reservoir containing the feeding. The rate is regulated by adjusting the height of the syringe. A typical feeding may take 15 to 30 minutes to complete.
5. Flush the tube with sterile water: 1 or 2 ml for small tubes; 5 to 15 ml or more for large ones.
6. Cap or clamp indwelling tubes to prevent loss of feeding. If the tube is to be removed, first pinch it firmly to prevent escape of fluid as the tube is withdrawn, then withdraw the tube quickly.
7. Position the child with the head elevated about 30 degrees and on the right side for at least 1 hour in the same manner as following any infant feeding to minimize the possibility of regurgitation and aspiration. If the child's condition permits, bubble the youngster after the feeding.
8. Record the feeding, including the type and amount of residual, the type and amount of formula, and the manner in which it was tolerated. For most infant feedings, any amount of residual fluid aspirated from the stomach is refed to prevent electrolyte imbalance. The amount is subtracted from the prescribed amount of feeding. For example, if the infant or child is to receive 30 ml, and 10 ml is aspirated from the stomach before the feeding, the 10 ml of aspirated stomach contents are refed, plus 20 ml of feeding. Another method in children is that if residual is more than one fourth of the last feeding, then aspirate is returned and rechecked in 30 to 60 minutes. When residual is less than one fourth of last feeding, give scheduled feeding. If high aspirates persist and the child is due for another feeding, notify the practitioner.
9. Between feedings, give infants pacifiers to satisfy oral needs.

NASODUODENAL AND NASOJEJUNAL TUBES

Children at high risk for regurgitation or aspiration such as those with gastroparesis, mechanical ventilation, or brain injuries may require placement of a postpyloric feeding tube. Insertion of a nasoduodenal or nasojejunal tube is done by a trained practitioner because of the risk of misplacement and potential for perforation in tubes requiring a stylet. Accurate placement is verified by radiography. Small-bore tubes may easily clog. Flush tube when feeding is interrupted, before and after medication administration, and routinely every 4 hours or as directed by institutional policy. Tube replacement should be considered monthly to ensure optimal tube patency.

Feeding Procedure

Continuous feedings are delivered by mechanical pump to regulate volume and rate. Bolus feeds are contraindicated. Tube displacement is suspected in the child showing signs of feeding intolerance such as vomiting. Stop feedings and notify practitioner.

GASTROSTOMY TUBES*

The gastrostomy tube is placed with the patient under general anesthesia or percutaneously using an endoscope with the patient under local anesthesia (typically known as percutaneous endoscopic gastrostomy [PEG]). The tube can be a Foley, skin level wing tip, or mushroom catheter G-button. Skin level/G-button devices are cosmetically pleasing in appearance, afford increased comfort and mobility to the child, are easy to care for, are fully immersible in water, and have a one-way valve that minimizes reflux and eliminates the need for clamping.

Feeding Procedure

Positioning and feeding of water, formula, and pureed foods are carried out in the same manner and rate as NG feedings. A mechanical pump may be used to regulate the volume and rate of feeding. With some skin-level devices that do not lock, the child must remain fairly still, because the tubing may easily disconnect from the device if the child moves. Some devices require a tube other than the feeding tube to be used for stomach decompression; some do not. After feedings, the infant or child is positioned on the right side or in Fowler position; the tube may be clamped or left open between feedings, depending on the child's condition.

*See Patient and Family Education, p. 551.

If the skin-level device is used, insert the extension tube (or decompression tube, in some devices) to remove air in the stomach. This will reduce leaking.

If a Foley catheter is used as the gastrostomy tube, very slight tension is applied and the tube securely taped to maintain the balloon at the gastrostomy opening. This prevents leakage of gastric contents and the tube's progression toward the pyloric sphincter, where it may occlude the stomach outlet. As a precaution, the length of the tube should be measured postoperatively and remeasured each shift to be sure it has not slipped. A mark can be made above the skin level to further ensure its placement. Tube holders are available commercially to assist with tube stabilization.

EVIDENCE-BASED PRACTICE

Assessing Correct Placement of Nasogastric or Orogastric Tubes in Children

Marilyn J. Hockenberry

Ask the Question

Question

In children, how do we assess for correct placement of nasogastric or orogastric tubes?

Background

Tube placement errors occur frequently in children and can cause serious problems. Tubes that are properly placed can become dislodged and need to be checked for continued proper placement. Auscultation, the method frequently used by nurses to confirm tube placement, is unreliable. Aspiration pneumonia is the most common complication resulting from incorrect tube placement.

Objective

To evaluate the evidence on methods to ensure correct placement of nasogastric or orogastric tubes

Search for Evidence

Search Strategies

Search selection criteria included English language publications within the past 10 years, research-based articles (level 3 or lower), children or adult populations, comparisons to gold standard (x-ray examination).

Databases Used

PubMed, Cochrane Collaboration, MD Consult, Joanna Briggs Institute, National Guideline Clearinghouse (AHQR), TRIP Database Plus, PedsCCM, BestBETs

Critical Appraisal of the Evidence

Studies compared various methods used to evaluate placement of the tube with the gold standard: x-ray examination. Eight (level 3) articles were found, five adult and four child sample populations.

- pH-assisted feeding tubes, child (Krafte-Jacobs, Persinger, Carver, and others, 1996)
- Bilirubin, adult and child (Westhus, 2004; Metheny, Stewart, Smith, and others, 1999; Metheny, Smith, and Stewart, 2000)
- Enzyme tests, child and adult (Westhus, 2004; Metheny, Stewart, Smith and others, 1997)
- Bedside sonography for tube placement, adult (Hernandez-Socorro, Marin, Ruiz-Santana, and others, 1996)
- Aspiration of insufflated air for tube placement, adult (Neumann, Meyer, Dutton and others, 1995; Harrison, Clay, Grant, and others, 1997)

Most reliable tests for determining tube placement in the nine published studies (other than the gold standard of x-ray examination) were the combination of:

- pH testing
- Visual inspection of aspirate
- Bilirubin and enzyme tests

Bilirubin and enzyme measures are not currently available at the bedside.

Sensitivity and specificity of the bedside tests for children need further evaluation.

Auscultation is an unreliable method to confirm tube placement because of the similarity of sounds produced by air in the bronchus, esophagus, or pleural space.

Apply the Evidence: Nursing Implications

- Use x-ray to confirm initial placement. Document pH and color of aspirate with initial placement.
- A pH of 5 or less supports the conclusion that the tip of the tube is in a gastric location (Huffman, Jarczyk, O'Brien, and others, 2004; Metheny, Stewart, Smith, and others, 1999; Westhus, 2004; Gharpure, Meert, Sarnaik, and others, 2000).
- A pH greater than 5 does not reliably predict the correct distal tip location. It may indicate respiratory or esophageal placement, or presence of medications to suppress acid secretion.
- If pH is greater than 5, use other measures to evaluate tube placement. If bilirubin and enzyme testing is not available, check color of aspirate. Gastric contents are clear, off-white, or tan; may be brown-tinged if blood is present. Respiratory secretions may look the same. Intestinal contents are often bile stained, light to dark yellow, or greenish brown. May also need to obtain an x-ray.

EVIDENCE-BASED PRACTICE

Assessing Correct Placement of Nasogastric or Orogastric Tubes in Children—cont'd

- A change in pH may indicate tube dislodgment. Check external markings and tube length to ensure tube has not moved. If uncertain about placement, need to obtain an x-ray.
- pH and color of aspirate can be checked before medication or feeding. For continuous feedings, it is recommended that tube placement be checked every 4 hours.
- A *Visual Bilirubin Scale,* effective in determining bilirubin content in feeding tube aspirates, has been published (Metheny, Smith, Stewart, 2000). Evaluation of the accuracy of the scale is needed with children.
- Risk factors for improper tube placement are comatose or semicomatose state, swallowing problems, and recurrent retching or vomiting.
- Experience of the individual inserting the tube is always important.

References

Gharpure V, Meert KL, Sarnaik AP, and others: Indicators of postpyloric feeding tube placement in children, *Crit Care Med* 28(8):2962-2966, 2000.

Harrison AM, Clay B, Grant MJ, and others: Nonradiographic assessment of enteral feeding tube position, *Crit Care Med* 25(12):2055-2059, 1997.

Hernandez-Socorro CR, Marin J, Ruiz-Santana S, and others: Bedside sonographic-guided versus blind nasoenteric feeding tube placement in critically ill patients, *Crit Care Med* 24(10):1690-1694, 1996.

Huffman S, Jarczyk KS, O'Brien E, and others: Methods to confirm feeding tube placement: application of research in practice, *Pediatr Nurs* 30(1):10-13, 2004.

Krafte-Jacobs B, Persinger M, Carver J, and others: Rapid placement of transpyloric feeding tubes: a comparison of pH-assisted and standard insertion techniques in children, *Pediatrics* 98(2 Pt 1):242-248, 1996.

Metheny NA, Smith L, Stewart BJ: Development of a reliable and valid bedside test for bilirubin and its utility for improving prediction of feeding tube location, *Nurs Res* 49(6):302-309, 2000.

Metheny NA, Stewart BJ, Smith L, and others: pH and concentration of bilirubin in feeding tube aspirates as predictors of tube placement, *Nurs Res* 48(4):189-197, 1999.

Metheny NA, Stewart BJ, Smith L, and others: pH and concentrations of pepsin and trypsin in feeding tube aspirates as predictors of tube placement, *JPEN J Parenteral Enteral Nutr* 21:279-285, 1997.

Neumann MJ, Meyer CT, Dutton JL, and others: Hold that x-ray: aspirate pH and auscultation prove tube placement, *J Clin Gastroenterol* 20(4):293-295, 1995.

Westhus N: Methods to test feeding tube placement in children, *MCN Am J Maternal/Child Nurs* 29(5):282-291, 2004.

Ostomy Care Procedures

This is a brief overview of ostomy care procedures. Consult a Wound/Ostomy/Continence (WOC) nurse for more information or see the resource list later in this chapter for additional literature.

Changing Ostomy Pouch

MATERIALS NEEDED

Ostomy pouch—One- or two-piece pouches of appropriate type and size and indication (fecal ostomy vs urostomy). A urostomy pouch has a spout opening at the bottom and is appropriate for urine and liquid stool. A drainable ostomy pouch has a large opening at the bottom for thicker stool.

Ostomy closure—Disposable closure provided in box of pouches or reusable clamp to close pouch. Some pouches have a built-in closure so that no additional closure is needed.

Ostomy pattern or measuring guide and marker—This can be a paper backing from a previous pouch that was cut out or a measuring guide found in a box of pouches.

Curved ostomy scissors—Can also use manicure scissors if there is not a starter hole in the pouch wafer.

Barrier paste/strips/rings—Caulking pectin barrier that fills in crevices and skin folds to flatten pouching surface or is placed around the stoma to prevent leaking. Stoma paste usually contains alcohol and may sting if skin is irritated; paste strips and rings may not contain alcohol.

Liquid skin barrier—Skin sealant or barrier wipes protect the peristomal skin from epidermal stripping by applying a clear film to the skin and may improve pouch adhesion in high humidity. Many contain alcohol and can sting denuded skin. Use an alcohol-free skin sealant for infants.

Washcloth or soft paper towel—To cleanse skin with warm water. Do not use a baby wipe to cleanse the skin because many of these contain lanolin, which interferes with the pouch adhering.

Mild soap—Use a mild soap that does not contain moisturizers, lotions, or deodorizers, which can leave a film on the skin and interfere with the pouch adhering.

Stoma powder (optional)—Apply only if peristomal skin is broken, reddened, or denuded. Dust off excess amount before pouching, leaving a thin layer of powder. May use a liquid skin barrier to pat over the powder to assist pouch to seal.

PROCEDURE

Place child supine, and empty pouch.

If the pouch is leaking, note where the leak is coming from under the wafer.

Using a warm cloth, gently *push* down on the child's abdomen and *pull* up a corner of the pouch. Work your way circumferentially around the stoma, removing the pouch.

Discard the pouch, saving the ostomy closure if it is a plastic reusable type clamp.

Gently cleanse the peristomal skin with warm water and soap if needed. It is normal for the stoma to bleed a little when the cloth rubs against it; this does *not* hurt the child. Allow area to dry thoroughly.

Assess the stoma for color, edema, retraction, bleeding, and prolapse. Assess the peristomal skin to decide what additional products are needed to treat any sign of irritation.

Measure the stoma with a previous pattern or measuring guide, and place the pattern on the pouch wafer to trace. The stoma opening can be cut off-center to move the pouch away from umbilicus or an incision if needed. Do not cut beyond the cutting guide printed on the pouch wafer. The stoma's measurements may change for up to 6 weeks after surgery.

Cut out the pouch wafer, taking care to lay it over the stoma repeatedly until the wafer fits completely and easily over the stoma without more than ⅛ inch of peristomal skin exposed.

If skin is reddened or denuded, apply stoma powder to dry peristomal skin and dust off excess.

Apply a liquid skin barrier to protect peristomal skin and let dry (optional).

Peel pouch wafer paper and apply barrier paste, strips, and rings directly around opening cut out for stoma. A syringe may be used to deliver the stoma paste in a thin bead closely around the opening on an infant or toddler ostomy pouch. Barrier paste and strips may also be placed directly on the child's skin to fill in deep crevices, skin folds, or problematic areas for leakage.

Turn the pouch over and place the pouch on the skin. Ensure the skin is clean and dry. If stool has seeped onto the skin, clean off with a moist cloth and let dry. It is helpful to apply the pouch at an angle away from the body with the opening down toward the feet if the child is in diapers. If the child is up walking, the pouch can be placed straight down or angled inward for ease in emptying between the legs into the toilet.

Press the wafer down around the stoma to ensure it is sealed, and place your hand over the wafer for 1 to 2 minutes to warm it and allow it to melt into the skin. The pouch can also be warmed between the hands before peeling off the paper backing and applying.

Apply the pouch closure and put supplies away. If using a disposable bendable closure, wrap pouch end around the closure three or four times and bend ends tightly. If using a plastic reusable clamp, fold end of pouch *one time* over the smooth end of the clip and snap closed. Save new paper pattern from pouch wafer if needed.

POUCHING TIPS

Empty the child's pouch when it is ⅓ to ½ full to prevent it from becoming too heavy and pulling off or leaking.

Choose a quiet time to change an infant's ostomy pouch, such as when the infant is sleepy, or have someone hold the infant's hands while the pouch is changed.

Release gas (flatus) build-up in pouch by opening bottom of pouch or apply filter to pouch. If pouch gets too taut, it may pull away and leak.

Deodorizing ostomy drops and powders may be placed inside the pouch. Do *not* spray a nonostomy deodorizer inside the pouch, but it can be used in the room away from the child's face.

If the child has a candidal (yeast) rash around the stoma, apply an antifungal powder in place of a stoma powder. Remove pouch every 48 hours, and retreat for 7 to 10 days.

Warm soapy water may be placed inside a small squirt bottle and flushed up inside the pouch to cleanse the pouch of its contents.

Cuffing the bottom of the pouch before emptying the pouch will help keep the ends clean and free of odor. Clean the pouch ends with toilet paper or moist toilet cloths or baby wipes. The pouches are odor proof.

Pediatric ostomy pouches are designed to adhere for 2 to 3 days. Adult ostomy pouches usually adhere for 5 to 7 days.

Incorporate the child in his or her own care as much as possible, as appropriate for age.

Measure a growing child's stoma weekly or whenever a previous pattern is no longer effective.

Urostomy pouches can be attached to a urinary collection container at night.

Bathing and Hygiene

The child can bathe with the ostomy pouch on or off. If the pouch is left on, ensure the edges are dried thoroughly when the bathing is finished. If the pouch is taken off, soap and water will not harm the stoma. The stoma may become active during the bath, but to limit this occurrence, bathe 1 hour before or 2 hours after the child eats. Dry the skin thoroughly before replacing the pouch.

Clothing

There are no restrictions regarding types of clothing. The child can wear items that are form-fitting or loose. Tighter clothing that contains Spandex or Lycra and nylons do not harm the stoma nor hinder the stool output. Do make sure belts and elastic waistbands do not rub across the stoma. One-piece bathing suits with skirts are flattering for girls, and one-piece wetsuits work well for boys. Onesies for infants, overalls for toddlers, and one-piece sleepers keep hands away from pouches and prevent pouches from getting pulled off. Place pouch inside diaper to help keep pouch secure and prevent it from catching on clothing or getting pulled off.

Diet and Medications

There are no diet restrictions for an infant. There are no diet restrictions for an older child if he or she has a colostomy.

If an older child has an ileostomy, there are specific foods that are fibrous and difficult to digest that can cause a blockage. Instruct the child to eat slowly and chew well, cut food up into small pieces, and encourage plenty of fluids to help prevent blockages.

Foods that commonly cause blockages include:

- Raw fruits and vegetables, especially celery
- Peelings of apples and potatoes
- Meat with casing (bologna, sausage)
- Popcorn
- Seeds in fruit and vegetables
- Peanuts and other nuts

Consult a WOC nurse regarding additional information on foods that cause blockages, how to treat a blockage, and foods that cause excess gas and odors.

Children with an ileostomy are at risk for becoming dehydrated because they do not have a colon to reabsorb water back into the body. Instruct parents on signs and symptoms of dehydration that can occur from diarrhea, vomiting, or sweating and when to call the doctor or go to the emergency room. Encourage plenty of fluids that replenish sodium and potassium, such as oral rehydration solutions and sport drinks.

Time-released medications may not be absorbed if the child has an ileostomy. Encourage the parent to let their pharmacist know that their child has an ileostomy each time they fill a new prescription.

Activities and School

There are no activity restrictions for infants with ostomies. Infants can lie and play on their stomach and can be hugged and held against an adult without concern of harming the stoma. Keep the pouch tucked into a diaper or under clothing so it is not pulled off while the child is crawling.

All activities including swimming and playing sports are generally allowed for children after obtaining a release from the surgeon. A WOC nurse can be consulted for more information about extra protective gear (stoma cups and pouch belts) during contact sports. Waterproof ostomy tape can be used to "picture frame" the edges of the wafer for extra security when swimming or during sports.

Carry extra pouching supplies in a diaper bag, fanny pack, or small backpack and store in a cool, dry place. The extra supplies should include a pouch that is already cut out to fit and a plastic bag to dispose of the soiled pouch. Pouches cannot be flushed!

Encourage the family to meet with the school nurse to discuss the child's ostomy. The family should find out if there is a private bathroom at school available for the child to use if the pouch needs to be changed or emptied. Have the child keep an extra change of clothes in a backpack, a school locker, or the nurse's office for emergencies.

Discharge

Ensure that the family has information regarding how to reorder ostomy supplies once the child is discharged from the hospital. The family should reorder pouches when they open the last box so they will not run out of supplies.

Resources

Pull-Thru Network—Quarterly newsletter for parents and families with children who have had ostomies
2312 Savoy St.
Hoover AL 35226-1528
(205) 978-2930
http://www.pullthrough.org

NIDDK—National Institute of Diabetes and Digestive and Kidney Disease
http://www.digestive.niddk.nih.gov

Coloplast—Pediatric ostomy literature, Tipster coloring books: "When I met Tipster…A child's story about living with an ostomy"
(800) 533-0464

Hollister—Pediatric ostomy literature and ostomy "Shadow Buddies" dolls for teaching
(800) 323-4060

Convatec—Pediatric ostomy literature
(800) 442-8811

WOCN—*Pediatric Ostomy Care: Best Practice Guideline*
4700 W. Lake Ave.
Glenview, IL 60025-1485
(800) 224-9626
http://www.wocn.org

Procedures Related to Maintaining Cardiorespiratory Function

Oxygen Therapy

Methods include use of a mask, hood, nasal cannula, face tent, or oxygen tent.

Method is selected on the basis of the following:

- Concentration of inspired oxygen needed
- Ability of the child to cooperate in its use

Oxygen is a drug and is administered only as prescribed by dose.

Concentration is regulated according to the needs of the child (usually 40% to 50%, or 4- to 6-L flow).

Oxygen is dry; therefore it must be humidified.

Use the following precautions with an oxygen hood:

- Do not allow oxygen to blow directly on the infant's face.
- Position hood to avoid rubbing against the infant's neck, chin, or shoulders.

Use the following precautions with an oxygen tent:

- Plan nursing activities so tent is opened as little as possible.
- Tuck open edges of tent carefully to reduce oxygen loss (oxygen is heavier than air).
- Check temperature inside tent frequently.
- Keep child warm and dry.
- Make certain cooling mechanism is functioning.
- Examine bedding and clothing periodically, and change as needed.
- Inspect any toys placed in the tent for safety and suitability.
  - Any source of sparks (e.g., from mechanical or electrical toys) is a potential fire hazard.
- Monitor child's color, respirations, and O_2 saturation.
- Periodically analyze oxygen concentration at a point near the child's head, and adjust oxygen flow rate to maintain desired concentration.

Provide comfort and reassurance to the child. Make sure the child is able to see someone nearby.

3 - EVIDENCE-BASED PEDIATRIC NURSING INTERVENTIONS

Invasive and Noninvasive Oxygen Monitoring

An essential goal in managing sick or injured children is to ensure the continuous delivery of adequate oxygen to vital organs. Although life-saving, oxygen therapy can cause a number of serious sequelae. To monitor oxygen therapy, blood oxygen levels are routinely measured.

ARTERIAL BLOOD GAS

Direct sampling of the blood's oxygen content (measured as partial pressure of oxygen [PO_2]) can be done on blood obtained from an indwelling arterial catheter or from arterial puncture (Atraumatic Care box).

ATRAUMATIC CARE

Blood Gas Monitoring

For continuous monitoring of blood gases, noninvasive measurements are used whenever possible. Oximetry should be used before arterial punctures are performed when information about O_2 saturation is sufficient to evaluate the child's condition.

Arterial blood gases may also be drawn via an umbilical arterial catheter in neonates, and a radial arterial catheter is sometimes used for blood sampling. These arterial catheters have inherent dangers, and sampling for arterial blood gases must follow stringent institutional policy to minimize complications.*

Arterial Blood Gas Analysis

Subtle and extreme changes in a patient's status need evaluation by a tool that helps give the "big picture" quickly. Arterial blood gas (ABG) analysis results are rapidly available and provide a baseline to determine a patient's current respiratory and metabolic status and needs.

Interpretation of these variables allows the practitioner to assess the degree to which the patient is able to maintain the most essential of bodily functions: airway and breathing (how well the body provides oxygen to the lungs and eliminates carbon dioxide end-products) and circulation (how well the body carries that oxygen to vital end-organs). Interpretation of ABGs is directed at determining whether the blood pH value—an important determinant of how effectively cellular

*For specific guidelines, see Webster HF: Bioinstrumentation: principles and techniques. In Hazinski MF: *Nursing care of the critically ill child*, ed 2, St Louis, 1992, Mosby.

processes occur—has been affected by a lung problem (respiratory acidosis or alkalosis) or kidney problem (metabolic acidosis or alkalosis).

Blood gases are obtained from an artery either via arterial puncture or from an indwelling arterial line. Ice is used to preserve the blood sample for accurate analysis if it cannot be processed within 15 minutes. Delays in analysis may cause inaccuracies owing to separation of blood cells from plasma.

Blood gas interpretation is based on assessing the arterial serum levels of the following variables:

ABG Component	Normal Levels
pH	7.35 to 7.45
$Paco_2$	35 to 45 mm Hg
HCO_3	22 to 26 mEq/liter
Pao_2	90 to 110 mm Hg

CONSISTENT APPROACH IS KEY

In order to make an interpretation based on the individual ABG values, a consistent sequence of steps should be followed:

1. Evaluate pH to determine presence of acidosis or alkalosis. The lungs and kidneys regulate the hydrogen ion status within the plasma. Alterations in these systems affect the acid-base balance, causing pH changes that affect multiple body systems.
   - Within normal limits (WNL) indicates normal or compensated state
   - Outside normal limits
     <7.35: Acidosis—Acidosis may cause pulmonary vasoconstriction leading to decreased pulmonary blood flow. Acidosis may also cause vasoconstriction to cerebral blood vessels.
     >7.45: Alkalosis—Alkalosis may diminish cellular metabolism, depress myocardial function, and dilate pulmonary blood vessels.
2. Evaluate $Paco_2$ to assess the alveolar ventilation status. In an uncompensated acidosis or alkalosis, an abnormal $Paco_2$ level will generally indicate that origin of the pH imbalance is respiratory rather than metabolic.
   - Within normal limits—Adequate ventilation
   - Outside normal limits
     >45: Hypercarbia—Hypoventilation leads to an increase in $Paco_2$, which in turn lowers the pH, resulting in a respiratory acidosis.
     <30: Hypocarbia—Hyperventilation leads to decreased $Paco_2$, which in turn raises the pH, resulting in a respiratory alkalosis.
3. Evaluate HCO_3 to assess the effectiveness of renal regulation of blood pH. In an uncompensated acidosis or alkalosis, an abnormal HCO_3 level will generally indicate that origin of the pH imbalance is metabolic rather than respiratory.
   - Within normal limits—Normal renal function
   - Outside normal limits
     <22: Decreased bicarbonate—Renal mechanisms lead to increased excretion of bicarbonate and a lower serum bicarbonate level. Owing to the absence of normal levels of bicarbonate to buffer serum H^+ (acid), the pH lowers and metabolic acidosis is the result.
     >29: Increased bicarbonate—Renal mechanisms lead to increased retention of bicarbonate. Owing to the higher levels of bicarbonate, more serum H^+ (acid) is buffered, the pH increases, and metabolic alkalosis is the result.
4. Look for signs of compensation—With prolonged abnormalities in pH, the body tries to return the pH to normal through respiratory compensation (adjusting $Paco_2$ levels) or metabolic compensation (adjusting HCO_3 levels). In a compensated acidosis or alkalosis, the pH will be normal, but the $Paco_2$ and HCO_3 will both be abnormal in the same "direction" (increased or decreased).
   The following table below may be used to assist with differentiation of respiratory versus metabolic acid-base imbalances, including presence of compensation:

Interpretation	pH	$Paco_2$	HCO_3
Acidosis			
Respiratory	<7.35	>45	WNL
Compensated respiratory	WNL	>45	>29
Metabolic	<7.35	WNL	<22
Compensated metabolic	WNL	<30	<22
Alkalosis			
Respiratory	>7.45	<30	WNL
Compensated respiratory	WNL	<30	<22
Metabolic	>7.45	WNL	>29
Compensated metabolic	WNL	>45	>29

WNL, Within normal limits.

5. Evaluate Pao_2 to assess the oxygenation status. It is important to be aware of a patient's specific "normal" values. Patients with certain cardiac or pulmonary conditions may have "acceptable" Pao_2 that is below normal limits. Assess each patient's unique needs and treat accordingly.
   - Within normal limits—Adequate oxygenation
   - Outside normal limits
     55-85: Mild hypoxemia
     40-55: Moderate hypoxemia
     <40: Severe hypoxemia

PULSE OXIMETRY

Measures arterial hemoglobin oxygen saturation (Sao_2) by passage of two different wavelengths of light through blood-perfused tissues to a photodetector. Sao_2 and heart rate are displayed on digital readout.

Attach sensor to earlobe, finger, or toe (Figure 3-14); make certain light source and photodetector are in opposition.

Avoid sites with restricted blood flow (e.g., distal to a blood pressure cuff or indwelling arterial catheter).

Secure sensor cord with self-adhering wrap or tape to avoid interference by patient movement. Shield sensor from bright light. Keep extremity warm (e.g., use a sock over foot or hand if extremity is cool).

Avoid IV dyes; green, purple, or black nail polish; non-opaque synthetic nails; and possibly footprint ink, which may cause erroneous readings.

Change placement of sensor every 4 to 8 hours. Inspect skin at sensor site in compromised children, and change sensor more frequently if needed to prevent pressure necrosis.

Advantages:

- Noninvasive technique
- No complicated preparation or calibration of sensor
- No special skin care needed
- Convenient sites can be used

Disadvantages:

- Requires peripheral arterial pulsation
- Limited use in hypotension or with vasoconstricting drugs
- Sensor affected by movement (Safety Alert)

SaO_2 is related to PO_2, but the values are not the same. As a rule of thumb, an SaO_2 of:

98% = PO_2 of 100 mm Hg or greater
90% = PO_2 of 60 mm Hg
80% = PO_2 of 45 mm Hg
60% = PO_2 of 30 mm Hg

- See Figure 3-15.
- In general, normal range is 95% to 99%. A consistent SaO_2 less than 95% should be investigated, and an SaO_2 of 90% signifies developing hypoxia.

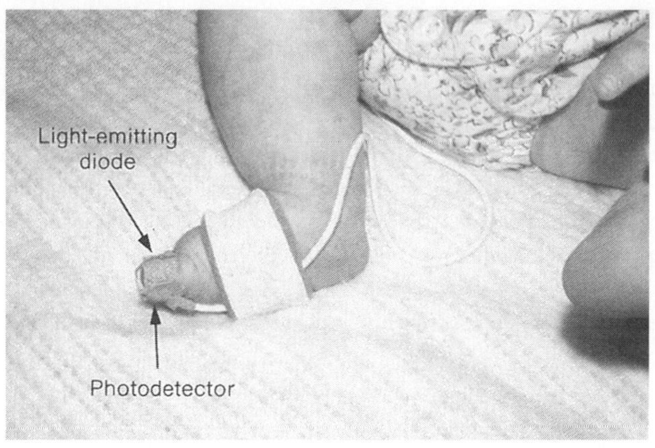

FIGURE **3-14** Oximeter sensor on great toe. Note that sensor is positioned with light-emitting diode opposite photodetector. Cord is secured to foot with self-adhering band (not tape) to minimize movement of sensor.

SAFETY ALERT

For the Infant

Tape the sensor securely to the great toe. Do not apply additional tape to the disposable sensors because it can cause a false reading if the sensor becomes disconnected but remains unnoticed. Place a snugly fitting sock over the foot.

For the Child

Tape the sensor securely to the index finger, and tape the wire to the back of the hand. Use self-adhering Ace-type wrap (e.g., CoFlex) around the finger and/or hand to further secure the sensor and cord.

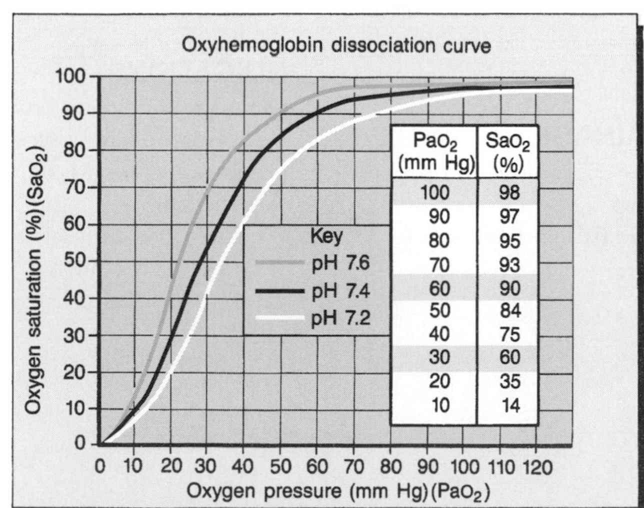

PaO_2 (mm Hg)	SaO_2 (%)
100	98
90	97
80	95
70	93
60	90
50	84
40	75
30	60
20	35
10	14

FIGURE **3-15** Oxyhemoglobin dissociation curve. Changes in the affinity of hemoglobin for oxygen shift the position of the oxyhemoglobin dissociation curve. Standard curve *(middle curve):* Assumes normal pH (7.4), temperature, PCO_2, and 2,3-DPG levels. Shift to left *(left curve):* Increases O_2 affinity of Hb; decreased pH; and increased temperature, PCO_2, and 2,3-DPG. Shift to right *(right curve):* Decreases O_2 affinity of Hb; decreased pH, and increased temperature, PCO_2, and 2,3-DPG.

TRANSCUTANEOUS OXYGEN MONITORING

Measures transcutaneous partial pressure of oxygen in arterial blood ($tcPaO_2$) (amount of oxygen dissolved in blood). An electrode attached to the skin causes local hyperemia and arterialization of blood within the capillaries beneath the electrode. A current, created as oxygen diffuses from the capillaries through the skin and a semipermeable membrane, is measured and converted to partial pressure of oxygen (PO_2). This is displayed on a digital readout. Place electrode on an area with good blood flow but thin subcutaneous skin.

Children—Place on chest.
Newborns and young infants—Place on chest, abdomen, or back.
Thin infants—Place center of sensor over an intercostal space on chest.

Avoid any pressure on electrode (e.g., infant lying on sensor).
Keep temperature of electrode at 44° or 45° C for term infants.
Change placement of electrode every 3 to 4 hours; change more frequently if needed to prevent superficial burns.
Recalibrate electrode each time it is moved.

Aerosol Therapy

The purpose is the inhalation of a solution in droplet (particle) form for direct deposition in the tracheobronchial tree.
Aerosols consist of liquid medications (e.g., bronchodilators, steroids, mucolytics, decongestants, antibiotics, antiviral agents) suspended in a particulate form in air.
Aerosol generators propelled by air or air-oxygen mixtures generally fall into three categories:

- Small-volume jet nebulizers or hand-held nebulizers
- Ultrasonic nebulizers for sterile water or saline aerosol only
- Metered-dose inhalers (MDIs) (sometimes with a "spacer" device that acts as a reservoir and simplifies use of the inhaler; devices such as the Rotohaler or Turbuhaler eliminate the need for a spacer device and are easier for young children to use)

Deposition of aerosol is maximized by instructing the child to breathe through the mouth with slow, deep inhalations, followed by holding the breath for 5 to 10 seconds, then slow exhalations while in an upright position.
Using an incentive spirometer can help a cooperative child learn this ventilatory pattern.
For infants and young children, activities to produce deep breathing and coughing include feet tapping, tactile stimulation, and crying. The infant must be held upright.
Assessment of breath sounds and work of breathing is performed before and after treatments.

Bronchial (Postural) Drainage*

The purpose is to facilitate drainage and expectoration of lung and bronchial secretions from specific areas by correct positioning of the patient, using gravity as an aid (Figures 3-16 and 3-17).

AIDS TO FACILITATE DRAINAGE

Consistency of lung secretions is changed from viscid to more liquid by use of the following:

- Maintenance of adequate fluid balance (oral or IV)
- Medication (mucolytics)
- Percussion and vibration
- Cough stimulation
- Breathing exercises

INDICATIONS

Pulmonary conditions: bronchitis, cystic fibrosis, pneumonia, asthma, lung abscess, obstructive lung disease
Postoperative prophylaxis: thoracotomy, stasis pneumonia
Prophylaxis in:

- Prolonged artificial ventilation
- Paralytic conditions
- Unconscious patient

*See Patient and Family Education, pp. 567-569.

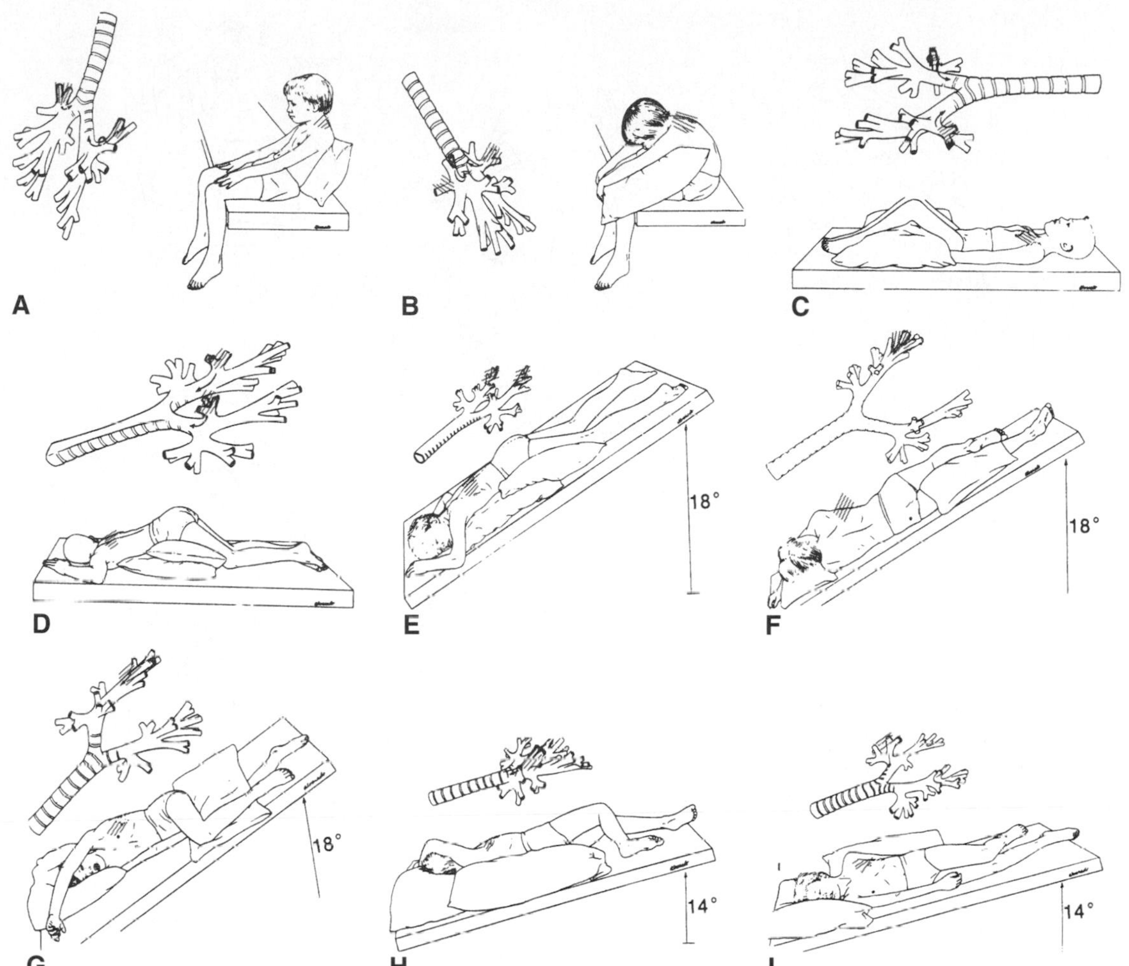

FIGURE **3-16** Bronchial drainage positions for all major lung segments of child. For each position, model of tracheobronchial tree is projected beside child to show segmental bronchus *(striped)*. Drainage platform is horizontal unless otherwise noted. Striped area on child's chest indicates area to be cupped or vibrated by therapist. **A,** Apical segment of right upper lobe and apical subsegment of apical-posterior segment of left upper lobe. **B,** Posterior segment of right upper lobe and posterior subsegment of apical-posterior segment of left upper lobe. **C,** Anterior segments of both upper lobes; child should be rotated slightly away from side being drained. **D,** Superior segments of both lower lobes. **E,** Posterior basal segments of both lower lobes. **F,** Lateral basal segments of right lower lobe; left lateral basal segment would be drained by mirror image of this position (right side down). **G,** Anterior basal segment of left lower lobe; right anterior basal segment would be drained by mirror image of this position (left side down). **H,** Medial and lateral segments of right middle lobe. **I,** Lingular segments (superior and inferior) of left upper lobe (homologue of right middle lobe). (From Chernick V, editor: *Kendig's disorders of the respiratory tract of children*, ed 6, Philadelphia, 1998, Saunders.)

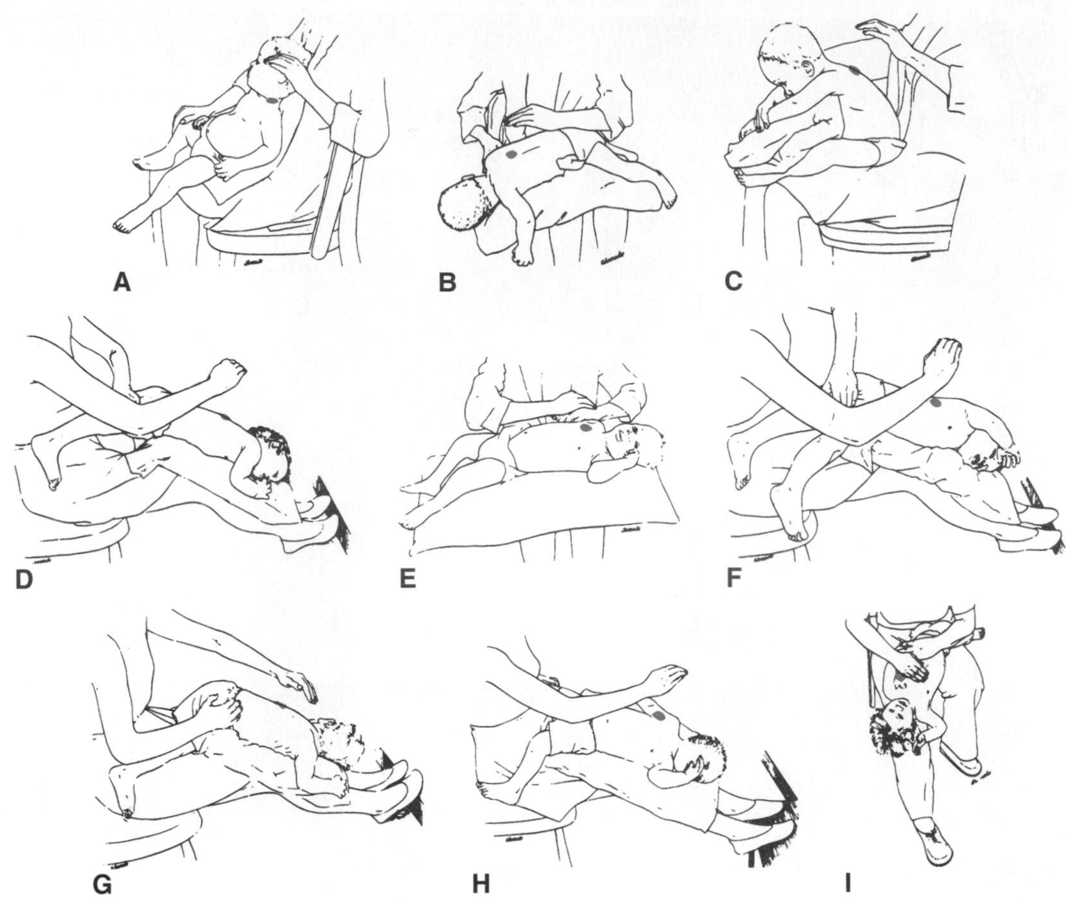

FIGURE **3-17** Bronchial drainage positions for all major lung segments of infant. Procedure is most easily carried out in therapist's lap. Therapist's hand indicates area to be cupped or vibrated. **A,** Apical segment of left upper lobe. **B,** Posterior segment of left upper lobe. **C,** Anterior segment of left upper lobe. **D,** Superior segment of right lower lobe. **E,** Posterior basal segment of right lower lobe. **F,** Lateral basal segment of right lower lobe. **G,** Anterior basal segment of right lower lobe. **H,** Medial and lateral segments of right middle lobe. **I,** Lingular segments (superior and inferior) of left upper lobe. (Modified from Cystic Fibrosis Foundation: *Infant segmental bronchial drainage*, Rockville, Md, The Foundation.)

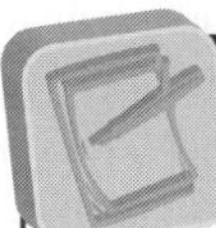

GUIDELINES

Use of a Peak Expiratory Flow Meter (PEFM)

1. Before each use, make sure the sliding marker or arrow on the PEFM is at the bottom of the numbered scale.
2. Stand up straight.
3. Remove gum or any food from the mouth.
4. Close your lips tightly around the mouthpiece. Be sure to keep your tongue away from the mouthpiece.
5. Blow out as hard and as quickly as you can, a "fast, hard puff."
6. Note the number by the marker on the numbered scale.
7. Perform entire routine three times, but wait at least 30 seconds between each routine.
8. Record the *highest* of the three readings, not the average.
9. Measure your peak expiratory flow rate (PEFR) at close to the same time and in the same way each day (e.g., morning and evening; before and 15 minutes after taking medication).
10. Keep a chart of your PEFRs.

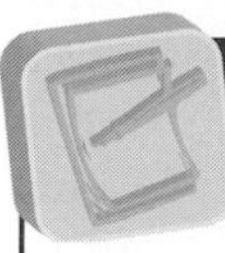

GUIDELINES

Use of a Metered-Dose Inhaler (MDI)

Steps for Checking How Much Medicine Is in the Canister

1. If the canister is new, it is full.
2. If the canister has been used repeatedly, it might be empty. (Check product label to see how many inhalations should be in each canister.)
3. The most accurate way to determine how many doses remain in an MDI is to count and record each actuation as it is used.
4. Many dry powder inhalers have a dose-counting device or dose indicator on the canister to let you know when the canister is empty.
5. Placing dry powder inhalers or MDIs with hydrofluoroalkanes in water will destroy these inhalers.

Steps for Using the Inhaler*

1. Remove the cap, and hold inhaler upright.
2. Shake the inhaler.
3. Tilt the head back slightly, and breathe out slowly.
4. With the inhaler in an upright position, insert the mouthpiece:
   - About 3-4 cm from the mouth *or*
   - Into an aerochamber *or*
   - Into the mouth, forming an airtight seal between the lips and the mouthpiece
5. At the end of a normal expiration, depress the top of the inhaler canister firmly to release the medication (into either the aerochamber or the mouth), and breathe in slowly (about 3 to 5 seconds). Relax the pressure on the top of the canister.
6. Hold the breath for at least 5 to 10 seconds to allow the aerosol medication to reach deeply into the lungs.
7. Remove the inhaler, and breathe out slowly through the nose.
8. Wait 1 minute between puffs (if additional one is needed).

Modified from Nurses' Asthma Education Working Group: *Nurses: partners in asthma care,* NIH Publication No. 95-3308, Bethesda, Md, 1995, National Heart Lung and Blood Institute, National Institutions of Health.

*NOTE: Inhaled dry powder such as Pulmicort requires a different inhalation technique. To use a dry powder inhaler, the base of the device is turned until a click is heard. It is important to close the mouth tightly around the mouthpiece of the inhaler and inhale rapidly.

Tracheostomy Care

Tracheostomy is a surgical opening in the trachea between the second and fourth tracheal rings (Figure 3-18). Congenital or acquired structural defects, such as subglottic stenosis, tracheomalacia, and vocal cord paralysis, account for many long-term tracheostomies. A tracheostomy may be required in an emergency situation for epiglottitis, croup, or foreign body aspiration. These tracheostomies remain in place for a short time. An infant or child requiring long-term ventilatory support may also have a tracheostomy.

Pediatric tracheostomy tubes are usually made of plastic or Silastic (Figures 3-19 and 3-20). The most common types are the Hollinger, Jackson, Aberdeen, and Shiley tubes. These tubes are constructed with a more acute angle than adult tubes, and they soften at body temperature, conforming to the contours of the trachea. Because these materials resist the formation of crusted respiratory secretions, they are made without an inner cannula. Some children require a metal tracheostomy tube (usually made of sterling silver or stainless steel), which contains an inner cannula. The principal advantages of metal tubes are their nonreactivity and decreased chance for an allergic reaction.

TRACHEOSTOMY SUCTIONING

The practice of instilling sterile saline in the tracheostomy tube before suctioning (Figure 3-21) is not supported by research and is no longer recommended by many institutions. Suctioning should require no more than 5 seconds. Counting 1, one thousand, 2, one thousand, 3, one thousand, and so on while suctioning is a simple means for monitoring the time. Without a safeguard, the airway may be obstructed for too long. Hyperventilating the child with 100% O_2 before and after suctioning (using a bag-valve-mask or increasing the FiO_2 ventilator setting) is also performed to prevent hypoxia.

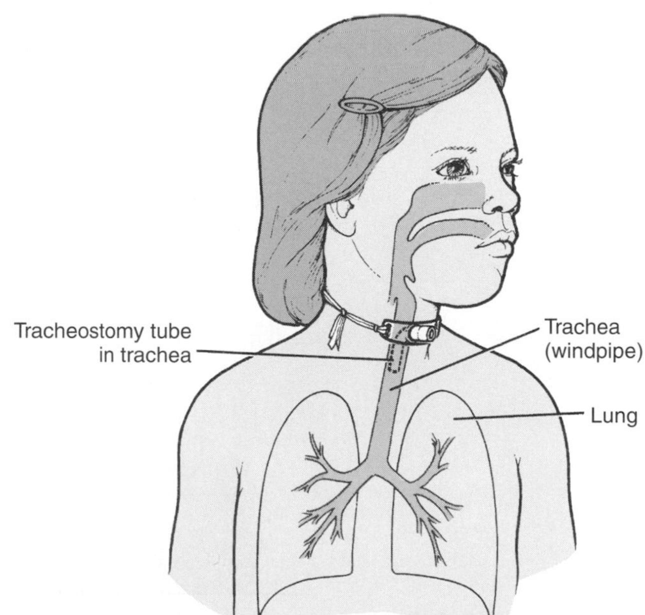

FIGURE **3-18** Tracheostomy tube in trachea and securely tied with cloth tape.

Closed tracheal suctioning systems that allow for uninterrupted O_2 delivery may also be used. In a closed suction system a suction catheter is directly attached to the ventilator tubing. This system has several advantages. First, there is no need to disconnect the patient from the ventilator, which allows for better oxygenation. Second, the suction catheter is enclosed in a plastic sheath, which reduces the risk of exposure to the patient's secretions.

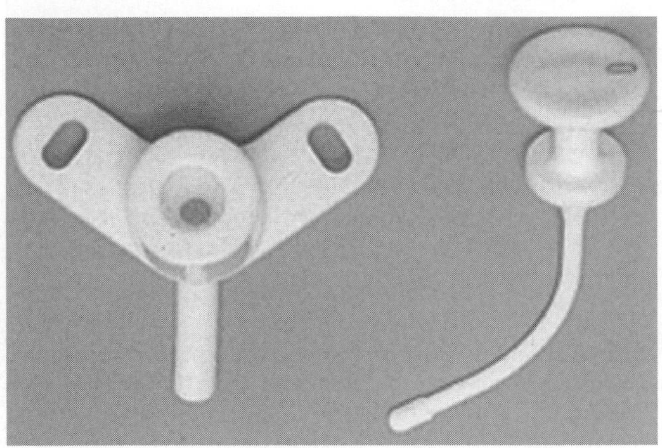

FIGURE **3-19** Silastic pediatric tracheostomy tube and obturator.

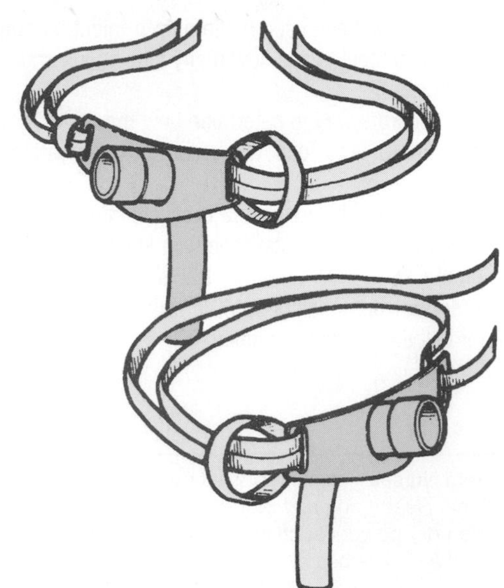

FIGURE **3-20** Pediatric tracheostomy tube. **A,** Cloth tape secured at both sides to be tied in back. **B,** Cloth tape secured on one side and looped through other side to be tied at side.

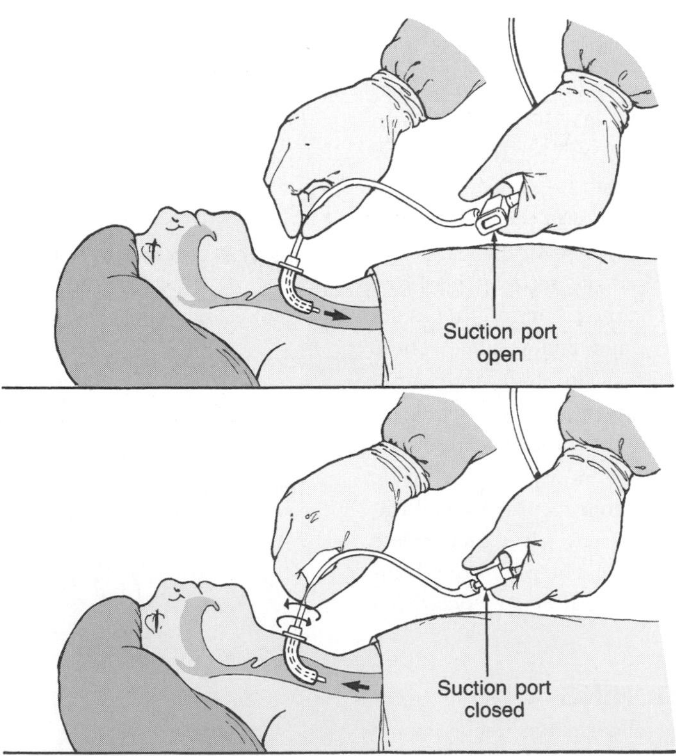

FIGURE **3-21** Tracheostomy suctioning. **A,** Insertion, port open. **B,** Withdrawal, port occluded. Note that catheter is inserted just slightly beyond end of tracheostomy tube.

EVIDENCE-BASED PRACTICE

Normal Saline Instillation Before Suctioning—Helpful or Harmful?

Marilyn J. Hockenberry

Ask the Question

Question

In intubated children and those with tracheostomy, is normal saline instillation before suctioning helpful or harmful?

Background

Removal of secretions to maintain a patent airway often requires endotracheal (ET) suctioning in children. A common technique is to instill 3 to 10 ml of normal saline into the ET tube before suctioning. This review explores the evidence on this technique.

Objective

To evaluate the evidence on normal saline instillation before suctioning

Search for Evidence

Search Strategies

Searched all literature within the child population

Databases Used

PubMed, Cochrane Collaboration, MDConsult, BestBETs, PedsCCM

Critically Analyze the Evidence

- Instillation of normal saline before ET tube suctioning has been used for years as a method to loosen and dilute secretion, lubricate the suction catheter, and promote cough. In recent years the possible adverse effects of this procedure have been explored. Adult studies have found decreased oxygen saturation, increased frequency of nosocomial pneumonia, and increased intracranial pressure after instillation of normal saline before suctioning (O'Neal, Grap, Thompson, and others, 2001; Kinlock, 1999; Hagler and Traver, 1994; Reynolds, Hoffman, Schlichtig, and others, 1990; Ackerman, 1993; Ackerman and Gugerty, 1990; Bostick and Wendelgass, 1987).
- Two of the first research studies evaluating the effect of normal saline instillation before suctioning in neonates found no deleterious effects. Shorten, Byrne, and Jones (1991) found no significant differences in oxygenation, heart rate, or blood pressure before or after suctioning in a group of 27 intubated neonates.
- In a second study of nine neonates acting as their own controls, no adverse effects on lung mechanics were found after normal saline instillation and suctioning (Beeram and Dhanireddy, 1992).
- A recent study evaluating the effects of normal saline instillation before suctioning in children found results similar to those in the previously published adult studies. Ridling, Martin, and Bratton (2003) evaluated the effects of normal saline instillation before suctioning in a group of 24 critically ill children, ages 10 weeks to 14 years (level 1 evidence). A total of 104 suctioning episodes were analyzed. Children experienced significantly greater oxygen desaturation after suctioning if normal saline was instilled.
- The American Thoracic Society's (2005) official position statement on the care of children with tracheostomies now states that normal saline should not be instilled before suctioning.

Apply The Evidence: Nursing Implications

Studies support that the adverse effects of normal saline instillation before suctioning in children are similar to those found for adults. This technique causes a significant reduction in oxygen saturation that can last up to 2 minutes after suctioning. The evidence does not support the use of normal saline instillation before ET suctioning in children.

References

Ackerman MH: The effect of saline lavage prior to suctioning, *Am J Crit Care* 2(4):326-330, 1993.

Ackerman MH, Gugerty B: The effect of normal saline bolus instillation in artificial airways, *The Journal,* Spring:14-17, 1990.

American Thoracic Society: Care of the child with a chronic tracheostomy, 2005, Retrieved April 17, 2006, from *http://www.thoracic.org/sections/publications/statements/pages/respiratory-disease-pediatric/childtrach1-12.html.*

Beeram MR, Dhanireddy R: Effects of saline instillation during tracheal suction on lung mechanics in newborn infants, *J Perinatol* 12(2):120-123, 1992.

Bostick J, Wendelgass ST: Normal saline instillation as part of the suctioning procedure: effects of Pa_{O_2} and amount of secretions, *Heart Lung* 16(5):532-537, 1987.

Hagler DA, Traver GA: Endotracheal saline and suction catheters: sources of lower airway contamination, *Am J Crit Care* 3(6):444-447, 1994.

Kinlock D: Instillation of normal saline during endotracheal suctioning: effects on mixed venous oxygen saturation, *Am J Crit Care* 8(4):231-240, 1999.

O'Neal PV, Grap MJ, Thompson C, and others: Level of dyspnoea experienced in mechanically ventilated adults with and without saline instillation prior to endotracheal suctioning, *Intensive Crit Care Nurs* 17(6):356-363, 2001.

Reynolds P, Hoffman LA, Schlichtig R, and others: Effects of normal saline instillation on secretion volume, dynamic compliance, and oxygen saturation (abstract), *Am Rev Respir Dis* 141:A574, 1990.

Ridling DA, Martin LD, Bratton SL: Endotracheal suctioning with or without instillation of isotonic sodium chloride in critically ill children, *Am J Crit Care* 12(3):212-219, 2003.

Shorten DR, Byrne PJ, Jones RL: Infant responses to saline instillations and endotracheal suctioning, *J Obstet Gynecol Neonatal Nurs* 20(6):464-469, 1991.

Suctioning, Catheter Length, and Saline

Traditional technique for suctioning ET or tracheostomy tubes recommends advancing a suction catheter into the tube until it meets resistance, then withdrawing it slightly and applying suction. However, studies indicate that this approach causes trauma to the tracheobronchial wall. This trauma can be avoided by inserting the catheter and advancing it to the premeasured depth of just to the tip (especially in infants) or no more than 0.5 cm beyond the tube (Kleiber, Krutzfield, and Rose, 1988).

Calibrated catheters are easier to use for premeasured suctioning technique, but unmarked catheters can also be used. To measure the length for catheter insertion, place the catheter near a sample ET or tracheostomy tube (same size as child's tube), with the end of the catheter at the correct position. Grasp the catheter with a sterile-gloved hand to mark the length, and insert the catheter until the hand reaches the stoma.

It has been common practice to instill a bolus of NS into the tube before suctioning. However, this technique may contribute to lower airway colonization and nosocomial pneumonia through repeated washing of organisms from the tube's surface into the lower airway (Hagler and Traver, 1994). The use of saline has been shown to have an adverse effect on SaO_2, and it should not be used routinely in patients receiving mechanical ventilation who have a pulmonary infection (Ackerman, 1998). Although the pediatric research is scarce, routine use of NS with ET tube suctioning should be avoided (Curley and Moloney-Harmon, 2001).

Cardiopulmonary Resuscitation

PROCEDURES FOR CARDIOPULMONARY RESUSCITATION

Methods of cardiopulmonary resuscitation (CPR) for health care workers are discussed in Figure 3-22. Figure 3-23 shows procedures for airway obstruction. Several changes were made in 2005 by the American Heart Association, including different hand positioning for two-rescuer infant CPR and a change in the age definition of children by health care providers. A single compression/ventilation ratio of 30:2 was also adopted for one-rescuer CPR for all ages except newborns. CPR for lay people is in the Patient and Family Education on pp. 576 to 580.

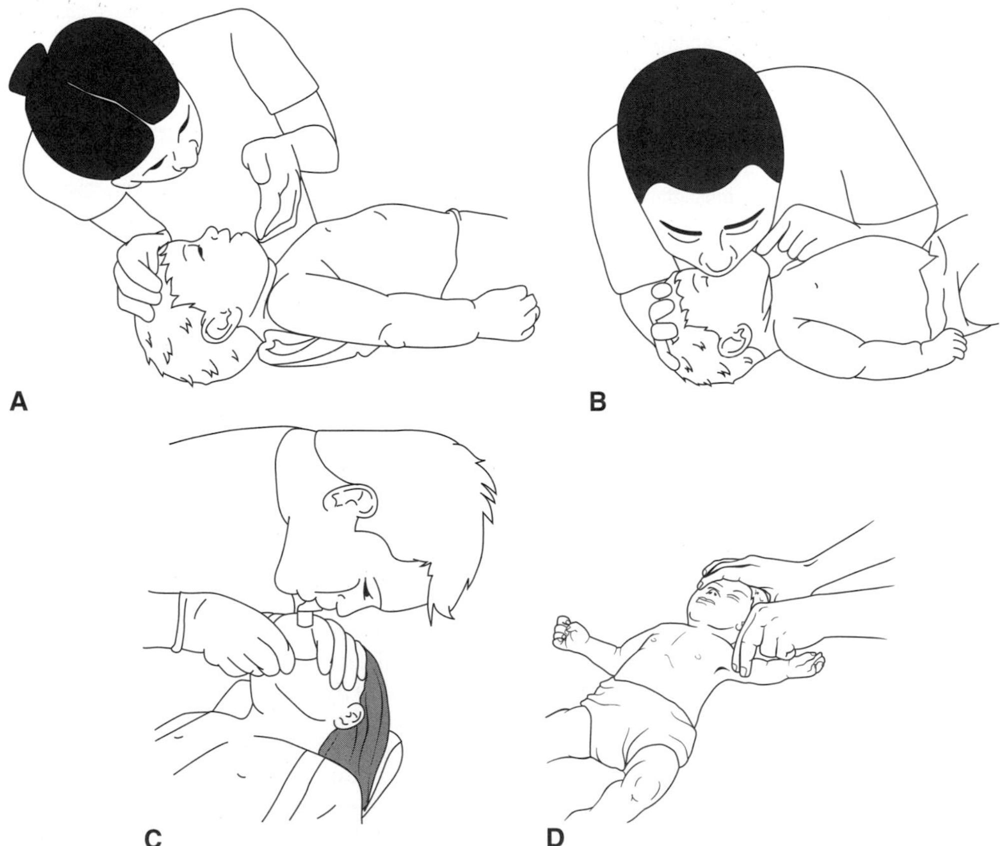

FIGURE **3-22** CPR guidelines. **A,** Open airway and check breathing. **B,** Mouth-to-mouth-and-nose breathing for an infant. **C,** Mouth-to-barrier breathing for child; mask covers nose and mouth. **D,** Locating and palpating the brachial pulse.

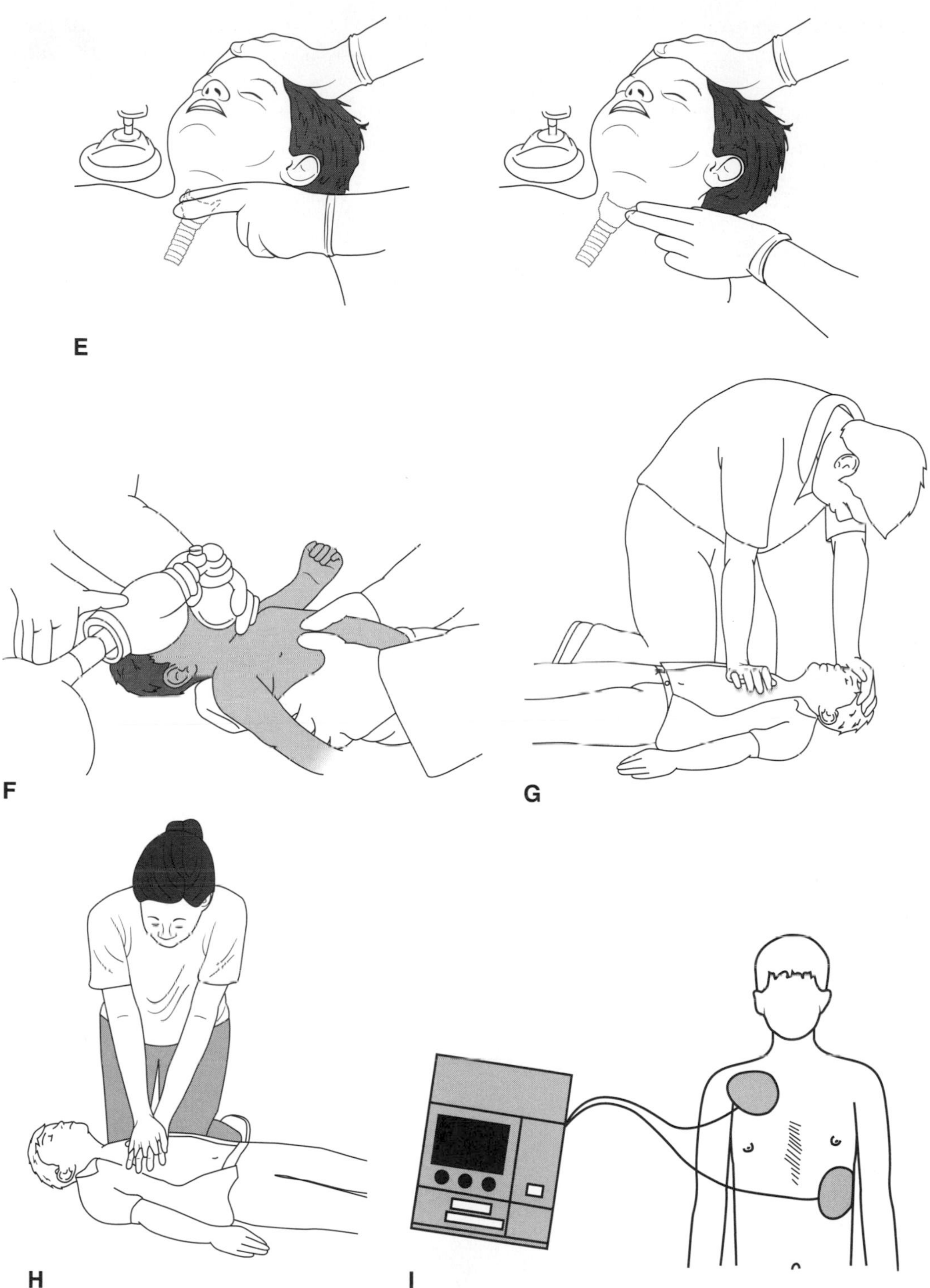

FIGURE **3-22, cont'd** CPR guidelines. **E,** Locating *(left)* and palpating *(right)* the carotid artery pulse. **F,** Two-rescuer chest compression technique in infant. **G,** One-handed chest compressions in a child. **H,** Two-handed chest compressions in a child or adult. **I,** Placement of the AED on a child.

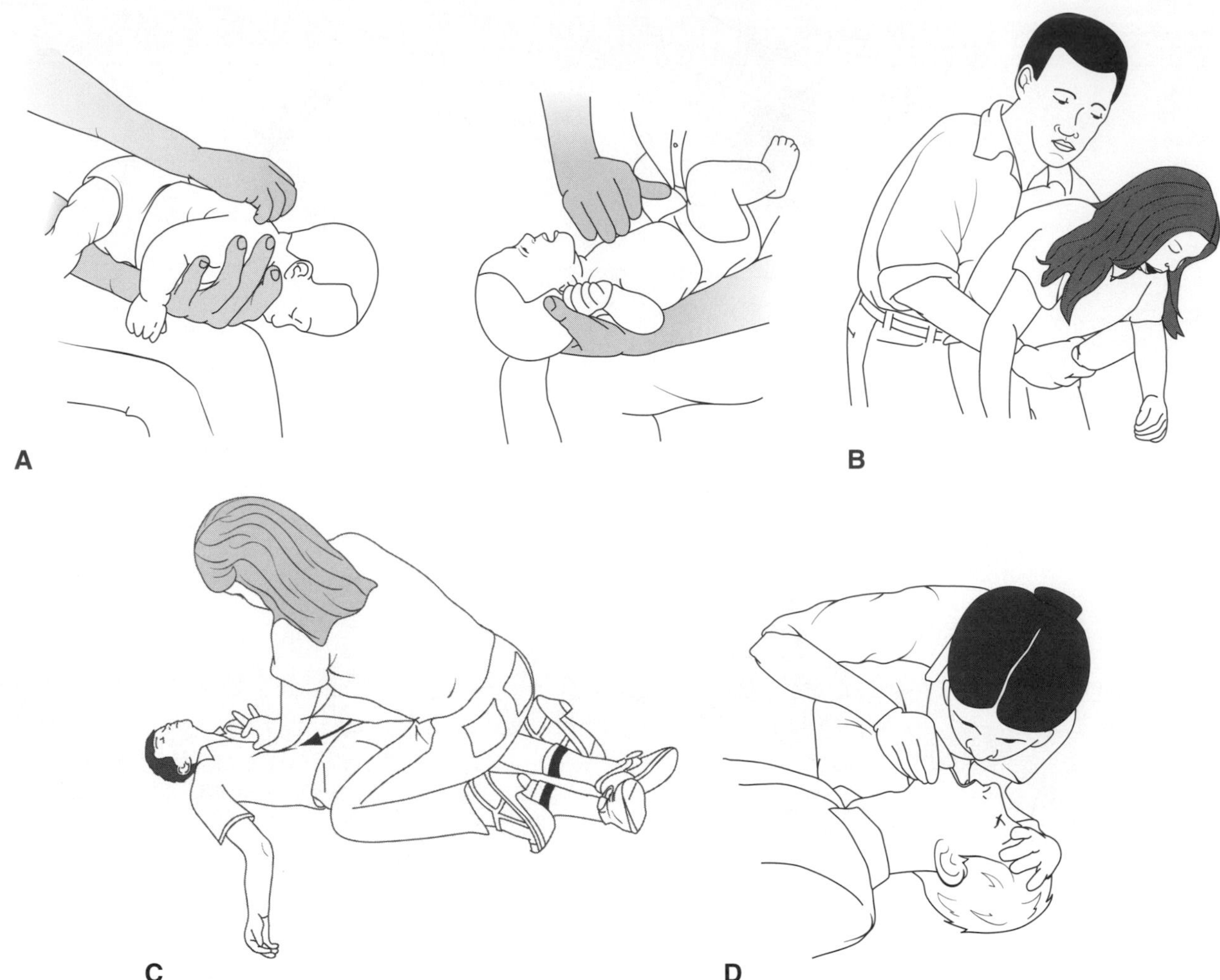

FIGURE **3-23** Procedures for airway obstruction. **A,** Relief of choking in the infant. *Left,* Back slaps. *Right,* Chest thrusts. **B,** Abdominal thrusts in standing choking child. **C,** Abdominal thrusts in supine choking child. **D,** Open airway and look for object.

Summary of Basic Life Support Maneuvers for Infants, Children, and Adults*

Maneuver	Adult **Lay rescuer:** ≥8 years **HCP:** Adolescent and older	Child **Lay rescuer:** 1-8 years **HCP:** 1 year to adolescence	Infant <1 year of age
Activate Emergency response Number (1 rescuer)	Activate when victim found unresponsive **HCP:** If asphyxial arrest likely, call after 5 cycles (2 minutes) of CPR	Activate after performing 5 cycles of CPR For sudden, witnessed collapse, activate after verifying that victim unresponsive	
Airway	Head tilt–chin lift (**HCP:** suspected trauma, use jaw thrust)		
Breaths Initial	2 breaths at 1 sec/breath	2 effective breaths at 1 sec/breath	
HCP: Rescue breathing without chest compressions	10-12 breaths/min (approximately 1 breath every 5-6 seconds)	12-20 breaths/min (approximately 1 breath every 3-5 seconds)	
HCP: Rescue breaths for CPR with advanced airway	8-10 breaths/min (approximately 1 breath every 6-8 seconds)		
Foreign-body airway obstruction	Abdominal thrusts		Back slaps and chest thrusts
Circulation **HCP:** Pulse check (≤10 seconds)	Carotid (**HCP** can use femoral in child)		Brachial or femoral
Compression landmarks	Center of chest, between nipples		Just below nipple line
Compression method Push hard and fast Allow complete recoil	**2 Hands:** Heel of 1 hand, other hand on top	**2 Hands:** Heel of 1 hand with second on top *or* **1 Hand:** Heel of 1 hand only	**1 Rescuer:** 2 fingers **HCP, 2 rescuers:** 2 thumb encircling hands
Compression depth	1½-2 inches	Approximately ⅓-½ the depth of the chest	
Compression rate	Approximately 100/min		
Compression-ventilation ratio	30:2 (1 or 2 rescuers)	30:2 (1 rescuer) **HCP:** 15:2 (2 rescuers)	
Defibrillation			
AED	Use adult pads. Do not use child pads/child system. **HCP:** For out-of-hospital response, may provide 5 cycles/2 minutes of CPR before shock if response >4-5 minutes and arrest not witnessed.	**HCP:** Use AED as soon as available for sudden collapse and in-hospital. **All:** After 5 cycles of CPR (out-of-hospital). If available, use child pads/child system for child 1-8 years. If pads/system not available, use adult AED pads.	No recommendation for infants <1 year of age.

From American Heart Association: 2005 American Heart Association guidelines for cardiopulmonary resuscitation and emergency cardiovascular care, *Circulation* 112:IV-12–IV-18, 2005.
HCP, Maneuvers used only by health care provider; *AED,* automated external defibrillator.
*Newborn/neonatal information not included.

DRUGS FOR PEDIATRIC CARDIOPULMONARY RESUSCITATION

Drug and Dose	Action	Implication
Epinephrine HCl* IV/IO: 0.01 mg/kg (1:10,000) Repeat doses: 0.01 mg/kg (1:10,000) Endotracheal tube (ET): 0.1 mg/kg (1:1000)	Adrenergic Acts on both α- and β-receptor sites, especially heart and vascular and other smooth muscle	Most useful drug in cardiac arrest Disappears rapidly from bloodstream after injection; instill 5 ml saline after ET administration May produce renal vessel constriction and decreased urine formation
Sodium bicarbonate IV/IO: 1 mEq/kg dose Newborn: 0.5 mEq/ml (4.2%)	Alkalinizer Buffers pH	Infuse slowly and only when ventilation is adequate; flush with saline before and after administration Do not mix with catecholamines or calcium
Atropine sulfate* 0.02 mg/kg/dose Minimum dose: 0.1 mg Maximum single dose: infants and children, 0.5 mg; adolescents, 1 mg	Anticholinergic-parasympatholytic Increases cardiac output, heart rate by blocking vagal stimulation in heart	Used to treat bradycardia after ventilatory assessment Always provide adequate ventilation and monitor O_2 saturation Produces pupillary dilation, which constricts with light
Calcium chloride 10% 20 mg/kg IV/IO 0.2 mg/kg/dose q10min	Electrolyte replacement Needed for maintenance of normal cardiac contractility	Used only for hypocalcemia, calcium blocker overdose, hyperkalemia, or hypermagnesemia Administer slowly; very sclerosing; administer in central vein Incompatible with phosphate solutions
Lidocaine HCl* 1 mg/kg/dose	Antidysrhythmic Inhibits nerve impulses from sensory nerves	Used for ventricular arrhythmias only
Amiodarone IV: 5 mg/kg over 30 min followed by continuous infusion Starting at 5 mcg/kg/min May increase to maximum 10 mcg/kg/min	Antidysrhythmic agent Inhibits adrenergic stimulation; prolongs action potential and refractory period in myocardial tissues; decreased atrioventricular (AV) conduction and sinus node function	Recommended as first choice for shock-refractory ventricular tachycardia Contraindicated in severe sinus node dysfunction, marked sinus bradycardia, 2nd- and 3rd-degree AV block Monitor ECG and blood pressure
Adenosine 0.1-0.2 mg/kg as a rapid IV bolus Maximum single initial dose: 6-12 mg (given over 1-2 sec) May repeat administration: double initial dose (maximum dose = 12 mg) repeat Follow with 5 ml normal saline flush	Antidysrhythmic, for supraventricular tachycardia Causes temporary block through AV node and interrupts reentry circuits	Administer by rapid IV push followed by saline flush May cause transient bradycardia

IO, Intraosseous; *IV,* intravenous.

*These drugs may be administered via ET tube if IV/IO is not available; IV/IO is the preferred route.

†Dose of naloxone to reverse respiratory depression without reversing analgesia from opioids is 0.5 mcg/kg in children <40 kg (88 lb) (American Pain Society, 1999).

Drug and Dose	Action	Implication
Naloxone (Narcan)* mg/kg/dose† May repeat q2-3min	Reverses respiratory arrest caused by excessive opiate administration	Evaluate level of pain after administration because analgesic effects of opioids are reversed with large doses of naloxone
Magnesium sulfate 25-50 mg/kg IV/IO Maximum: 2 g	Inhibits calcium channels and causes smooth muscle relaxation	Given by rapid IV infusion for suspected hypomagnesemia Have calcium gluconate (IV) available as antidote
Infusions		
Epinephrine HCl infusion 0.05 mcg/kg/min	Adrenergic See above	Titrated to desired hemodynamic effect
Dopamine HCl infusion 2 mcg/kg/min	Agonist Acts on alpha receptors, causing vasoconstriction Increases cardiac output	Titrated to desired hemodynamic response
Dobutamine HCl infusion 2 mcg/kg/min	Adrenergic direct-acting β_2-agonist Increases contractility and heart rate	Titrated to desired hemodynamic response Little vasoconstriction, even at high rates
Lidocaine HCl infusion 20-50 mcg/kg/min	Antidysrhythmic Increases electrical stimulation threshold of ventricle	See above Lower infusion dose used in shock

EVIDENCE-BASED PRACTICE

Family Presence During Resuscitation of a Child

David Wilson

Ask the Question

Question

Is family presence at the resuscitation of a child perceived by the family as a positive event?

Objective

To evaluate the evidence on the effect of family presence during a respiratory or cardiac arrest

Background

For families whose child has a respiratory or cardiac arrest, support is aimed at keeping the family informed of the child's status and helping them to cope with a near-death experience or an actual death. Uncertainty regarding the outcome—both mortality and morbidity—is a primary concern. In the past, few acute care facilities have allowed parents to remain during CPR or a "code." The traditional thinking was that this experience would be upsetting to parents and that family members would require care that would interfere with resuscitation efforts. Traditionally, family members have not been allowed to be present during resuscitation efforts. However, there is increasing evidence in the literature that family presence during adult resuscitation is entirely acceptable and rapidly becoming the standard of care. The topic continues to be controversial among health care workers.

Search for Evidence

Search Strategies

The literature was searched to obtain information regarding the presence of family members during the resuscitation of a child family member. The literature published between 1994 and 2005 was searched.

Databases Used

PubMed, CINAHL, professional organization websites

Critically Analyze the Evidence

A number of studies in adult patients indicate that family presence during invasive procedures and resuscitation alleviates the family's anger about being separated from the patient during a crisis, reduces their anxiety, eliminates doubts about what was done to help the patient, facilitates the grieving process, increases the perception of the patient as an individual and ascribed respect for the patient, lessens the family's feelings of helplessness, allows closure and affords a chance to say good-bye, facilitates a relationship between the medical staff and family through increased communication, and helps family understand the gravity or severity of the child's condition (Meyers, Eichhorn, Guzzetta, and others, 2000; Powers and Rubenstein, 1999; Sacchetti, Lichenstein, Caraccio, and others, 1996; Eichhorn, Meyers, Mitchell, and others, 1996; Tucker, 2002). In many cases family members expressed that it was their right to be present when a family member receives emergent treatment or resuscitation.

Interviews with 39 English-speaking family members and 96 health care providers who were present in the emergency department (ED) during invasive procedures or CPR (Meyers and others, 2000) revealed that their presence at the procedure was helpful and found that they would do it again. Ninety-six percent of the nurses and 79% of the attending physicians supported family presence and felt it should be continued at the hospital. Family members said they wanted to be at the patient's side during the ED visit that involved resuscitation; 80% wanted to be present during the patient's resuscitation when given the choice. The sample consisted mostly of adult patients, and only the mean age of the group is provided (44.5 ± 23.1 years).

In a survey of parents with children admitted to the ED for invasive procedures and possibly CPR, family members responded favorably to being present if the child was conscious (less favorably if child was unconscious) on admission to the ED, and 83 % of the respondents expressed a desire to be present if the child was likely to die (Boie, Moore, Brummett, and others, 1999). The survey consisted of five case scenarios with increasing level of invasiveness, and the parent was asked to respond whether or not he or she would want to be present at the family member's bedside during the procedure.

Professional organizations support the presence of family members during CPR. The Emergency Nurses Association (2001) has developed national guidelines for family presence during invasive procedures and CPR. These guidelines include recommendations for assessing family members to determine if family presence is appropriate and the use of a family facilitator (e.g., a nurse, child-life specialist, social worker, or chaplain) who remains with the family during resuscitation to answer questions, clarify information, and offer comfort.

The American Heart Association (2000) recommended that providers offer families the option to remain with the loved one during resuscitation. Likewise, the *PALS Provider* (Pediatric Advanced Life Support) *Manual* (Hazinski, Zaritsky, Nadkarni, and others, 2002) supports the presence of family during the child's CPR with the presence of a family support facilitator. Protocols to prepare and support family presence should be implemented; a sample protocol based on the recommendations of the Association for Care of Children's Health may be found in Meyers, Eichhorn, Guzzetta, and others' publication (2000).

Some studies addressed health care workers' attitudes about family presence during resuscitation of a child (O'Brien, Creamer, Hill, and others, 2002; Mangurten, Scott, Guzzetta, and others, 2005; Sacchetti, Carraccio, Leva, and others, 2000; Tsai, 2002), or adult family member (Sanford, Pugh, and Warren, 2002). Health care workers' attitudes about family presence during resuscitation vary considerably. Sixty percent of the HCWs (nurses and physicians) surveyed said they felt comfortable performing resuscitation procedures with a family member present; there was no distinction made between adult or child patient (Mangurten and others, 2005). ED staff with previous experience in having family members present during pediatric resuscitation favored the practice whereas the staff without prior exposure to family presence were against the practice (Sacchetti and others, 2000). Tsai (2002) asserted that most physicians and nurses do not favor family members' presence during resuscitation procedures, and in O'Brien and colleagues' (2002)

EVIDENCE-BASED PRACTICE

Family Presence During Resuscitation of a Child—cont'd

survey of pediatricians, nurses, and residents, 65% said they would not allow family presence during pediatric CPR.

Two critical reviews of the presence of family members during resuscitation include articles by Moreland (2005) and Nibert and Ondrejka (2005). Moreland's (2005) review of 23 studies on family presence during resuscitation and invasive procedures emphasizes the differing aspects of each study reviewed; mixed research methodologies make conclusions difficult to draw for the general population, and most were based on sample interviews and questionnaires following the event. Moreland (2005) concludes that the issue of family presence needs further research to evaluate the long-term effects of family presence on family members and health care providers. Nibert and Ondrejka (2005) concluded that there is no research supporting the exclusion of family from resuscitation events; that many clinician beliefs and practices on the topic are not evidence-based, and that families want to be consulted regarding their presence during the resuscitation of a child.

Conclusions

The studies reviewed included information regarding family presence during invasive procedures and resuscitation, not solely pediatric resuscitation.

There were no studies in this review that evaluated the responses of family members actually present during a pediatric resuscitation in the ED.

Most of the studies published to date did not address the issue of family presence during resuscitation in areas other than the ED (general pediatric floor, pediatric intensive care unit [PICU], outpatient settings). Three studies identified family presence in the PICU as being important for invasive procedures and end-of-life decisions, but family presence during resuscitation and subsequent reactions to the event as being positive or negative was not addressed (Anderson, McCall, Leversha, and others, 1994; Meyer, Burns, Griffith, and others, 2002; Powers and Rubenstein, 1999).

Studies addressed the reactions and opinions of the health care workers regarding family presence during the resuscitative event. Health care worker beliefs and opinions for or against the practice of family presence during resuscitation were not a part of this review.

There is no evidence to support excluding the presence of family members during a child's resuscitation unless a facilitator is unavailable to communicate with the family during the process.

Further research is needed to validate the effects of family presence in childhood resuscitation events.

Apply the Evidence: Nursing Implications

- The presence of family at the resuscitation of a child can be beneficial, provided that a facilitator is present to communicate with the family.
- Provide the family the option of being present during a pediatric resuscitation.
- Health care workers should encourage family presence during resuscitation when appropriate.
- Protocols for family presence during resuscitation should be developed and implemented in institutions where children and families are served.

References

American Heart Association: Guidelines 2000 for cardiopulmonary resuscitation and emergency cardiovascular care, *Circulation* 102(Suppl I):1-374, 2000.

Anderson B, McCall E, Leversha A, and others: A review of children's dying in a paediatric intensive care unit, *N Z Med J* 107(985):345-347, 1994.

Boie T, Moore GP, Brummett C, and others: Do parents want to be present during invasive procedures performed on their children in the emergency department? A survey of 400 parents, *Ann Emerg Med* 34(1):70-74, 1999.

Eichhorn DJ, Meyers TA, Mitchell TG, and others: Opening the doors: family presence during resuscitation, *J Cardiovasc Nurs* 10(4):59-70, 1996.

Emergency Nurses Association: *Position Statement: Family presence at the bedside during invasive procedures and resuscitation,* Des Plaines, Ill, 2001, The Association, retrieved June 27, 2005, from *http://www.ena.org/about/position.*

Hazinski MF, Zaritsky AL, Nadkarni VM, and others: *PALS provider manual,* Dallas, 2002, American Heart Association.

Mangurten JA, Scott SH, Guzzetta CE, and others: Family presence: making room, *Am J Nurs* 105(5):40-48, 2005.

Meyer EC, Burns JP, Griffith JL, and others: Parental perspectives on end-of-life care in the pediatric intensive care unit, *Crit Care Med* 30(1): 226-231, 2002.

Meyers TA, Eichhorn DJ, Guzzetta CE, and others: Family presence during invasive procedures and resuscitation, *Am J Nurs* 100(2):32-42, 2000.

Moreland P: Family presence during invasive procedures and resuscitation in the emergency department: a review of the literature, *J Emerg Nurs* 31(1):58-72, 2005.

Nibert L, Ondrejka D: Family presence during pediatric resuscitation: an integrative review of evidence-based practice, *J Pediatr Nurs* 20(2):145-147, 2005.

O'Brien M, Creamer KM, Hill EE, and others: Tolerance of family presence during pediatric cardiopulmonary resuscitation: a snapshot of military and civilian pediatricians, nurses, and residents, *Pediatr Emerg Care* 18(6):409-413, 2002.

Powers KS, Rubenstein JS: Family presence during invasive procedures in the pediatric intensive care unit: a prospective study, *Arch Pediatr Adolesc Med* 153(9):955-958, 1999.

Sacchetti A, Carraccio C, Leva E, and others: Acceptance of family member presence during pediatric resuscitations in the emergency department: effects of personal experiences, *Pediatr Emerg Care* 16(2):85-87, 2000.

Sacchetti A, Lichenstein R, Caraccio CA, and others: Family member presence during pediatric emergency department procedures, *Pediatr Emerg Care* 12(4):268-271, 1996.

Sanford M, Pugh D, Warren NA: Family presence during CPR: new decisions in the twenty-first century, *Crit Care Nurs Q* 25(2):61-66, 2002.

Tsai E: Should family members be present during cardiopulmonary resuscitation? *N Engl J Med* 346(13):1019-1021, 2002.

Tucker T: Family presence during resuscitation, *Crit Care Nurs Clin North Am* 14(2):177-185, 2002.

Intubation Procedures

INDICATIONS FOR INTUBATION

Respiratory failure or arrest, agonal or gasping respirations, apnea
Upper airway obstruction
Significant increase in work of breathing, use of accessory muscles
Potential for developing partial or complete airway obstruction—respiratory effort with no breath sounds, facial trauma, and inhalation injuries
Potential for or actual loss of airway protection, increased risk for aspiration
Anticipated need for mechanical ventilation related to chest trauma, shock, increased intracranial pressure
Hypoxemia despite supplemental oxygen
Inadequate ventilation

INTUBATION PROCEDURE

Gather supplies needed for intubation.

- Suction, large bore tonsil tip or Yankauer, and sterile suction catheter
- ET tube of appropriate size plus 0.5 mm larger and 0.5 mm smaller. Length based charts are most reliable for determining appropriate ET size. Estimation formulas for children 1 year of age are:
  - Uncuffed ET tube size in mm = (age in years/4) + 4
  - Cuffed ET tube size in mm = (age in years/4) + 3
- Stylet to fit the selected ET
- Laryngoscope and blade
- Light source (ensure it is functioning)
- Bag and mask
- Oxygen source
- Adhesive tape and skin barrier or securement device
- End-tidal carbon dioxide detector
- NG tube and catheter tip syringe
- Gloves and eye protection for universal precautions
- Emergency cardiopulmonary resuscitation equipment including medications

Monitor cardiac rhythm, heart rate, and pulse oximetry continuously with audible tones.
Preoxygenate with 100% oxygen using appropriately sized bag and mask.
Administer preintubation medications.

- Sedative, if conscious
- Short-acting muscle relaxant
- Muscarinic anticholinergic

Assist with intubation by providing supplies and monitoring patient.
Verify placement by:

- Visualization of bilateral chest expansion
- Auscultation over the epigastrium (breath sounds should not be heard) and the lung fields bilaterally (breath sounds should be equal and adequate)
- Color change on end-tidal carbon dioxide detector
- Chest radiograph

Apply protective skin barrier, and secure ET tube with tape or securement device.
Insert NG tube and verify placement.

ONGOING ASSESSMENT

Chest rise and fall, symmetry
Bilateral breath sounds
Pulse oximetry
End-tidal carbon dioxide
Vital signs

- Heart rate too fast or too slow is a possible indication of hypoxemia, air leak, or low cardiac output.
- Hypotension or hypertension may be indicative of hypoxemia or hypovolemia.

Capillary refill and skin color
Level of consciousness
Intake and output
Blood gas
ET tube stabilization and patency
Skin integrity

PATIENT COMFORT AND SAFETY PROCEDURES

Skin Integrity

Reposition at least every two hours, as patient condition tolerates.
Apply a hydrocolloid barrier to protect facial cheeks.
Place gel pillows under pressure points such as occiput, heels, elbows, shoulders.
Allow no tubes, lines, wires, or wrinkles in bedding under patient.
Provide meticulous skin care.

Comfort

Provide analgesia and sedation as needed
Use a system for communication including sign boards, pointing, opening and closing eyes
Provide oral care every 2 hours

Safety

Use soft restraints if necessary to maintain a critical airway
Continuously assess for complications:

- Tube dislodgment caused by position change, agitation, or transport
- Tube occlusion caused by excessive secretions or biting on ET tube
- Pneumothorax or other air leaks
- Equipment failure or disconnection from ventilator

PROCEDURES TO PREVENT VENTILATOR-ASSOCIATED PNEUMONIA

Use aggressive hand hygiene.
Provide enteral nutrition to decrease risk of bacterial translocation.

Minimize aspiration potential with enteral feeds.
Elevate the head of the bed between 30 and 45 degrees unless contraindicated.
Routinely verify the appropriate placement of the feeding tube.
Routinely assess the patient's intestinal motility (e.g., by auscultating for bowel sounds and measuring residual gastric volume or abdominal girth), and adjust the rate and volume of enteral feeding to avoid regurgitation.
Use postpyloric (duodenal or jejunal) feeding in high-risk patients (decreased gag reflex, delayed gastric emptying, gastroesophageal reflux, severe bronchospasm).
Provide aggressive oral care every 2 hours with an approved oral care regimen.
Suction hypopharynx before suctioning the ET tube, before repositioning the ET tube, and before repositioning the patient to prevent the aspiration of pooled secretions. Use closed Endotracheal suctioning. Eliminate saline instillation.
Prevent ventilator circuits' condensate from entering ET tube or in-line medication nebulizers.
Use orotracheal or orogastric tubes to prevent nosocomial sinusitis.
If cuffed ET tubes are used, inflate them to maintain cuff pressure no greater than 20 cm H_2O.
Provide peptic ulcer prophylaxis, as ordered.
Avoid neuromuscular blockade.
Assess readiness to extubate daily.

- Underlying condition improved
- Hemodynamically stable
- Able to clear and maintain secretions
- Mechanical support no longer necessary

EXTUBATION PROCEDURE

Assess level of consciousness and ability to maintain a patent airway by mobilizing pulmonary secretions through effective coughing.
Maintain nothing by mouth (NPO) status 4 hours before extubation.
Preoxygenate.
Place patient in a semi-Fowler's position.
Suction the ET tube and the oropharynx. Suction down to the cuff when using a cuffed ET tube.
Remove tape or ET tube securement device.
If cuff is present, deflate and ask the patient to cough if developmentally appropriate.
Remove ET tube.
Provide oxygen via facemask or nasal cannula.
Perform chest x-ray examination after extubation as ordered.
Monitor for postextubation respiratory distress, which could develop within minutes or hours after extubation:

- Unstable vital signs
- Desaturations
- Stridor
- Hoarseness
- Increased work of breathing

Pericardiocentesis

Pericardiocentesis is a procedure performed to remove the fluid of a pericardial effusion (PCE). A PCE is an accumulation of fluid in the pericardial space that surrounds the heart. Therapeutic indications for pericardiocentesis include the relief of cardiac tamponade or the prevention of cardiac compression by a moderate to large PCE. Pericardiocentesis is also performed to assist in diagnosis of neoplasms, rheumatologic conditions, and infections.

Sedatives and analgesics are administered before the procedure. The xyphoid area is prepped with antiseptic, a needle is introduced into the pericardial space by a physician, and the catheter is then placed. Pericardial fluid is aspirated via the catheter until most of the fluid has been evacuated. The catheter is then secured to the skin with sutures, and the drainage bag is attached. In emergent situations, a 60-ml Luer-Lok syringe attached to a stopcock and an 18-gauge Angiocath may be used to tap the pericardial space and aspirate fluid (Figure 3-24).

PREPARATION FOR PROCEDURE

Gather supplies. Many institutions stock pre-packaged pericardiocentesis kits that will include the supplies needed for the procedure. Be familiar with these kits so that items not included can be obtained from floor stock supplies.

- Sterile gloves, mask, gown, and cap
- Sterile drapes and towels
- Sterile gauze (variety of sizes)
- Sterile drainage bag
- Sterile saline flush
- Sterile specimen container
- Skin antiseptic, per hospital policy
- Three- or four-way stopcock
- Luer-Lok syringes in a variety of sizes (10, 15, 30, 60 ml)
- Straight or pigtail catheter with side holes (request style and size from physician)

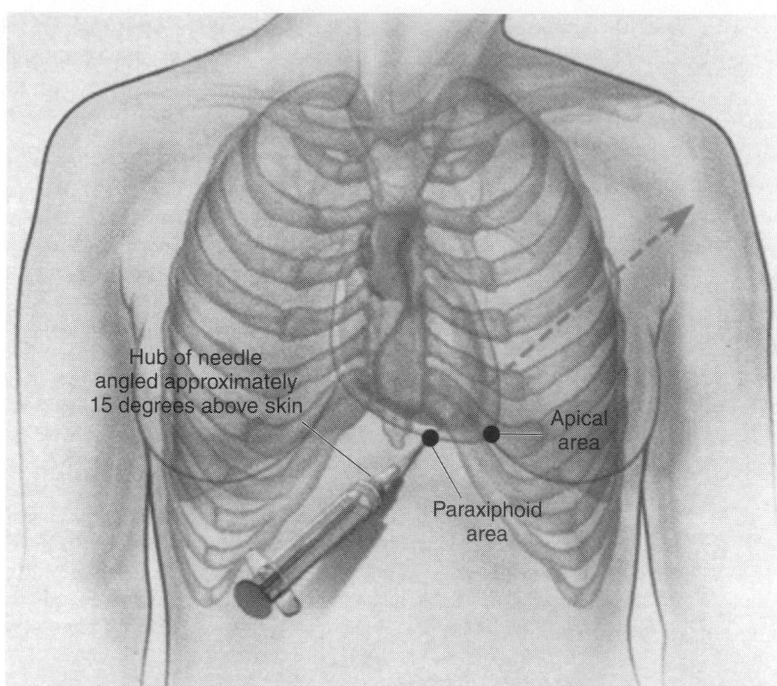

FIGURE **3-24** Pericardiocentesis.

- 18-gauge needle (6 inches long) or 18-gauge Angiocath (physician preference)
- 1% or 2% lidocaine for local anesthesia
- Suture material (physician preference)
- Scalpel blade
- Fluid for volume resuscitation as needed
- Emergency equipment nearby

Ensure the patient has well functioning venous access.

Administer pain and sedation medication as ordered.

Attach patient to monitoring equipment (electrocardiogram [ECG] at a minimum).

PROCEDURAL SUPPORT

Position the patient with the head of the bed elevated 30 to 45 degrees.

Assist physician with preparation of the sterile field as directed.

Provide sterile supplies to the physician as directed.

Monitor airway, breathing, circulation, and cardiac rhythm throughout the procedure.

Send specimens to laboratory as ordered. Ask the physician before discarding fluid.

Place dressing over catheter insertion site per hospital policy.

Obtain chest radiograph to confirm placement of catheter.

AFTER THE PROCEDURE

Ensure daily chest radiographs are scheduled to monitor placement of the pericardial drain.

Assess for signs and symptoms of infection around the catheter insertion site throughout the duration of pericardial drain placement.

Assess drainage for color, consistency, and quantity. If quantity of drainage significantly decreases, assess area around the insertion site for drainage.

Notify the physician of any changes in quality or quantity of drainage.

Chest Tube Procedures

A chest tube is placed to remove fluid or air from the pleural or pericardial space. Chest tube drainage systems collect air and fluid while inhibiting backflow into the pleural or pericardial space. Indications for chest tube placement include pneumothorax, hemothorax, chylothorax, empyema, pleural or pericardial effusion, and prevention of accumulation of fluid in the pleural and pericardial space after cardiothoracic surgery. Nursing responsibilities include assisting with chest tube placement, managing chest tubes, and assisting with chest tube removal.

CHEST TUBE INSERTION PROCEDURE

Before procedure, assess hematologic and coagulation studies for any risk of bleeding during the procedure. Notify the physician of abnormal findings.

Gather supplies.

- Appropriately sized chest tube with or without trocar, as desired by inserter
- Disposable chest drainage system (pediatric or adult size)
- Connecting tubing
- Vacuum suction
- Skin antiseptic such as chlorhexidine or povidone-iodine, per hospital policy
- Scalpel, blade, suture, needle driver, clamps
- 1% or 2% lidocaine for local anesthesia
- Selection of syringes and needles
- Tape
- Sterile gloves, mask, gown, and cap
- Sterile drapes and towels
- Sterile gauze (variety of sizes)
- Sterile specimen container
- Sterile water

Attach monitoring equipment (pulse oximeter at a minimum) to patient.

Administer pain and sedation medications as ordered.

Follow Universal Protocol for Preventing Wrong Site, Wrong Procedure, Wrong Person Surgery (Time-Out Procedure) as guided by hospital policy.

Prepare drainage system with sterile water as described in package insert (some systems may not require this step).

Monitor airway, breathing, and circulation throughout the procedure.

Once the chest tube is inserted and secured, hand the physician the drainage system tubing while keeping the open end sterile. The physician will join the chest tube to the drainage system with the patient tube connector. Secure tubing so it does not become disconnected.

If suction is required, use connection tubing to join the drainage system to a wall suction adapter, and adjust suction on drainage system as ordered (usually −10 to −20 cm H_2O). There should be gentle, continuous bubbling in the suction control chamber.

Place occlusive dressing over chest tube insertion site per hospital policy. Note date, time, and your initials on the dressing. If gauze is used, use presplit gauze; "homemade" split gauze may leave loose threads in the wound.

Ensure that the drainage system is positioned below the patient's chest.

Obtain a chest radiograph to confirm placement of the chest tube. Ensure daily chest radiographs are scheduled to monitor placement of the chest tube as well as the resolution of the pneumothorax or effusion.

CHEST DRAINAGE SYSTEM MANAGEMENT PROCEDURE

Disposable chest drainage systems typically consist of three chambers next to one another in one drainage unit (Figure 3-25). The fluid collection chamber collects drainage from the patient's pleural or pericardial space. The water seal chamber is directly connected to fluid collection chamber and acts as a one-way valve, protecting patients from air returning to the pleural or pericardial space. The suction chamber may be a dry suction or calibrated water chamber and is connected to external vacuum suction set to the amount of suction ordered and controls the amount of suction patients experience.

Closely monitor the patient's cardiorespiratory status.

Provide adequate analgesia.

Secure the drainage system to the floor or bed.

Ensure all connections are tight.

Keep drainage tubing free of dependent loops.

Assess for blood clots and fibrin strands in tubes with sanguinous or serosanguineous drainage, and ensure that there are no obstructions to drainage in the tube. Maintain chest tube clearance per hospital policy. Milking or stripping of chest tubes is not recommended for chest tube clearance because of the high negative intrathoracic pressure that is created. However, there are special circumstances that warrant chest tube clearance with these methods, such as maintaining chest tube patency while a patient is bleeding. Notify the physician immediately if chest tube obstruction is suspected.

Generally, chest tubes should not be clamped. However, it may be necessary to clamp a chest tube when exchanging the collection chamber or to determine the site of an air leak.

Assess the drainage in the collection chamber.

- Type (sanguinous, serosanguineous, serous, chylous, empyemic), color, amount, consistency. If there is a marked decrease in the amount of drainage, assess for drainage around the chest tube insertion site.
- Notify the physician of any changes in the quantity or quality of drainage.
- If 3 ml/kg/hr or greater of sanguinous drainage occurs for 2 to 3 consecutive hours after cardiothoracic surgery, it may indicate active hemorrhaging and warrants immediate attention of the physician.
- If the collection chamber is almost full, exchange existing drainage system with a new one per manufacturer's instructions using sterile technique.

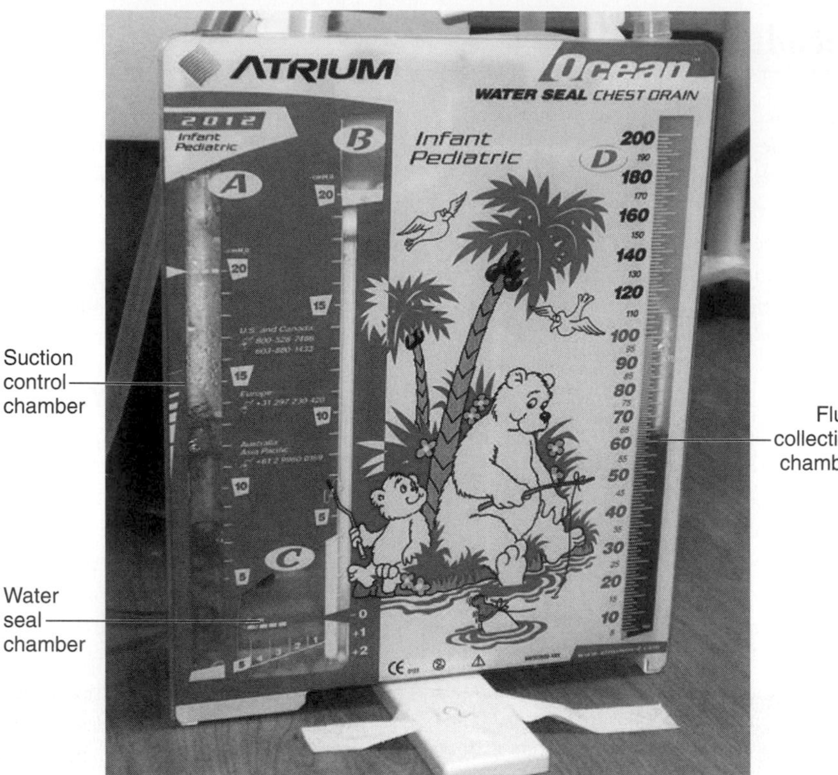

FIGURE 3-25 Chest tube drainage system.

Assess the suction control chamber.
- Ensure the prescribed amount of suction is being applied to the patient.

Assess the water seal chamber.
- Water level is at 2 cm. If the water column is too high, the flow of air from the chest may be impeded. To lower the water column, depress the manual vent on the back of the unit until the water level reaches 2 cm. *Do not depress the filtered manual vent when the suction is not functioning or connected.*
- Bubbling in the water seal chamber is normal if the chest tube was placed to evacuate a pneumothorax. The bubbling will stop when the pneumothorax has resolved.
- If evacuation of a pneumothorax was not the indication for placement of the chest tube, bubbling in the water seal chamber may be the result of a break in the chest drainage system. Identify the break in the system by briefly clamping the system between the drainage unit and the patient. When the clamp is placed between the unit and the break in the system, the bubbling will stop. Tighten any loose connections. If the air leak is suspected to be at the patient's chest wall, notify the physician.
- Fluctuations may be seen in the water column because of changes in intrathoracic pressure. Substantial fluctuations may reflect changes in a patient's respiratory status.

Assess and maintain the chest tube insertion site.
- Change dressing and perform site care per hospital policy. Typically a minimal, occlusive dressing is applied.
- Ensure that chest tube sutures are intact.
- Dressing should be clean, dry, and intact.
- Assess skin for signs and symptoms of infection or skin breakdown.
- Palpate for the presence of subcutaneous air.

Encourage patient ambulation. Secure chest tube drainage system to prevent chest tube dislodgment from patient or disconnection from drainage system.

Obtain samples from the chest tube per hospital infection control policy.

Prepare a syringe with a 20-gauge (or smaller) needle.

Form a temporary dependent loop, and, using aseptic technique, insert the needle at an angle into the dependent loop.

Aspirate amount of drainage required.

CHEST TUBE REMOVAL PROCEDURE

Administer pain medication before procedure.

Gather supplies: gloves, suture removal kit, sterile gauze (2×2 or 4×4), and tape.

Assist in removal of the chest tube. The chest tube is removed on patient exhalation to prevent a pneumothorax.

Apply dressing and perform site care per hospital policy.

Obtain a chest radiograph as ordered to confirm that a pneumothorax has not occurred after chest tube removal.

Closely monitor patient's respiratory status.

Cardioversion Procedures

Supraventricular tachycardia (SVT) is the most common tachydysrhythmia in children. SVT is a rapid, regular rhythm of over 200 beats per minute. Because cardiac output is a product of heart rate and stroke volume, prolonged SVT can cause hemodynamic compromise. Signs and symptoms of SVT in infants include irritability, poor feeding, sweating, and pallor. Older children may complain of dizziness, chest pain, or a feeling that their heart is racing.

Whenever SVT is suspected, assess the adequacy of the patient's airway and ventilatory effort. Check for a pulse. If the patient does not have a pulse or adequate respirations, proceed with cardiopulmonary resuscitation. If a patient does have a pulse, assess the patient's perfusion. Notify the physician if SVT is suspected. Choosing the appropriate type of treatment depends on accurate evaluation of the patient's cardiac output and hemodynamic status.

The treatment of SVT is cardioversion, or converting an abnormal heart rhythm into a normal one. There are three types of cardioversion: mechanical, chemical, and electrical. *Mechanical* refers to the use of vagal maneuvers such as ice to the face, one sided carotid massage, or Valsalva maneuvers. *Chemical* refers to the use of medications, and *electrical* refers to the use of electrical energy delivered to a patient to convert the tachydysrhythmia to a normal rhythm. A physician should be present for all forms of cardioversion.

If the patient has adequate perfusion, anticipate the need for a 12 lead ECG and pediatric cardiology consult (if available). Proceed with mechanical cardioversion, then chemical, if needed. Elective synchronized cardioversion may also be required.

If the patient has poor perfusion, mechanical cardioversion may be attempted but should not delay treatment. Chemical cardioversion may be attempted if reliable IV access in a large vein, such as antecubital, is immediately available. Electrical cardioversion should be employed if reliable IV access is not available or chemical cardioversion is unsuccessful. Administer sedation or analgesia before chemical or electrical cardioversion.

MECHANICAL CARDIOVERSION

Administer oxygen, as ordered.

Attach an ECG monitor and pulse oximeter to the patient.

Vagal maneuvers such as ice to the face, one-sided carotid massage, and the Valsalva maneuver may be attempted to cardiovert the patient.

Ice to the face is the most effective vagal maneuver. Place crushed ice in a glove or bag and apply to the face for 10-15 seconds, being careful not to obstruct the nose or mouth. If a Valsalva maneuver is desired, one method is to have a child blow in an occluded straw.

Assess the patient's cardiac rhythm, breathing, pulse, and perfusion.

If cardioversion is unsuccessful and the patient remains stable with adequate perfusion, additional attempts at mechanical cardioversion may be considered before advancing to chemical cardioversion.

CHEMICAL CARDIOVERSION

Adenosine is the drug of choice for chemical conversion of SVT. It works by blocking electrical conduction through the AV node. To be effective, adenosine must be delivered rapidly because it is metabolized quickly in the bloodstream.

Administer oxygen, as ordered.

Attach the ECG monitor component of a defibrillator to the patient. Also attach a pulse oximeter.

Check patency of IV or start IV in large vein, such as antecubital.

Have several syringes of saline flush available.

Prepare the dose of adenosine based on the patient's weight.

Rapidly administer adenosine using two syringes connected to a T-connector or stopcock; give adenosine rapidly with one syringe and immediately flush with 5 ml of NS with the other.

Assess the patient's cardiac rhythm, breathing, pulse, and perfusion.

Because adenosine blocks conduction through the AV node, patients may have asystole for 1 to 2 seconds after adenosine administration. Closely monitor the patient; if asystole does not resolve, proceed with cardiopulmonary resuscitation.

SYNCHRONIZED ELECTRICAL CARDIOVERSION

Electrical cardioversion for SVT is synchronized. This means that the electrical impulses delivered to the patient are coordinated with the patient's own rhythm. This is very important because delivering electrical impulses that are not synchronized can cause the patient to develop a more dangerous dysrhythmia. Ensure that the "sync mode" is always used.

Administer oxygen, as ordered.

Attach the ECG monitor of a defibrillator to the patient. Attach a pulse oximeter to the patient.

Place appropriately sized pads or paddles on the patient.

Select the sync mode.

Set the appropriate amount of energy to be delivered. The starting dose is 0.5 to 1 joules/kg.

Deliver energy to patient.

Assess the patient's cardiac rhythm, breathing, pulse, and perfusion.

Advance to 2 joules/kg if the first dose is ineffective.

Assess the patient's cardiac rhythm, breathing, pulse, and perfusion.

Throughout all cardioversion procedures, monitor the patient's airway, breathing, circulation. Continuously monitor the patient's heart rhythm. Intervene with cardiopulmonary resuscitation if warranted at any point.

Procedures Related to Maintaining Neurologic Function

Increased Intracranial Pressure Management

A neurologic pressure monitoring system is used to measure intracranial pressure (ICP). Causes of increased ICP include accidental and abusive head trauma, hydrocephalus, tumor, edema, and subarachnoid or other intracranial hemorrhage. The system may be used to alleviate increased ICP by draining cerebral spinal fluid (CSF) from the ventricular system. A decrease in cerebral oxygen delivery related to hypotension, hypoxemia, cerebral edema, intracranial hypertension, or abnormalities in cerebral blood flow may precipitate a secondary injury. General nursing care activities and environmental stimuli can present a challenge to the patient with increased ICP. If ICP is increasing, then further nursing activities should be delayed if possible. Care must be individualized based on the patient's responses. The optimal rest period is at least 1 hour between nursing care interventions.

POSITIONING

Maintain neutral or midline head and neck alignment.

Elevate the head of bed (HOB) 15 to 30 degrees to promote venous drainage.

Closely evaluate the effect of HOB elevation on ICP, cerebral perfusion pressure (CPP), and mean arterial pressure (MAP).

Avoid extreme hip flexion, as this can increase intraabdominal pressure and restrict movement of the diaphragm and impede respiratory effort.

Reposition the patient by using logrolling technique.

ENDOTRACHEAL SUCTIONING

Preoxygenate per intensive care unit (ICU) routine. Use of hyperventilation is controversial, can reduce cerebral blood flow to ischemic levels, and may cause loss of autoregulation.

Premedicate as ordered. Adequate sedation may prevent movement and coughing during suctioning and prevent decreases in CPP.

Administer lidocaine intravenously or via endotracheal tube to attenuate possible ICP increases that occur with endotracheal suctioning.

Limit each pass of the suction catheter to 10 seconds or less.

TEMPERATURE

Maintain normothermia (37° C). Core temperatures greater than 37.5° are associated with increased cerebral metabolic rate, increased oxygen consumption, and increased ICP.

Moderate hypothermia is reserved for children with refractory intracranial hypertension that is not responsive to traditional therapies.

SEDATION AND NEUROMUSCULAR BLOCKING AGENTS

Use of sedatives and analgesics should be based on the patient's ICP and response to the sedation being administered. Protocols vary from institution to institution.

Cautious use of neuromuscular blocking agents is recommended. Neuromuscular assessment is altered (with the exception of pupillary response) with the use of neuromuscular blockade, sedation, and analgesia. This is an important consideration when assessing the patient's ICP response and neurologic status. Continuous electroencephalographic (EEG) monitoring may be indicated for patients at risk for seizures and receiving neuromuscular blocking agents. The risk for ventilator-acquired pneumonia is also increased with the use of neuromuscular blocking agents.

When neuromuscular blocking agents are used, sedation and analgesia should always be considered.

TOUCH AND FAMILY VISITATION

ICP does not generally increase significantly or decrease with family presence or with physical touch.

NURSING ESSENTIALS

Normal Intracranial Pressure Ranges

ICP: 0 to 15 mm Hg or 0 to 20 mm H_2O.

CPP represents the pressure drop between the arterial pressure and the venous pressure. Normal CPP is not delineated in the pediatric population. The thought is that if a CPP is greater than 50 mm Hg, then there is adequate cerebral perfusion; if CPP is less than 40 mmHg, cerebral perfusion is compromised. CPP is calculated by subtracting the ICP from the MAP: CPP = MAP − ICP.

Hemodynamic Monitoring

Arterial line—necessary for consistent blood pressure monitoring and obtaining MAP for calculation of CPP.

Central venous left atrium line—necessary for monitoring of central venous pressure (CVP).

Pulmonary artery pressure monitoring—if indicated.

Patient and Family Preparation

Placement of ICP monitoring systems may be performed at the bedside or in the operating room.

Family should be aware that the patient may remain intubated for an extended period of time if the neurologic status is compromised.

Explain the monitor and the waveforms and that the patient will be continually monitored for increased ICP.

Intracranial Pressure Monitoring Systems

Fluid-coupled systems—An intraventricular catheter (IVC) is placed in the anterior horn of the lateral ventricle; this is the most accurate and reliable method of monitoring. This system allows for CSF drainage and measurement of ICP when attached to an external fluid filled transducer (not simultaneously). Must be zeroed to atmosphere and maintained at a fixed point such as the foramen of Monroe.

Fiberoptic—Placed in intraventricular, intraparenchymal, subarachnoid and subdural spaces. These catheters are light-sending and light-receiving systems and respond to the movement of a diaphragm at the tip of the catheter. Zeroed to atmospheric pressure just before insertion. No leveling or rezeroing is necessary because the transducer is located in the catheter tip.

Internal strain gauge or microchip transducer—Placed in intraparenchymal, subarachnoid, and subdural spaces. A miniature strain-gauge pressure sensor is positioned at the tip of the catheter; when pressure is exerted an electrical signal is generated and pressure is measured. Catheter is zeroed to atmosphere before insertion and never rezeroed after the catheter is inserted.

External Ventricular Drain Procedures

Children with external ventricular drains (EVDs) may be hospitalized in an ICU, step-down unit, or acute care floor. EVDs are used to temporarily control ICP by draining CSF from the ventricles, most often in shunt infections, brain tumors, and intracranial bleeds. The drainage is dependent on gravity, and the level of the flow chamber determines the amount of CSF flow. Proper positioning, maintenance of patency, infection prevention, and patient monitoring are important aspects of care.

POSITIONING OF EXTERNAL VENTRICULAR DRAINS

Raising the flow chamber too high results in decreased CSF flow into the external reservoir and increased intracranial pressure. Positioning a flow chamber too low results in too much drainage of CSF and potential collapse of the ventricles. The zero reference point is the foramen of Monro, usually aligned with the external auditory canal. The level of the flow chamber is prescribed by a physician. A level and measure is then used to set the collection device at the prescribed height, often 20 cm H_2O. Physicians will lower a chamber to increase drainage and reduce intracranial pressure and raise the height as the patient's condition improves. The drain will be removed when normal intracranial pressures have been sustained and a temporary condition has resolved. Internal ventriculoperitoneal shunts are placed when hydrocephaly continues, infection clears, and protein amounts are low enough to maintain shunt tubing patency.

PATENCY OF EXTERNAL VENTRICULAR DRAINS

Keep the tubing free from kinks. Observe for oscillation of CSF in the tubing. Do not milk or strip EVD tubing. Keep the air filter on the collection chamber dry. Change the bag when three-quarters full using aseptic technique.

INFECTION PREVENTION: EXTERNAL VENTRICULAR DRAIN DRESSING CHANGES

Dressings should be changed when damp, loose, or soiled. Report damp dressings caused by CSF leak immediately. Dressing change frequency is established by each institution.

Clamp ventriculostomy drainage system.

Allow the child to choose a position of comfort as long as head control and sterility of supplies and dressing area can be maintained.

Open sterile dressing kit using sterile technique. Prepare sterile supplies on sterile drape.

Don clean gloves. Remove all components of the dressing.

Assess insertion site for redness, edema, drainage from site, and intact sutures.

Remove clean gloves and don sterile gloves.

Clean skin around ventriculostomy insertion site with alcohol swabstick. Start at the insertion site, making concentric circles around the ventriculostomy 3 inches in diameter. Conclude by cleaning the length of the tubing that was coiled, if applicable. Repeat two times.

Clean skin around ventriculostomy insertion site with povidone-iodine swabstick. Use appropriate alternative if allergic to iodine. Start at the insertion site, making concentric circles around the ventriculostomy 3 inches in diameter. Conclude by cleaning the length of the tubing that was coiled, if applicable. Repeat two times.

Place 1-inch antimicrobial disk around drain at insertion site.

Using forceps, place 2×2 split gauze on ventriculostomy with catheter between the split. Place 2×2 gauze over split gauze.

Carefully coil remainder of catheter, if applicable, on top of 2×2 gauze. Prevent pressure ulcers by padding hub of catheter with additional 2×2 gauze.

Place 2×2 gauze on top of coiled ventriculostomy tubing. Place 4-inch clear occlusive dressing on top of gauze dressing.

Remove sterile gloves.

Position the patient for comfort. Ensure the collection chamber is at the level ordered, and unclamp ventriculostomy drainage system.

PATIENT MONITORING

Record CSF hourly. Report excessive drainage or a sudden cessation in drainage immediately. Document color, and report any changes in color (milky, cloudy, blood-tinged).

Monitor neurologic status including verbal, motor, and pupillary assessments hourly.

Abnormal findings include irritability, confusion, lethargy, headache, and vomiting. Changes in blood pressure (increased), heart rate (decreased), respiratory pattern (periods of apnea), and pupils (dilated, sluggish, or nonreactive) are later signs of increased intracranial pressure.

PATIENT ACTIVITY OR CLAMPING OF THE EXTERNAL VENTRICULAR DRAIN SYSTEM

Nurses should assist the child with all position changes and ensure the proper height of the collection chamber at all times the tubing is unclamped.

Clamp for short periods of time, not to exceed 30 minutes. Clamping is generally done to allow position changes, during transport to other areas of the hospital, and during patient ambulation.

Pediatric Coma Rating Scale

NEUROLOGIC ASSESSMENT

Pupils	Right	Size	
		Reaction	
	Left	Size	
		Reaction	

++ = Brisk
\+ = Sluggish
– = No reaction
C = Eye closed by swelling

Pupil scale (mm): 1, 2, 3, 4, 5, 6, 7, 8

GLASGOW COMA SCALE

Eyes open	Spontaneously	4	
	To speech	3	
	To pain	2	
	None	1	
Best motor response	Obeys commands	6	
	Localizes pain	5	
	Flexion withdrawal	4	
	Flexion abnormal	3	
	Extension	2	
	None	1	

Usually record best arm or age-appropriate response

	>2 years		<2 years
Best response to auditory and/or visual stimulus	Orientation	5	5 Smiles, listens, follows
	Confused	4	4 Cries, consolable
	Inappropriate words	3	3 Inappropriate persistent cry
	Incomprehensible words	2	2 Agitated, restless
	None	1	1 No response
	Endotracheal tube or trach	T	

COMA SCALE TOTAL	

HAND GRIP:
Equal
Unequal
R____L
Weakness

LOC:
Alert/oriented x4
Sleepy
Irritable
Comatose
Disoriented
Combative
Lethargic
Awake
Sleeping
Drowsy
Agitated

MUSCLE TONE:
Normal
Arching
Spastic
Flaccid
Weak
Decorticate
Decerebrate
Other ________

EYE MOVEMENT:
Normal
Nystagmus
Strabismus
Other ________

FONTANEL/ WINDOW:
Soft
Flat
Sunken
Tense
Bulging
Closed
Other ________

MOOD/AFFECT:
Happy
Content
Quiet
Withdrawn
Sad
Flat
Hostile

References

Ackerman MH: Instillation of normal saline before suctioning in patients with pulmonary infections: a prospective randomized controlled trial, *Am J Crit Care* 7(4): 261-266, 1998.

Anand KJS, International Evidence-Based Group for Neonatal Pain: Consensus statement for the prevention and management of pain in the newborn, *Arch Pediatr Adolesc Med* 155(2):173-179, 2001.

Barrier G, Attia J, Mayer MN, and others: Measurement of postoperative pain and narcotic administration in infants using a new clinical scoring system, *Anesthesiology* 67(3A): A532, 1987.

Beyer JE, Denyes MJ, Villarruel AM: The creation, validation and continuing development of the Oucher: a measure of pain intensity in children, *J Pediatr Nurs* 7(5):335-346, 1992.

Blauer T, Gerstmann D: A simultaneous comparison of three neonatal pain scales during common NICU procedures, *Clin J Pain* 14(1):39-47, 1998.

Cline ME, Herman J, Shaw ER, and others: Standardization of the visual analogue scale, *Nurs Res* 41(6):378-380, 1992.

Curley MAQ, Moloney-Harmon PA: *Critical care nursing of infants and children*, ed 2, Philadelphia, 2001, Saunders.

Eland JA, Banner W: Analgesia, sedation, and neuromuscular blockage in pediatric critical care. In Hazinski ME, editor: *Manual of pediatric critical care,* St Louis, 1999, Mosby.

Geyer J, Ellsbury D, Kleiber C, and others: An evidence-based multidisciplinary protocol for neonatal circumcision pain management, *J Obstet Gynecol Neonatal Nurs* 31(4):403-410, 2002.

Hagler DA, Traver GA: Endotracheal saline and suction catheters: sources of lower airway contamination, *Am J Crit Care* 3(6):444-447, 1994.

Hannallah RS, Broadman LM, Belman AB, and others: Comparison of caudal and ilioinguinal/iliohypogastric nerve blocks for control of post-orchiopexy pain in pediatric ambulatory surgery, *Anesthesiology* 66:832-834, 1987.

Hester NO, Foster RL, Jordan-Marsh M, and others: Putting pain measurement into clinical practice. In Finley GA, McGrath PJ, editors: *Measurement of pain in infants and children,* vol 10, Seattle, 1998, International Association for the Study of Pain Press.

Hjelle JJ, Grauer GF: Acetaminophen-induced toxicosis in dogs and cats, *J Am Vet Med Assoc* 188(7):742-749, 1986.

Hodgkinson K, Bear M, Thorn J, and others: Measuring pain in neonates: evaluating an instrument and developing a common language, *Austral J Adv Nurs* 12(1):17-22, 1994.

Jordan-Marsh M, Yoder L, Hall D, and others: Alternate Oucher form testing gender ethnicity and age variations, *Res Nurs Health* 17:111-118, 1994.

Joyce BA, Schade JG, Keck JF, and others: Reliability and validity of preverbal pain assessment tools, *Issues Comp Pediatr Nurs* 17:121-135, 1994.

Kleiber C, Krutzfield N, Rose EF: Acute histologic changes in tracheobronchial tree associated with different suction catheter insertion techniques, *Heart Lung* 17:10-14, 1988

Krechel SW, Bildner J: CRIES: a new neonatal postoperative pain measurement score: initial testing of validity and reliability, *Pediatr Anaesth* 5:53-61, 1995.

Lawrence J, Alcock D, McGrath P, and others: The development of a tool to assess neonatal pain, *Neonat Netw* 12(6):59-66, 1993.

Luffy R, Grove SK: Examining the validity, reliability, and preference of three pediatric pain measurement tools in African-American children, *Pediatr Nurs* 29(1):54-60, 2003.

McGrath PJ, Johnson G, Goodman JT, and others: The CHEOPS: a behavioral scale to measure postoperative pain in children. In Fields H, Dubner R, Cervero F, editors: *Advances in pain research and therapy,* New York, 1985, Raven Press.

Merkel SI, Voepel-Lewis T, Shayevitz JR, and others: The FLACC: a behavioral scale for scoring postoperative pain in young children, *Pediatr Nurs* 23(3):293-297, 1997.

Prescott LF: *Paracetamol (acetaminophen): a critical bibliographic review*, Bristol, 1996, Taylor & Francis.

Puchalski M, Hummel P: The reality of neonatal pain, *Adv Neonatal Care* 2(5):233-244, 2002.

Razmus I, Dalton M, Wilson D: Pain management for newborn circumcision, *Pediatr Nurs* 20(5):414-417, 427, 2004.

Robieux I, Kumar R, Radhakrishnan S, and others: Assessing pain and analgesia with a lidocaine-prilocaine emulsion in infants and toddlers during venipuncture, *J Pediatr* 118(6):971-973, 1991.

Schade JG, Joyce BA, Gerkensmeyer J, and others: Comparison of three preverbal scales for postoperative pain assessment in a diverse pediatric sample, *J Pain Symptom Manage* 12(6):348-359, 1996.

Selekman J, Snyder B: Institutional policies on the use of physical restraints on children, *Pediatr Nurs* 23(5):531-537, 1997.

Serour F, Mandelberg A, Mori J: Slow injection of local anesthetic will decrease pain during dorsal penile nerve block, *Acta Anesthesiol Scand* 42:926-928, 1998.

Smith DP, Gjellum M: The efficacy of LMX versus EMLA for pain relief in boys undergoing office meatotomy, *J Urol* 172(4 Pt 2):1760-1761, 2004.

Stang H, Snellman LW, Condon LM, and others: Beyond dorsal penile nerve block: a more humane circumcision, *Pediatrics* 100(2):E3, 1997, retrieved from *http://www.pediatrics.org/cgi/content/full/100/2/e3.*

Stevens B: Development and testing of a pediatric pain management sheet, *Pediatr Nurs* 16(6):543-548, 1990.

Stevens B, Johnston C, Petryshen P, and others: Premature Infant Pain Profile: development and initial validation, *Clin J Pain* 12:13-22, 1996.

Taddio A, Nulman I, Koren BS, and others: A revised measure of acute pain in infants, *J Pain Symptom Manage* 10(6):456-463, 1995.

Taddio A, Pollock N, Gilbert-MacLeod C, and others: Combined analgesia and local anesthesia to minimize pain during circumcision, *Arch Pediatr Adolesc Med* 154(5):620-623, 2000.

Tesler MD, Savedra MC, Holzemer WL, and others: The word-graphic rating scale as a measure of children's and adolescents' pain intensity, *Res Nurs Health* 14:361-371, 1991.

Villarruel AM, Denyes MJ: Pain assessment in children: theoretical and empirical validity, *Adv Nurs Sci* 14(2):32-41, 1991.

Wong D: Topical local anesthetics: two products for pain relief during minor procedures, *Am J Nurs* 103(6):42-45, 2003.

Wong DL, Baker CM: Pain in children: comparison of assessment scales, *Pediatr Nurs* 14(1):9-17, 1988.

Zerwekh JV: Do dying patients really need IV fluids? *Am J Nurs* 3:26-30, 1997.

Bibliography

Broadman LM, Hannallah RS, Belman AB, and others: Post-circumcision analgesia: a prospective evaluation of subcutaneous ring block of the penis, *Anesthesiology* 67:339-402, 1987.

Howard CR, Howard FM, Weitzman ML: Acetaminophen analgesia in neonatal circumcision: the effect on pain, *Pediatrics* 93(4):641-646, 1994.

Lander J, Brady-Fryer B, Metcalfe JB, and others: Comparison of ring block, dorsal penile nerve block, and topical anesthesia for neonatal circumcision, *JAMA* 278:2157-2162, 1997;

Mintz MR, Grillo R: Dorsal penile nerve block for circumcision, *Clin Pediatr* 28:590-591, 1989.

Spencer DM, Miller KA, O'Quinn M, and others: Dorsal penile nerve block in neonatal circumcision: chloroprocaine versus lidocaine, *Am J Perinatol* 9(3):214-218, 1992;

Stevens B, Taddio A, Ohlsson A, and others: The efficacy of sucrose for relieving procedural pain in neonates—a systematic review and meta-analysis, *Acta Paediatr* 86:837-842, 1997.

Taddio A, Stevens B, Craig K, and others: Efficacy and safety of lidocaine-prilocaine cream (EMLA) for pain during circumcision, *N Engl J Med* 336(17):1197-1201, 1997.

UNIT 4

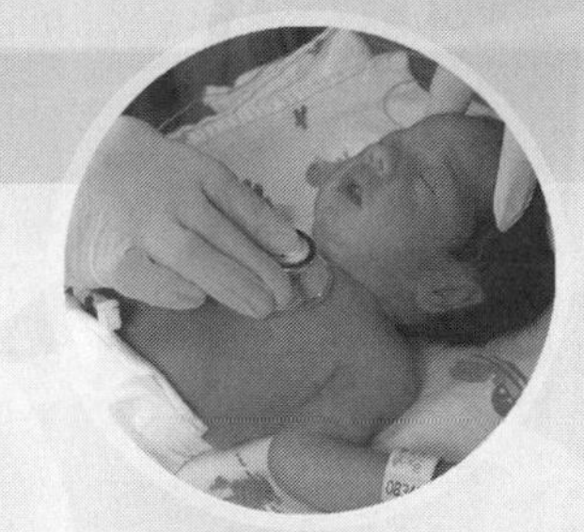

Nursing Care Plans

The Process of Nursing Infants and Children

The care of sick children and their families requires the same systematic decision-making approach that is applied to nursing care for all patients. This problem-solving process involves both cognitive and operational skills and consists of five phases:

1. **Assessment**—The analysis and synthesis of collected data
2. **Problem identification**—The determination of the actual or potential problem or need stated as a nursing diagnosis
3. **Plan formulation**—A design of action sometimes stated as nursing orders, nursing interventions, or nursing functions
4. **Implementation**—The performance or execution of the plan
5. **Evaluation**—A measure of the outcome of nursing action(s) that either completes the nursing process or serves as a basis for reassessment

The American Nurses Association has established Standards of Practice (use of the nursing process):

1. **Assessment**—The nurse collects comprehensive data pertinent to the patient's health or the situation.
2. **Diagnosis**—The nurse analyzes assessment data to determine the diagnoses or issues.
3. **Outcomes identification**—The nurse identifies expected outcomes for a plan individualized to the patient or the situation.
4. **Planning**—The nurse develops a plan of care that prescribes strategies and alternatives to attain expected outcomes.
5. **Implementation**—The nurse implements the identified plan.
6. **Evaluation**—The nurse evaluates progress toward attainment of outcomes.

Nursing Diagnoses

The nursing diagnosis is the naming of the cue clusters that are obtained during the assessment phase. The North American Nursing Diagnosis Association's (NANDA) currently accepted definition of the term nursing diagnosis is "a clinical judgment about individual, family, or community responses to actual and potential health problems/life processes. Nursing diagnoses provide the basis for selection of nursing interventions to achieve outcomes for which the nurse is accountable."

Nursing diagnoses do not describe everything that nursing does. Nursing practice consists of three types of activity: dependent, interdependent, and independent. The differences reside in the source of authority for the action. Dependent activities are those areas of nursing practice that hold the nurse accountable for implementing the prescribed medical regimen. Interdependent activities are those areas of nursing practice in which medical and nursing responsibility and accountability overlap and require collaboration (labeled *Collaborative* in care plan) between the two disciplines. Independent activities are those areas of nursing practice that are the direct responsibility of the individual nurse. Nursing diagnoses should reflect the interdependent and independent dimensions of nursing.

The nursing diagnoses used in this segment are those compiled and approved by NANDA and organized according to priority. Those selected for inclusion in this unit represent only one interpretation (Box 4-1). Some diagnoses are closely related, and it is often difficult to determine which diagnostic category best represents any given goal. The diagnoses selected for inclusion and nursing interventions serve as a general guide for nursing care of children with health problems; therefore others must be added by the user to individualize care for a specific child and family.

Both NANDA and Marjory Gordon have developed frameworks for nursing diagnoses. NANDA bases its framework on nine human response patterns; and Gordon bases hers on 11 functional health patterns. In clinical practice the classification systems, especially Gordon's patterns, serve as a framework for organizing a nursing assessment and standardizing data collection. Additional research is needed to broaden the list of nursing diagnoses, especially for specialty areas such as pediatrics, and to define a universally accepted taxonomy.

BOX 4-1 | NANDA NURSING DIAGNOSES 2007-2008

Activity Intolerance
Activity Intolerance, Risk for
Airway Clearance, Ineffective
Allergy Response, Latex
Allergy Response, Risk for Latex
Anxiety
Anxiety, Death
Aspiration, Risk for
Attachment, Risk for Impaired Parent/Child
Autonomic Dysreflexia
Autonomic Dysreflexia, Risk for
Behavior, Risk-Prone Health
Body Image, Disturbed
Body Temperature, Risk for Imbalanced
Bowel Incontinence
Breastfeeding, Effective
Breastfeeding, Ineffective
Breastfeeding, Interrupted
Breathing pattern, Ineffective
Cardiac Output, Decreased
Caregiver Role Strain
Caregiver Role Strain, Risk for
Comfort, Readiness for Enhanced
Communication, Impaired Verbal
Communication, Readiness for Enhanced
Conflict, Decisional
Conflict, Parental Role
Confusion, Acute
Confusion, Chronic
Confusion, Risk for Acute
Constipation
Constipation, Perceived
Constipation, Risk for
Contamination
Contamination, Risk for
Coping, Compromised Family
Coping, Defensive
Coping, Disabled Family
Coping, Ineffective
Coping, Ineffective Community
Coping, Readiness for Enhanced
Coping, Readiness for Enhanced Community
Coping, Readiness for Enhanced Family
Death Syndrome, Risk for Sudden Infant
Decision Making, Readiness for Enhanced
Denial, Ineffective
Dentition, Impaired
Development, Risk for Delayed
Diarrhea
Dignity, Risk for Compromised Human
Distress, Moral
Disuse Syndrome, Risk for
Diversional Activity, Deficient
Energy Field, Disturbed
Environmental Interpretation Syndrome, Impaired
Failure to Thrive, Adult
Falls, Risk for
Family Processes: Alcoholism, Dysfunctional
Family Processes, Interrupted
Family Processes, Readiness for Enhanced
Fatigue
Fear
Fluid Balance, Readiness for Enhanced
Fluid Volume, Deficient
Fluid Volume, Excess
Fluid Volume, Risk for Deficient
Fluid Volume, Risk for Imbalanced
Gas Exchange, Impaired
Glucose, Risk for Unstable Blood
Grieving
Grieving, Complicated
Grieving, Risk for Complicated
Growth and Development, Delayed
Growth, Risk for Disproportionate
Health Maintenance, Ineffective
Health-Seeking Behaviors
Home Maintenance, Impaired
Hope, Readiness for Enhanced
Hopelessness
Hyperthermia
Hypothermia
Identity, Disturbed Personal
Immunization Status, Readiness for Enhanced
Incontinence, Functional Urinary
Incontinence, Overflow Urinary
Incontinence, Reflex Urinary
Incontinence, Stress Urinary
Incontinence, Total Urinary
Incontinence, Urge Urinary
Incontinence, Risk for Urge Urinary
Infant Behavior, Disorganized
Infant Behavior, Risk for Disorganized
Infant Behavior, Readiness for Enhanced Organized
Infant Feeding Pattern, Ineffective
Infection, Risk for
Injury, Risk for
Injury, Risk for Perioperative Positioning
Insomnia
Intracranial Adaptive Capacity, Decreased
Knowledge, Deficient
Knowledge, Readiness for Enhanced
Lifestyle, Sedentary
Liver Function, Risk for Impaired
Loneliness, Risk for
Memory, Impaired
Mobility, Impaired Bed

From North American Nursing Diagnosis Association International: *Nursing diagnoses: definitions and classification 2007-2008,* Philadelphia, 2007, NANDA International.

Continued

BOX 4-1 | NANDA Nursing Diagnoses 2007-2008—cont'd

Mobility, Impaired Physical
Mobility, Impaired Wheelchair
Nausea
Neglect, Unilateral
Noncompliance
Nutrition: Less Than Body Requirements, Imbalanced
Nutrition: More Than Body Requirements, Imbalanced
Nutrition, Readiness for Enhanced
Nutrition: More Than Body Requirements, Risk for Imbalanced
Oral Mucous Membrane, Impaired
Pain, Acute
Pain, Chronic
Parenting, Readiness for Enhanced
Parenting, Impaired
Parenting, Risk for Impaired
Peripheral Neurovascular Dysfunction, Risk for
Poisoning, Risk for
Post-Trauma Syndrome
Post-Trauma Syndrome, Risk for
Power, Readiness for Enhanced
Powerlessness
Powerlessness, Risk for
Protection, Ineffective
Rape-Trauma Syndrome
Rape-Trauma Syndrome: Compound Reaction
Rape-Trauma Syndrome: Silent Reaction
Religiosity, Impaired
Religiosity, Readiness for Enhanced
Religiosity, Risk for Impaired
Relocation Stress Syndrome
Relocation Stress Syndrome, Risk for
Role Performance, Ineffective
Self-Care, Readiness for Enhanced
Self-Care Deficit, Bathing/Hygiene
Self-Care Deficit, Dressing/Grooming
Self-Care Deficit, Feeding
Self-Care Deficit, Toileting
Self-Concept, Readiness for Enhanced
Self-Esteem, Chronic Low
Self-Esteem, Situational Low
Self-Esteem, Risk for Situational Low
Self-Mutilation
Self-Mutilation, Risk for
Sensory Perception, Disturbed
Sexual Dysfunction
Sexuality Pattern, Ineffective
Skin Integrity, Impaired
Skin Integrity, Risk for Impaired
Sleep Deprivation
Sleep, Readiness for Enhanced
Social Interaction, Impaired
Social Isolation
Sorrow, Chronic
Spiritual Distress
Spiritual Distress, Risk for
Spiritual Well-Being, Readiness for Enhanced
Stress Overload
Suffocation, Risk for
Suicide, Risk for
Surgical Recovery, Delayed
Swallowing, Impaired
Therapeutic Regimen Management, Effective
Therapeutic Regimen Management, Ineffective
Therapeutic Regimen Management, Ineffective Community
Therapeutic Regimen Management, Ineffective Family
Therapeutic Regimen Management, Readiness for Enhanced
Thermoregulation, Ineffective
Thought Processes, Disturbed
Tissue Integrity, Impaired
Tissue Perfusion, Ineffective
Transfer Ability, Impaired
Trauma, Risk for
Urinary Elimination, Impaired
Urinary Elimination, Readiness for Enhanced
Urinary Retention
Ventilation, Impaired Spontaneous
Ventilatory Weaning Response, Dysfunctional
Violence, Risk for Other-Directed
Violence, Risk for Self-Directed
Walking, Impaired
Wandering

Nursing Care of Common Problems of Ill and Hospitalized Children

NURSING CARE PLAN

The Child with Elevated Body Temperature

Nursing Diagnosis	Expected Patient Outcomes	Nursing Interventions	Rationale
Ineffective Thermoregulation related to inflammatory process, elevated environmental temperature (fever)	Child will maintain body temperature within normal limits	Monitor temperature.	To determine effectiveness of treatment
		Administer antipyretic drug in appropriate dosage for child's weight.	To lower child's temperature
Child's/Family's Defining Characteristics *(Subjective and Objective Data)* Clinical manifestations of fever: • Increase in body temperature above normal range (set point) • Flushed skin • Skin warm to touch • Glassy look to eyes • Increased respiratory rate or tachycardia	**The Following NOC Concept Applies to These Outcomes** Thermoregulation	Use the following cooling measures, preferably 1 hour after administering antipyretic: • Increase air circulation. • Reduce environmental temperature. • Place in lightweight clothing. • Expose skin to air. • Apply cool compress to skin (e.g., forehead).	To lower the child's temperature
		Avoid chilling; if child shivers, apply more clothing or blankets.	To prevent shivering that increases the body's metabolic rate
		The Following NIC Concepts Apply to These Interventions Temperature Regulation Vital Signs Monitoring Heat/Cold Application Bathing Fluid Management Malignant Hyperthermia Precautions Medication Administration Medication Management	
Hyperthermia related to increased heat production	Child will maintain body temperature within normal limits	Monitor temperature.	To prevent excessive body cooling
		Apply cooling blanket or mattress.	To decrease temperature
Child's/Family's Defining Characteristics *(Subjective and Objective Data)* Body temperature exceeds normal range (e.g., heat stroke, aspirin toxicity, hyperthyroidism) Febrile seizures	**The Following NOC Concepts Apply to These Outcomes** Thermoregulation Vital Signs Comfort Level	Avoid chilling. • Give tepid water bath of 20-30 minutes' duration. (Exact temperature range for tepid water bath has not been established; it is usually best to start with warm water and gradually add cooler water until a temperature is reached that is beneficial but does not cause chilling.) • Apply cool, moist towels or washcloths; expose only one area of body at a time; change as needed; continue approximately 30 minutes.	To prevent excess body cooling

Continued

NURSING CARE PLAN

The Child with Elevated Body Temperature—cont'd

Nursing Diagnosis	Expected Patient Outcomes	Nursing Interventions	Rationale
Hyperthermia related to increased heat production—cont'd		Never use isopropyl rubbing alcohol in bath or for sponging.	To prevent neurotoxic effects
		Explain to family that antipyretics are of no value in hyperthermia.	To increase understanding
		The Following NIC Concepts Apply to These Interventions Fever Treatment Temperature Regulation Heat/Cold Applications Seizure Precautions	

NURSING CARE PLAN

The Child with Fluid and Electrolyte Disturbances

Nursing Diagnosis	Expected Patient Outcome	Interventions	Rationale
Fluid Volume Deficit related to active fluid loss from renal, gastrointestinal (vomiting, diarrhea, gastric suction), or respiratory (hyperventilation) tracts; or from skin (wounds, diaphoresis) Fluid Volume Deficit related to failure of regulatory mechanisms such as renal or hypothalamus (hyperthermia) **Child's/Family's Defining Characteristics** ***(Subjective and Objective Data)*** Dry oral mucosa Capillary refill >3 seconds Urinary output <1 ml/kg/hr Tachycardia Urine specific gravity 1.030 Weakness	Fluid (water) and electrolyte balance will be restored ***Evidence (Measurable)*** Moist mucous membranes Na^+ 135-145 mEq Voiding (>1 ml/kg/hr) Capillary refill 1-3 sec (brisk) Skin turgor brisk and without tenting Activity level as before illness Vital signs appropriate for age **The Following NOC Concepts Apply to These Outcomes** Fluid Balance Hydration Nutritional Status: Food & Fluid Intake	Assess and record hydration status.	To provide baseline assessment of clinical status
		Describe to parents (and child as age appropriate) plan for interventions (lab, IV fluids, hydration over several hours and monitoring).	To provide accurate information regarding plan of care for child's illness
		Obtain necessary laboratory samples by peripheral vein (collaborative).	To evaluate degree of fluid deficit
		Place topical analgesic on IV site before laboratory draw (collaborative).	To reduce pain
		Establish IV access.	To administer fluids and medications
		Administer antiemetic such as ondansetron (Zofran) (collaborative).	To stop nausea and vomiting
		Administer 0.9% NS bolus 20 ml/kg IV over 20 minutes (collaborative).	To replace fluid losses
		Monitor IV site for erythema, edema, pain, streaking every 1 hr.	To prevent fluid extravasation into tissues To detect signs of phlebitis
		Monitor vital signs every 2 hr or as status change requires.	To prevent further complications and intervene if status changes
		Monitor fluid intake and output.	To assess hydration status
		Offer small sips of oral hydration solution (Pedialyte), 5 ml (1 tsp) every 5-10 minutes after first fluid bolus and 30 min after antiemetic administration.	To rehydrate and assess tolerance to oral fluids

		Monitor urinary output.	To assess renal function and adequacy of hydration interventions
		Monitor laboratory values per protocol (collaborative).	To assess hydration status after initial fluid bolus and/or oral fluid administration and interventions
		The Following NIC Concepts Apply to These Interventions Intravenous (IV) Therapy Laboratory Data Interpretation Vital Signs Monitoring Fluid Monitoring Electrolyte Monitoring	
Risk for Deficient Fluid Volume related to loss of appetite, self-care deficit, immobility, altered sensorium, NPO status, prolonged diagnostic test ***Risk Factors*** Medications (diuretics, chemotherapeutic) Knowledge deficit related to fluid volume	Child exhibits evidence of adequate hydration **The Following NOC Concepts Apply to These Outcomes** Fluid Balance Hydration Risk Control	Administer antiemetic medication	To decrease nausea and vomiting
		Decrease stimuli which may make child anorexic (odors, environmental stimuli).	To reduce nausea
		Provide small amounts of fluids—5 to 10 ml—in flavored form; ice popsicle (freezer pops); flavored (sugar-free) Kool Aid; flavored oral hydration solution such as Pedialyte.	To encourage fluid intake
		Monitor urinary output.	To assess hydration status
		Monitor laboratory values as necessary.	
		Establish IV access as required by assessment data.	To administer fluids
		The Following NIC Concepts Apply to These Interventions Fluid Management Electrolyte Monitoring Intravenous (IV) Therapy	
Fluid Volume Excess related to overhydration, excess free water intake, failure of regulatory mechanism, iatrogenic causes **Child's/Family's Defining Characteristics** ***(Subjective and Objective Data)*** Weight gain over short period of time Intake that exceeds output Edema Changes in respiratory pattern, dyspnea, shortness of breath, abnormal breath sounds, pulmonary congestion, pleural effusion	Child exhibits evidence of fluid and electrolyte balance Child avoids precipitous free water intake **The Following NOC Concepts Apply to These Outcomes** Fluid Balance Hydration Urinary Elimination Nutritional Status: Food & Fluid Intake	Regulate IV fluid intake closely; administer IV fluids via an infusion pump. Check pump hourly for appropriate function.	To prevent excess fluid intake
		Administer diuretics on schedule.	To eliminate excess water (fluid)
		Monitor response to diuretic therapy.	To assess hydration status and renal function
		Monitor urinary output closely. Insert Foley catheter as appropriate to monitor fluid output	To implement appropriate therapy for water reduction or prevention of complications related to water overload
		Monitor serum electrolytes.	To monitor electrolyte stability
		Monitor vital signs including auscultation of lungs, presence of edema (tibial and periorbital in infants; ankle, facial in older child), pulse oximeter, blood pressure.	To assess for edema

Continued

NURSING CARE PLAN

The Child with Fluid and Electrolyte Disturbances—cont'd

Nursing Diagnosis	Expected Patient Outcome	Interventions	Rationale
Fluid Volume Excess related to overhydration, excess free water intake, failure of regulatory mechanism, iatrogenic causes—cont'd		Observe infant for seizure activity and altered sensorium and institute seizure precautions.	To prevent bodily harm
		For Infants	
		Teach parents how to mix powder formula with water.	To avoid unnecessary free water administration
		Teach parents to avoid free water intake, especially in hot weather.	
		Observe child swimming to see if gulping excessive amounts of water.	To monitor for excess water intake
		The Following NIC Concepts Apply to These Interventions Neurologic Monitoring Vital Signs Monitoring Electrolyte Monitoring Medication Administration Urinary Elimination Management Parent Education: Infant	

NURSING CARE PLAN

The Child in Pain

Nursing Diagnosis	Expected Patient Outcomes	Nursing Interventions	Rationale
Pain related to (specify acute or chronic) **Child's/Family's Defining Characteristics** ***(Subjective and Objective Data)*** Facial expression changes Physiologic changes: Increased heart rate and blood pressure, increased respirations, crying, sweating, decreased oxygen saturation, dilation of pupils, flushing or pallor, nausea, muscle tension in the early onset of acute pain that subsides in continuing and chronic pain, making these symptoms unreliable indicators of persistent acute and chronic pain	Experiences either no pain or a reduction of pain to level acceptable to child (equal to or less than comfort or function goal) when receiving analgesics **The Following NOC Concepts Apply to These Outcomes** Comfort Level Pain Control Pain Level Pain: Disruptive Effects	Use QUESTT pain assessment: *Q*uestion the child. *U*se pain rating scales. *E*valuate behavior and physiologic changes. *S*ecure parents' involvement. *T*ake cause of pain into account. *T*ake action and assess its effectiveness.	Child's self-report of pain is most important factor in assessment
		Ask parents about child's behavior when in pain by taking a pain history before pain is expected.	To evaluate the child's pain history
		Obtain information regarding current pain, such as duration, type, and location. Asses for influencing factors that may include (1) precipitating events (those that cause or increase the pain), (2) relieving events (those that lessen the pain, e.g., medications), (3) temporal events (times when the pain is relieved or increased), (4) positional events (standing, sitting, lying down), and (5) associated events (meals, stress, coughing). Have parent or child describe pain in terms of interruption of daily activities.	

Occurrence of specific behaviors (e.g., pulling ears, rolling head from side to side, lying on side with legs flexed, limping, refusing to move a body part) that indicate location of body pain	Use pain assessment scales to promote accurate assessment.	To promote accurate assessment
Occurrence of improvement in behavior when pain medication is given (e.g., less irritability, cessation of crying or playing)	Have child locate pain by marking body part on a human figure drawing or pointing to area with one finger on self, doll, stuffed animal, or "where Mommy or Daddy would put a bandage."	To ensure accurate assessment, because children as young as toddler age, or even children who have difficulty understanding pain scales, can usually locate pain on a drawing or on their bodies
Occurrence of coping strategies child uses during painful procedure (e.g., talking, moaning, lying rigidly still, squeezing hand)	Be aware of reasons why children may deny or not tell the truth about pain.	To decrease fear of receiving an injection if they admit to discomfort; belief that suffering is punishment for some misdeed; lack of trust in telling a stranger (but readily admitting to parent that they are hurting)
	Use a variety of words to describe pain (e.g., "ouch," "owie," "boo-boo," "hurt," "ow ow"). Use appropriate foreign language words (e.g., in Spanish, pain is "duele," "le le," "dolor," or "ai ai"). Use translations of pain rating scale.	To assess pain in a young child who may not know what the word *pain* means and may need to describe pain using familiar language.
	Use pain rating scales.	To provide subjective and quantitative measures of pain intensity
	Select a scale that is suitable to the child's developmental or cognitive age, abilities, and preference (e.g., scales using numbers require an understanding of numeric value, such as knowing that 5 is larger than 3).	To promote accuracy, because some scales are more appropriate for younger children than other scales
	Use pain assessment record or adapt existing form to include pain assessment (e.g., fifth vital sign on vital sign sheet) to document effectiveness of interventions.	To give practitioners objective documentation of pain, rather than opinion, is more likely to lead to favorable change in analgesic orders
	Encourage parents to participate in assessing current pain by using the pain assessment record.	To involve parents in their child's care
	Plan to administer prescribed analgesic before procedure.	To ensure that the peak effect coincides with painful event
	Plan preventive schedule of medication around the clock (ATC) or, if analgesic is ordered PRN, administer it at regular intervals when pain is continuous and predictable (e.g., postoperatively).	To maintain steady blood levels of analgesic
	Administer analgesia by least traumatic route whenever possible; avoid intramuscular or subcutaneous injections.	To avoid causing additional pain
	Prepare child for administration of analgesia by using supportive statements (e.g., "This medicine I am putting in the IV will make you feel better in a few minutes").	To minimize fear and anxiety
	Reinforce the effect of the analgesic by telling the child that he or she will begin to feel better in the appropriate amount of time, according to drug used; use a clock or timer to measure onset of relief with the child; reinforce the cause and effect of pain-analgesic.	To promote expectations of pain relief

Continued

NURSING CARE PLAN

The Child in Pain–cont'd

Nursing Diagnosis	Expected Patient Outcomes	Nursing Interventions	Rationale
Pain related to (specify acute or chronic)—cont'd		If an injection must be given, avoid saying, "I am going to give you an injection for pain"; if the child refuses an injection, explain that the little hurt from the needle will take away the bigger hurt for a long time.	To minimize fear and anxiety, because an injection causes pain
		Avoid statements such as, "This is enough medicine to take away anyone's pain," or "By now you shouldn't need so much pain medicine"	To prevent a judgmental attitude
		Give the child control whenever possible (e.g., using patient-controlled analgesia, choosing which arm for a venipuncture, taking bandages off, or holding the tape or other equipment).	To promote participation in self-care
		Administer prescribed analgesic. Nonopioids, including acetaminophen (Tylenol, paracetamol) and nonsteroidal. antiinflammatory drugs (NSAIDs), are suitable for mild to moderate pain. Opioids are needed for moderate to severe pain. A combination of the two analgesics may be given to provide increased analgesia.	To treat pain at the peripheral nervous system and at the central nervous system and provides increased analgesia without increased side effects
Risk for Injury related to sensitivity, excessive dose, decreased gastrointestinal motility **Child's/Family's Defining Characteristics** ***(Subjective and Objective Data)*** Behavioral or physiologic changes may indicate physical conditions or emotions other than pain (e.g., respiratory distress, fear, anxiety, constipation)	Child will not develop constipation and will receive treatment for other opioid-related side effects Child will feel less distress about the painful experience by using appropriate nonpharmacologic strategies **The Following NOC Concepts Apply to These Outcomes** Pain: Adverse Psychological Response Bowel Elimination Depression Self-Control Risk Detection Risk Control	After intervention, assess child's response to pain relief measures. Determine timing of assessment based on expected onset and peak effect of intervention. IV analgesic: assess after 5 minutes and 15 minutes.	To evaluate response to pain medication
		Titrate (adjust) dosage for maximum pain relief with minimal side effects. Begin with recommended dosage for age and weight.	To promote maximum pain relief
		Increase dosage and/or decrease interval between dosages if pain relief is inadequate.	To manage pain most effectively
		If using parenteral route, change to oral route as soon as possible using equianalgesic (equal analgesic effect) dosages. Convert directly by giving next dose of analgesic orally in equivalent dosage without parenteral form of the same drug, or convert gradually to oral using the following steps: • Convert half parenteral dose to oral. • Administer half the parenteral dose and the oral dose. • Assess pain relief in 30-60 minutes. • If pain relief is inadequate, increase the oral dose as needed. • If sedation occurs, decrease the oral dose of opioid and request order for addition of nonopioid (e.g., Tylenol).	To consider the first-pass effect (an oral opioid is rapidly absorbed from the gastrointestinal tract and enters the portal or hepatic circulation, where it is partially metabolized before reaching the systemic circulation; therefore oral dosages must be larger) To ensure adequate pain management

	• When the parenteral and oral doses are effective, discontinue the parenteral dose and give twice the oral dose.	
Child will exhibit normal respiratory function	Avoid combining opioids with so-called *potentictors*.	To prevent risk of sedation and respiratory depression without increasing analgesia by combining drugs such as promethazine (Phenergan) and chlorpromazine (Thorazine)
	Do not use placebos in the assessment or treatment of pain.	To prevent use of placebos, because they do not provide useful information about the presence or severity of pain, can cause side effects similar to those of opioids, can destroy child's and family's trust in the health care staff
	Monitor rate and depth of respirations and level of sedation.	To prevent depression of these functions, which can lead to apnea
	Have emergency drugs and equipment ready in case of respiratory depression from opioids.	To begin therapy as soon as needed
	Administer bolus IV push every 2 minutes until effect is obtained	
	Closely monitor patient.	To prevent apnea
	• If respiratory depression is a result of benzodiazepines (e.g., diazepam, midazolam), administer flumazenil. Pediatric dosing experience suggests 0.01 mg/kg (0.1 ml/kg) as loading dose; if inadequate within 1-2 minutes, repeat as needed at 1-minute intervals for maximum dose of 1 mg (10 ml).	
	Decrease opioid dose by 25% to determine if this dose decreases side effects (except constipation) while relieving pain.	To decrease side effects of opioids
	Administer laxative (with or without stool softener).	To prevent constipation
	Stop or decrease medication if evidence of rash (urticaria) occurs.	To minimize histamine release from opioids such as morphine
	Advise family that urticaria or pruritus alone is not a sign of allergic reaction to opioid.	To prevent misinformation that can prevent child from receiving opioids
	Administer antipruritic.	To decrease pruritus
	Administer antiemetic.	To decrease nausea and vomiting
	Encourage child to lie quietly until nausea subsides.	To decrease nausea and vomiting
	Recognize signs of tolerance (e.g., decreasing pain relief, decreasing duration of pain relief).	To ensure adequate pain management

Continued

NURSING CARE PLAN

The Child in Pain–cont'd

Nursing Diagnosis	Expected Patient Outcomes	Nursing Interventions	Rationale
Risk for Injury related to sensitivity, excessive dose, decreased gastrointestinal motility—cont'd		Recognize signs of withdrawal after discontinuation of drug (physical dependence).	To ensure adequate management, because these signs and symptoms are involuntary, physiologic responses that occur from prolonged use of opioids
		Help treat tolerance and physical dependence appropriately. Treat tolerance by increasing opioid dose. Suggested guidelines for preventing withdrawal syndrome in patients with physical dependence: • Gradually reduce dose (similar to tapering of steroids). • Give one half of previous daily dose every 6 hours for first 2 days. • Then reduce dose by 25% every 2 days. • Continue this schedule until total daily dose of 0.6 mg/kg/day of morphine (or equivalent) is reached. • After 2 days on this dose, discontinue opioid.	
		May also switch to oral methadone, using one fourth of equianalgesic dose as initial weaning dose and proceeding as described above.	To promote effective management
		Never refer to child who is tolerant or physically dependent as *addicted.*	To prevent labeling the child
		Use nonpharmacologic interventions to supplement, not replace, pharmacologic interventions.	To emphasize that treatment of pain is with analgesics
		Assess the appropriateness of using nonpharmacologic interventions; used alone, they are not appropriate for moderate to severe pain.	To emphasize that they are most useful for mild pain and when pain is reasonably well controlled with analgesics
		Employ nonpharmacologic strategies to help child manage pain.	To encourage techniques such as relaxation, rhythmic breathing, and distraction, which can make pain more tolerable
		Use strategy that is familiar to child, or describe several strategies and let child select one.	To facilitate the child's learning and use of strategy
		Involve parent in selection of strategy. Select appropriate person(s), usually parent, to assist child with strategy.	To promote family involvement
		Teach child to use specific nonpharmacologic strategies before pain occurs or before it becomes severe.	To prevent pain when possible
		Assist or have parent assist child with using strategy during actual pain.	To promote parent coaching

		The Following NIC Concepts Apply to These Interventions Airway Management Analgesic Administration Respiratory Monitoring Fluid Management Constipation/Impaction Management Pain Management Distraction Behavior Management Coping Enhancement Art Therapy Music Therapy Active Listening Medication Management	

NURSING CARE PLAN

The Child with a Fracture

Nursing Diagnosis	Expected Patient Outcomes	Nursing Interventions	Rationale
Risk for Injury related to presence of immobilization device (cast, traction), tissue swelling.	Child's neurologic and circulatory status in immobilized extremity remains intact; toes and fingers are warm, pink, responsive to touch, pulses are palpable, and capillary refill is brisk.	Elevate extremity: Place leg cast on pillows with leg supported without pressure.	To decrease swelling, because elevation increases venous return
		Place arm on pillows or support in stockinette sling (supported by IV pole) or a triangular arm sling for lesser elevation or support.	
Child's/Family's Defining Characteristics ***(Subjective and Objective Data)*** Increased pain at cast site Increased swelling at cast site Increased discoloration, pallor, or cyanosis Decreased pulses Decreased warmth at cast site Decreased sensation at cast site Decreased ability to move *External:* Cast *Internal:* Tissue injury Altered mobility Developmental age (physiological and psychological)	Cast integrity is maintained; plaster cast dries evenly and remains clean and intact.	Assess exposed part for pain, swelling, discoloration (cyanosis or pallor), pulsation, warmth, sensation, and ability to move.	To asses for changes in pain; cyanosis, pallor, and decreased sensation may indicate a problem such as compartmental syndrome
	Child will not experience increased swelling from cast or injury	Cover rough edges with adhesive tape petals (plaster).	To prevent indenting, which can cause pressure areas
		Keep wet cast uncovered (plaster).	To protect cast edges and prevent skin irritation and to allow drying inside out
	The Following NOC Concepts Apply to These Outcomes Fall Prevention Behavior Immune Status Parenting: Psychosocial Safety Personal Safety Behavior Risk Control Safe Home Environment	Change position of body cast or spica cast (plaster) periodically.	To prevent consequences of prolonged immobilization such as loss of muscle function
		Elevate injured tissue.	To reduce edema To reduce pain from edema
		The Following NIC Concepts Apply to These Interventions Neurologic Monitoring Positioning Skin Surveillance	

Continued

NURSING CARE PLAN

The Child with a Fracture—cont'd

Nursing Diagnosis	Expected Patient Outcomes	Nursing Interventions	Rationale
Impaired Physical Mobility related to musculoskeletal impairment **Child's/Family's Defining Characteristics** ***(Subjective and Objective Data)*** *Subjective* Decreased movement because of cast or traction *Objective* Inability to move because of cast or traction *External:* Cast or traction *Internal:* Prolonged bed rest, fear of pain with movement from one bed position to another Developmental age—physiologic and psychologic mobility level	Child engages in activities Muscle tone in affected extremity remains optimal **The Following NOC Concepts Apply to These Outcomes** Ambulation Mobility Self-Care: Activities of Daily Living (ADL) Transfer Performance	Encourage participation in muscle strengthening ROM (passive or active). Perform passive ROM if unable to move independently. Remove toys, hazardous floor rugs, pets, or items that might cause a stumble. Encourage ambulation with assistive device. Teach child to use crutches. Encourage activities: child life projects, playroom if possible. Position for comfort; use pillows to elevate and support dependent areas. Avoid powder or lotions inside cast. **The Following NIC Concepts Apply to These Interventions** Positioning Cast Care: Maintenance	To prevent consequences of prolonged immobilization such as loss of muscle function To prevent pain To prevent falls To establish independent ambulation To use time spent in bed and keep up cognitive development To minimize pain and discomfort To prevent skin irritation
Risk for Impaired Skin Integrity related to immobilization device, insensate areas of skin resulting from artificial covering (cast, traction) **Child's/Family's Defining Characteristics** ***(Subjective and Objective Data)*** *Subjective* Altered nutritional status Impaired mobility Moisture Mechanical factors such as shearing forces Altered sensation Altered circulation *Objective* Pressure ulcer staging Braden or Modified Braden Risk Assessment	Skin remains intact without evidence of irritation Cast (plaster) dries evenly and remains clean and intact **The Following NOC Concepts Apply to These Outcomes** Immobility Consequences: Physiological Tissue Integrity: Skin & Mucous Membranes	Protect cast with plastic film during bathing unless synthetic cast is waterproof. Protect rim of cast around perineal area with plastic film. After cast is removed soak and gently wash skin; avoid scrubbing. Use lotion to help loosen dead skin. Turn every 2 hours if patient is unable to move site by himself or herself. Assess skin as part of ongoing nursing assessment based on severity of illness. **The Following NIC Concepts Apply to These Interventions** Incision Site Care Pressure Ulcer Care Skin Care: Topical Treatment Skin Surveillance Wound Care	To prevent cast from getting wet To prevent soiling during toileting To prevent skin breakdown To prevent pressure sore development To identify early signs of skin breakdown Modified Braden Q is a skin scale for children The more critical the child's condition, the more at risk the child is for skin breakdown

Nursing Care of the Newborn

NURSING CARE PLAN

The Newborn with Jaundice

Nursing Diagnosis	Expected Patient Outcomes	Nursing Interventions	Rationale
Risk for Injury related to abnormal blood profile (increased breakdown of products of red blood cells), developmental age (immature blood-brain barrier and immature liver function)	Newborn will receive appropriate therapy to enhance bilirubin excretion	Initiate breast-feeding within first hour of life in delivery room.	To promote breast milk intake and stooling
	Newborn will remain injury-free	If formula-feeding, assist parents in initiation of early feeding.	To promote milk intake and stooling
	The Following NOC Concept Applies to These Outcomes	Assess skin for jaundice every 4 hr.	To detect evidence of clinical jaundice and rising bilirubin levels
Child's/Family's Defining Characteristics	Risk Control	Observe for development of jaundice, especially within 24 hr of birth.	To institute treatment and prevent complications
(Subjective and Objective Data)	Risk Detection	Monitor transcutaneous bilirubin levels per institution protocol or at least every 6 to 8 hours.	To detect rising levels of bilirubin for institution of appropriate therapy
Clinical jaundice evident within 24 hr of birth		Obtain serum bilirubin (collaborative intervention).	
Altered breast-feeding (ineffective latch-on, nurses less than 6-8 times in 24-hr period)		Monitor intake and output with each occurrence.	To evaluate effectiveness of breast-feeding or formula intake by measuring urinary and stool output
Altered stooling pattern (less than 1 stool in 24 hr)		Maintain accurate record of urine and stool output and assist parents in same.	To provide accurate record of output to evaluate effectiveness of feedings
		Monitor vital signs per unit protocol or at least every 8 hr. Report signs of poor transition to extrauterine life.	To evaluate transitional events and ensure infant is making an effective transition without cardiorespiratory, metabolic, thermoregulatory, or other physiologic problems
		Instruct parents regarding newborn care, including jaundiced appearance, its significance, importance of follow-up visit to practitioner within 2-3 days of discharge, feeding methods, and noting stooling and voiding patterns.	To promote physical care of newborn and decrease parents' anxiety related to home care
		The Following NIC Concepts Apply to These Interventions Risk Identification Nutrition Management Breastfeeding Assistance Lactation Counseling Newborn Monitoring Newborn Care Fluid Monitoring	

Continued

NURSING CARE PLAN

The Newborn with Jaundice—cont'd

Nursing Diagnosis	Expected Patient Outcomes	Nursing Interventions	Rationale
Readiness for Enhanced Parenting related to birth of a new family member	Parent(s) of newborn assume responsibility for emotional and physical care and well-being of the new family member	Initiate skin-to-skin contact between mother and newborn and father and newborn in delivery room within first hour of birth.	To enhance parent-infant interaction and acquaintance with newborn
Child's/Family's Defining Characteristics ***(Subjective and Objective Data)***	**The Following NOC Concepts Apply to These Outcomes**	Encourage early breast-feeding in first hour of birth.	To enhance breast-feeding and parent-infant interaction and to promote early stooling and bilirubin clearance
Parent(s) express willingness to enhance parenting	Parent-Infant Attachment	Perform physical assessment with parents present, and show typical newborn characteristics. Point out state traits such as quiet awake and cues to feeding readiness.	To promote parents' knowledge of infant physical characteristics and behavior
Emotional support of child is evident; bonding or attachment is evident	Parenting: Psychosocial Safety	Encourage parent participation in care behaviors such as diapering, formula feeding (as applicable), and bathing.	To promote familiarity with behaviors and decrease parental anxiety To enhance parental feeling of contribution as newborn's primary caretakers
	Caregiver Home Care Readiness	Encourage sibling visitation and participation in care and holding of newborn as age-appropriate.	To promote sibling participation in care and acceptance of new family member
		The Following NIC Concepts Apply to These Interventions Anxiety Reduction Family Support Family Process Maintenance Parent Education: Infant	

NURSING CARE PLAN

The Infant with Bronchopulmonary Dysplasia (BPD)

Nursing Diagnosis	Expected Patient Outcomes	Nursing Interventions	Rationale
Ineffective Breathing Pattern related to pulmonary, vascular, and alveolar tissue damage **Child's/Family's Defining Characteristics** ***(Subjective and Objective Data)*** Decreased minute ventilation Use of accessory muscles to breathe Nasal flaring Tachypnea Altered chest excursion Decreased vital capacity Increased work of breathing* Persistent respiratory rate >60/min* High caloric needs and restricted growth* Hypoxemia and prolonged O_2 dependence* Hypercarbia* In some cases reactive airway disease and wheezing*	Infant maintains effective ventilation status **The Following NOC Concepts Apply to These Outcomes** Respiratory Status: Airway Patency Vital Signs	Position to facilitate airway expansion and prevent collection of secretions (prone position may be preferred initially in preterm infant to increase chest expansion and oxygenation).	To allow oxygen entry into bronchial tree and alveoli
		Closely monitor for deviations from desired breathing pattern—pulse oximetry, arterial blood gases, clinical signs of poor oxygenation, grunting, nasal flaring, apnea, tachypnea, retractions, cyanosis.	To implement appropriate therapy such as supplemental oxygen, mechanical ventilation, or change of position and facilitate proper oxygenation
		Administer supplemental oxygen (established unit protocols may be used to maintain oxygen saturations within given parameters).	To prevent lung damage, hypoxemia and hyperoxemia
		Monitor vital signs for change in condition or status such as decreased cardiac output (poor perfusion, mottling, deteriorating ventilation status).	To implement appropriate therapy such as suctioning, supplemental oxygen, or vasopressor drugs
		Suction oropharynx, nasopharynx, trachea or endotracheal tube only as necessary and based on respiratory assessment.	To remove secretions that may interfere with adequate ventilation and oxygenation
		Perform gentle chest percussion, vibration, and postural drainage based on assessed need and infant tolerance to same.	To facilitate drainage of secretions and removal
		Administer bronchodilators such as caffeine citrate, albuterol, or other.	To expand airways and prevent hypoxia
		Administer diuretics such as aldosterone, furosemide (Lasix).	To promote fluid excretion
		Implement neurodevelopmental care including skin-to-skin holding by parent(s), positioning with borders, provision of quiet time with no handling, pain management, altered lighting, and others as appropriate.	To promote appropriate neurodevelopmental growth To prevent complications related to poor state regulation
		Encourage parent(s) to assume responsibility for as much of the infant's care as possible while in NICU.	To prevent sense of helplessness and enhance parental involvement in care
		Teach family and assist with respiratory syncytial virus (RSV) infection and upper respiratory infection (URI) prevention; prevent contact with those possibly exposed to RSV.	To prevent contraction of RSV, which can result in serious respiratory illness in infant with BPD
		At discharge, assist and teach family to prevent exposure to infected contacts.	
		Assist with RSV prophylaxis— administer palivizumab (Synagis) once monthly in high-risk exposure months (usually November to March).	To prevent RSV infection

*Gracey K, Talbot D, Lankford R, Dodge P: The changing face of bronchopulmonary dysplasia: Part 1, *Adv Neonatal Care* 2(6):327-338, 2002.

Continued

NURSING CARE PLAN

The Infant with Bronchopulmonary Dysplasia (BPD)—cont'd

Nursing Diagnosis	Expected Patient Outcomes	Nursing Interventions	Rationale
Ineffective Breathing Pattern related to pulmonary, vascular, and alveolar tissue damage—cont'd		Assist with teaching care of monitor and reinforcing proper use of home apnea monitor as indicated for infant's condition.	To allay parental anxiety related to alarms and infant's condition
		Teach parent(s) to evaluate infant's color and activity if alarm is activated. Assist with familiarization with equipment and meaning of false alarms.	To allay parent(s) anxiety regarding use of equipment and alarms, which can be quite stressful
		Teach parent(s) infant CPR and procedure for removal of foreign body obstruction.	To educate parent(s) on how to resuscitate infant if required and to decrease fear of helplessness if infant's condition is poor; to give parents confidence in caring for child with chronic illness
		The Following NIC Concepts Apply to These Interventions Oxygen Therapy Positioning Respiratory Monitoring Vital Signs Monitoring Acid-Base Management Ventilation Assistance Medication Management Fluid Management Developmental Care Infection Control	
Imbalanced Nutrition: Less Than Body Requirements **Child's/Family's Defining Characteristics** ***(Subjective and Objective Data)*** Inadequate weight gain Restricted physical growth	Achieves and maintains adequate physical growth **The Following NOC Concepts Apply to These Outcomes** Nutritional Status: Food & Fluid Intake Nutritional Status: Nutrient Intake Child Development: 2 Months Child Development: 4 Months Child Development: 6 Months Child Development: 12 Months	Encourage mother to feed expressed breast milk (EBM) with human milk fortifier (HMF); when infant is able to suckle at breast, encourage breastfeeding; assist mother with latch-on.	To promote breast milk as the best nutritional source for preterm infants; has immune properties; HMF enhances caloric and micronutrient (vitamins, minerals, amino acids) intake; mothers need assistance with preterm infants, who are not as vigorous feeders as healthy term infants
		Provide nonnutritive sucking (NNS) opportunities at breast. Provide NNS opportunities for infant who is gavage-fed.	To encourage NNS, because it is essential in the development of preterm infants and enhances eventual progression to (breast or bottle) nipple feeding
		Ensure infant receives adequate amount of calories/nutrients per feeding (projected need 120-140 cal/kg/day).	Provide adequate calories
		Avoid excess fluid intake from medication dilutions, free water administration.	To prevent fluid overload which may exacerbate BPD and cause complications such as patent ductus arteriosus (PDA)
		Gavage- or bottle-feed preterm specialty formula feedings as appropriate to capabilities.	To provide adequate caloric and nutrient intake

		Maintain adequate thermoregulation as per illness requirements and infant's physiologic status (incubator or crib with extra blanket and head covering as needed).	To prevent cold stress, which can increase oxygen and glucose requirements, further compromising infant's respiratory and metabolic status
		Monitor oxygenation status during feedings, and use supplemental O_2 as required to maintain saturation parameters.	To monitor tolerance to feeding process and provide alternate method as necessary
		Weigh daily.	To monitor physical growth
		Measure head circumference and length weekly.	To monitor physical and brain growth
		Discharge planning: Assist parents with special equipment and supplies needed to provide for infant's nutritional care at home (as required).	To provide necessary supplies and equipment to facilitate continuation of feeding plan at home (for adequate caloric and nutrient intake)
		Teach parent(s) gavage-feeding or special feeding (gastrostomy) regimen, and encourage return demonstration in NICU; encourage full participation in care.	To facilitate transition to home and maintain feeding protocol for adequate growth to occur after discharge To promote parent familiarization with feeding technique and allay anxiety regarding feeding method (specialized)
		Ensure follow-up examinations for eye, developmental, and hearing assessments.	To assess infants with BPD, who often have special needs related to eye development and disease (retinopathy of prematurity [ROP]), hearing impairment, and developmental delays To provide adequate early intervention for any deficits
		The Following NIC Concepts Apply to These Interventions Nutritional Monitoring Lactation Counseling Fluid Management Vital Signs Monitoring Bottle Feeding Laboratory Data Interpretation	
Risk for Caregiver Role Strain related to assuming home care of an infant with a chronic illness **Child's/Family's Defining Characteristics *(Subjective and Objective Data)*** Preterm birth Child requires complex or multiple caregiving tasks	Parent(s) assume responsibility for infant's home care. **The Following NOC Concepts Apply to These Outcomes** Caregiver Well-Being Caregiver Performance: Direct Care Caregiver Emotional Health Risk Control	Encourage parent(s) to be involved in care of infant in NICU in such activities as holding (skin-to-skin contact), feeding (breast or bottle), diapering, dressing infant in regular clothing, encouraging other family members to visit such as grandparents and siblings (as allowed by unit).	To facilitate parent involvement in infant's care To promote feelings of success in caring for infant To allay anxiety related to infant's perceived fragile or vulnerable status To promote sense of personal investment in child's well-being To promote parent-infant attachment and bonding
		Encourage parent to focus on the positive attributes and physical characteristics of the infant.	To promote personal nature of child as valuable human being
		Encourage and engage parent in a discussion of feelings regarding the care of the infant in the home	To permit open discussion of feelings and concerns regarding childrearing and the challenges in a therapeutic setting

Continued

NURSING CARE PLAN

The Infant with Bronchopulmonary Dysplasia (BPD)–cont'd

Nursing Diagnosis	Expected Patient Outcomes	Nursing Interventions	Rationale
Risk for Caregiver Role Strain related to assuming home care of an infant with a chronic illness—cont'd		Encourage open discussion of how lifestyle alterations will affect personal and family functioning.	To promote open discussion of potential problems in being the parent of a child with a chronic illness
Infant may require oxygen therapy, special feedings, apnea monitoring, and medication administration at home		Assess the resources available to the parent and family for home care of child with a chronic illness.	To provide financial and physical resources for assistance
Infant requires frequent medical visits for follow-up		Discuss available family and friend resources to assist with the care of the infant in the home.	To provide respite for continual care of child with chronic illness and for emotional and social support of family and parent(s) of child
Parent and family lifestyle disruption		Encourage involvement in parent-to-parent support group before and after discharge.	To allow parents to see what parents with similar challenges face and how they deal with the responsibility of caring for an infant with chronic illness
		Discuss plans for infant's care in home in relation to home modifications, special equipment, lifestyle changes, potential for assistance with daily care, transportation with special equipment, managing other children's childrearing, and support needs.	To promote mutual decision making regarding infant's care and address realistic concerns before they occur (anticipate problems and corrective action)
		Arrange for interview with home health care nurse (as appropriate) before discharge for care considerations.	To encourage discussion of home care needs
		See also nursing interventions in previous diagnosis section related to discharge and home care: oxygen, monitor use, CPR, and nutrition needs.	
		The Following NIC Concepts Apply to These Interventions Coping Enhancement Support System Enhancement Emotional Support Decision-Making Support Family Support Home Maintenance Assistance Abuse Protection Support: Child Parent Education: Infant	

Nursing Care of the Child with Respiratory Dysfunction

NURSING CARE PLAN

The High-Risk Infant with Respiratory Distress

Nursing Diagnosis	Patient Outcomes	Nursing Interventions	Rationale
Ineffective Breathing Pattern related to pulmonary, neurologic, vascular, alveolar, and muscular immaturity	High-risk infant will maintain patent airway and ventilatory status adequate for oxygenation.	Position to facilitate airway expansion and prevent collection of secretions (prone position may be preferred in preterm infant to increase chest expansion and oxygenation).	To allow oxygen entry into bronchial tree and alveoli
Child's/Family's Defining Characteristics ***(Subjective and Objective Data)***	**The Following NOC Concepts Apply to These Outcomes**	Closely monitor for deviations from desired breathing pattern—pulse oximetry, arterial blood gases, clinical signs of poor oxygenation, grunting, nasal flaring, apnea, tachypnea, retractions, cyanosis.	To facilitate proper oxygenation by implementing appropriate therapy such as supplemental oxygen, mechanical ventilation, or change of position
Decreased inspiratory/expiratory pressure	Respiratory Status: Ventilation	Monitor vital signs for change in condition or status such as decreased cardiac output (poor perfusion, mottling, deteriorating ventilation status).	To implement appropriate therapy such as suctioning, supplemental oxygen, or vasopressor drugs
Decreased minute ventilation	Respiratory Status: Gas Exchange	Assist with exogenous surfactant administration and monitor patient tolerance or change in status.	To increase alveolar expansion and enhance oxygen–carbon dioxide exchange
Use of accessory muscles to breathe	Tissue Perfusion: Pulmonary	Suction oropharynx, nasopharynx, trachea, or endotracheal tube only as necessary and based on respiratory assessment.	To remove secretions that may interfere with adequate ventilation and oxygenation
Nasal flaring		Perform gentle chest percussion, vibration, and postural drainage based on assessed need and infant tolerance.	To facilitate drainage and removal of secretions
Grunting		**The Following NIC Concepts Apply to These Interventions**	
Apnea		Vital Signs Monitoring	
Tachypnea		Newborn Monitoring	
Altered chest excursion		Acid-Base Management	
Respiratory rate: <20 or >60 breaths/min		Airway Management	
		Chest Physiotherapy	
		Oxygen Therapy	
		Airway Suctioning	
		Energy Management	
		Respiratory Monitoring	

Continued

NURSING CARE PLAN

The High-Risk Infant with Respiratory Distress—cont'd

Nursing Diagnosis	Patient Outcomes	Nursing Interventions	Rationale
Ineffective Thermoregulation related to immature neurologic and metabolic temperature control	Infant will maintain stable body temperature (specify range for age).	Place newborn in a thermally controlled incubator or radiant warmer.	To control environmental temperature and keep infant's temperature stable
		Place knitted or cloth cap on head.	To prevent heat loss from exposed scalp
	The Following NOC Concept Applies to These Outcomes	Use environmental controls for decreasing body heat loss—plastic heat shield, increased ambient temperature, servo-control on warmer or incubator.	To regulate body temperature within acceptable range and minimize heat loss
Child's/Family's Defining Characteristics *(Subjective and Objective Data)*	Thermoregulation: Newborn	Monitor axillary temperature as often as necessary or per unit protocol.	To detect necessity for environmental temperature regulation and to determine infant's response to environmental thermoregulation
Reduction in body temperature below normal range		Check temperature of newborn in relation to environmental temperature and temperature of heating element.	To detect change in thermoregulatory status, which may indicate a significant disease process such as sepsis
Prolonged capillary refill		Monitor vital signs and skin color, perfusion, pulses, and respiratory status.	To detect changes in status that require additional intervention for stabilization
Cool skin Increased respiratory rate		Monitor for signs of hyperthermia (flushing, tachycardia, altered level of consciousness) and hypothermia (decreased activity; respiratory distress [deterioration]; cool, mottled extremities).	To prevent untoward effects of hyperthermia (fluctuating cerebral perfusion, apnea, increased metabolism with decreased available glucose for vital functions) or hypothermia (increased glucose utilization, lactic acidosis, respiratory compromise).
Tachycardia		Monitor serum glucose levels as necessary or per unit protocol.	To ensure euglycemia is maintained
		The Following NIC Concepts Apply to These Interventions Environmental Management Hypothermia Treatment	
Risk for Impaired Parent-Infant Attachment	Parent(s) will form emotional bond or attachment with newborn.	Encourage parent(s) to hold and make eye contact with newborn as physical status allows.	To minimize effects of physical separation from newborn
		Encourage parent-newborn skin-to-skin contact as condition of newborn allows.	To facilitate parent-infant interaction, which is meaningful and comforting
Risk Factors Separation	**The Following NOC Concept Applies to These Outcomes**	Explain to parents the newborn's illness in simple terms and expectations for recovery.	To enhance parental knowledge and decrease potential fear of unknown regarding infant's survival and recovery
Preterm infant		Encourage parents to name newborn.	To provide child individual identity
Physical barriers	Parent-Infant Attachment	Encourage parent participation in newborn care activities such as touching infant, expressing and storing maternal breast milk, and talking to infant.	To facilitate parental involvement in attaining the role of parents and decrease feelings of hopelessness
		The Following NIC Concepts Apply to These Interventions Infant Care Breastfeeding Assistance Anxiety Reduction Parent Education: Infant	

NURSING CARE PLAN

The Child with Acute Respiratory Infection

Nursing Diagnosis	Expected Patient Outcomes	Nursing Interventions	Rationale
Ineffective Breathing Pattern related to inflammatory process **Child's/Family's Defining Characteristics** ***(Subjective and Objective Data)*** Use of accessory muscles to breathe Dyspnea Shortness of breath Nasal flaring Altered chest excursion Assumption of three-point position (tripod) Respiratory rate is outside normal parameter for child's age (increased or decreased rate)	Child's ventilatory status is adequate for oxygenation **The Following NOC Concepts Apply to These Outcomes** Respiratory Status: Airway Patency Respiratory Status: Ventilation	Position for maximal ventilatory efficiency and airway patency. Position to facilitate drainage of secretions. Provide humidified oxygen as necessary. Monitor oxygenation status, including vital signs for changes in condition. Suction airway (nose, trachea) as necessary. Provide gentle chest percussion and physiotherapy as necessary. Administer bronchodilator medications. Administer anti inflammatory medications. Administer antibiotics (if bacterial). **The Following NIC Concepts Apply to These Interventions** Aspiration Precautions Positioning Respiratory Monitoring Surveillance Oxygen Therapy Airway Suctioning Vital Signs Monitoring Cough Enhancement	To allow increased chest expansion To maintain patent airway and prevent airway obstruction To improve oxygenation To determine need for additional interventions To remove secretions and maintain airway patency To facilitate secretion removal To promote bronchodilation and improve ventilation To decrease airway inflammation To decrease inflammatory response
Ineffective Airway Clearance related to inflammation, mechanical obstruction, increased secretions **Child's/Family's Defining Characteristics** ***(Subjective and Objective Data)*** Dyspnea Difficulty vocalizing Orthopnea Adventitious breath sounds (crackles, wheezing, rhonchi) Cough ineffective or absent Restlessness Changes in respiratory rate and rhythm	Child's airways remain patent **The Following NOC Concepts Apply to These Outcomes** Aspiration Prevention Respiratory Status: Airway Patency	Position to facilitate drainage of secretions. Perform chest physiotherapy. Suction airway as necessary. Provide humidified oxygen. Assist with coughing (as developmentally or age appropriate). Avoid throat examination if epiglottitis suspected. Assure child (as appropriate) all measures will be taken to ensure adequate airway is maintained. Implement comfort measures such as allowing parental presence, parental holding, favorite blanket or stuffed animal at side; explain all procedures beforehand. **The Following NIC Concepts Apply to These Interventions** Cough Enhancement Positioning Chest Physiotherapy Vital Signs Monitoring Anxiety Reduction	To prevent airway obstruction To loosen and remove secretions To remove secretions To moisten secretions and prevent airway drying To remove secretions To prevent airway compromise To allay anxiety To promote anxiety reduction and decrease effects of medical therapy, including hospitalization if required

Continued

NURSING CARE PLAN

The Child with Acute Respiratory Infection–cont'd

Nursing Diagnosis	Expected Patient Outcomes	Nursing Interventions	Rationale
Risk for Injury related to presence (only as indicated) of infective organisms	Child remains free from complications of infection	Maintain aseptic environment using sterile suction equipment and technique.	To prevent spread of infectious organisms in child and family
		Implement and practice Standard Precautions.	
		Implement contact and/or airborne precautions as necessary.	
Child's/Family's Defining Characteristics	**The Following NOC Concept Applies to These Outcomes**	Obtain (secretion, tissue, or blood) specimen as indicated.	To identify infective organism
(Subjective and Objective Data)	Risk Control	Encourage child and family contacts to practice frequent handwashing and avoid hand-to-eye and mouth contact.	To prevent spread of infection
Tissue hypoxia Abnormal blood profile People or provider (nosocomial agents)		Teach child (as age appropriate) and family how to decrease spread of organisms by covering mouth when coughing and disposing of secretions to avoid cross-contamination.	To prevent spread of infection
Mode of transport		Administer antibiotic or antiviral medications.	To treat infection source
Developmental age		Administer fever reduction medication(s) as appropriate.	To promote comfort if fever is present
		Monitor and assess for signs and symptoms of secondary complications: hypoxia, skin breakdown, poor nutrient and fluid intake, increased work of breathing, deteriorating cardiorespiratory status.	To implement therapy for prevention of secondary complications
		The Following NIC Concepts Apply to These Interventions Risk Identification Environmental Management Infection Control Parent Education: Childrearing Family	
Interrupted Family Processes related to child's illness and/or hospitalization, medical therapeutic regimen	Family demonstrates ability to cope with child's illness	Allow family to remain with child.	To decrease effects of separation
		Promote family-centered care. Explain procedures and therapeutic regimen to family.	To provide accurate information regarding therapy and child's condition
		Keep family informed of child's status. Encourage family involvement in child's care.	To promote family sense of control and involvement in care
Child's/Family's Defining Characteristics ***(Subjective and Objective Data)*** Communication patterns Participation in decision making Availability for emotional support Expressions of conflict within family Patterns and rituals	**The Following NOC Concepts Apply to These Outcomes** Family Functioning Family Normalization Parenting Performance	Provide support and referral for continued support as necessary. **The Following NIC Concepts Apply to These Interventions** Caregiver Support Family Support Coping Enhancement Emotional Support Financial Resource Assistance	

NURSING CARE PLAN

The Child with Asthma

Nursing Diagnosis	Expected Patient Outcomes	Nursing Interventions	Rationale
Risk for Suffocation related to interaction between individual and triggering factors (allergens, respiratory infection, exercise, irritants, emotions, temperature changes)	Child will have adequate airway exchange	Assist child and family to recognize factors such as allergens, irritants, temperature changes, and upper respiratory infections (URIs) that trigger asthma symptoms.	To avoid asthma exacerbations
	Family and child assume responsibility for asthma symptom management	Assist child (according to developmental age) and family to recognize early signs of an asthmatic episode (use peak expiratory flow meter [PEFM]).	To control symptoms with medication
Child's/Family's Defining Characteristics	**The Following NOC Concepts Apply to These Outcomes**	Educate child and family in the use of inhaled corticosteroids and bronchodilator.	To control symptoms and minimize shortness of breath
(Subjective and Objective Data)		Educate child and family regarding proper use of rescue medications in case of disease exacerbation.	To prevent illness exacerbations and hospitalization; to prevent side effects from improper use of certain asthma drugs
Wheezing Dry cough Labored respirations Dyspnea Intercostal retractions Complains of tightness in chest, shortness of breath Bronchial inflammation and airway constriction	Asthma Self-Management Anxiety Self-Control Knowledge: Child Physical Safety	Educate child and family regarding the proper use of MDI inhaler with spacer, aerosolized nebulizer, and PEFM (know child's personal best).	To help child and family effectively manage asthma symptoms independently
		The Following NIC Concepts Apply to These Interventions Respiratory Monitoring Medication Administration: Inhalation Risk Identification Family Integrity Promotion Energy Management Coping Enhancement Environmental Management	
Interrupted Family Processes related to child with a chronic illness	Family copes with effects of the disease	Provide family and child (as age appropriate) with explanations about the disease and management.	To provide adequate knowledge To provide realistic expectations
	Family provides child an appropriate protective environment	Cooperate with family to develop a written action plan for asthma management.	To provide family and child sense of control
Child's/Family's Defining Characteristics ***(Subjective and Objective Data)***		Discuss facilitators and barriers to effective asthma management.	To assist family members in understanding their role as being vital in the management of asthma
Anxiety Family interactions with child and members are disrupted	**The Following NOC Concepts Apply to These Outcomes**	Encourage family and child (age appropriate) to discuss the impact of the illness on the family's lifestyle.	To provide opportunity to verbalize frustrations and challenges of having a child with a chronic illness
Family conflicts Inadequate child support Child's health status is ignored Family ignores other members' needs for those of the child with asthma	Family Functioning Family Normalization	Evaluate family resources for asthma management in relation to the following: • Access to health care • Medication availability in home and school (or daycare, as appropriate) • Allergen exposure control and eradication	To enhance family coping with chronic illness

Continued

NURSING CARE PLAN

The Child with Asthma–cont'd

Nursing Diagnosis	Expected Patient Outcomes	Nursing Interventions	Rationale
Interrupted Family Processes related to child with a chronic illness—cont'd		**The Following NIC Concepts Apply to These Interventions** Emotional Support Anticipatory Guidance Family Involvement Promotion Financial Resource Assistance Decision-Making Support Mutual Goal Setting	

NURSING CARE PLAN

The Child with Cystic Fibrosis

Nursing Diagnosis	Expected Patient Outcomes	Nursing Interventions	Rationale
Ineffective Airway Clearance related to thick, tenacious mucus	Child will maintain a patent airway at all times	Auscultate breath sounds every 2-4 hours.	To assess respiratory status
		Assist child to cough and expectorate mucus.	To promote airway clearance
		Monitor respiratory patterns: rate, depth, and effort.	To decrease viscosity of mucus and improve pulmonary function tests
Child's/Family's Defining Characteristics *(Subjective and Objective Data)*	**The Following NOC Concepts Apply to These Outcomes**	Provide nebulization with appropriate solution and equipment as prescribed.	To loosen secretions
Meconium Ileus (newborn) Abdominal distention, vomiting, failure to pass stools, rapid development of dehydration	Aspiration Prevention	Suction if needed to clear secretions.	To loosen secretions
Gastrointestinal Large, bulky loose, frothy extremely foul-smelling stools, voracious appetite (early in disease), loss of appetite (later in disease), weight loss, marked tissue wasting, failure to grow, sallow skin, thin extremities, evidence of deficiency of fat-soluble vitamins	Respiratory Status: Airway Patency	Perform chest physiotherapy.	To facilitate removal of mucus
		Teach child how to use flutter clearance device.	To help loosen secretions
	Respiratory Status: Ventilation	Teach child and family how to use therapy vest.	To promote air movement
	Symptom Control	Teach child and family how to administer bronchodilator medications.	To help loosen secretions and open airways
Endocrine Elevated serum glucose levels; development of cystic fibrosis–related diabetes		Teach child and family how to administer mucolytic medications.	To liquefy secretions
		Teach child and family how to assess airway status using peak flow meter.	To promote compliance at home

Respiratory **Initial manifestations** • Wheezy respirations • Dry, nonproductive, chronic cough **Eventually** • Increased dyspnea, paroxysmal cough; evidence of obstructive emphysema and patchy areas of atelectasis • Progressive involvement • Overinflated, barrel-shaped chest, cyanosis, clubbing of fingers and toes, repeated episodes of bronchitis and bronchopneumonia, chronic nasal congestion, rhinitis, chronic sinusitis, nasal polyps		Help family set up a timetable for medication administration. **The Following NIC Concepts Apply to These Interventions** Airway Management Airway Suction Medication Administration Cough Enhancement	To encourage optimal therapy
Imbalanced Nutrition: Less Than Body Requirements related to inability to digest nutrients, loss of appetite (advanced disease) **Child's/Family's Defining Characteristics *(Subjective and Objective Data)*** Immature or inappropriate activity level for developmental age or stage Evidence of physical handicap Weight loss with adequate food intake Steatorrhea Abdominal cramping Hyperactive bowel sounds	Will exhibit signs of adequate digestion Will exhibit appropriate height and weight for age **The Following NOC Concepts Apply to These Outcomes** Nutritional Status: Nutrient Intake Nutritional Status: Food & Fluid Intake Weight Control	Administer pancreatic enzymes with meals and snacks as prescribed. Teach child and family proper administration of pancreatic enzymes. Take with meals or snacks. Capsules can be swallowed whole or opened and sprinkled on food but not crushed or chewed. Encourage high protein diet, which includes small frequent meals. Consider nutritional consultation if not meeting dietary requirements for age. Observe frequency and nature of stools. Monitor child's physical growth (height and weight). **The Following NIC Concepts Apply to These Interventions** Nutritional Counseling Weight Management Nutritional Monitoring Medication Management	To replace enzymes necessary for digestion to occur in the child with pancreatic insufficiency To prevent destroying enteric coating that results in inactivation of enzymes and excoriation of oral mucosa To promote optimal digestion To determine need for supplemental nutritional program (e.g., night tube feedings) To assess for potential nutritional problems To determine trends in growth and development
Knowledge Deficit related to child and family unfamiliarity with chronic disease management **Child's/Family's Defining Characteristics *(Subjective and Objective Data)*** Child does not take medications Child and family do not follow treatment plan Child and family verbalize lack of understanding of treatment regimen	Will verbalize understanding of management of cystic fibrosis. **The Following NOC Concepts Apply to These Outcomes** Knowledge: Personal Safety	Begin discharge planning as soon as possible. Assess need for assistive support systems and assistive devices. Arrange for community or home health services to visit child and family and teach how to use inhalant or nebulizer. Instruct on reporting effectiveness of treatments and medications to physician.	To facilitate transition to home management To promote transition to home To determine adherence to medical regimen. Inappropriate use of medications (too much or too little) can influence amount of respiratory secretion To encourage realistic expectations that may prevent activities that exceed energy level

Continued

NURSING CARE PLAN

The Child with Cystic Fibrosis—cont'd

Nursing Diagnosis	Expected Patient Outcomes	Nursing Interventions	Rationale
Knowledge Deficit related to child and family unfamiliarity with chronic disease management—cont'd	Knowledge: Infection Control	Involve child in self-care.	To promote lifelong health promotion behaviors
	Knowledge: Health Behavior	Encourage child's involvement in routine activities such as school and sports.	To support socialization with peers, which is a developmental task for school-age children
	Knowledge: Illness Care	In adolescent children discuss activities, limitations, and goal setting.	To promote age-appropriate behaviors
	Knowledge: Treatment Procedure(s)	Teach child to recognize signs and symptoms of inadequate therapy and need for practitioner follow-up.	To prevent long-term sequelae related to poor response to treatment
		Teach importance of setting realistic expectations such as gradual increase in activity and exercise routine, attendance at school, and possibility of hospitalization.	To promote age-appropriate behaviors
		The Following NIC Concepts Apply to These Interventions Health Education Teaching: Disease Process Teaching: Procedure/Treatment Parent Education: Childrearing Family Support System Enhancement	

NURSING CARE PLAN

The Child with Respiratory Failure

Nursing Diagnosis	Expected Patient Outcomes	Nursing Interventions	Rationale
Impaired Gas Exchange related to altered oxygen supply, altered pulmonary flow, alveolar-capillary membrane changes **Child's/Family's Defining Characteristics *(Subjective and Objective Data)*** Visible retractions with respirations, intercostal, subcostal, substernal, or nasal flaring with respirations Dry nonproductive, productive, or chronic cough Increased dyspnea, paroxysmal cough; evidence of obstructive emphysema and patchy areas of atelectasis Overinflated, barrel-shaped chest, cyanosis, repeated episodes of bronchitis and bronchopneumonia, chronic nasal congestion, rhinitis, chronic sinusitis, nasal polyps	Child will exhibit signs of improved ventilatory capacity and gas exchange. Child will maintain an open airway. **The Following NOC Concepts Apply to These Outcomes** Aspiration Prevention Respiratory Status: Ventilation Respiratory Status: Gas Exchange Tissue Perfusion: Pulmonary Vital Signs	Auscultate breath sounds every 2-4 hours or more often as needed.	To assess respiratory status
		Monitor respiratory pattern: rate, depth, and effort.	To implement treatment and anticipate changes in ventilation
		Provide nebulization with appropriate solution and equipment as prescribed.	To decrease viscosity of mucus and improve pulmonary function tests
		Administer supplemental oxygen (nasal prongs, mist tent, incubator, hood or mechanical ventilator) as prescribed or needed.	To promote air movement To improve oxygenation
		Maintain child on NPO status if necessary.	To prevent aspiration
		Assist child to cough and expectorate mucus.	To remove secretions
		Suction oropharynx or trachea as needed to clear secretions.	To remove secretions
		Perform chest physiotherapy.	To promote airway clearance To facilitate removal of mucus
		Position for optimum lung expansion (in infant, position for maximum airway maintenance as well). • Elevate head of bed unless contraindicated. • Have child sit upright or lean forward when possible. • Maintain proper body alignment.	To increase lung expansion
		Closely monitor arterial blood gas measurements and pulse oximeter and transcutaneous oxygen readings to detect changes in oxygenation.	To detect changes in oxygenation and implement further therapy
		Anticipate possible need for intubation, tracheostomy, and mechanical ventilation (have equipment appropriate for child's age and size on hand).	To prevent delay in treatment
		Assess for and manage fever.	To decrease potential for increased oxygen consumption caused by fever
		Assess for and manage pain.	To decrease potential for increased oxygen consumption caused by pain
		Organize activities to allow for rest.	To decrease oxygen consumption
		Implement measures that reduce fear and anxiety, such as explaining all procedures.	To decrease respiratory efforts and oxygen consumption
		Teach child and family how to use therapy vest.	To help loosen secretions
		Teach child and family how to administer bronchodilator medications.	To promote air movement
		Teach child and family how to administer mucolytic medications.	To help loosen secretions
		Teach child and family how to assess airway status using peak flow.	To promote compliance at home
		Help family set up a timetable for medication administration.	To encourage optimal therapy
		The Following NIC Concepts Apply to These Interventions Airway Management Airway Suction Medication Administration	

Continued

NURSING CARE PLAN

The Child with Respiratory Failure—cont'd

Nursing Diagnosis	Expected Patient Outcomes	Nursing Interventions	Rationale
Risk for Suffocation related to mechanical or functional obstruction to airflow	Child's airway remains patent	Position for maximum airway opening (e.g., sitting up if older child is in respiratory distress).	To maximize airway patency
		Administer supplemental oxygen (humidified) via nasal cannula or mask per assessment.	To improve oxygenation
Child's/Family's Defining Characteristics ***(Subjective and Objective Data)***	**The Following NOC Concepts Apply to These Outcomes**	Monitor vital signs, including blood pressure and oxygen saturation with pulse oximetry, every 30 minutes until stable.	To implement treatment
Internal Risk Factors	Aspiration Prevention	Anticipate possible need for intubation, tracheotomy, and mechanical ventilation (have equipment appropriate for child's age and size on hand).	To prevent delay in treatment
Reduced motor abilities	Respiratory Status: Ventilation	Administer bronchodilator medications collaboratively.	To expand airways
Disease or injury process		Monitor child's response to bronchodilator medications.	To implement further therapy
		Maintain NPO status if child demonstrates diminished capacity to swallow effectively.	To prevent aspiration
		Initiate and maintain peripheral intravenous access.	To prevent dehydration
		Suction airway as needed.	To clear mucus
		The Following NIC Concepts Apply to These Interventions Airway Management Airway Suctioning Vital Signs Monitoring Aspiration Precautions	
Interrupted Family Processes related to situational crisis (seriously ill child)	Family exhibits evidence of coping with child's illness	Keep family informed of child's progress.	To promote understanding of condition by family
	Family provides child emotional support	Explain procedures and therapies so family may understand child's illness and treatments.	
		Reinforce information regarding child's condition.	To promote adjustment to situational crisis
Child's/Family's Defining Characteristics ***(Subjective and Objective Data)***	**The Following NOC Concepts Apply to These Outcomes**	Encourage expression of feelings, especially about the severity of the condition and prognosis.	To facilitate transition to home management
Changes In:	Family Coping	Begin discharge planning as soon as possible.	To promote transition to home
Mutual support	Social Support	Assess need for assistive support systems and assistive devices.	To determine adherence to medical regimen
Patterns and rituals	Parent-Infant Attachment	Arrange for community or home health services to visit child and family and teach how to use inhalant or nebulizer.	To prevent inappropriate use of medications (too much or too little); can influence amount of respiratory secretion
Participation in problem solving		Instruct on reporting effectiveness of treatments and medications to practitioner.	To support realistic expectations; may prevent activities that exceed energy level
Communication patterns			To maintain most appropriate plan of care
Availability for emotional support		Involve child in self-care.	To promote lifelong health promotion behaviors
Expressions of conflict within family		Encourage child's involvement in routine activities such as school and sports.	To support socialization with peers, which is a developmental task for school-age children

Nursing Diagnosis	Expected Patient Outcomes	Nursing Interventions	Rationale
		With adolescents, discuss activities, limitations, and goal setting.	To promote age-appropriate behaviors
		Teach child to recognize signs and symptoms of inadequate therapy and need for practitioner follow-up.	To prevent long-term sequelae related to poor response to treatment
		Teach importance of setting realistic expectations such as gradually increasing activity and exercise routine, attendance at school, and possibility of hospitalization.	To promote age-appropriate behaviors
		The Following NIC Concepts Apply to These Interventions Attachment Promotion Developmental Care	

NURSING CARE PLAN

The Infant with Bronchiolitis and Respiratory Syncytial Virus (RSV) Infection

Nursing Diagnosis	Expected Patient Outcomes	Nursing Interventions	Rationale
Ineffective Breathing Pattern related to inflammatory process and narrowing airways **Child's/Family's Defining Characteristics** ***(Subjective and Objective Data)*** Decreased inspiratory/expiratory pressure Nasal flaring Use of accessory muscles to breathe Dyspnea Respiratory rate <20 or >60 Wheezing Cough Decreased minute ventilation Apnea Tachypnea Grunting Cyanosis	Respirations are effective **The Following NOC Concepts Apply to These Outcomes** Respiratory Status: Airway Patency Respiratory Status: Ventilation Vital Signs	Instill nasal saline in nares, and suction nose.	To clear airway of mucus
		Collect nasopharyngeal mucus sample for diagnostic evaluation.	To establish diagnosis
		Administer humidified oxygen as necessary to maintain oxygen saturation ≥92 %.	To prevent hypoxia and drying of airways
		Administer aerosolized bronchodilator (as prescribed).	To relieve constricted airways
		Monitor vital signs including oxygen saturation.	To determine need for intervention
		Position in semireclining position.	To facilitate breathing and mucous drainage
		Monitor hydration status and fluid intake and output.	To determine need for additional oral or intravenous hydration
		Administer small amounts of fluid by mouth; 1-2 tsp every 10-15 minutes as necessary.	To maintain adequate hydration
		Implement and maintain Standard Precautions and Contact Precautions (gloves, mask, gown) for infant with illness and between infant and other ill patients, especially those who are immunocompromised.	To prevent spread of virus to others
		Teach parents use of aerosolized nebulizer treatments for home care as indicated.	To provide for home care management of symptoms (most infants do not require hospitalization if breathing is effective after aerosolized bronchodilator treatment and infant is adequately hydrated)
		Teach parents to recognize signs of dehydration (dry mucous membranes, decreased urinary output).	To alleviate parental anxiety over care of infant at home
		Teach parents signs of deteriorating respiratory status: increased work of breathing, grunting, nasal flaring, intercostal retractions, poor fluid intake, altered activity level and sensorium, color changes (cyanosis).	To provide sense of control in decision making

Continued

NURSING CARE PLAN

The Infant with Bronchiolitis and Respiratory Syncytial Virus (RSV) Infection–cont'd

Nursing Diagnosis	Expected Patient Outcomes	Nursing Interventions	Rationale
Ineffective Breathing Pattern related to inflammatory process and narrowing airways—cont'd		**The Following NIC Concepts Apply to These Interventions** Respiratory Monitoring Positioning Vital Signs Monitoring Airway Suctioning Fluid Management Airway Management	
Interrupted Family Processes related to illness and/or hospitalization of infant **Child's/Family's Defining Characteristics** ***(Subjective and Objective Data)*** ***Changes in*** Patterns and rituals Participation in decision making Communication patterns Mutual support Expressions of conflict within family	Family functioning is maintained intact **The Following NOC Concepts Apply to These Outcomes** Family Coping Family Normalization Family Functioning	Recognize parental concern for infant's illness and need for information and support. Explain infant's illness, therapy, and plan for managing symptoms. Encourage family to be involved in infant's care. Encourage discussion of problems related to managing illness in home setting. Assess family functioning and ability to cope with infant's illness. Discuss available family resources. Provide referral for resources as needed. **The Following NIC Concepts Apply to These Interventions** Family Process Maintenance Family Involvement Promotion Emotional Support	To involve family and keep informed To alleviate fear and anxiety related to unknown prognosis and outcome of illness To promote family involvement in infant's care To promote mutual decision-making process To determine need for additional emotional support and counseling To provide additional resources for home care
Ineffective Infant Feeding Pattern related to increased mucous production, inability to breathe through nose and mouth and suck and swallow at same time **Child's/Family's Defining Characteristics** ***(Subjective and Objective Data)*** Decreased oral intake Pulls away from breast or bottle when offered Abundant nasal secretions	Infant breast-feeds or bottle-feeds successfully Infant maintains adequate hydration status **The Following NOC Concepts Apply to These Outcomes** Breastfeeding Maintenance Hydration Nutritional Status: Food & Fluid Intake	Assist breast-feeding mother; encourage more frequent feeding, and demonstrate nasal saline irrigation procedure before feeding. Encourage parents to offer small amounts of fluids, including breast milk and formula; offer 1-2 tsp every 5-10 minutes. Monitor fluid intake, urinary output, and hydration status. Teach parents how to recognize potential signs of dehydration: decreased oral intake and urinary output. **The Following NIC Concepts Apply to These Interventions** Infant Care Nutrition Management	To encourage breast-feeding and maintain milk supply To prevent accompanying infection, because breast milk has antiinfective properties To maintain adequate fluid intake To prevent dehydration To determine need for additional treatment: IV hydration To prevent dehydration and need for IV hydration

Nursing Care of the Child with Gastrointestinal Dysfunction

NURSING CARE PLAN

The Child with Appendicitis

Nursing Diagnosis	Expected Patient Outcomes	Nursing Interventions	Rationale
Acute Pain related to inflamed appendix **Child's/Family's Defining Characteristics** ***Subjective and Objective Data*** Crying, guarding abdomen, limited movement, withdrawal, refusal to eat or drink, fever, increased pulse	No pain or reduction of pain to level acceptable to child **The Following NOC Concepts Apply to These Outcomes** Comfort Level Pain Control Pain: Disruptive Effects	Allow position of comfort (usually legs flexed). Provide small pillow for abdomen. Administer analgesia per orders. **The Following NIC Concepts Apply to These Interventions** Analgesic Administration Positioning Presence Coping Enhancement Pain Management	To allow child to choose most comfortable position To splint the abdomen To provide pain relief
Risk for Infection related to possibility of rupture **Child's/Family's Defining Characteristics** ***(Subjective and Objective Data)*** Abdominal pain, fever, rebound tenderness, nausea, vomiting, anorexia, increased white blood cell count, fluid around the appendix visualized on ultrasound imaging	Child is free of signs and symptoms of peritonitis Signs of peritonitis are recognized early **The Following NOC Concepts Apply to These Outcomes** Infection Severity Wound Healing: Primary Intention Risk Detection	Keep child NPO. Establish and maintain IV. Closely monitor vital signs. Assess pain with vital signs. Administer antibiotics as prescribed. **The Following NIC Concepts Apply to These Interventions** Medication Management Vital Signs Monitoring Infection Protection	To prevent further GI distress To provide hydration To detect status change To intervene in case of rupture To determine possible rupture and implement pain management To prevent spread of infection

Continued

NURSING CARE PLAN

The Child with Appendicitis–cont'd

Nursing Diagnosis	Expected Patient Outcomes	Nursing Interventions	Rationale
Risk for Deficient Fluid Volume related to decreased intake and losses secondary to loss of appetite, vomiting **Child's/Family's Defining Characteristics** ***(Subjective and Objective Data)*** Dry mucous membranes Loss of skin turgor Sunken eyes, rapid thready pulse, rapid breathing, lethargy	Child receives sufficient fluids to replace losses Child exhibits signs of adequate hydration (specify) **The Following NOC Concepts Apply to These Outcomes** Electrolyte & Acid/Base Balance Fluid Balance	Maintain NPO status. Maintain integrity of infusion site for IV fluids. Administer IV fluids and electrolytes as prescribed. Monitory intake and output. **The Following NIC Concepts Apply to These Interventions** Acid-Base Monitoring Electrolyte Monitoring Fluid Monitoring Fluid Management Intravenous (IV) Therapy Laboratory Data Interpretation Vital Signs Monitoring	To minimize losses through vomiting and minimize abdominal distention To infusion fluids and electrolytes To replace losses To assess hydration
Surgical recovery, delayed because of absence of bowel motility **Child's/Family's Defining Characteristics** ***(Subjective and Objective Data)*** Abdominal distention, nausea, vomiting, absence of bowel sounds, abdominal tenderness, no passage of stools	Child will not experience abdominal distention or vomiting caused by decreased bowel mobility **The Following NOC Concepts Apply to These Outcomes** Immobility Consequences: Physiological Ambulation	Maintain NPO status in early postoperative period. Maintain nasogastric tube decompression. Assess abdomen for distention, tenderness, presence of bowel sounds. Monitor passage of flatus and stool. **The Following NIC Concepts Apply to These Interventions** Bowel Management Flatulence Reduction Positioning	To prevent abdominal distention and vomiting To rest bowel until motility returns To assess presence of peristalsis To assess for an indicator of bowel motility

NURSING CARE PLAN

The Child with Acute Diarrhea (Gastroenteritis)

Nursing Diagnosis	Expected Patient Outcomes	Nursing Interventions	Rationale
Deficient Fluid Volume related to diarrhea (gastrointestinal) losses, inadequate intake **Child's/Family's Defining Characteristics *(Subjective and Objective Data)*** Dry mucous membranes Loss of skin turgor Sunken eyes, sunken fontanel, rapid thready pulse, rapid breathing, lethargy Weakness	Child exhibits signs of adequate hydration **The Following NOC Concepts Apply to These Outcomes** Nutritional Status: Food & Fluid Intake Weight Control Hydration	Administer oral rehydration solutions (ORS) for both rehydration and replacement of (GI) stool losses.	To rehydrate and replace stool losses
		Give ORS frequently (every 5-10 minutes) in small amounts (1-2 tsp), especially if child is vomiting (vomiting, unless severe, is not a contraindication to using ORS).	To rehydrate, because vomiting, unless severe, is not a contraindication to use of ORS
		Administer and monitor IV fluids as prescribed (for severe dehydration and vomiting).	To treat severe dehydration and vomiting
		Administer antimicrobial agents as prescribed to treat specific pathogens causing excessive GI losses.	To treat specific identified pathogens causing excessive GI losses
		After rehydration, offer child regular diet as tolerated.	To support early reintroduction of normal diet is beneficial in reducing number of stools and weight loss and shortening duration of illness
		Alternate ORS with a low-sodium fluid such as water, breast milk, lactose-free formula, or half-strength lactose-containing formula for maintenance fluid therapy.	To provide maintenance fluid therapy
		Maintain strict record of fluid intake and output (urine, stool, and emesis).	To evaluate effectiveness of intervention
		Monitor urine specific gravity every 8 hours or as indicated to assess hydration, and weigh patient daily.	To assess hydration status
		Assess vital signs including temperature, skin turgor, mucous membranes, and mental status every 4 hours or as indicated	
		Administer antipyretics for fever.	To promote fever reduction and comfort maintenance
		Discourage intake of (clear) fluids such as fruit juices, carbonated soft drinks, and gelatin (these fluids usually are high in carbohydrates, are low in electrolytes, and have a high osmolality); gelatin may be given once the child is rehydrated.	To restrict fluids high in carbohydrates, low in electrolytes, and with a high osmolality
		Instruct family in providing appropriate therapy, monitoring intake and output, and assessing for signs of dehydration to ensure optimum results and improve compliance with the therapeutic regimen.	To ensure optimum results and improve compliance with the therapeutic regimen
		The Following NIC Concepts Apply to These Interventions Nutrition Therapy Nutritional Counseling Nutritional Monitoring Fluid Management Fever Treatment Diarrhea Management	

Continued

NURSING CARE PLAN

The Child with Acute Diarrhea (Gastroenteritis)—cont'd

Nursing Diagnosis	Expected Patient Outcomes	Nursing Interventions	Rationale
Risk for Infection related to microorganisms invading GI tract **Child's/Family's Defining Characteristics** ***(Subjective and Objective Data)*** Loose stools, fever, lethargy, decreased appetite, vomiting, stomach pain	Child will not exhibit signs of gastrointestinal infection Infection does not spread systemically or to others **The Following NOC Concepts Apply to These Outcomes** Infection Severity Risk Control Risk Detection Self Care: Hygiene	Implement Standard Precautions and Contact Precautions, including appropriate disposal of stool and laundry and appropriate handling of specimens. Maintain frequent and careful hand washing. Use super absorbent disposable diapers. Obtain stool sample for cultures, ova, and parasites as prescribed. Attempt to keep infants and small children from placing hands to mouth and eyes (and objects in diaper area). Teach children, when possible, protective measures such as hand washing after using toilet. Instruct family members and visitors in Contact Precautions, especially hand washing. **The Following NIC Concepts Apply to These Interventions** Communicable Disease Management Environmental Management Skin Surveillance	To reduce risk of spreading infection To reduce risk of spreading infection To contain feces and decrease chance of diaper dermatitis To identify organism causing illness To reduce risk of spreading infection To prevent spread of infection To reduce risk of spreading infection
Impaired Skin Integrity related to irritation caused by frequent, loose stools **Child's/Family's Defining Characteristics** ***(Subjective and Objective Data)*** Excoriated skin, skin breakdown, pain	Child exhibits no evidence of skin breakdown **The Following NOC Concept Applies to These Outcomes** Tissue Integrity: Skin & Mucous Membranes	Change diaper frequently. Cleanse buttocks gently with bland, nonalkaline soap and water or immerse child in a bath for gentle cleansing. Apply barrier ointment such as zinc oxide to area. Expose slightly reddened intact skin to air whenever possible. Avoid using commercial baby wipes containing alcohol on excoriated skin. Observe buttocks and perineum for infection. Apply appropriate antifungal medication if fungal infection is present. **The Following NIC Concepts Apply to These Interventions** Infection Control Infection Protection Skin Care: Topical Treatment Medication Administration: Skin Skin Surveillance Teaching: Procedure/Treatment	To keep skin clean and dry To prevent bacteria in diarrheal stools that are highly irritating to skin To protect skin from irritation To promote healing To prevent stinging To initiate appropriate therapy To treat fungal infection of skin

NURSING CARE PLAN

The Infant with Gastrointestinal Dysfunction, Obstructive

Nursing Diagnosis	Expected Patient Outcome	Nursing Intervention	Rationale
Risk for Injury related to partial or complete mechanical bowel obstruction, altered bowel function (peristalsis), or abnormal fetal bowel development	Infant's bowel tissue remains protected and intact	For any diagnosed or suspected bowel obstructive condition, put infant on NPO status.	To avoid intake of nutrients
		Establish peripheral IV access.	To administer fluids, glucose, and medication
	Infant's bowel function is reestablished	Monitor fluid intake and urinary output closely.	To replace fluids
		Insert nasogastric tube for gastric decompression; ensure adequate function of drainage system.	To remove gastric contents
Child's/Family's Defining Characteristics	**The Following NOC Concepts Apply to These Outcomes**	Offer pacifier when child is on NPO status.	To promote nonnutritive sucking and comfort
(Subjective and Objective Data)		Position for aspiration prevention if emesis occurs.	To prevent aspiration complications
Risk Factors			
Internal: Physical (broken skin)	Risk Detection	Monitor vital signs (specify frequency), including blood pressure.	To assess hemodynamic status and implement therapy
Embryonic developmental defect	Risk Control		
Disrupted bowel function	Aspiration Prevention	Observe color and consistency of stool.	To assess stool for blood, mucus
Tissue hypoxia		Monitor pattern and frequency of emesis (with obstruction).	To evaluate need for fluid replacement
		For abdominal wall defect: cover defect with moist warm saline.	To maintain exposed bowel tissue integrity
		Maintain thermoneutrality (e.g., place in radiant warmer or incubator).	To prevent respiratory compromise and tissue hypoxia
		Assist with diagnostic procedures such as contrast studies.	To accurately perform diagnostic process
		Encourage parents to hold and console infant as condition allows.	To promote parent-infant bonding
		Explain diagnostic and therapeutic procedures.	To keep parents informed of infant's condition and allay fears, anxiety
		The Following NIC Concepts Apply to These Interventions	
		Fluid Management	
		Airway Management	
		Positioning	
		Vital Signs Monitoring	
		Gastrointestinal Intubation	
		Environmental Management	
		Intravenous (IV) Therapy	

Continued

4 - NURSING CARE PLANS

NURSING CARE PLAN

The Infant with Gastrointestinal Dysfunction, Obstructive—cont'd

Nursing Diagnosis	Expected Patient Outcome	Nursing Intervention	Rationale
Risk for Deficient Fluid Volume related to abnormal fluid loss via gastrointestinal tract (emesis, third spacing, exposed bowel)	Infant remains adequately hydrated	Establish peripheral IV access.	To replace fluids lost as a result of condition, NPO status, nasogastric drainage
		Monitor fluid infusion carefully.	To maintain electrolyte balance
	The Following NOC Concepts Apply to These Outcomes	Monitor urinary output carefully.	
Child's/Family's Defining Characteristics		Monitor NG tube drainage carefully.	To adjust fluid intake as condition warrants or changes
(Subjective and Objective Data)	Fluid Balance	Monitor serum electrolytes as appropriate.	
Excessive fluid losses through normal routes	Electrolyte & Acid/Base Balance	Observe for and report signs of fluid and electrolyte imbalance: skin turgor, mucous membrane status, capillary refill, urinary output, seizure activity, decreased or altered activity level; monitor vital signs.	To implement therapy if status changes
Loss of fluids through abnormal routes (third spacing)	Hydration	Maintain warm, moist dressings over any exposed bowel.	To prevent tissue drying and injury
Factors influencing fluid needs	Nausea & Vomiting Severity	Weigh infant daily.	To detect fluid gains or losses
		Maintain infant in thermoneutral environment.	To prevent respiratory or metabolic compromise
		The Following NIC Concepts Apply to These Interventions Vital Signs Monitoring Intravenous (IV) Therapy Environmental Management Electrolyte Monitoring Fluid Management	
Interrupted Family Processes related to infant's physical defect, required surgical intervention, long-term acute or home care	Family exhibits effective coping strategies and integrates infant into family	Explain diagnostic and therapeutic procedures to family in simple language; encourage questions.	To provide accurate information
		Explain infant's condition and short-term standard care procedures, including surgery.	To decrease fear of the unknown
		Allow family to express feelings regarding infant's condition.	To allow grief work to begin
Child's/Family's Defining Characteristics	**The Following NOC Concepts Apply to These Outcomes**	Allow family to hold infant as condition allows.	To promote parent-infant interaction
(Subjective and Objective Data)		Assist family to mobilize sources of support (emotional, spiritual or religious, financial).	To promote family resources for emotional and physical support
Changes in patterns and rituals		Encourage family to be involved in infant's care to the extent that the child's status allows.	To decrease sense of helplessness
Changes in mutual support	Family Functioning		
Changes in communication patterns	Family Normalization	When appropriate, expose family to other family in unit whose infant has similar or same condition and surgery.	To help family express emotions, feelings about their own child
		The Following NIC Concepts Apply to These Interventions Normalization Promotion Family Involvement Promotion Family Support Decision-Making Support Family Process Maintenance	

NURSING CARE PLAN

The Child with Cleft Lip and/or Cleft Palate (CL/CP)

Nursing Diagnosis	Expected Patient Outcomes	Nursing Interventions	Rationale
Preoperative period, CL/CP Impaired Swallowing related to impaired sucking and palatal cleft **Child's/Family's Defining Characteristics *(Subjective and Objective Data)*** Choking Gagging Spitting breast milk or formula through nose and mouth	Infant breast-feeds or bottle-feeds successfully **The Following NOC Concepts Apply to These Outcomes** Aspiration Prevention Swallowing Status: Esophageal Phase Swallowing Status: Oral Phase	Suction nose and mouth with bulb syringe.	To maintain patent airway
		Position on right side with head of bed elevated 30 degrees.	To facilitate drainage of secretions and/or feeding
		Assist mother with breast-feeding, if so desired.	To provide emotional and physical support
		Assess infant's ability to suckle at breast and maintain effective latch-on.	To promote optimum nutrition
		Use special CL/CP feeder such as CL/CP Nurser (Mead Johnson), Ross Gravity Flow, Pigeon bottle, or Haberman feeder as necessary; place device to back of oral cavity and adjust flow to infant's ability to swallow.	To ensure adequate intake of formula if not breast-feeding; to prevent choking and spitting up
		For feeding, position infant in semi-reclining position facing caregiver.	To minimize spitting up and assess tolerance of fluid intake
		The Following NIC Concepts Apply to These Interventions Parent Education: Infant Airway Suctioning Airway Management Positioning Risk Identification	
Risk for Impaired Parent-Infant Attachment **Child's/Family's Defining Characteristics *(Subjective and Objective Data)*** Infant with visible facial defect	Parents demonstrate attachment behaviors and willingness to nurture infant **The Following NOC Concepts Apply to These Outcomes** Parenting Performance Parent-Infant Attachment	Discuss with parents the infant's physical characteristics and positive attributes.	To promote acceptance of infant
		Provide nursing care as with any other infant.	To demonstrate acceptance of infant with birth defect
		Encourage parents to interact with infant through verbalizations and eye contact.	To promote normalization of infant
		Involve parents in infant caregiving activities without restrictions or limitations.	To promote acceptance of infant as important family member
		Provide lactation consult and feeding assistance. Assist with feedings as necessary.	To promote nutrition and fluid intake
		Encourage parents to discuss feelings related to infant's appearance.	To allow feelings to be discussed in the open and assess areas for intervention
		Assess parents and other family members for signs of inadequate coping.	To provide early intervention as necessary
		Encourage siblings (as age appropriate) and other family members to visit and interact with infant.	To promote family integration

Continued

NURSING CARE PLAN

The Child with Cleft Lip and/or Cleft Palate (CL/CP)–cont'd

Nursing Diagnosis	Expected Patient Outcomes	Nursing Interventions	Rationale
Risk for Impaired Parent-Infant Attachment—cont'd		**The Following NIC Concepts Apply to These Interventions** Infant Care Kangaroo Care Normalization Promotion Anxiety Reduction Family Process Maintenance	
Imbalanced Nutrition: Less Than Body Requirements related to palatal defect **Child's/Family's Defining Characteristics** ***(Subjective and Objective Data)*** Reported food intake less than RDA Body weight 20% or more under ideal Weakness of muscles required for swallowing	Infant regains birth weight by 10-14 days of life and maintains steady weight gain of 10-30 g/day (0.2-0.6 lb/day) until surgical repair of cleft occurs **The Following NOC Concepts Apply to These Outcomes** Nutritional Status: Food & Fluid Intake Weight Control Nutritional Status: Food & Fluid Intake	Weigh daily; use consistency in weighing process—same time of day, dry diaper only, and same scales.	To monitor weight gain or loss
		Assist parents with feeding; breast-feeding may require lactation consultation; different positions may be required to achieve latch-on.	To promote parental involvement and adequate nutrient intake
		Bottle-feed using specialized nipple (soft versus hard) such as Haberman, Ross Gravity Flow, or Mead Johnson CL/CP Nurser.	To optimize feeding ability
		Teach parents use of special feeding techniques or apparatus.	To promote involvement in care of infant
		Use patience and creativity during feeding.	To promote nutrient intake from mother and father
		Suction nose and mouth as necessary with bulb syringe or Yankauer suction set.	To maintain patent airway
		Encourage father's participation in feeding, whether via breast or bottle, by helping position infant's cheeks and lip for optimum seal.	To promote family involvement
		Monitor for signs and symptoms of dehydration (dry buccal membranes and lips, loose dry skin, tenting, prolonged capillary refill [>3 sec], hypernatremia).	To detect early signs requiring intervention
		Teach parents signs and symptoms of inadequate caloric and fluid intake, dehydration.	To involve parents in care and prevent complications
		If medically indicated, use gavage to feed infant prescribed amount of breast milk or formula.	To ensure adequate caloric and fluid intake
		Allow parent(s) to hold during gavage feeding, and allow infant non-nutritive sucking.	To promote parent involvement in care
		The Following NIC Concepts Apply to These Interventions Vital Signs Monitoring Nutrition Management Lactation Counseling Fluid Management	

<table>
<tr>
<td>Postoperative period, CL/CP
Risk for Trauma to surgical site related to surgical procedure, developmental age of child, skin and mucous membrane fragility

Child's/Family's Defining Characteristics
(Subjective and Objective Data)
Surgical sutures exposed
Skin delicate
Developmental phase of oral exploration and gratification</td>
<td>Tissue integrity at surgical site remains intact and undamaged

The Following NOC Concept Applies to These Outcomes
Tissue Integrity: Skin & Mucous Membranes</td>
<td>Protect surgical site by doing the following:
• Place infant supine.
• Avoid straws, hard utensils or objects (hard pacifier, suction catheter, tongue depressor) in mouth (especially in infant with CP).
• Use elbow restraints as indicated.
• Cup or spoon feed as indicated.
• Breast-feed as indicated (CL).
• Gavage feed as indicated.
Cleanse surgical site with normal saline and topical antibiotic ointment as indicated.
Teach parents care of surgical incision.

The Following NIC Concepts Apply to These Interventions
Skin Care: Topical Treatment
Infection Protection
Oral Health Maintenance
Nutrition Management</td>
<td>To promote healing of surgical repair site skin, mucosa
To prevent injury to sutures and surrounding skin, mucosa

To prevent infection

To promote parental involvement in infant's care</td>
</tr>
<tr>
<td>Acute Pain related to surgical repair of CL/CP

Child's/Family's Defining Characteristics
(Subjective and Objective Data)
Observed evidence
Objective pain scale evaluation indicative of pain
Sleep disturbance</td>
<td>Infant is comfortable and rests quietly

The Following NOC Concepts Apply to These Outcomes
Pain Control
Comfort Level</td>
<td>Administer oral or intravenous (as indicated) pain medication postoperatively on around-the-clock basis for 24-48 hr.
Use objective pain scale to quantify pain.

Encourage parents to use nonpharmacologic pain management measures such as rocking and cuddling, swaddling, singing, reading story.
Teach parents to administer oral pain medication such as acetaminophen at home.

The Following NIC Concepts Apply to These Interventions
Medication Administration: Oral
Analgesic Administration
Positioning
Presence
Environmental Management: Comfort</td>
<td>To achieve optimum pain relief

To ascertain requirement for additional dosage and strength of pain medication
To involve parents in infant's care

To manage infant's pain and promote parental involvement in infant's care</td>
</tr>
</table>

NURSING CARE PLAN

The Infant with Esophageal Atresia and Tracheoesophageal Fistula

Nursing Diagnosis	Expected Patient Outcomes	Nursing Interventions	Rationale
Preoperative period Risk for Suffocation related to abnormal opening between esophagus and trachea **Child's/Family's Defining Characteristics** ***(Subjective and Objective Data)*** Abundant mucus Choking Gagging and regurgitation Episodes of cyanosis Retractions	The child's airway remains patent and respirations are effective **The Following NOC Concepts Apply to These Outcomes** Aspiration Prevention Respiratory Status: Ventilation Family Coping Parenting Performance	Suction as necessary to clear mucus. Position supine or on right side with head elevated to at least 30 degrees. Monitor airway patency. Monitor vital signs, including pulse oximetry. Place on cardiorespiratory monitor. Administer oxygen as needed per unit protocol. Keep child on NPO status until cause of distress is determined. Insert double-lumen nasogastric tube and place to low suction. Establish peripheral IV access. Keep parents informed of infant's status. Encourage parents to visit and touch (or hold) child as permissible. **The Following NIC Concepts Apply to These Interventions** Airway Suctioning Airway Management Vital Signs Monitoring Environmental Management: Safety Fluid Monitoring	To relieve obstruction To facilitate mucous drainage into stomach To detect signs of airway occlusion To determine oxygenation status To monitor cardiac and respiratory status To prevent hypoxia To prevent airway obstruction and hypoxia To decompress stomach or remove mucus from blind pouch (diagnosis dependent) To maintain hydration and administer medications as necessary To decrease parents' anxiety; establish open lines of communication and trust To promote attachment
Risk for Altered Parenting related to infant's physical defect and environmental factors causing parent-infant separation. **Child's/Family's Defining Characteristics** ***(Subjective and Objective Data)*** Infant is placed in an intensive care unit for care	Parents form an emotional bond with infant and demonstrate willingness to nurture infant **The Following NOC Concepts Apply to These Outcomes** Parenting Performance Parenting: Psychosocial Safety Parent-Infant Attachment	Encourage parents and siblings (per unit protocol) to visit infant. Encourage parents to hold and touch infant as condition permits. Involve parents in infant's care as much as possible in the preoperative and postoperative phase of care. Keep parents informed of infant's progress, complications, and care needs. Involve parents in decisions regarding infant's care. Educate parents on infant's home care needs, any special procedures required such as gastrostomy feedings, and potential complications or adverse effects to be alert for in care of infant in home. Teach infant CPR and foreign body obstruction management.	To promote bond with parents and siblings To promote sense of closeness To promote participation in nurturing child To maintain parental involvement in decision-making To provide necessary information for home care To promote child's well-being and possibly relieve parents' anxiety

		The Following NIC Concepts Apply to These Interventions Attachment Promotion Caregiver Support Anticipatory Guidance Infant Care Family Integrity Promotion	
Postoperative period Risk for Altered Growth related to inadequate nutritional intake secondary to surgical repair of tracheoesophageal fistula (TEF) **Child's/Family's Defining Characteristics** ***(Subjective and Objective Data)*** Infant unable to take in adequate amounts of calories by mouth Swallowing impaired Lack of weight gain	Infant achieves growth and developmental milestones for age **The Following NOC Concepts Apply to These Outcomes** Child Development: 6 Months Child Development: 12 Months Knowledge: Infant Care	Weigh daily. Provide nonnutritive sucking (NNS). If infant is fed via gastrostomy or nasogastric tube, provide NNS during feeding. Ensure infant receives amount of calories prescribed at each feeding. Monitor for signs of feeding intolerance such as choking, spitting up, pneumonia (which may indicate an esophagotracheal fistula). Provide age-appropriate developmental care (specify). Involve parents in provision of developmental care interventions. **The Following NIC Concepts Apply to These Interventions** Risk Identification Bottle Feeding Parent Education: Infant Nutritional Monitoring Aspiration Precautions Breastfeeding Assistance Lactation Counseling	To monitor growth To promote and enhance oral and emotional satisfaction To provide oral satisfaction and prevent food refusal when able to take foods by oral route To promote growth To detect complications and implement therapy To promote development, attachment, and parental involvement in decision making

NURSING CARE PLAN

The Child with Tonsillectomy or Myringotomy

Nursing Diagnosis	Expected Patient Outcome	Nursing Interventions	Rationale
Risk for Injury from hemorrhage related to raw, denuded surfaces of tonsil sockets **Child's/Family's Defining Characteristics** ***(Subjective and Objective Data)*** Surgery for removal of tonsils Assess for evidence of hemorrhage: • More than usual frequency of swallowing (note frequency when child is sleeping) • Frequent clearing of throat • Vomiting of bright red (fresh) blood, blood-tinged mucus expected; may be small amounts of dark red or brown (old) blood • Increased pulse • Decreased blood pressure (late sign) • Pallor • Restlessness • Agitation • Increased respiratory rate • Progressive cyanosis	Child will exhibit no evidence of bleeding Child does not aggravate the operative site If bleeding occurs, it is quickly assessed and appropriate interventions are implemented **The Following NOC Concepts Apply to These Outcomes** Tissue Integrity: Skin & Mucous Membranes Risk Detection Risk Control	Discourage child from coughing frequently or clearing throat. Avoid use of gargles or vigorous toothbrushing. Avoid foods that are irritating (high-acid fruit juices, dry toast, raw vegetables) or highly seasoned. Encourage cool liquids or semi-soft foods. Avoid placing hard objects in mouth (straws, toys). Assess child for evidence of bleeding or hemorrhage. Notify practitioner immediately if continuous bleeding is suspected. Have suction equipment at the bedside; when suctioning is necessary, suction carefully. Explain to parents that any sign of bleeding requires immediate medical attention. Have emergency equipment and medications readily available. Monitor laboratory values for evidence of an infection. Notify primary care practitioner of abnormal lab values or changes in assessment. Monitor respiratory status as postoperative vital signs indicate and as needed. Monitor intake and output. **The Following NIC Concepts Apply to These Interventions** Medication Administration Bleeding Precautions Airway Management Postanesthesia Care	To prevent bleeding from surgical site To prevent interference with wound healing To prevent interference with wound healing To promote intake of foods that do not irritate surgical site To avoid trauma to the operative site To provide prompt treatment To provide prompt initiation of treatment To provide prompt treatment To provide prompt treatment To provide prompt treatment of infection To assess for increased swelling and compromise to airway. To ensure adequate fluid and electrolyte balance postoperatively.
Acute Pain related to surgical site ***Objective Data*** Physiologic or verbal indication of pain Elevated pain score on objective pain scale	Child exhibits minimal level of discomfort **The Following NOC Concepts Apply to These Outcomes** Pain Control Comfort Level	Administer analgesia as prescribed. Regularly scheduled pain medication is recommended for at least the first 24 hours. Administer mild sedative as prescribed. Administer antiemetic (transdermal form may be available). Specify. Use nonpharmacologic pain reduction techniques. Specify. Delay prevention education until child's condition stabilizes. Encourage parents to remain with child. **The Following NIC Concept Applies to These Interventions** Medication Administration	To reduce irritability and to lessen crying, which may irritate operative site, thus increasing chance of bleeding To prevent vomiting To enhance healing To promote positive learning experience To decrease stress related to separation

Risk for Infection from myringotomy tubes and tonsillectomy	Child exhibits no evidence of infection	Educate family about care of child with tubes.	To ensure appropriate care after surgery
	Laboratory values within normal limits	Educate family on how to administer medication or eardrops at home.	To ensure proper administration
Child's/Family's Defining Characteristics	Ear is free of purulent discharge	Educate family on how to care for ears around water.	To prevent water from entering ear canal and becoming a source of infection
(Subjective and Objective Data)		Educate family on how to treat ears if exposed to water.	To prevent possible source of infection
Risk Factors:		Educate family on signs and symptoms of infection based on age and location of surgery.	To ensure prompt treatment of infection
Placement of myringotomy tubes	**The Following NOC Concept Applies to These Outcomes**	**The Following NIC Concepts Apply to These Interventions**	
Postoperative status	Tissue Integrity: Skin & Mucous Membranes	Medication Administration Risk Control	

Nursing Care of the Child with Cardiovascular Dysfunction

NURSING CARE PLAN

The Child with Congestive Heart Failure (CHF)

Nursing Diagnosis	Expected Patient Outcomes	Nursing Interventions	Rationale
Decreased Cardiac Output related to structural defect, myocardial dysfunction, altered hemodynamics	Child will have adequate cardiac output as evidenced by: • Heart rate within acceptable range (state specific range) • Respiratory rate within acceptable range (state specific range) • Skin warm to touch • Strong and equal peripheral pulses • Blood pressure normal for age • Brisk capillary refill within 2-3 seconds • Lack of distended neck veins • Normal sinus rhythm • Lack of edema • Adequate urine output (state specific; 1-2 ml/kg/hr)	Assess and record heart rate (HR), respiratory rate (RR), blood pressure (BP), and any signs and symptoms of decreased cardiac output (listed under defining characteristics) every 2 to 4 hours and as needed (PRN).	To assess for changes in vital signs and child's physical status that reflect altered cardiac output
Child's/Family's Defining Characteristics ***(Subjective and Objective Data)***		Administer cardiac drugs on schedule. Assess for and record any side effects or any signs or symptoms of toxicity. Follow hospital protocol for administration.	To improve heart function, drugs should be given on time; dangerous if not given as prescribed and without careful assessment before administration
Tachycardia Tachypnea		Keep accurate record of intake and output.	To assess for CHF, which causes decreased urinary output
Ineffective peripheral circulation, cool extremities Hypotension		Weigh child or infant on same scale at same time of day. Document results and compare with previous weight.	To observe for weight increase that may indicate excess fluid accumulation
Rapid, weak peripheral pulses Prolonged capillary refill, longer than 2-3 seconds	Child will have age-appropriate weight gain on standardized growth curve.	Administer diuretics on schedule. Assess and record effectiveness and any side effects noted.	To prevent fluid retention, which commonly occurs with CHF; diuretics are used to eliminate excess water
Narrow pulse pressure	Infant will demonstrate successful feeding.	Elevate head of bed at a 30- to 45-degree angle.	To promote maximum chest expansion

Continued

NURSING CARE PLAN

The Child with Congestive Heart Failure (CHF)—cont'd

Nursing Diagnosis	Expected Patient Outcomes	Nursing Interventions	Rationale
Decreased Cardiac Output related to structural defect, myocardial dysfunction, altered hemodynamics—cont'd Distended neck veins in older children Cardiomegaly revealed on chest x-ray film Gallop rhythm Edema Rapid weight gain Feeding difficulty Irritability	Child and/or family will be able to state at least four characteristics of congestive heart failure such as: • Rapid heart rate • Fast breathing • Cool extremities • Puffiness (edema) • Fussiness • Decreased appetite Child and/or family will be able to state knowledge of care regarding: • Medication administration • Head elevated positioning • Sufficient rest periods • Monitoring intake and output • When to contact health care provider **The Following NOC Concepts Apply to These Outcomes** Cardiac Pump Effectiveness Knowledge: Illness Care Tissue Perfusion: Cardiac	Offer small frequent feedings to infant's or child's tolerance. Organize nursing care to allow child/infant uninterrupted rest. Educate child and family about characteristics of CHF. Assess and record teaching session. Educate child and family about care such as medication administration. Assess and record results and family's participation in care. **The Following NIC Concepts Apply to These Interventions** Cardiac Care Fluid Management Medication Administration Positioning Vital Signs Monitoring Respiratory Monitoring	To prevent fatigue during feeding; metabolic rate is greater because of poor cardiac function To account for decreases energy level and lower tolerance to activity To provide parent education that can promote measures to improve cardiac function and decrease demands To educate on proper medication administration can promote safety and minimize medication side effects
Ineffective Breathing Pattern related to pulmonary congestion, decreased cardiac output **Child's/Family's Defining Characteristics** ***(Subjective and Objective Data)*** Tachypnea Dyspnea Retractions Crackles Shortness of breath Cyanosis Pallor Mottling Nasal flaring	Child will have effective breathing pattern as evidenced by: • Respiratory rate within acceptable range (state specific range) • Clear and equal breath sounds bilaterally anterior and posterior • Pink or tan color • Absence of nasal flaring, retractions, cough, and head bobbing • Unlabored breath sounds • Tolerance of activities appropriate for age Child and/or family will be able to state four characteristics of ineffective breathing pattern such as: • Color change from pink or tan to pale, dusky, or blue	Assess and record RR, breath sounds, and any signs and symptoms of ineffective pattern (listed under characteristics) every 2 to 4 hours and PRN. Administer humidified oxygen in correct amount and using correct route of delivery. Record percent of oxygen and route of delivery. Assess and record child's response to therapy. Keep head of bed elevated at a 30- to 45-degree angle. Suction if child has ineffective cough or is unable to manage secretions. Assess and record amount and characteristics of secretions. Assess and record oxygen saturation every 2 to 4 hours and PRN.	To assess for respiratory changes that can be indicators of worsening CHF To provide oxygen, which can reduce respiratory distress by easing respiratory effort To promote maximum chest expansion To maintain patent airway to promote respiratory expansion To evaluate pulmonary function

Grunting Head bobbing Cough Use of accessory muscles Activity intolerance	• Fast breathing • Change in amount and/or characteristics of secretions • Retractions, head bobbing • Ineffective cough • Decreased or altered activity level Child and/or family will be able to state knowledge of care regarding: • Positioning to facilitate respiratory effort • Oxygen administration • When to contact healthcare provider **The Following NOC Concepts Apply to These Outcomes** Activity Tolerance Knowledge: Illness Care Respiratory Status: Gas Exchange Tissue Perfusion: Pulmonary	Educate child and family about characteristics of ineffective breathing pattern. Assess and record results. Educate child and family about care. Assess and record results and family participation in care. **The Following NIC Concepts Apply to These Interventions** Airway Management Airway Suctioning Chest Physiotherapy Family Involvement Promotion Health Education	To provide parent education that can promote measures to improve breathing effort To promote family support

NURSING CARE PLAN

The Child with Rheumatic Fever (RF)

Nursing Diagnosis	Expected Patient Outcomes	Nursing Interventions	Rationale
Risk for Injury related to presence of streptococcal organisms, susceptibility to recurrence of RF, and bacterial endocarditis	Child will comply with therapeutic regimen	Assist with diagnostic procedures and tests (e.g., electrocardiography; throat culture; blood analysis for increased erythrocyte sedimentation rate, c-reactive protein, antistreptolysin-O titer).	To promote early detection
Child's/Family's Defining Characteristics *(Subjective and Objective Data)*	Child will experience no or minimal complications or discomfort	Ask family and older child if child has ever had an allergic reaction to penicillin.	To prevent allergic reaction
Evidence of antecedent streptococcus infections Observe for manifestations of rheumatic fever		Administer penicillin, or erythromycin in penicillin-sensitive child, as ordered therapeutically and prophylactically.	To eradicate hemolytic streptococci and prevent recurrence of RF and bacterial endocarditis
General Positive throat culture or rapid streptococcal antigen test	**The Following NOC Concepts Apply to These Outcomes**	Teach family and older child proper administration of antibiotic.	To ensure proper treatment
Elevated or rising streptococcal antibody titer Low-grade fever, usually spiking in late afternoon		Institute measures to encourage compliance with therapeutic regimen.	To ensure proper treatment
Unexplained epistaxis Abdominal pain Arthralgia without arthritic changes	Risk Control Comfort Level Pain Control	Explain to child and family importance of ongoing, long-term health supervision.	To increase family understanding

Continued

NURSING CARE PLAN

The Child with Rheumatic Fever (RF)—cont'd

Nursing Diagnosis	Expected Patient Outcomes	Nursing Interventions	Rationale
Risk for Injury related to presence of streptococcal organisms, susceptibility to recurrence of RF, and bacterial endocarditis—cont'd	Pain: Disruptive Effects Risk Detection	Explain to child and family need for antibiotic prophylaxis for dental work, infection, and invasive procedures.	To promote understanding
Weakness, fatigue		Encourage adequate rest and nutrition.	To support the body's natural defenses
Pallor Loss of appetite Weight loss		Administer salicylates as ordered.	To control the inflammatory process and reduce fever and discomfort
Specific Manifestations		Administer prednisone, if ordered.	To treat pancarditis and valvulitis
Carditis Tachycardia out of proportion to degree of fever		If carditis is present, explain to child and family any activity restrictions and help them choose less strenuous activities.	To promote recovery
Cardiomegaly New murmur or change in preexisting murmur		Recognize that chorea, if present, is usually disturbing and frustrating to child and family.	To increase understanding
Muffled heart sounds Precordial friction rub Precordial pain		Explain that chorea is a manifestation of RF, because it may be misinterpreted by child, family, and others (e.g., teachers).	To increase understanding
Changes in ECG (especially prolonged P-R interval) Migratory polyarthritis		Stress that chorea is involuntary and transitory and that all manifestations eventually disappear.	
• Swollen, hot, red, painful joint(s)		Give child and family opportunity to verbalize feelings.	To facilitate positive coping
• After 1-2 days affects different joint(s) • Favors large joints—knees, elbows, hips, shoulders, wrists		**The Following NIC Concepts Apply to These Interventions**	
Subcutaneous nodes • Non tender swelling • Located over bony prominences • May persist for some time, then gradually resolve Chorea (St. Vitus dance, Sydenham chorea) • Sudden, aimless, irregular movements of extremities • Involuntary facial grimaces • Speech disturbances • Emotional lability • Muscle weakness (can be profound)		Infection Control Health Education Health Screening Learning Facilitation Learning Readiness Enhancement Risk Identification Analgesic Administration Positioning Pain Management Medication Administration	
• Muscle movements exaggerated by anxiety and attempts at fine motor activity; relieved by rest, especially sleep Erythema marginatum • Erythematous macules with clear center and wavy, well-demarcated border • Transitory • Non pruritic • Primarily affects trunk and proximal extremities (inner surfaces)			

NURSING CARE PLAN

The Child in Shock (Cardiovascular Failure)

Nursing Diagnosis	Expected Patient Outcomes	Nursing Interventions	Rationale
Ineffective Tissue Perfusion (Cardiopulmonary) related to reduced blood flow, decreased blood volume, and reduced vascular tone	Child will exhibit signs of adequate cardiac output and circulation.	Monitor vital signs, central venous pressure (CVP), capillary filling, intake and output, and cardiac function, on admission and continuously or very frequently as condition warrants.	To assess efficacy of therapy and provide prompt treatment
Child's/Family's Defining Characteristics ***(Subjective and Objective Data)*** Shock and circulatory failure—a clinical syndrome characterized by tissue perfusion that is inadequate to meet the metabolic demands of the body, resulting in cellular dysfunction and eventual organ failure Compensated shock—vital organ function is maintained, microcirculation is uneven or maldistributed; signs and symptoms include apprehensiveness, irritability, unexplained tachycardia, normal blood pressure, thirst, pallor, diminished urinary output, reduced perfusion of extremities Decompensated shock—efficiency of the cardiovascular system gradually diminishes and microcirculation becomes marginal despite compensatory efforts; signs and symptoms include confusion and somnolence, tachypnea, tachycardia, moderate metabolic acidosis, oliguria, cool and pale extremities, decreased skin turgor, poor capillary filling Irreversible or terminal shock—damage to vital organs, such as heart or brain, of such magnitude that the entire organism is disrupted despite therapeutic intervention; death occurs even if cardiac function returns to normal levels of therapy; signs and symptoms include thready, weak pulse, hypotension, periodic breathing or apnea, anuria, stupor, coma Types of shock—cardiogenic shock; distributive shock; hypovolemic shock	Vital signs within normal limits based on age and size. (refer to the inside front cover for vital signs reference table) **The Following NOC Concepts Apply to These Outcomes** Tissue Perfusion: Cardiac Circulation Status Cardiac Pump Effectiveness Vital Signs	Assist with diagnostic procedures and tests such as complete blood count (CBC), blood gases, pH, coagulation studies, renal function tests, blood cultures, electrolytes, electrocardiography.	To implement appropriate therapy
		Initiate and monitor IV infusion of prescribed fluid and plasma expander.	To administer fluid resuscitation as part of the Pediatric Advanced Life Support (PALS) protocol for shock To promote rapid restoration of blood volume
		Weigh child once daily.	To calculate accurate drug dosages and determine body fluid status
		Administer vasopressor medications as prescribed.	To improve cardiac output and circulation
		Monitor urinary output.	To evaluate renal function
		Apply lower compression stockings or vest as appropriate.	To improve venous return to the heart
		Position child flat on back with legs elevated.	To improve venous return to the heart
		The Following NIC Concepts Apply to These Interventions Circulatory Care: Arterial Insufficiency Circulatory Care: Venous Insufficiency Shock Management Positioning Vital Signs Monitoring Hemodynamic Regulation	

Continued

4 - NURSING CARE PLANS

NURSING CARE PLAN

The Child in Shock (Cardiovascular Failure)—cont'd

Nursing Diagnosis	Expected Patient Outcomes	Nursing Interventions	Rationale
Impaired Gas Exchange related to diminished oxygen needed for tissue perfusion **Child's/Family's Defining Characteristics *(Subjective and Objective Data)*** Tachycardia Abnormal arterial blood gases Hypoxia Hypoxemia Hypercarbia Abnormal rhythm, rate, depth of breathing	Child will exhibit signs of improved cardiac output and circulation as evidenced by oxygen saturation >95%; blood gases within normal limits **The Following NOC Concepts Apply to These Outcomes** Respiratory Status: Gas Exchange Electrolyte & Acid-Base Balance	Administer oxygen as necessary with mask or nasal cannula to maintain oxygen saturation (specify target). Position to maintain open airway (neck in neutral or sniffing position). Suction airway as needed. Be prepared for endotracheal intubation. Monitor artificial airway and mechanical ventilation (if implemented). Monitor arterial blood gases (ABGs) as needed. Attach monitor and asses for apnea, cardiac status, and oxygenation. Administer anxiolytics, analgesics as necessary (intubated). Administer volume expanders as required. Keep family informed regarding child's status. **The Following NIC Concepts Apply to These Interventions** Acid-Base Monitoring Acid-Base Management Ventilation Assistance	To ensure adequate tissue oxygenation To promote open airway or loss To maintain airway and improve ventilation To provide ongoing assessment of the child To ascertain acid-base status of child and implement appropriate therapy To decrease child's anxiety (if intubated) To support blood pressure To decrease family anxiety during an uncertain situational crisis
Interrupted Family Processes related to a child in a life-threatening condition **Child's/Family's Defining Characteristics *(Subjective and Objective Data)*** Child separated from family because of acuity and medical treatments Family in waiting room and not with child during tests or procedures	Child will receive emotional support from family and health care workers **The Following NOC Concepts Apply to These Outcomes** Family Coping Social Support Parent-Infant Attachment Parenting: Psychosocial Safety Personal Safety Behavior	Arrange for someone to remain with family and serve as liaison between them and the critical care area (if possible). Allow family to see child as soon as feasible. Encourage expression of feelings, especially regarding severity of condition and prognosis. Arrange for presence of family support systems (friends, clergy if possible). Involve family in child's care as much as feasible. Involve in age-appropriate activities such as activity therapy and recreation therapy, once acute phase has passed. **The Following NIC Concepts Apply to These Interventions** Family Support Counseling Family Process Maintenance Anticipatory Guidance	To support family To reassure family of the child's status To relieve anxiety To allow family to be a part of the child's recovery and to minimize sense of helplessness To prevent developmental regression during hospitalization

Nursing Care of the Child with Hematologic/ Immunologic Dysfunction

NURSING CARE PLAN

The Child with Anemia

Nursing Diagnosis	Expected Patient Outcomes	Nursing Interventions	Rationale
Anxiety/Fear related to diagnostic procedures or transfusion	Child and family will become knowledgeable about the disorder, diagnostic tests, and treatment	Prepare child for tests.	To relieve anxiety and fear
		Assist with diagnostic tests (e.g., analysis of blood elements).	
Child's/Family's Defining Characteristics ***(Subjective and Objective Data)***		Allow child to play with the equipment on a doll and/or participate in the actual procedure (e.g., cleanse own finger with alcohol swab).	
Occurrence of:	**The Following NOC Concepts Apply to These Outcomes**	Remain with child during tests and initiation of transfusion.	To provide support and observe for possible complications
• Muscle weakness • Easy fatigability, frequent resting • Shortness of breath • Poor feeding (infants) • Pale skin; waxy pallor seen in severe anemia • Pica (eating of nonfood substances such as clay, ice, or paste) • Headache or dizziness • Light-headedness or irritability • Slowed thought processes • Decreased attention span • Apathy, depression • Shock (blood loss anemia) • Poor peripheral perfusion • Skin moist and cool • Low blood pressure and central venous pressure • Increased heart rate	Anxiety Self-Control Fear Self-Control Nutritional Status: Nutrient Intake Circulation Status	Explain purpose of blood components. **The Following NIC Concepts Apply to These Interventions** Anxiety Reduction Therapeutic Play Calming Technique Coping Enhancement Medication Administration Teaching: Procedure/Treatment Laboratory Data Interpretation Medication Management Nutrition Therapy	To increase understanding of disorder, diagnostic tests, and treatment

Continued

NURSING CARE PLAN

The Child with Anemia–cont'd

Nursing Diagnosis	Expected Patient Outcomes	Nursing Interventions	Rationale
Activity Intolerance related to generalized weakness, diminished oxygen delivery to tissues **Child's/Family's Defining Characteristics** ***(Subjective and Objective Data)*** Occurrence of: • Tachycardia, palpitations, tachypnea • Dyspnea, shortness of breath, hyperpnea, breathlessness • Dizziness, light-headedness • Sweating • Change in skin color • Fatigue (sagging, limp posture, slow, strained movements, inability to tolerate additional activity) • Poor feeding in infants	Child will receive adequate rest	Anticipate and assist in activities of daily living that may be beyond child's tolerance.	To plan appropriately for rest periods To prevent exertion
		Provide diversional play activities.	To promote rest and quiet but prevent boredom and withdrawal
		Choose appropriate roommate of similar age and interests who requires restricted activity.	To encourage compliance with need for rest
		Plan nursing activities.	To provide sufficient rest
	Child will exhibit normal respirations	Maintain high Fowler position.	To promote optimum air exchange
		Administer supplemental oxygen, if needed.	To increase oxygen to tissues
		Take vital signs during periods of rest	To establish baseline for comparison during periods of activity
	Child will experience minimal emotional stress	Anticipate child's irritability, short attention span, and fretfulness by offering to assist child in activities rather than waiting for a request for help.	To prevent unneeded exertion
		Encourage parents to remain with child.	To minimize stress of separation
		Provide comfort measures (e.g., pacifier, rocking, music).	To minimize stress
		Encourage child to express feelings.	To minimize anxiety and fear
	Child will receive appropriate blood elements	Administer blood, packed cells, platelets as prescribed.	To replace blood cells and clotting components
		Administer hematopoietic growth factors as prescribed.	To stimulate blood cell formation
	The Following NOC Concepts Apply to These Outcomes Activity Tolerance Endurance Circulation Status	**The Following NIC Concepts Apply to These Interventions** Energy Management Environmental Management Teaching: Prescribed Activity/Exercise Health Screening Oxygen Therapy Vital Signs Monitoring Blood Products Administration	

Imbalanced Nutrition: Less Than Body Requirements related to reported inadequate iron intake (less than recommended dietary allowance [RDA]); deficient knowledge regarding iron-rich foods	Child will receive adequate supply of iron	Provide dietary counseling to caregiver, especially in regard to the following: • Food sources of iron (e.g., meat, liver, fish, egg yolks, green leafy vegetables, legumes, nuts, whole grains, iron-fortified infant cereal, and dry cereal)	To ensure that child receives adequate supply of iron
Child's/Family's Defining Characteristics ***(Subjective and Objective Data)*** Less than minimal intake of daily requirement of iron		Milk as supplemental food in infant's diet after solids are begun	To prevent excess milk in diet, because excess milk decreases child's intake of iron-rich solid foods
		Teach older child about importance of adequate iron in the diet.	To encourage compliance
	Child will consume iron supplements	Administer iron preparations as prescribed.	To ensure adequate iron intake
		Instruct family regarding correct administration of oral iron: • Give in divided doses (specify).	To promote maximum absorption
		• Give between meals.	To increase absorption in upper gastro-intestinal tract
		• Administer with citrus fruit or juice preparation.	To promote absorption, because vitamin C reduces iron to its most soluble state
		• Do not give with milk or antacids.	To decrease the absorption of iron
		• Do not give with tea.	To ensure adequate absorption, because tannins in tea form an insoluble complex with iron from foods other than meat and because some herbal teas may affect iron absorption
		• Administer liquid preparation with dropper, syringe, or straw.	To avoid iron contact with teeth and possible staining
		Describe characteristics of stools.	To assess compliance, because adequate dosage of oral iron turns stool a tarry green color
		Store iron preparation safely away from reach of children, and keep no more than a 1-month supply in the home.	To prevent poisoning, because iron can be toxic
	The Following NOC Concepts Apply to These Outcomes Activity Tolerance Endurance Nutritional Status Nutritional Status: Nutrient Intake	**The Following NIC Concepts Apply to These Interventions** Energy Management Teaching: Prescribed Diet Teaching: Prescribed Activity/Exercise Nutrition Management Health Screening Nutritional Counseling	

NURSING CARE PLAN

The Child with Sickle Cell Disease

Nursing Diagnosis	Expected Patient Outcomes	Nursing Interventions	Rationale
Risk for Injury related to abnormal hemoglobin, decreased ambient oxygen. **Child's/Family's Defining Characteristics** ***(Subjective and Objective Data)*** Shortness of breath, dyspnea, fatigue, headache, pallor, icteric sclera or jaundice, systolic murmur, cyanosis, increased pulse	Child will avoid situations that reduce tissue oxygenation and will allow for adequate tissue oxygenation **The Following NOC Concepts Apply to These Outcomes** Risk Control Parenting: Early/Middle Childhood Physical Safety	Explain measures to minimize complications related to physical exertion and emotional stress. Prevent infection. Avoid low-oxygen environment (e.g., high altitudes, nonpressurized airplane flights). **The Following NIC Concepts Apply to These Interventions** Health Education Behavior Modification	To avoid additional tissue oxygen needs To avoid additional tissue oxygen needs To prevent a decrease in oxygenation
Risk for Fluid Volume Deficit related to decreased fluid intake, fluid losses **Child's/Family's Defining Characteristics** ***(Subjective and Objective Data)*** Dry mucous membranes Loss of skin turgor Sunken eyes, absent or diminished tears, sunken fontanel, dark-colored urine, rapid thready pulse, rapid breathing, lethargy, weakness	Child takes adequate amounts of fluids and shows no signs of dehydration **The Following NOC Concepts Apply to These Outcomes** Fluid Balance Electrolyte & Acid/Base Balance	Calculate recommended daily fluid intake (1600 ml/m^2/day), and base child's fluid requirements on this amount. Increase fluid intake above minimum requirements during physical exercise and emotional stress and during a crisis. Give parents written instructions regarding specific quantity of fluid required daily. Encourage child to drink. Stress importance of avoiding overheating. Teach family signs of dehydration. **The Following NIC Concepts Apply to These Interventions** Fluid Monitoring Fluid/Electrolyte Management	To ensure adequate hydration To compensate for additional fluid needs To encourage compliance To encourage compliance To minimize fluid loss To avoid delay in rehydration therapy
Acute Pain related to tissue anoxia (vasoocclusive crisis) **Child's/Family's Defining Characteristics** ***(Subjective and Objective Data)*** Pain can occur in any location in the body, can be acute in onset and severe, can be localized or generalized; low grade fever may be present; localized swelling can occur over joints with arthralgia	Child will experience no or minimal pain **The Following NOC Concepts Apply to These Outcomes** Comfort Level Pain Control	Discuss preventive schedule of medication around the clock with parents. Encourage high level of fluid intake. Recognize that various analgesics, including opioids and medication schedules, may need to be tried. Reassure child and family that analgesics including opioids are medically indicated, and that although high doses may be needed, children rarely become addicted. Apply heat, or massage affected area. Avoid applying cold compresses. Instruct parents to seek medical attention immediately for sudden, persistent headache, weakness on one side of the body, sudden gait or speech problems, or altered mental status.	To prevent pain To promote hydration To achieve satisfactory pain relief To prevent suffering that may result from their unfounded fears To sooth To prevent vasoconstriction that may enhance sickling To recognize acute central nervous system (CNS) events to prevent progressive CNS damage

		Stress importance of adequate nutrition; routine immunizations, including pneumococcal and meningococcal vaccines; protection from known sources of infection; and frequent health evaluation, with regularly scheduled comprehensive evaluation. **The Following NIC Concepts Apply to These Interventions** Medication Management Pain Management Patient-Controlled Analgesia	
Risk for Infection related to compromised immune status **Child's/Family's Defining Characteristics** ***(Subjective and Objective Data)*** Fever, chills, pain, redness, lethargy, increased pallor, listlessness, irritability, increased pulse and respiration, history of prior sepsis	Child will remain free of infection **The Following NOC Concepts Apply to These Outcomes** Infection Severity Knowledge: Infection Control Risk Detection	Report any signs of infection immediately. Promote compliance with prophylactic antibiotic therapy. Instruct parents regarding signs and symptoms of splenic sequestration including palpating the spleen regularly. **The Following NIC Concepts Apply to These Interventions** Environmental Management Communicable Disease Management Medication Prescribing Medication Administration Medication Management	To ensure preventive measures that decrease risk for infection exposure To prevent and to treat infection To provide early recognition of splenic sequestration crisis
Knowledge Deficit related to understanding of sickle cell disease and its management **Child's/Family's Defining Characteristics** ***(Subjective and Objective Data)*** Lack of understanding, inability to identify signs and symptoms of painful crises, inability to follow disease management guidelines, difficulty describing treatment plan, improper medication administration	Child and family demonstrate understanding of the disease, its cause, and its treatment **The Following NOC Concepts Apply to These Outcomes** Family Coping Knowledge: Illness Care	Teach family and children characteristics of basic genetic defect and measures to minimize complications. Stress importance of informing significant health personnel of child's disease. Explain signs of developing complications such as fever, pallor, respiratory distress, persistent headaches, and pain. Reinforce basic information regarding trait transmission, and refer to genetic counseling services. Teach parents to be advocates for their child Educate the school and teachers regarding etiology of sickle cell disease and measures to avoid complications within the classroom. Stress with educators the need to provide tutorials and to allow time to make up schoolwork during medically related absences. **The Following NIC Concepts Apply to These Interventions** Teaching: Disease Process Teaching: Prescribed Medication	To minimize complications of sickling To ensure prompt and appropriate treatment To avoid delay in treatment To allow for informed decision making To provide support To provide support and prevent complications To provide support and prevent complications

NURSING CARE PLAN

The Child with Hemophilia

Nursing Diagnosis	Expected Patient Outcomes	Nursing Interventions	Rationale
Risk for Injury related to hemorrhage **Child's/Family's Defining Characteristics** ***(Subjective and Objective Data)*** Evidence of the disease in male relatives Observe for manifestations of hemophilia: • Prolonged bleeding anywhere from or in the body • Hemorrhage after any trauma (e.g., loss of deciduous teeth, circumcision, cuts, epistaxis, injections) • Excessive bruising, even from a slight injury such as a fall • Subcutaneous and intramuscular hemorrhages • Hemarthrosis (bleeding into the joint cavities), especially of the knees, ankles, and elbows • Hematomas with pain, swelling, and limited motion • Spontaneous hematuria	Child will experience minimum or no bleeding	Perform a physical assessment.	To ensure accurate diagnosis
		Assist with diagnostic procedures and tests (e.g., coagulation tests, determination of specific factor deficiency, deoxyribonucleic acid [DNA] testing).	
		Prepare and administer factor VIII concentrate or, for mild hemophilia, DDAVP (1-deamino-8-D-arginine vasopressin) as needed.	To prevent bleeding
		Teach home administration of blood factor replacement.	To promote early treatment without delay, which results in more rapid recovery and decreased complications
		Institute supportive measures.	To control bleeding
		Apply pressure to area for 10-15 minutes.	To allow for clot formation
		Immobilize and elevate area above level of heart.	To decrease blood flow
		Apply cold, and encourage family to have plastic bags of ice or cold packs ready in freezer.	To promote vasoconstriction
	Child will experience decreased risk of injury	Make environment as safe as possible with close supervision.	To minimize injuries without hampering development.
		Encourage pursuit of intellectual and creative activities.	To provide safe alternatives
		Encourage noncontact sports (e.g., swimming) and use of protective equipment (e.g., padding, helmet).	To decrease risk of injury
		Encourage older child to choose activities but to accept responsibility for his or her own safety.	To encourage independence and sense of responsibility
		Involve teachers and school nurse in planning school activities.	To promote normalization while decreasing risk of injury
		Discuss with parents appropriate limit-setting patterns.	To emphasize child's need for normal development, which is considered in addition to need for safety
		Teach methods of dental hygiene. Use soft, small toothbrush or sponge-tipped disposable toothbrush. Soften toothbrush in warm water before brushing. Use water-irrigating device.	To minimize trauma to gums and prevent bleeding
		Encourage adolescent to use electric shaver.	To decrease risk of trauma
		Avoid passive range-of-motion exercises after an acute episode of bleeding.	To prevent the joint capsule from being stretched and causing bleeding
		Advise patient to wear medical identification.	To facilitate prompt, appropriate emergency care
		Encourage older children to recognize situations in which disclosing their condition is important (e.g., dental care, injections).	To receive appropriate care
		Discuss dietary considerations.	To prevent excessive body weight that can increase strain on joints and predispose to hemarthrosis

		Advise not to take aspirin or aspirin-containing products.	To prevent products from inhibiting platelet function
		Use acetaminophen or ibuprofen for fever or discomfort.	
		Teach family and older child how to recognize and control bleeding.	To ensure that prompt, appropriate care is instituted
		Take special precautions during nursing procedures such as injections (e.g., there is less bleeding after venipuncture than from finger and heel punctures; subcutaneous route is substituted for intramuscular injections when possible).	To minimize bleeding
	The Following NOC Concepts Apply to These Outcomes Blood Loss Severity Personal Safety Behavior Risk Detection	**The Following NIC Concepts Apply to These Interventions** Bleeding Precautions Bleeding Reduction Hemorrhage Control Emergency Care Surveillance: Safety Home Maintenance Assistance Physical Restraint Medication Administration Medication Management	
Impaired Physical Mobility related to effects of hemorrhages into joints and other tissues **Child's/Family's Defining Characteristics** ***(Subjective and Objective Data)*** Decreased mobility, swollen joints and other tissues	Child will experience reduced risk of impaired physical mobility **The Following NOC Concepts Apply to These Outcomes** Mobility Body Mechanics Performance Pain Level Joint Movement: Knee Joint Movement: Ankle Joint Movement: Elbow	Assess need for pain management. Administer replacement therapy and use local measures. Elevate and immobilize joint during bleeding episodes. Institute active range-of-motion exercises after acute phase. Exercise unaffected joints and muscles. Consult with physical therapist concerning exercise program. Refer to public health nurse or physical therapist for supervision at home. Explain to family serious long-range consequences of hemarthrosis. Discuss dietary considerations. **The Following NIC Concepts Apply to These Interventions** Exercise Therapy: Joint Mobility Environmental Management Surveillance: Safety Positioning	To increase ease of mobility. To control bleeding To minimize swelling To allow child to control the degree of exercise according to level of discomfort To maintain mobility To promote maximum function of joint and unaffected body parts To ensure prompt treatment is instituted for bleeding episodes To prevent excessive body weight that can increase strain on joints and predispose to hemarthrosis

Continued

NURSING CARE PLAN

The Child with Hemophilia—cont'd

Nursing Diagnosis	Expected Patient Outcomes	Nursing Interventions	Rationale
Interrupted Family Processes related to a child with a serious disease	Family will receive adequate support	Refer for genetic counseling, including identification of carrier offspring and other female relatives.	To ensure appropriate education of parents
		Refer to special groups and agencies offering services to families with hemophilia.	To support family
Child's/Family's Defining Characteristics *(Subjective and Objective Data)*	**The Following NOC Concepts Apply to These Outcomes**	**The Following NIC Concepts Apply to These Interventions**	
History of hemophilia within family	Family Functioning	Coping Enhancement	
Lack of disease understanding	Family Coping	Family Process Maintenance	
Inability to understand treatment	Family Participation in Professional Care	Normalization Promotion	
Lack of family support	Knowledge: Treatment Regimen	Family Involvement Promotion	
		Home Maintenance Assistance	
		Teaching: Disease Process	
		Teaching: Procedure/Treatment	

NURSING CARE PLAN

The Child or Adolescent with Human Immunodeficiency Virus (HIV) Infection

Nursing Diagnosis	Expected Patient Outcomes	Nursing Interventions	Rationale
Risk for Infection related to impaired body defenses, presence of infective organisms	Child will experience minimized risk of secondary opportunistic infection	Use thorough hand-washing technique.	To minimize exposure to infective organisms
		Advise visitors to use good hand-washing technique.	To minimize exposure to infective organisms
		Place child in room with noninfectious children or in private room.	To minimize exposure to infective organisms
		Obtain an immunization history.	To assess risk for infectious disease
	Child will not spread virus to others	Restrict contact with persons who have infections, including family members, other children, friends, and members of staff; explain that child is highly susceptible to infection.	To encourage cooperation and understanding
Child's/Family's Defining Characteristics *(Subjective and Objective Data)*	**The Following NOC Concepts Apply to These Outcomes**	Observe medical asepsis as appropriate.	To decrease risk of infection
		Encourage good nutrition and adequate rest.	To promote the body's remaining natural defenses
Exposure in utero to HIV-infected mother	Immune Status	Explain to family and older child importance of contacting health professional if exposed to childhood illnesses (e.g., chickenpox, measles).	To ensure appropriate immunizations can be given
Recipients of blood products, especially children with	Infection Severity	Administer appropriate immunizations as prescribed.	To prevent infectious diseases
	Risk Control: Sexually Transmitted Diseases (STD)	Administer antibiotics as prescribed.	To treat infections
		Implement and carry out Standard Precautions.	To prevent spread of virus

hemophilia (before testing began in 1985) Adolescents engaging in high-risk behaviors Recurrent bacterial infections Pulmonary diseases (especially *Pneumocystis carinii* pneumonia, lymphocytic interstitial pneumonitis, pulmonary lymphoid hyperplasia)	Knowledge: Infection Control	Instruct others (e.g., family, members of staff) in appropriate precautions; clarify any misconceptions about communicability of virus. Teach affected children protective methods (e.g., hand washing, handling genital area, care after using bedpan or toilet). Assess home situation, and implement protective measures as feasible in individual circumstances. **The Following NIC Concepts Apply to These Interventions** Infection Control Infection Prevention Communicable Disease Management Health Education Medication Management Medication Prescribing Health Screening Immunization/Vaccination Management Infection Protection Medication Administration	To ensure adequate knowledge To prevent spread of infection To prevent spread of infection
Impaired Nutrition: Less Than Body Requirements related to recurrent illness, diarrheal losses, loss of appetite, oral candidiasis **Child's/Family's Defining Characteristics *(Subjective and Objective Data)*** Observe for manifestations of acquired immunodeficiency syndrome (AIDS) in children: • Failure to thrive • Lymphadenopathy • Hepatosplenomegaly • Oral candidiasis • Recurrent bacterial infections • Chronic or recurrent diarrhea	Child will receive optimum nourishment **The Following NOC Concepts Apply to These Outcomes** Nutritional Status Nutritional Status: Food & Fluid Intake Sensory Function: Taste & Smell Symptom Control	Provide high-calorie, high-protein meals and snacks. Provide foods child prefers. Fortify foods with nutritional supplements (e.g., powdered milk, commercial supplements). Provide meals when child is most likely to eat well. Use creativity to encourage child to eat. Monitor child's weight and growth. Administer antifungal medication as ordered. **The Following NIC Concepts Apply to These Interventions** Nutritional Counseling Nutritional Monitoring Nutrition Management Fluid Monitoring Self-Care Assistance: Feeding Teaching: Prescribed Diet Medication Administration	To meet the body's requirements for metabolism and growth To encourage eating To maximize quality of intake To promote oral intake To promote additional nutritional interventions that can be implemented if growth begins to slow or weight drops To treat oral candidiasis

Continued

NURSING CARE PLAN

The Child or Adolescent with Human Immunodeficiency Virus (HIV) Infection–cont'd

Nursing Diagnosis	Expected Patient Outcomes	Nursing Interventions	Rationale
Impaired Social Interaction related to physical limitations, hospitalizations, social stigma toward HIV	Child will participate in peer-group and family activities	Assist child in identifying personal strengths.	To facilitate coping
		Educate school personnel and classmates about HIV.	To ensure child is not unnecessarily isolated
		Encourage child to participate in activities with other children and family.	
	The Following NOC Concepts Apply to These Outcomes	Encourage child to maintain phone contact with friends during hospitalization.	To decrease isolation
Child's/Family's Defining Characteristics *(Subjective and Objective Data)*	Social Interaction Skills	**The Following NIC Concepts Apply to These Interventions**	
Neurologic features are: • Developmental delay • Loss of previously achieved motor milestones • Possible microcephaly • Abnormal neurologic examination	Play Participation	Behavior Modification: Social Skills Recreation Therapy Socialization Enhancement Family Integrity Promotion	
Ineffective Sexuality Patterns related to risk of disease transmission	Adolescent exhibits healthy sexual behavior	Educate adolescent about the following: • Sexual transmission • Risks of perinatal infection • Dangers of promiscuity • Abstinence, use of condoms • Avoidance of high-risk behaviors	To ensure that adolescent has adequate information to identify safe, healthy expressions of sexuality
Child's/Family's Defining Characteristics *Subjective and Objective Data*	**The Following NOC Concepts Apply to These Outcomes**	Encourage adolescent to talk about feelings and concerns related to sexuality.	To facilitate coping
Perinatal infection Promiscuity High-risk sexual behaviors	Personal Well-Being Risk Control: Sexually Transmitted Diseases (STD) Child Development: Adolescence	**The Following NIC Concepts Apply to These Interventions** Behavior Management: Sexual Sexual Counseling Infection Protection Teaching: Safe Sex	

Chronic Pain related to disease process (e.g., encephalopathy, treatments) **Child's/Family's Defining Characteristics *(Subjective and Objective Data)*** Irritability Moaning Rigid position Refusal to eat or drink Abnormal neurologic examination	Child will exhibit minimal or no evidence of pain or irritability **The Following NOC Concepts Apply to These Outcomes** Comfort Level Pain Control Pain: Disruptive Effects	Assess pain. Use nonpharmacologic strategies. For infants, may try general comfort measures (e.g., rocking, holding, swaddling, reducing environmental stimuli [may or may not be effective because of encephalopathy]). Use pharmacologic strategies. Plan preventive schedule if analgesics are effective in relieving continuous pain. Encourage use of premedication for painful procedures (e.g., use of EMLA). Child may benefit from use of adjunctive analgesics (e.g., antidepressants) that are effective against neuropathic pain. Use pain assessment record. **The Following NIC Concepts Apply to These Interventions** Analgesic Administration Pain Management	To ensure adequate intervention To help child to manage pain To minimize pain To treat pain To prevent pain To minimize discomfort To treat neuropathic pain as needed To evaluate the effectiveness of pharmacologic and nonpharmacologic interventions
Interrupted Family Processes related to having a child with a dreaded and life-threatening disease **Child's/Family's Defining Characteristics *(Subjective and Objective Data)*** Family members verbalize: • Fear of child's death • Lack of understanding of disease • Inability to understand treatment plan	Family will receive adequate support and will be able to meet needs of child **The Following NOC Concepts Apply to These Outcomes** Family Coping Family Normalization Caregiver Emotional Health Parenting Performance Family Functioning Hope Fear Self-Control Knowledge: Treatment Regimen	Recognize family's concerns and need for information. Assess family's understanding of diagnosis and plan of care. Reinforce and clarify explanation of child's condition, procedures, and therapies, as well as the prognosis. Use every opportunity to increase family's understanding of the disease and therapy. Repeat information as often as necessary. Help family interpret infant's or child's behaviors and responses. Set up an appointment time for patient/family education and discussion of concerns. **The Following NIC Concepts Apply to These Interventions** Family Support Counseling Family Involvement Promotion Coping Enhancement Family Process Maintenance Caregiver Support Emotional Support Spiritual Support	To increase understanding To increase adherence to treatment schedule

Continued

NURSING CARE PLAN

The Child or Adolescent with Human Immunodeficiency Virus (HIV) Infection—cont'd

Nursing Diagnosis	Expected Patient Outcomes	Nursing Interventions	Rationale
Anticipatory Grieving related to having a child with a potentially fatal illness	Family will receive adequate support and will be able to meet needs of child	**The Following NIC Concepts Apply to These Interventions** Family Support Counseling Family Integrity Promotion Emotional Support Grief Work Facilitation	
Child's/Family's Defining Characteristics *(Subjective and Objective Data)* Unstable emotions Depression Withdrawn behavior Aggressiveness	**The Following NOC Concepts Apply to These Outcomes** Family Coping Family Normalization Caregiver Emotional Health Parenting Performance Family Functioning Grief Resolution Dignified Life Closure		

Nursing Care of the Child with Renal Dysfunction

NURSING CARE PLAN

The Child with Nephrotic Syndrome

Nursing Diagnosis	Expected Patient Outcomes	Nursing Interventions	Rationale
Fluid Volume Excess (Total Body) related to fluid accumulation in tissues and third spaces **Child's/Family's Defining Characteristics *(Subjective and Objective Data)*** Manifestations of nephrotic syndrome: • Weight gain • Edema ○ Puffiness of face, especially around the eyes, which is apparent on arising in the morning and subsides during the day ○ Abdominal swelling (ascites) ○ Respiratory difficulty (pleural effusion) ○ Labial or scrotal swelling ○ Diarrhea (caused by edema of intestinal mucosa)	Child will exhibit no or minimal evidence of fluid accumulation **The Following NOC Concepts Apply to These Outcomes** Fluid Balance Electrolyte & Acid/Base Balance Kidney Function	Assess intake relative to output. Measure and record intake and output accurately Weigh daily (or more often if indicated). Assess changes in edema. Measure abdominal girth at umbilicus. Monitor edema around eyes and dependent areas. Note degree of pitting if present. Note color and texture of skin. Test urine for specific gravity and albumin. Collect specimens for laboratory examination. Administer corticosteroids as prescribed (and immunosuppressive drugs if ordered). Administer diuretics if ordered, and limit fluids as indicated. **The Following NIC Concepts Apply to These Interventions** Fluid Management Fluid Monitoring Fluid/Electrolyte Management	To evaluate renal excretory function To assess fluid retention To assess ascites To evaluate common sites of edema To assess for hyperalbuminuria, because it is a manifestation of nephrotic syndrome To reduce excretion of urinary protein To provide temporary relief from edema To treat massive edema
Risk for (Intravascular) Fluid Volume Deficit related to protein and fluid loss, edema **Child's/Family's Defining Characteristics *(Subjective and Objective Data)*** Rapid thready pulse, rapid breathing, lethargy Weakness	Child exhibits no or minimal evidence of intravascular fluid loss or hypovolemic shock **The Following NOC Concepts Apply to These Outcomes** Fluid Balance Risk Detection	Monitor vital signs to detect physical evidence of fluid depletion. Assess pulse quality and rate. Measure blood pressure. Report any deviations from normal so that prompt treatment is instituted. Administer salt-poor albumin if prescribed. **The Following NIC Concepts Apply to These Interventions** Fluid Management Fluid Monitoring Hypovolemia Management	To assess for signs of hypovolemic shock To assess for signs of hypovolemic shock To assess rapid identification of changes in status To provide a plasma expander for severe edema

Continued

NURSING CARE PLAN

The Child with Nephrotic Syndrome—cont'd

Nursing Diagnosis	Expected Patient Outcomes	Nursing Interventions	Rationale
Risk for Infection related to lowered body defenses, fluid overload **Child's/Family's Defining Characteristics** ***(Subjective and Objective Data)*** Occurrence of fever, swelling, redness or skin breakdown, cough, shortness of breath, abdominal pain, diarrhea	Child and family apply good health practices Child exhibits no evidence of infection **The Following NOC Concepts Apply to These Outcomes** Infection Severity Immune Status Knowledge: Infection Control	Protect child from contact with infected persons. Place in room with noninfectious children. Restrict contact with persons who have infections, including family, other children, friends, and staff members. Teach visitors appropriate preventive behaviors (e.g., hand washing). Observe medical asepsis. Use good hand washing. Keep child warm and dry. Monitor temperature. Teach parents signs and symptoms of infection. **The Following NIC Concepts Apply to These Interventions** Infection Protection Skin Surveillance	To minimize exposure to infective organisms To assess for early evidence of infection To provide early assessment of infection
Imbalanced Nutrition: Less Than Body requirements related to restricted diet **Child's/Family's Defining Characteristics** ***(Subjective and Objective Data)*** Weight loss, inadequate growth, poor nutritional intake	Child consumes an adequate amount of appropriate foods Child shows no evidence of deficiencies or weight loss **The Following NOC Concepts Apply to These Outcomes** Nutritional Status: Nutrient Intake Nutritional Status: Food & Fluid Intake Weight Control	Provide dietary instructions for foods that reduce excretory demands on kidney and provide sufficient calories and protein for growth. Limit phosphorus, salt, and potassium as prescribed. Encourage intake of carbohydrates and foods high in calcium. Arrange for renal dietitian to meet with family to review allowable foods and assist in dietary planning. Help hemodialysis patient to fill out menu requests for meals. **The Following NIC Concepts Apply to These Interventions** Teaching: Prescribed Diet Vital Signs Monitoring Fluid Management Nutrition Management Nutrition Therapy Nutritional Monitoring	To provide appropriate diet that can reduce kidney demands To promote adequate nutrition To provide calories for growth and calcium to prevent bone demineralization To promote family needs and understanding of the child's dietary needs To promote appropriate food choice decisions

Risk for Impaired Skin Integrity related to edema, lowered body defenses **Child's/Family's Defining Characteristics** ***(Subjective and Objective Data)*** Occurrence of erythema, swelling, skin breakdown	Child's skin displays no evidence of redness or irritation **The Following NOC Concept Applies to These Outcomes** Tissue Integrity: Skin & Mucous Membranes	Provide meticulous skin care. Avoid tight clothing. Cleanse and powder opposing skin surfaces several times per day. Separate opposing skin surfaces with soft cotton. Support edematous organs, such as scrotum. Cleanse edematous eyelids with warm saline wipes. Change position frequently; maintain good body alignment. Use pressure-relieving or pressure-reducing mattresses or beds as needed. **The Following NIC Concepts Apply to These Interventions** Bed Rest Care Pressure Management	To prevent pressure areas To prevent skin breakdown To prevent skin breakdown To relieve pressure areas To prevent skin breakdown To promote movement, because a child with massive edema is usually lethargic, easily fatigued, and content to lie still To prevent ulcers
Disturbed Body Image related to change in appearance **Child's/Family's Defining Characteristics** ***(Subjective and Objective Data)*** Occurrence of depression, sadness, withdrawal from others, lack of participation in activities, lack of communication with others	Child discusses feelings and concerns Child engages in activities appropriate to interests and abilities **The Following NOC Concept Applies to These Outcomes** Body Image	Explore feelings and concerns regarding appearance. Point out positive aspects of appearance and evidence of diminished edema. Explain to child and family that signs and symptoms associated with steroid therapy will subside when medication is discontinued. Encourage activity within limits of tolerance. Encourage socialization with persons without active infection. Provide positive feedback. Explore areas of interest, and encourage their pursuit. **The Following NIC Concept Applies to These Interventions** Body Image Enhancement	To facilitate coping To promote understanding To encourage child To prevent loneliness and isolation To encourage child To promote acceptance
Risk for Activity Intolerance **Defining Characteristics** ***(Subjective and Objective Data)*** Occurrence of fatigue, tiredness, lack of attention, inability to participate in activities	Child receives adequate rest and sleep. Child engages in activities appropriate to capabilities. **The Following NOC Concepts Apply to These Outcomes** Activity Tolerance Endurance Energy Conservation	Maintain bed rest initially if severely edematous. Balance rest and activity when ambulatory. Plan and provide quiet activities. Instruct child to rest when he or she begins to feel tired. Allow for periods of uninterrupted sleep. **The Following NIC Concepts Apply to These Interventions** Energy Management Exercise Promotion: Strength Training	To support rest To prevent fatigue To encourage rest To prevent fatigue To encourage rest

NURSING CARE PLAN

The Child with Acute Renal Dysfunction

Nursing Diagnosis	Expected Patient Outcomes	Nursing Interventions	Rationale
Risk for Injury related to accumulated electrolytes and waste products **Child's/Family's Defining Characteristics** ***(Subjective and Objective Data)*** Excesses in potassium, sodium and phosphorus Evidence of hyperkalemia, hyperphosphatemia, uremia Excess blood urea nitrogen	Child exhibits no evidence of waste product accumulation **The Following NOC Concept Applies to These Outcomes** Risk Control	Assist with renal dialysis. Administer Kayexalate. Provide diet low in potassium, sodium, and phosphorus. Observe for evidence of accumulated waste products. Increase water intake. **The Following NIC Concepts Apply to These Interventions** Risk Identification Medication Administration Surveillance Teaching: Disease Process	To maintain renal excretory function To reduce serum potassium levels To reduce excretory demand on kidneys To ensure prompt treatment To increase waste excretion by kidneys
Imbalanced Nutrition: Less Than Body Requirements related to restricted diet **Child's/Family's Defining Characteristics** ***(Subjective and Objective Data)*** Weight loss, inadequate growth, poor nutritional intake	Child consumes an adequate amount of appropriate foods Child shows no evidence of deficiencies or weight loss **The Following NOC Concepts Apply to These Outcomes** Nutritional Status: Nutrient Intake Nutritional Status: Food & Fluid Intake Weight Control	Provide dietary instructions for foods that reduce excretory demands on kidney and provide sufficient calories and protein for growth. Limit phosphorus, salt, and potassium as prescribed. Encourage intake of carbohydrates and foods high in calcium. Arrange for renal dietitian to meet with family to review allowable foods and assist in dietary planning. Help hemodialysis patient to fill out menu requests for meals. **The Following NIC Concepts Apply to These Interventions** Teaching: Prescribed Diet Vital Signs Monitoring Fluid Management Nutrition Management Nutrition Therapy Nutritional Monitoring	To provide an appropriate diet can that reduce kidney demands To promote adequate nutrition To provide calories for growth and calcium to prevent bone demineralization To promote understanding of the child's dietary needs To promote appropriate food choice decisions

Nursing Care of the Child with Neurologic Dysfunction

NURSING CARE PLAN

The Child with Seizure Disorder

Nursing Diagnosis	Expected Patient Outcomes	Nursing Interventions	Rationale
Risk for Injury related to central nervous system (CNS) dysfunction and inability to control self (motor) secondary to type of seizure **Child's/Family's Defining Characteristics** ***(Subjective and Objective Data)*** Change in level of consciousness (LOC), disorientation, clonic movements, automatisms, aura, postictal impairment (dependent on the type of seizure)	Child will not experience physical injury as a result of seizure activity **The Following NOC Concepts Apply to These Outcomes** Risk Control Personal Safety Behavior Safe Home Environment Falls Occurrence	Administer antiepileptic medication (AED).	To prevent seizure activity
		Teach family and child, as appropriate, the purpose of AED medication, action, potential side effects, and administration of medications.	To prevent seizure activity and encourage self-care
		Monitor for side effects of AED as well as therapeutic levels according to child's growth, illness factors that affect metabolism, and effects of drug.	To prevent secondary effects of AED and prevent seizure from subtherapeutic drug levels
		Stress importance of compliance with medication regimen even if child has no evidence of seizure activity.	To prevent seizure activity
		Avoid situations that are known to precipitate a seizure (e.g., blinking lights, fatigue, excess activity or exercise, physical factors).	To prevent exposure to situations that may cause a seizure
		Assess home care environment for risk factors that may produce childhood physical injury: loose rugs, unprotected stairway, access to water buckets, pool, or standing water.	To prevent physical harm
		Teach parents by anticipatory guidance risk factors for injury in environment based on child's developmental age and type of seizure (e.g., not leaving child in bathtub without adult supervision).	
		Counsel female patients of childbearing age taking AEDs about contraception and birth defects associated with AEDs.	To prevent birth defects in offspring of women taking AEDs
		In the event of a tonic-clonic seizure: • Place child on side. • Time seizure. • Protect child during seizure. • Do not attempt to restrain child or use force. • If child is standing or sitting in wheelchair at beginning of episode, ease child to floor. • Do not put anything in child's mouth. • Place small cushion or blanket under child's head. • Remove eyeglasses. • Loosen clothing. • Prevent child from hitting head on objects. • Remove hazards. • Pad objects such as crib, side rails, or wheelchair.	To prevent injury and trauma To prevent aspiration and maintain a patent airway

Continued

NURSING CARE PLAN

The Child with Seizure Disorder—cont'd

Nursing Diagnosis	Expected Patient Outcomes	Nursing Interventions	Rationale
Risk for Injury related to central nervous system (CNS) dysfunction and inability to control self (motor) secondary to type of seizure—cont'd		• Keep side rails raised when child is sleeping, resting, or having a seizure. • Allow seizure to end without interference. Teach parent/caregiver care of child during seizure and in postictal state. Protect child after seizure (postictal period). • Time the period. • Maintain child in a side-lying or recovery position. • Call EMS as necessary or ensure child receives medical evaluation after seizure. **The Following NIC Concepts Apply to These Interventions** Surveillance: Safety Environmental Management: Safety Medication Administration Teaching: Disease Process Neurologic Monitoring Seizure Precautions	To protect child and caregiver from injury To prevent trauma and implement therapeutic intervention
Risk for Aspiration and Ineffective Breathing Pattern related to impaired motor activity, loss of consciousness, and loss of airway protection (tonic-clonic seizure) **Child's/Family's Defining Characteristics** ***(Subjective and Objective Data)*** Reduced LOC Depressed cough reflex Apnea Decreased inspiratory pressure	Child's airway will remain patent Child will have effective ventilations **The Following NOC Concepts Apply to These Outcomes** Aspiration Prevention Respiratory Status: Airway Patency Respiratory Status: Ventilation	In the event of a seizure, place child in a side-lying position on a flat surface such as floor or bed. Remain with child. Remove secretions, food, liquids from mouth when seizure subsides. If child has emesis, place on side. In postictal state monitor oxygenation status. Administer oxygen as necessary to maintain pulse oximeter >89%. Suction oropharynx once seizure subsides as necessary to clear mucus or food. Administer medications intended to stop seizure (Diastat, rectal dilantin; IV dilantin). **The Following NIC Concepts Apply to These Interventions** Risk Identification Aspiration Precautions Oxygen Therapy Medication Administration	To prevent aspiration and protect airway To determine need for emergency care To prevent choking, aspiration To prevent choking, aspiration To determine need for oxygen To prevent hypoxia To prevent aspiration To prevent continued seizure activity

Risk for Injury related to impaired consciousness and automatisms **Child's/Family's Defining Characteristics** ***(Subjective and Objective Data)*** Immediate loss of consciousness, tonic rigidity replaced by intense jerking movements, may become incontinent of urine and feces, postictal impairment Change in vital signs, respiratory status, color, presence of vomiting	Child will not experience physical injury and will remain calm **The Following NOC Concepts Apply to These Outcomes** Risk Control Safe Home Environment Personal Safety Behavior Physical Injury Severity Falls Occurrence	Time seizure. Protect child during seizure. Do not attempt to restrain child or use force. Remove hazards in immediate environment. Redirect child to safe area, especially away from windows, stairs, heating elements, or sources of water. Do not agitate; rather talk in calm voice and reassuring manner. Watch to see if seizure generalizes into a tonic-clinic seizure. Protect child after seizure (postictal period). Time the period. Stay with child until fully alert. **The Following NIC Concepts Apply to These Interventions** Risk Identification Environmental Management: Safety Surveillance Seizure Precautions	To establish duration and possible need for emergency care To prevent injury to child or self To prevent injury To prevent injury from falls, burns, and drowning To prevent further agitation To determine type of seizure To provide support, because child may be confused and frightened
Anxiety/Fear, (Parent) related to child having life-threatening and incapacitating seizure activity* **Child's/Family's Defining Characteristics** ***(Subjective and Objective Data)*** Anguish Fright Feelings of inadequacy and hopelessness Worry, apprehension Panic Excitement	Parent copes with child's condition and receives adequate support **The Following NOC Concepts Apply to These Outcomes** Anxiety Self-Control Coping Fear Self-Control	Allow parent(s) to remain with child during seizure. Instruct parent on proper protection interventions during child's seizure activity: positioning, safety, airway maintenance, reassurance techniques, emergency medication administration. Provide information regarding nature (type) of seizure, therapeutic interventions, and lifestyle modifications. Encourage family involvement in daily care of child, with goal of normalization and promotion of optimal growth and development of child. Involve parents in discussion of fears and anxieties; discuss resource and support options available to family. **The Following NIC Concepts Apply to These Interventions** Support Group Coping Enhancement Anxiety Reduction Family Process Maintenance Active Listening Counseling Decision-Making Support Family Involvement Promotion	To decrease fear of unknown and allow parent to see measures taken to protect child To promote parent participation and to promote sense of control over situation To promote knowledge of condition; parental intervention; sense of control To provide hope and promote family functioning and coping To promote family integrity and functioning

*Nursing diagnosis may also apply to child in the postictal phase, depending on type of seizure and child's understanding and cognitive level

NURSING CARE PLAN

The Unconscious Child

Nursing Diagnosis	Expected Patient Outcome	Nursing Interventions	Rationale
Risk for Suffocation related to depressed sensorium, impaired motor function, inability to protect airway **Child's/Family's Defining Characteristics *(Subjective and Objective Data)*** Reduced Motor abilities Altered level of consciousness Increased secretions	Child will maintain patent airway **The Following NOC Concepts Apply to These Outcomes** Respiratory Status: Airway Patency Aspiration Prevention	Position for optimum ventilation. Insert oral airway if indicated. Position supine with neck slightly extended and nose in "sniffing" position. Avoid neck hyperextension. Place in semiprone or side-lying position. Remove accumulated secretions promptly. Provide routine care of endotracheal tube or tracheostomy as appropriate. **The Following NIC Concepts Apply to These Interventions** Airway Management Aspiration Precautions Positioning Vital Signs Monitoring Airway Suctioning	To open airway To prevent airway obstruction To prevent aspiration To maintain patent airway
Decreased Intracranial Adaptive Capacity **Child's/Family's Defining Characteristics *(Subjective and Objective Data)*** ***Risk Factors*** Altered mobility Decreased level of consciousness Inability to protect airway Temperature instability Seizures Sensory dysfunction	Child will maintain stable intracranial pressure (ICP) **The Following NOC Concepts Apply to These Outcomes** Tissue Perfusion: Cerebral Neurological Status	Elevate head of bed 15-30 degrees, with child's head in midline position. Avoid positions or activities that increase ICP. • Pressure on neck veins • Turning side-to-side • Flexion or hyperextension of neck • Head rotation • Valsalva maneuver • Painful stimuli • Respiratory procedures (especially suctioning, percussion) Administer stool softener as prescribed. Closely monitor bowel elimination when child is receiving codeine. Cluster nursing activities for minimum disturbance. Minimize emotional stress and crying. • Provide quiet, subdued environment. • Use therapeutic touch. • Avoid emotionally stressful conversation (e.g., about pain, condition, prognosis). • Administer sedation, as ordered, for extreme agitation or restlessness. Provide adequate pain relief measures	To facilitate venous drainage and avoid jugular venous compression To decrease risk of increased ICP To prevent elevated ICP To prevent constipation To minimize stimulation To minimize stress, because it can cause increased ICP To decrease pain that can cause increased ICP

	Closely observe child for signs of pain, especially changes in behavior (e.g., agitation); increased heart rate, respiratory rate, and blood pressure; and decreased oxygen saturation.	To implement therapeutic pain management strategies
	Observe child's response during times of induced or suspected pain	To provide accurate assessment for ongoing therapy
	Observe child's response after a painful procedure or the administration of analgesia.	
	Use objective pain assessment tool.	To quantify pain and implement appropriate pain management
	Schedule disturbing procedures to take advantage of therapies that reduce ICP (e.g., bathe child after sedation or osmotherapy).	To prevent elevated ICP
	Maintain patent airway.	To prevent respiratory obstruction that leads to cardiac arrest
Child will exhibit no signs of cerebral hypoxia	Provide oxygen as necessary.	To prevent cerebral hypoxia
	Monitor blood gases and pH.	To assess oxygenation status
	If child is on mechanical ventilation: • Monitor for correct settings, proper functioning. • Prepare to provide artificial ventilation in case of ventilatory failure; have manual resuscitation bag at bedside.	
	Maintain IV fluids as prescribed.	To maintain hydration status
Child will exhibit no evidence of cerebral edema	Avoid overhydration.	To prevent cerebral edema
	Monitor intake and output, electrolyte balance, and specific gravity: • Administer hyperosmolar fluids as prescribed. • Administer corticosteroids as ordered.	To detect signs of hypernatremia and hyperosmolality, because diabetes insipidus and the syndrome of inappropriate antidiuretic hormone commonly occur with CNS diseases and trauma.
Child exhibits no seizure activity	Avoid stimulation that precipitates undesirable responses.	To prevent seizures
	Administer antiepileptic drugs (AEDs) per order/protocol.	To prevent seizures
Body temperatures remains within safe limits	Administer antipyretics if prescribed. Apply and monitor hypothermia blanket if indicated and ordered.	To maintain stable temperature
	Turn frequently (at least every 2 hours, as tolerated) unless contraindicated by increased ICP.	To promote lung perfusion
Child will exhibit no evidence of respiratory tract infection	Keep persons with upper respiratory tract infection away from child.	To prevent infection
	Use good hand-washing technique. Keep all equipment in contact with child clean or sterile. Provide good oral hygiene	To promote good hygiene that decreases risk of infection

Continued

NURSING CARE PLAN

The Unconscious Child–cont'd

Nursing Diagnosis	Expected Patient Outcome	Nursing Interventions	Rationale
Decreased Intracranial Adaptive Capacity—cont'd	**The Following NOC Concepts Apply to These Outcomes** Tissue Perfusion: Cerebral Immobility Consequences: Physiological Neurological Status Respiratory Status: Ventilation Seizure Control Thermoregulation Respiratory Status: Airway Patency	**The Following NIC Concepts Apply to These Interventions** Cerebral Edema Management Cerebral Perfusion Promotion Intracranial Pressure (ICP) Monitoring Neurologic Monitoring Vital Signs Monitoring Medication Administration Intravenous (IV) Therapy Fluid Management Fluid Monitoring Fluid/Electrolyte Management	
Risk for Impaired Skin Integrity related to immobility, bodily secretions, invasive procedures	Child's skin remains intact	Closely monitor child's temperature.	To assess for temperature elevations that often occur with CNS dysfunction
		Remove excess coverings.	To minimize temperature elevation
	Child will experience no corneal abrasion	Assess eyes carefully.	To identify early signs of irritation or inflammation
Child's/Family's Defining Characteristics *(Subjective and Objective Data)* Risk Factors: Immobility Poor nutritional status Disrupted physiologic integrity		Patch eyes, if indicated.	To protect the eyes
Feeding, Bathing/Hygiene, Toileting, Self-Care Deficits related to physical immobility, perceptual and cognitive impairment	Child will receive proper hygienic care	Keep lids completely closed.	To protect corneas when corneal reflexes are absent
		Instill artificial tears.	To lubricate eyes
		Provide meticulous mouth care.	To prevent infection
		Avoid drying products (e.g., lemon, glycerin, alcohol).	To prevent dry mouth or mouth coated with mucus

Child's/Family's Defining Characteristics ***(Subjective and Objective Data)*** Decreased muscle strength/tone and endurance Disuse atrophy/loss of muscle mass Difficulty performing self-care activities	Child will experience no physical injury	Keep side rails up.	To prevent falls
		Pad hard surfaces.	To prevent injury to extremities during spontaneous or involuntary movements
		Perform passive range-of-motion exercises. Reposition frequently. Place small, rolled pad in palms.	To prevent contractures To reduce contractures To maintain proper position of fingers
	Child will maintain limb flexibility and full range of motion	Use foot board or ankle-high shoes.	To prevent footdrop
		Splint joints, if needed.	To prevent severe contractures of wrists, knees, and ankles
	The Following NOC Concepts Apply to These Outcomes Mobility Tissue Integrity: Skin & Mucous Membrane Immobility Consequences: Physiological Joint Movement: Elbow Joint Movement: Knee Joint Movement: Ankle Joint Movement: Wrist Joint Movement: Neck	**The Following NIC Concepts Apply to These Interventions** Fever Treatment Temperature Regulation Vital Signs Monitoring Medication Administration Malignant Hyperthermia Precautions Positioning Chest Physiotherapy Airway Management Eye Care Oral Health Maintenance Pressure Ulcer Prevention Fall Prevention Environment Management: Safety Exercise Promotion: Stretching Exercise Therapy: Joint Mobility Exercise Therapy: Muscle Control Activity Therapy Positioning	
Disturbed Sensory Perception (Specify: Visual, Auditory, Kinesthetic, Gustatory, Tactile, Olfactory) related to central nervous system (CNS) impairment, bed rest	Child receives sensory stimulation as tolerated Child appears relaxed and rests quietly Stimulation does not induce seizures or increase ICP	Place child on pressure-reducing surface.	To prevent tissue breakdown and pressure necrosis
		Change position frequently unless contraindicated. Protect pressure points (e.g., trochanter, sacrum, ankle, heels, shoulder, occiput).	To prevent pressure ulcers
		Inspect skin surfaces regularly for signs of irritation, redness, and evidence of pressure. Cleanse skin regularly, at least once daily. Protect skinfolds and surfaces that rub together. Keep clothing and linen clean, dry, and free of wrinkles. Carry out good perineal care.	To observe for breakdown To prevent infection To prevent skin excoriation To prevent skin breakdown To prevent infection

Continued

NURSING CARE PLAN

The Unconscious Child–cont'd

Nursing Diagnosis	Expected Patient Outcome	Nursing Interventions	Rationale
Disturbed Sensory Perception (Specify: Visual, Auditory, Kinesthetic, Gustatory, Tactile, Olfactory) related to central nervous system (CNS) impairment, bed rest—cont'd	**The Following NOC Concepts Apply to These Outcomes**	Gently massage skin with lotion or other lubricating substance (unless on existing reddened pressure areas).	To stimulate circulation and prevent drying
	Mobility	Protect lips with cream or ointment.	To prevent drying and cracking
	Immobility Consequences: Physiological	**The Following NIC Concepts Apply to These Interventions** Exercise Therapy: Muscle Control Activity Therapy Positioning Pressure Management Skin Care: Topical Treatment Simple Massage Surveillance	
Child's/Family's Defining Characteristics *(Subjective and Objective Data)*	Child will receive optimum nutrition	Provide nourishment in manner suitable to child's condition.	To promote nutrition
Diminished environmental stimuli		Monitor IV fluids when ordered.	To assess fluid status
Feelings of isolation and boredom		Record intake and output.	To assess nutritional status
		Feed prescribed formula by means of nasogastric or gastrostomy tube.	To promote intake
		Weigh daily or as ordered.	To assess weight stability
		The Following NIC Concepts Apply to These Interventions Feeding Nutrition Management Weight Management Nutritional Counseling	

NURSING CARE PLAN

The Child with Bacterial Meningitis

Nursing Diagnosis	Expected Patient Outcomes	Nursing Interventions	Rationale
Risk for Injury related to presence of harmful bacteria	Child exhibits evidence of diminishing symptoms	Administer antibiotics as soon as lumbar puncture and blood cultures are obtained.	To implement bactericidal therapy
Child's/Family's Defining Characteristics ***(Subjective and Objective Data)*** ***Risk Factors*** External: Chemical Internal: Immune-autoimmune dysfunction Physical: Abnormal blood (and cerebrospinal fluid [CSF]) profile	**The Following NOC Concepts Apply to These Outcomes** Risk Control Physical Injury Severity	Initiate and maintain isolation precautions—private room, standard and droplet-mask, gown, gloves (droplet for at least 24 hr after initiation of antibiotics).	To prevent spread of infection
		Maintain IV access for administration of fluids and medications.	To maintain adequate tissue hydration and increase effectiveness of medications
		Explain all procedures to child at age-appropriate level.	To decrease child's fear of the unknown
		Monitor child closely for signs of complications such as increased intracranial pressure (ICP), shock, seizure activity, respiratory distress. Observe child for signs such as change in level of consciousness (LOC), appearance of petechiae, spontaneous bleeding.	To implement therapy and prevent life-threatening complications
		Monitor and record fluid intake and output.	To evaluate tissue hydration status
		Implement seizure precautions.	To prevent bodily harm in the event of seizure activity
		Help child achieve position of comfort and reduce environmental stimuli as necessary.	To decrease stimuli that may be irritating to the child's neurologic system
		The Following NIC Concepts Apply to These Interventions Risk Identification Support System Enhancement Environmental Management: Safety Infection Protection Medication Administration Seizure Precautions Vital Signs Monitoring	
Acute Pain related to inflammatory process	Child exhibits no or minimum signs of pain	Allow child to assume position of comfort.	To reduce discomfort
		Elevate head of bed 15 to 30 degrees.	To reduce ICP
		Administer analgesic or other pain reliever.	To manage pain by reduction or removal of pain
Child's/Family's Defining Characteristics ***(Subjective and Objective Data)*** Verbal report Guarding behavior Observed evidence Sleep disturbance	**The Following NOC Concept Applies to These Outcomes** Pain Control	Use nonpharmacologic pain management such as distraction.	To manage pain
		Allow child's parent to stay with child at all times.	To reduce fear and provide support
		Allow child to keep favorite stuffed animal, doll, or pillow from home.	To promote comfort and emotional security
		Monitor for indications of increased ICP, meningeal irritation.	To institute therapies to reduce ICP (as necessary) or meningeal irritation and prevent further pain

Continued

NURSING CARE PLAN

The Child with Bacterial Meningitis—cont'd

Nursing Diagnosis	Expected Patient Outcomes	Nursing Interventions	Rationale
Acute Pain related to inflammatory process—cont'd ***Related Factors*** Changes in appetite and eating Autonomic responses (diaphoresis, changes in blood pressure, respiration, pulse)		Monitor IV site and lumbar puncture site for pain or discomfort. Monitor child's response to analgesic, and encourage child to request pain medication when pain begins; use objective pain scale such as FLACC or Faces Pain Scale (as developmentally appropriate). **The Following NIC Concepts Apply to These Interventions** Analgesic Administration Positioning Environmental Management: Comfort Teaching: Individual Pain Management Distraction	To implement pain-management strategies and reduce chance of physical trauma
Interrupted Family Processes related to child's serious illness, hospitalization, unfamiliar environment, change in pattern of routines **Child's/Family's Defining Characteristics *(Subjective and Objective Data)*** Changes in patterns and rituals ***Related Factor*** Shift in health status of a family member	Family function is maintained, and family assumes supportive role of child **The Following NOC Concepts Apply to These Outcomes** Family Coping Family Functioning Family Normalization	Educate parent(s) about child's illness. Educate parent(s), family regarding isolation precautions and encourage frequent hand washing by child and family members. Provide information about child's condition, progress during hospitalization, and treatment and procedures required. Allow parent to remain with child as much as possible. Encourage parent to participate in the child's care as much as feasible. Identify close contacts who may require prophylactic antibiotic therapy. Initiate discharge planning for home care. Encourage health maintenance activities such as routine childhood immunizations, including meningococcal vaccine for susceptible individuals. **The Following NIC Concepts Apply to These Interventions** Family Involvement Promotion Family Support Family Process Maintenance Normalization Promotion Family Integrity Promotion	To decrease fear of unknown To keep family informed of child's condition and prevent spread of infection To reduce anxiety To promote sense of control and decrease sense of helplessness of child To promote normalization of family and family functioning To prevent spread of infection in close contacts To involve family in child's care To prevent childhood illness and promote wellness

NURSING CARE PLAN

The Child with Cerebral Palsy

Nursing Diagnosis	Patient Outcomes	Nursing Interventions	Rationale
Impaired Physical Mobility related to neuromuscular impairment **Child's/Family's Defining Characteristics** ***(Subjective and Objective Data)*** Postural instability during performance of routine activities of daily living Limited ability to perform gross motor skills Limited range of motion Limited ability to perform fine motor skills Gait changes Movement-induced tremor Persistence of primitive reflexes	The infant or toddler will demonstrate active joint movement The child will have adequate mobility to perform activities of daily living to maximum potential **The Following NOC Concepts Apply to These Outcomes** Body Mechanics Performance Ambulation: Wheelchair Joint Movement: Elbow Joint Movement: Wrist Joint Movement: Neck Joint Movement: Knee Joint Movement: Hip Joint Movement: Ankle Joint Movement: Mobility	Carry out and teach family to perform stretching exercises on affected joints. Use assistive devices such as wheelchair, ankle-foot orthoses (AFOs), and wrist splints. Administer medications intended to decrease muscle spasticity. Encourage and teach parent(s) to use jaw control during feedings. Position child semi-upright during feedings. Encourage play exercises that involve joint movement and promote fine and gross motor skill acquisition and repetition. **The Following NIC Concepts Apply to These Interventions** Exercise Therapy: Joint Mobility Exercise Promotion: Stretching Self-Care Assistance	To prevent muscle contractures To increase mobility To minimize pain and decrease spasticity To facilitate eating To decrease chance of aspiration and facilitate mobilization of food and fluids through esophagus To promote joint movement To promote achievement of developmental milestones
Risk for Injury related to mobility limitation, neuromuscular impairment, and perception and cognition impairment **Child's/Family's Defining Characteristics** ***(Subjective and Objective Data)*** Physical factors: altered mobility Neuromuscular factors: • Limited perception of danger • Uncontrollable muscular movements	Child will remain injury free Home physical environment will be safe **The Following NOC Concepts Apply to These Outcomes** Personal Safety Behavior Falls Occurrence	Educate family regarding child's physical limitations that place her or him at greater risk for injury. Instruct family in steps to avoid injury: padded furniture, lowered bed or side rails as appropriate, gates on stairs, avoidance of throw rugs, thick carpeting. Position child in semi-upright position after feedings. Use jaw support as needed during feedings. Use appropriate mobilization devices and ensure they are safe for child's age. Encourage mobilization and play activities that stretch muscles. Teach child which activities of daily living are safe and appropriate to perform without assistance of another person. **The Following NIC Concepts Apply to These Interventions** Risk Identification Environmental Management: Safety Surveillance: Safety Physical Restraint Parent Education: Childrearing Family	To prevent accidental injury during mobilization To promote family involvement in injury prevention To prevent aspiration To prevent choking To prevent muscle contractures To promote personal safety To promote self-care

Continued

NURSING CARE PLAN

The Child with Cerebral Palsy—cont'd

Nursing Diagnosis	Patient Outcomes	Nursing Interventions	Rationale
Pain (chronic) related to involuntary muscle movements (spasticity) and treatments for muscle spasticity	Child's optimum comfort level will be maintained	Administer medications to control spasticity.	To prevent muscle spasm pain
		Perform stretching exercises after pain medication has been administered—60 minutes for oral medications.	To control pain impulses during exercises
	The Following NOC Concepts Apply to These Outcomes	Administer pain medications such as nonsteroidal antiinflammatory drugs.	To minimize pain
Child's/Family's Defining Characteristics **_(Subjective and Objective Data)_**	Comfort Level Pain: Disruptive Effects Depression Level	For treatments such as botulinum toxin type A (Botox) injections, apply topical analgesic such as EMLA (an eutectic mix of lidocaine and prilocaine) or LMX4 (4% lidocaine).	To decrease pain of injection at site
Observed evidence of guarded behavior, grimace, crying, restlessness		For postoperative pain, administer pain medications on an around-the-clock schedule for 48 to 72 hours; use patient-controlled analgesia pump as child's cognitive and motor skills allow.	To promote personal physical comfort
Atrophy of involved muscle group		Use objective pain scale to assess pain level.	To provide objective measure of pain for intervention
Altered ability to continue previous activities		Encourage child to verbalize effects of pain on activities of daily living.	To provide outlet for frustration related to chronic pain experience
		Use assistive devices such as AFOs.	To decrease muscle spasticity and contractures.
		Teach parent(s) and child appropriate positions to assume while sitting and recumbent to minimize effects of muscle spasticity.	To promote self-care
		The Following NIC Concepts Apply to These Interventions Medication Administration Analgesic Administration Emotional Support Splinting Environmental Management: Comfort Exercise Promotion	

NURSING CARE PLAN

The Child with Myelomeningocele

Nursing Diagnosis	Expected Patient Outcomes	Nursing Interventions	Rationale
Risk for Injury related to neuromuscular impairment, exposed spinal column and sac with cerebrospinal fluid (CSF), insensate skin, and latex exposure **Child's/Family's Defining Characteristics *(Subjective and Objective Data)*** Developmental delays Hydrocephalus may be associated with condition Irritability Lethargy Infant cries when picked up or handled Increased frontal-occipital circumference; separated sutures Change in level of consciousness (LOC) Child headache, apathy, confusion Paralysis of lower extremities Impaired circulation around sac Neuromuscular impairment secondary to lesion External: Injury Internal: Impaired mobility, altered thought processes Developmental age (young) (physiologic and psychological)	Infant or child will experience no physical injury Sac remains intact with no evidence of trauma to spinal cord or surgical site Child does not develop latex injury from repeated latex exposure while in the hospital Evidence of hydrocephalus is detected early Minimal risk of lower extremity deformity **The Following NOC Concepts Apply to These Outcomes** Fall Prevention Behavior Immune Status Parenting: Psychosocial Safety Personal Safety Behavior Risk Control Safe Home Environment	***Preoperatively***	
		Educate family about risk for injury in the hospital.	To decrease the risk for injury
		Discuss with family the child's capabilities, how to hold infant, and how to position infant. Position child so that child is not lying on the sac.	To prevent rupture of sac covering and entry of microorganisms into the exposed spinal column
		Keep bed items and clothing off of sac.	To prevent friction and shearing injuries to the skin
		Provide incentives to move. Use passive range-of-motion (ROM) exercises.	To reduce developmental delays associated with neuromuscular impairment
		Use latex-free products (catheters, gowns, IV catheters, tape, and other patient care supplies).	To reduce exposure to latex
		Have supplies on hand for anaphylaxis reaction. Post sign to other staff members to use latex-free products.	To reduce complications related to an allergic reaction to latex
		Postoperatively	
		Assess for signs and symptoms of increased ICP: • Bulging fontanel • Sunset eyes • Irritability • Decreased LOC	To provide immediate treatment (increased blood pressure is a primary determinant of increasing intracranial pressure)
		Minimize stressful events because they increase blood pressure, and that increases ICP.	To minimize complications associated with increased ICP
		Maintain hips in slight to moderate abduction.	To reduce occurrence of dislocating hips
		Use devices such as foam blocks.	To decrease skin breakdown and maintain abduction
		Older child: Encourage mobilization.	To increase independence in mobility
		Incorporate play that encourages desired behavior.	To keep the child doing tasks that maintain well-being.
		Involve school in performance of activites of daily living (ADLs).	Need for assistance in ADLs based on level of spinal cord paralysis
		Involve schools in latex avoidance.	To prevent latex reaction
		Teach parents bowel training program for a child >3 years of age.	To involve parents in ADLs
		Involve parents in discharge teaching: care of skin, contracture prevention, ROM devices, use of assistive and mobilization devices.	To facilitate positive transition to home
		Obtain physical therapy consultation when indicated.	To optimize neuromuscular development and prevent contractures

Continued

NURSING CARE PLAN

The Child with Myelomeningocele–cont'd

Nursing Diagnosis	Expected Patient Outcomes	Nursing Interventions	Rationale
Risk for Injury related to neuromuscular impairment, exposed spinal column and sac with cerebrospinal fluid (CSF), insensate skin, and latex exposure—cont'd		**The Following NIC Concepts Apply to These Interventions** Behavior Modification Health Education Patient Contracting Self-Modification Assistance Environmental Management: Safety	
Social Isolation related to hospitalization and surgical status **Child's/Family's Defining Characteristics** ***(Subjective and Objective Data)*** *Objective Data* Altered Mobility related to neuromuscular limitations Dependence on others for physical and psychologic activity Evidence of physical or mental handicap	Child will participate in cognitive and physical activities while in the hospital **The Following NOC Concepts Apply to These Outcomes** Social Support Social Involvement Play Participation	Use therapeutic play while caring for child. Encourage parents to involve child in normal activities for age and educational level. Involve in activities such as activity therapy, recreation therapy. Involve in animal therapy. Promote method of communication of needs. **The Following NIC Concepts Apply to These Interventions** Developmental Care Caregiver Support Family Therapy	To prevent developmental regression during hospitalization To decrease isolation To promote psychosocial development
Risk for Infection related to presence of infective organisms, nonepithelialized sac, lower extremity paralysis, and urinary stasis and retention **Child's/Family's Defining Characteristics** ***(Subjective and Objective Data)*** Open lesion along spinal cord External: Nosocomial agents Physical: Invasion of skin where sac is located Paralysis below lesion: Urinary retention Lack of perineal or bladder sensation	Child will exhibit no signs or symptoms of infection **The Following NOC Concepts Apply to These Outcomes** Immune Status Infection Severity	Handle sac carefully before surgical repair. Place under warmer as necessary, and clean sac with sterile normal saline as ordered. Teach parents to recognize signs and symptoms of urinary tract infection (UTI). Administer antibiotics for infection. Monitor of signs and symptoms of infection: increased temperature, irritability, lethargy, nuchal rigidly, and poor feeding. Teach parent and child (age appropriate) how to perform clean intermittent catheterization (CIC) on a regular basis. **The Following NIC Concepts Apply to These Interventions** Self-Care Assistance: Toileting Bed Rest Care Skin Surveillance Infection Protection Medication Administration Urinary Elimination Management	To prevent damage to meningeal sac To prevent damage to sac and to help child maintain a neutral thermal environment To prevent complications associated with untreated UTI To treat UTI To implement therapy and prevent adverse consequences from sepsis To drain bladder and prevent urinary stasis

Nursing Care of the Child with Metabolic Dysfunction

NURSING CARE PLAN

The Child with Diabetes Mellitus

Nursing Diagnosis	Expected Patient Outcomes	Nursing Interventions	Rationale
Risk for Injury related to insulin deficiency	Child demonstrates normal blood glucose levels	Obtain blood glucose level.	To determine most appropriate dose of insulin
		Administer insulin as prescribed.	To maintain normal blood glucose level
Child's/Family's Defining Characteristics *(Subjective and Objective Data)* Polyphagia Polydipsia Polyuria Weight loss Enuresis or nocturia Abnormal blood profile-glucose, insulin Irritability Shortened attention span Fatigue Dry Skin Blurred vision Headache Frequent infections Hyperglycemia Flushed skin	**The Following NOC Concepts Apply to These Outcomes** Blood Glucose Level Nutritional Status: Nutrient Intake	Understand the action of insulin: differences in composition, time of onset, and duration of action for the various preparations. Employ aseptic techniques when preparing and administering insulin. Rotate sites. **The Following NIC Concepts Apply to These Interventions** Health Education Hyperglycemia Management Hypoglycemia Management Nutrition Management Medication Administration	To ensure accurate insulin administration To prevent infection To enhance absorption of insulin
Risk for Injury related to hypoglycemia	Child will exhibit no evidence of hypoglycemia	Recognize signs of hypoglycemia early: Be alert at times when blood glucose levels are lowest (before meals and snacks; 2-4 AM; after bursts of physical activity without additional food; or with delayed, omitted, or incompletely consumed meal or snack.	To prevent hypoglycemia
Child's/Family's Defining Characteristics *(Subjective and Objective Data)* Shaky feeling; hunger; headache; dizziness; difficulty concentrating speaking, focusing; tremors; tachycardia; shallow respirations; can lead to convulsion, shock and coma	**The Following NOC Concept Applies to These Outcomes** Blood Glucose Level	Test blood glucose. Offer 10-15 g of readily absorbed carbohydrates, such as orange juice, hard candy, or milk. Follow with complex carbohydrate and protein, such as bread or cracker spread with peanut butter or cheese. Administer glucagons to unconscious or combative child.	To evaluate glucose level To elevate blood glucose level and alleviate symptoms of hypoglycemia To maintain blood glucose level To elevate blood glucose level; position child to minimize risk of aspiration, because vomiting may occur

Continued

NURSING CARE PLAN

The Child with Diabetes Mellitus—cont'd

Nursing Diagnosis	Expected Patient Outcomes	Nursing Interventions	Rationale
Risk for Injury related to hypoglycemia—cont'd		**The Following NIC Concepts Apply to These Interventions** Health Education Hypoglycemia Management	
Knowledge Deficit (Diabetes Management) related to care of a child with newly diagnosed diabetes mellitus **Child's/Family's Defining Characteristics** ***(Subjective and Objective Data)*** Lack of understanding, inability to prepare and administer insulin, inability to follow meal planning guidelines, difficulty describing treatment plan	Child and family have attitude conducive to learning	Select methods, vocabulary, and content appropriate to learner's level.	To maximize learning
		Allow time for family and child to begin to adjust to initial impact of the diagnosis.	To allow child and family to set pace
		Select an environment conducive to learning.	To promote learning
		Involve all senses and employ a variety of teaching strategies, especially participation.	To promote most-effective methods for learning
		Provide pamphlets or other supplementary materials.	To promote learning
	Child and family will demonstrate understanding of meal planning	Emphasize relationship between normal nutritional needs and the disease.	To encourage sense of normalcy
		Become familiar with family's culture and food preferences.	To include in meal planning
		Teach or reinforce learners' understanding of the basic food groups and the prescribed meal plan.	To reinforce existing knowledge base
		Help child and family estimate portion sizes by volume.	To provide a more practical method than weighing food
		Suggest low-carbohydrate snack items.	To promote appropriate food choices
		Guide family in assessing labels of food products for carbohydrate content.	To reinforce that consistency in carbohydrate portions is essential
	Child and family demonstrate knowledge of and ability to administer insulin	Teach child and family the characteristics of the insulins prescribed.	To increase understanding that there are several insulin preparations
		Teach proper mixing of insulins.	To prevent contaminating the vials
		Teach injection procedure.	To promote appropriate administration
		Teach basic techniques using an orange or similar item.	To allow for confidence building
		Use demonstration and return demonstration techniques on another before injecting child.	To prevent stress for the child
		Help families and child work out a set rotational pattern.	To ensure maximum absorption of insulin and prevention of hypertrophy at injection site
		Teach proper care of insulin and equipment.	To prevent contamination and minimize complications
	Child and family demonstrate ability to test blood glucose level	Teach family and child, if old enough, blood glucose monitoring or use of equipment, interpretation of results, and care and maintenance of equipment.	To ensure that child and family learn how to adjust insulin based on blood glucose level
	Child and family demonstrate knowledge of management of hyperglycemia and hypoglycemia	Instruct learners in how to recognize signs of hyperglycemia and hypoglycemia.	To prevent delay of treatment

	Explain relationship of insulin needs to illness, activity, and intense emotion.	To ensure appropriate treatment
	Teach how to adjust food, activity, and insulin at times of illness and during other situations that alter blood glucose levels.	To ensure appropriate treatment
	Suggest carrying source of carbohydrate, such as sugar cubes or hard candy, in pocket.	To prevent delay in treatment
	Instruct parents and child in how to treat hypoglycemia with food, simple sugars, or glucagons.	To establish health practices that last a lifetime
Child and family demonstrate understanding of proper hygiene	Emphasize importance of personal hygiene.	To stress importance for child's general health
	Encourage regular dental care and yearly ophthalmologic examinations.	To minimize risk of infection
	Teach proper care of cuts and scratches; teach proper foot care.	To prevent infection
The Following NOC Concepts Apply to These Outcomes Blood Glucose Level Knowledge: Medication Knowledge: Treatment Regimen	**The Following NIC Concepts Apply to These Interventions** Health Education Hyperglycemia Management Hypoglycemia Management	

NURSING CARE PLAN

The Child with Diabetic Ketoacidosis (DKA)

Nursing Diagnosis	Expected Patient Outcomes	Nursing Interventions	Rationale
Deficient Fluid Volume related to high blood glucose level, decreased oral fluid intake, acute illness	Child remains adequately hydrated	Establish intravenous access.	To administer fluids
		Administer bolus infusion of 20 ml/kg 0.9% normal saline initially then additional maintenance fluids as required and prescribed.	To hydrate tissues
Child's/Family's Defining Characteristics	**The Following NOC Concepts Apply to These Outcomes**	Monitor electrolyte status, especially potassium.	To detect alterations requiring electrolyte supplementation and fluid administration requirements
(Subjective and Objective Data)	Electrolyte & Acid/Base Balance	Monitor health status for acute illness.	To evaluate for acute illness that may alter fluid balance and may alter insulin and glucose levels
Weakness	Fluid Balance	Obtain baseline blood glucose level on admission then per unit protocol.	To identify intervention for maintaining blood glucose within acceptable limits
Thirst	Knowledge: Health Promotion	Monitor urinary output closely.	To determine renal function and need for intravenous fluids
Dry skin and mucous membranes		**The Following NIC Concepts Apply to These Interventions**	
Change in mental status		Fluid/Electrolyte Monitoring	
Electrolyte imbalance		Electrolyte Management	
Acute illness (e.g., fever, cough, rash, pain)		Fluid/Electrolyte Management	
		Intravenous (IV) Therapy	
		Fluid Monitoring	
		Laboratory Data Interpretation	
		Fluid Management	
		Health Education	
Risk for Injury related to insulin deficiency	Child exhibits normal blood glucose levels and normal urinalysis results	Administer insulin as prescribed.	To maintain blood glucose within acceptable parameters
		Monitor vital signs.	To determine patient's response to therapy and need for additional interventions
			To detect change in patient's condition
Patient's/Family's Defining Characteristics		Place on cardiac monitor.	To detect possible changes in cardiac function (related to hypokalemia)
(Subjective and Objective Data)	**The Following NOC Concept Applies to These Outcomes**	Observe (monitor) for signs of cerebral edema.	To prevent cerebral damage
Elevated blood glucose level	Knowledge: Diabetes Management	Provide family information regarding child's status and therapeutic intervention plans.	To increase family knowledge regarding child's status
Glycosuria		Involve family in child's care.	
Ketonuria		Reinforce diabetic teaching regarding activity, diet, and insulin dosage.	To promote control of diabetes
Acidosis (fruity breath)		Monitor glucose levels closely during illness, growth, and emotional upset.	To ensure accurate insulin administration

		The Following NIC Concepts Apply to These Interventions Vital Signs Monitoring Medication Administration Health Education	
Interrupted Family Processes related to separation from child, hospitalization, and child's health status **Child's/Family's Defining Characteristics** ***(Subjective and Objective Data)*** Changes in: • Communication patterns • Availability for affective responsiveness and intimacy • Availability for emotional support • Patterns and rituals	Family function is maintained intact **The Following NOC Concepts Apply to These Outcomes** Family Normalization Family Functioning	Allow family to be with child. Provide primary caretakers information regarding child's status and plans for intervention. Involve family members in child's care as much as possible. Provide family support and resources for maintaining functioning (financial, emotional, informational, spiritual, child care). Allow family to express concerns, frustrations regarding child's illness, family pattern disruption. **The Following NIC Concepts Apply to These Interventions** Home Maintenance Assistance Family Support Conflict Mediation Family Involvement Promotion Financial Resource Assistance Emotional Support Role Enhancement	To prevent effects of separation To prevent fear of the unknown and discourage sense of helplessness To promote family's sense of involvement in child's life To promote family functioning To promote expression of ideas and opinions

Nursing Care of the Child with Cancer

NURSING CARE PLAN

The Child with Cancer

Nursing Diagnosis	Expected Patient Outcomes	Nursing Interventions	Rationale
Risk for Injury related to chemotherapy treatment	Child exhibits no complications of chemotherapy Child will receive prompt, appropriate treatment of complications	Administer chemotherapeutic agents using established guidelines.	To minimize inappropriate administration techniques
		Assist with procedures for administration of chemotherapeutic agents.	To promote safer cancer treatment
		Administer medications around the clock to prevent nausea and vomiting before chemotherapy.	To minimize side effects of nausea and vomiting
Child's/Family's Defining Characteristics *(Subjective and Objective Data)*		Administer IV fluid as prescribed.	To maintain hydration
Anaphylaxis: wheezing, hypotension, urticaria, cyanosis		Encourage frequent intake of fluids in small amounts.	To promote hydration
Nausea, vomiting		Observe for signs of infiltration of intravenous site: pain, stinging, swelling redness.	To prevent infiltration when possible
IV infiltration: pain, redness, swelling at IV infusion site	**The Following NOC Concept Applies to These Outcomes** Risk Control	Institute policies to treat infiltration if it occurs.	To prevent complications
		Observe child for 20 minutes after infusion of drugs that are associated with risk of anaphylaxis.	To observe for signs of anaphylaxis
		Stop infusion of drug and flush IV line with normal saline is reaction if suspected.	To prevent further reaction
		Have emergency equipment and emergency drugs readily available.	To prevent delay in treatment
		The Following NIC Concepts Apply to These Interventions Chemotherapy Management Nausea Management	
Risk for Infection related to depressed body defenses	Child does not exhibit signs of infection Child does not come in contact with infected persons	Use good hand-washing technique.	To minimize exposure to infective organisms
		Screen all visitors and staff for signs of infection.	To decrease exposure to possible infective organisms
		Use aseptic technique for all invasive procedures.	To decrease chance of infection spread
		Monitor temperature.	To detect possible infection
Child's/Family's Defining Characteristics *(Subjective and Objective Data)*		Evaluate child for any potential sites of infection.	To evaluate needle puncture sites, mucosa for ulceration, minor abrasions for possible infection
Fever, altered vital signs, lethargy, change in behavior, septic shock	**The Following NOC Concepts Apply to These Outcomes** Risk Control Immune Status Infection Severity	Provide nutritionally complete diet.	To support body's natural defenses
		Avoid giving live attenuated virus vaccines.	To prevent overwhelming infection
		Give inactivated virus vaccines.	To prevent specific infections and to avoid placing the child at risk for acquiring the illness
		Administer antibiotics as prescribed.	To treat a specific infection
		Administer granulocyte colony-stimulating factor (G-CSF) as prescribed.	To promote production of infection-fighting cells
		The Following NIC Concepts Apply to These Interventions Infection Protection Infection Control Immunization/Vaccination Management	

Imbalanced Nutrition: Less Than Body Requirements related to loss of appetite **Child's/Family's Defining Characteristics *(Subjective and Objective Data)*** Weight loss, lack of appetite, nausea	Child's nutritional intake is adequate **The Following NOC Concepts Apply to These Outcomes** Nutritional Status: Food & Fluid Intake Nutritional Status: Nutrient Intake	Encourage parents to relax pressure placed on eating. Allow child any food tolerated. Explain expected increase in appetite if child will be taking steroids. Fortify foods with nutritious supplements. Allow child to be involved in food preparation and selection. Make food appealing. Monitor child's weight. **The Following NIC Concepts Apply to These Interventions** Nutrition Management Nutrition Therapy	To educate that loss of appetite is a consequence of chemotherapy To provide food; selections can improve once appetite increases To prepare child and family for this change To maximize quality of intake To encourage eating To encourage eating To monitor child's status
Pain (Specify: Acute, Chronic) related to diagnosis, treatment, physiologic effects of cancer **Child's/Family's Defining Characteristics *(Subjective and Objective Data)*** Crying, withdrawal, fear of procedures, reluctance to move, change in vital signs	Child will experience no pain or reduction of pain to level acceptable to the child **The Following NOC Concepts Apply to These Outcomes** Pain Level Pain: Disruptive Effects Pain Control	Use pharmacologic and nonpharmacologic interventions before painful procedures. Assess pain with each vital sign measurement. Evaluate effectiveness of pain relief. Administer analgesics as prescribed on preventive schedule (around the clock) when needed. **The Following NIC Concept Applies to These Interventions** Pain Management	To minimize discomfort To determine level of pain To determine effectiveness To prevent pain from recurring
Fear related to diagnostic tests, procedures, treatment **Child's/Family's Defining Characteristics *(Subjective and Objective Data)*** Worry and anxiety before procedures, withdrawal, lack of control, outbursts, anger, lack of cooperation	Child has reduced fear related to diagnostic procedures and treatment **The Following NOC Concepts Apply to These Outcomes** Fear Self-Control Pain Control	Explain procedures carefully at child's level of understanding. Explain what will take place and what child will feel, see, and hear. Listen to special requests of child when possible. Provide child with some means of involvement with procedures (e.g., holding a piece of equipment, helping put on bandage, counting). Implement distraction techniques and pain reduction interventions. **The Following NIC Concepts Apply to These Interventions** Pain Management	To reduce fear of unknown To provide sense of control To encourage cooperation To provide sense of control, encourage cooperation, and support child's coping skills To reduce pain

Continued

4 - NURSING CARE PLANS

NURSING CARE PLAN

The Child with Cancer–cont'd

Nursing Diagnosis	Expected Patient Outcomes	Nursing Interventions	Rationale
Body Image Disturbance related to changes caused by cancer and treatment **Child's/Family's Defining Characteristics *(Subjective and Objective Data)*** Sadness, depression, withdrawal, anger	Child will exhibit positive coping skills **The Following NOC Concept Applies to These Outcomes** Body Image	Encourage child to decide how he or she will cope with hair loss (e.g., wig, cap, scarf). Provide adequate covering during exposure to sunlight, wind, or cold. Explain that hair begins to regrow in 3 to 6 months and may be a different color and texture. Encourage good hygiene and grooming. Encourage rapid return to peer group and friends. Encourage visits from friends before discharge. **The Following NIC Concepts Apply to These Interventions** Counseling Body Image Enhancement	To promote early adjustment and preparation for hair loss To prevent exposure To reduce risk of infection To prepare child for reactions of others To prepare child for reactions of others
Altered (Interrupted) Family Processes related to having a child with a life-threatening disease **Child's/Family's Defining Characteristics *(Subjective and Objective Data)*** Lack of understanding of disease and treatment, inability to identify side effects of treatment, inability to understand child's treatment plan, lack of family support	Child and family demonstrate understanding of the disease and treatment **The Following NOC Concepts Apply to These Outcomes** Family Functioning Family Coping Family Normalization Knowledge: Illness Care	Teach parents and child about the disease, and explain all procedures. Advise family of expected side effects and toxicities; clarify which demand medical evaluation. Reassure family that reactions are complications of treatment. Prepare family for what to do when side effects occur. Interpret prognostic statistics carefully, realizing family's level of understanding. Schedule time for family to be together without interruptions. Help family plan for future. Encourage family to discuss feelings regarding child's disease. **The Following NIC Concepts Apply to These Interventions** Counseling Family Support	To promote understanding To prevent delay in treatment To provide support To prevent delay in treatment To promote understanding To encourage communication and expression of feelings To promote child's development To encourage expression of feelings

Nursing Care of the Child with Musculoskeletal Dysfunction

NURSING CARE PLAN

The Child with Idiopathic Scoliosis

Nursing Diagnosis	Expected Patient Outcome	Nursing Interventions	Rationale
Disturbed Body Image related to diagnosis of scoliosis and subsequent therapy and perceived defect in body structure	Adolescent copes effectively with therapy	Allow adolescent to verbalize feelings about wearing brace and how it affects her lifestyle.	To promote expression of negative feelings
		Discuss a plan of action for participation in activities with peers.	To encourage participation and prevent self-isolation
	The Following NOC Concepts Apply to These Outcomes	Discuss implications of not wearing brace and impact on appearance.	To provide information related to noncompliance
Child's/Family's Defining Characteristics *(Subjective and Objective Data)*	Psychosocial Adjustment: Life Change	Emphasize positive aspects of participation in activities of daily life with brace.	To promote positive reinforcement of treatment plan
Verbalization of change in lifestyle	Self-Esteem	Encourage self-care regarding activities of daily living; address with adjustments related to restrictions with brace, adjusting and removing brace.	To promote self-care
Expresses negative feelings about body		Encourage meeting periodically with other female adolescents who must wear brace.	To gain perspective and support of others like her who are affected by wearing brace
Verbalization of perceptions that reflect an altered view of one's body in appearance, structure, or function		Encourage meeting with peers as before and performing activities as tolerated with peers.	To promote acceptance by peers and self
		Assist parents and siblings with discussion of feelings about daughter's diagnosis, wearing of brace, and family's and siblings' feelings regarding therapy.	To provide emotional support
		Discuss with family and siblings how they can support adolescent through therapy.	To promote family functioning
		The Following NIC Concepts Apply to These Interventions Body Image Enhancement Socialization Enhancement Family Involvement Promotion Mutual Goal Setting Anticipatory Guidance	

Continued

NURSING CARE PLAN

The Child with Idiopathic Scoliosis—cont'd

Nursing Diagnosis	Expected Patient Outcome	Nursing Interventions	Rationale
Postoperative Period Risk for Injury related to neurologic surgical intervention on spinal column	Adolescent attains ambulation	Logroll with assistance.	To prevent injury
		Implement aspiration precautions.	To prevent aspiration while supine
		Administer pain medications and/or assist with patient-controlled anesthesia (PCA) pump infusion of pain medications.	To promote comfort
Child's/Family's Defining Characteristics *(Subjective and Objective Data)* Spinal immobilization Tissue and bone trauma	**The Following NOC Concepts Apply to These Outcomes** Risk Control Personal Safety Behavior Neurological Status: Spinal Sensory/Motor Function	Encourage isometric exercises of lower extremities as allowed.	To promote muscle movement and tone
		Assess neurologic signs as warranted or per protocol.	To assess signs indicating further intervention required to prevent neurologic injury
		Assist to a sitting position on side of bed and ambulation as allowed as soon as possible (depending on type of instrumentation and surgery performed); medicate for pain 30-45 minutes before ambulation.	To prevent side effects of immobilization
		Encourage patient to ambulate and assist with ambulation.	To prevent immobilization complications
		Assess pressure points if immobile for long period, and provide appropriate interventions (massage, special mattress, turning).	To prevent skin breakdown
		The Following NIC Concepts Apply to These Interventions Risk Identification Environmental Management: Safety Exercise Promotion Positioning Surveillance Vital Signs Monitoring Postanesthesia Care Skin Surveillance	

NURSING CARE PLAN

The Child with Arthritis (Juvenile Idiopathic Arthritis)

Nursing Diagnosis	Expected Patient Outcome	Nursing Interventions	Rationale
Chronic Pain related to joint inflammation **Child's/Family's Defining Characteristics *(Subjective and Objective Data)*** Verbal report of pain Guarding behavior Change in sleep pattern	Child is able to move (joints) and complete activities of daily living with no discomfort or minimal discomfort **The Following NOC Concepts Apply to These Outcomes** Comfort Level Pain Control Anxiety Self-Control Coping	Use pain rating scale to evaluate pain (discomfort) level. Administer antiinflammatory medications (NSAIDs) promptly on report of pain and around the clock (ATC) when discomfort is acute. Administer other rheumatic drugs such as slow-acting antirheumatic drugs (SAARDS). Schedule routine rest periods throughout the day. Encourage child to eat a well-balanced diet and exercise daily. Help child set up a routine of daily exercise. Encourage nonpharmacologic pain relief remedies such as use of heat pad, moist heat, and pool therapy. Encourage child to discuss effect of pain on lifestyle and activities. **The Following NIC Concepts Apply to These Interventions** Analgesic Administration Sleep Enhancement Exercise Promotion Medication Management Environmental Management: Comfort	To provide objective assessment of pain level To manage pain and prevent breakthrough pain To provided relief from inflammation To prevent obesity and promote wellness To prevent further joint stiffness To promote mobility of joints and relieve painful stiff joints To provide outlet for emotions such as anger, frustration, depression at having a chronic illness
Impaired Physical Mobility related to pain and swelling in joints **Child's/Family's Defining Characteristics *(Subjective and Objective Data)*** Limited ability to perform fine and gross motor skills Limited range of motion Verbal report of pain Measurable pain on pain scale	Child engages in activities of daily living **The Following NOC Concepts Apply to These Outcomes** Ambulation Body Mechanics Performance Rest Joint Movement: Ankle Joint Movement: Spine Joint Movement: Wrist Joint Movement: Knee Joint Movement: Hip Joint Movement: Elbow Joint Movement: Fingers	Encourage ambulation and performance of activities of daily living to maximal potential every day. Assist with range-of-motion exercises for child who is severely limited Encourage child to be as active as tolerated. Assist with planning and encourage rest periods during the day. Encourage taking pain medication such as NSAIDs before ambulation and activity. Use nonpharmacologic pain adjuncts such as heat pad, hydrotherapy. Encourage child to be active in self-care activities to maximal potential. **The Following NIC Concepts Apply to These Interventions** Energy Management Exercise Promotion: Stretching Exercise Therapy: Joint Mobility Self-Care Assistance Teaching: Prescribed Activity/Exercise	To keep joints limber and prevent disuse contractures To promote muscle movement and keep joints limber To promote independence To prevent fatigue To promote activity with minimal pain To decrease pain and encourage mobility of joints To enhance self-worth and independence

Nursing Care of the Child with Cognitive Impairment

NURSING CARE PLAN

The Child with Impaired Cognitive Function

Nursing Diagnosis	Expected Patient Outcomes	Nursing Interventions	Rationale
Delayed Growth and Development related to impaired cognitive functioning **Child's/Family's Defining Characteristics** ***(Subjective and Objective Data)*** Deprived environment Psychiatric disorders (e.g., autism) Infections, especially those involving the brain (e.g., meningitis, encephalitis, measles) or a high body temperature Chromosomal abnormality Nonresponsiveness to contact Poor eye contact during feeding Diminished spontaneous activity Decreased alertness to voice or movement Irritability Slow feeding	Child will achieve optimum growth and development potential Child will achieve optimum socialization **The Following NOC Concepts Apply to These Outcomes** Cognitive Orientation Communication: Receptive Social Interaction Skills Growth Role Performance Self-Care: Activities of Daily Living (ADL)	Perform a physical and developmental assessment. Assist with diagnostic tests (e.g., chromosome analysis, metabolic dysfunction, radiography, tomography, electroencephalography).	To further evaluate cognitive impairment
		Involve child and family in an early infant stimulation program.	To maximize child's development
		Assess child's developmental progress at regular intervals; keep detailed records to distinguish subtle changes in functioning.	To revise the plan of care as needed
		Help family determine child's readiness to learn specific tasks.	To screen for readiness, because it may not be easily recognized
		Help family set realistic goals for child.	To encourage successful attainment of goals and to support self-esteem
		Employ positive reinforcement for specific tasks or behaviors.	To improve motivation and learning
		Encourage learning of self-care skills as soon as child is ready.	To encourage independence
		Reinforce self-care activities.	To facilitate optimum development
		Encourage family to investigate special daycare programs and educational classes as soon as possible.	To promote development
		Emphasize that child has same needs as other children (e.g., play, discipline, social interaction).	To optimize development
		Before adolescence, counsel child and parents regarding physical maturation, sexual behavior, marriage, and childrearing. Encourage optimum vocational training	To promote the child's potential
		Encourage family to teach child socially acceptable behavior (e.g., saying "hello" and "thank you," manners, appropriate touch).	To encourage socialization
		Encourage grooming and age-appropriate dress.	To encourage acceptance by others and support self-esteem
		Recommend programs that provide peer relationships and experiences (e.g., mainstreaming, Boy Scouts, Girl Scouts, Special Olympics).	To promote optimum socialization
		Provide adolescent with practical sexual information and a well-defined, concrete code of conduct.	To decrease risk because of child's easy persuasion and lack of judgment
		Perform or assist with intelligence tests: • Bayley Scales of Infant Development • Mullen Scales of Early Learning • Wechsler Preschool and Primary Scales of Intelligence (WPPSI-R) (preschoolers)	To establish level of cognitive impairment

		• Wechsler Intelligence Scale for Children (WISC III) (school-age children) • Differential Ability Scales • Stanford-Binet Intelligence Scale, ed 4 • Kaufman Assessment Battery for Children Perform or assist with testing of adaptive behaviors • Vineland Social Maturity Scale • AAMR Adaptive Behavior Scale **The Following NIC Concepts Apply to These Interventions** Learning Readiness Enhancement Environmental Management Self-Esteem Enhancement Active Listening Developmental Enhancement: Child Family Involvement Promotion Behavior Modification: Social Skills Parent Education: Adolescent Attachment Promotion Parent Education: Infant Sibling Support Caregiver Support Self-Care Assistance Behavior Modification	
Interrupted Family Processes related to having a child with cognitive impairment **Child's/Family's Defining Characteristics** ***(Subjective and Objective Data)*** Family history of mental retardation or hereditary disorders with mental retardation Prenatal, perinatal, or postnatal trauma or physical injury Prenatal maternal infection (e.g., rubella), alcoholism, drug consumption Lack of disease understanding Inability to understand plan of treatment Lack of family support	Family will receive adequate information and support Family will be prepared for long-term care of child **The Following NOC Concepts Apply to These Outcomes** Family Resiliency Social Support Family Coping Family Functioning Parenting Performance Caregiver Lifestyle Disruption	Inform family at or as soon as possible after birth. Have both parents present at informing conference. Give family, when possible, written information about the condition (e.g., a specific syndrome or disease). Discuss with family members the pros and cons of home care and other placement options; allow them opportunities to investigate all residential alternatives before making a decision. Encourage family to meet other families that have a child with a similar diagnosis. Refrain from giving definitive answers about the degree of retardation; stress the potential learning abilities of each child, especially with early intervention. Demonstrate acceptance of child through own behavior. Emphasize normal characteristics of child. Encourage family members to express their feelings and concerns.	To prevent fears and concerns and provide immediate support To avoid problem of one parent having to relay complex information to the other parent and deal with the reaction To inform parent of disorder To increase understanding To receive additional support To encourage hope To demonstrate caring attitude of the professional To help family see child as an individual with strengths as well as weaknesses To promote adaptation process and effective collaboration

Continued

NURSING CARE PLAN

The Child with Impaired Cognitive Function–cont'd

Nursing Diagnosis	Expected Patient Outcomes	Nursing Interventions	Rationale
Interrupted Family Processes related to having a child with cognitive impairment—cont'd		Discuss with parents alternatives to home care, especially as child grows older and as parents near retirement or old age.	To optimize appropriate long-term care that can be provided
		Encourage family to consider respite care as needed.	To facilitate family's ability to cope with child's long-term care
		Help family investigate residential settings.	To provide the child's optimum care
		Encourage family to include affected member in planning and to continue meaningful relationships after placement.	To promote family development
		Refer to agencies that provide support and assistance.	To promote support
		The Following NIC Concepts Apply to These Interventions Counseling Caregiver Support Family Therapy Family Involvement Promotion Parenting Promotion Referral Coping Enhancement Insurance Authorization Anticipatory Guidance Support Group Decision-Making Support	

Nursing Care of the Child with Burns

NURSING CARE PLAN

The Child with Burns

Nursing Diagnosis	Expected Patient Outcomes	Nursing Interventions	Rationale
Ineffective Thermoregulation related to heat loss and disruption of skin's defense mechanisms to maintain body temperature	Maintain optimal thermal regulation as evidenced by (normal) body temperatures ranging from 36.5° C to 38.1° C (98.6° to 100.5° F).	Assess skin for coolness, color changes, and capillary refill (acrocyanosis, nail bed color, and mottling).	To identify vascular accommodation of heat loss
		Monitor vital signs, especially temperature.	To identify significant trends in temperature fluctuation
		Observe for chilling and shivering.	To evaluate signs of heat loss and provide comfort
		Avoid exposure to cold stress procedures (limit time in tub to 20 minutes, bundle child, cover the head of a child younger than 6 months of age, use artificial heat).	To maintain stable body temperature and prevent body heat loss
Child's/Family's Defining Characteristics *(Subjective and Objective Data)*	**The Following NOC Concept Applies to These Outcomes**	**The Following NIC Concepts Apply to These Interventions**	
Changes in skin temperature, capillary refill, and color Chilling and shivering Changes in temperature from cold exposure	Thermoregulation	Hypothermia Treatment Vital Signs Monitoring Environmental Management Fluid Monitoring Fever Management	
Risk for Fluid Volume Deficit related to normal fluid loss from tissues secondary to burn insult	Child will maintain adequate fluid hydration status during the acute postburn period	Administer crystalloid or colloid fluid per protocol, monitoring effect and maintaining intravenous line.	To replace fluid loss related to burn injury
		Assess fluid replacement status: Observe for changes in vital signs, mental status, urinary output.	To recognize appropriate fluid balance
		Monitor daily weights.	To evaluate status of fluid retention or excess fluid loss and possible diuresis
Child's/Family's Defining Characteristics *(Subjective and Objective Data)*	**The Following NOC Concepts Apply to These Outcomes**	Observe and monitor hemodynamic parameters for changes in stability related to hypovolemia or fluid overload.	To assess for change in blood pressure (a late sign of shock)
Decreased skin turgor Increased pulse Decreased urinary output Decreased circulation status Altered electrolyte status Restlessness	Electrolyte & Acid/Base Balance Fluid Balance	Monitor laboratory results.	To identify fluid and electrolyte imbalance
		Monitor for tissue edema.	To implement therapies to reestablish intravascular protein and prevent further tissue damage
		Administer potassium-rich or potassium-restricted fluids or foods if child is hypokalemic or hyperkalemic.	To supplement IV therapy as needed to maintain electrolyte balance and prevent sequelae from alteration in K^+ imbalance

Continued

NURSING CARE PLAN

The Child with Burns–cont'd

Nursing Diagnosis	Expected Patient Outcomes	Nursing Interventions	Rationale
Risk for Fluid Volume Deficit related to normal fluid loss from tissues secondary to burn insult—cont'd Disorientation Pulmonary congestion Pulmonary edema		**The Following NIC Concepts Apply to These Interventions** Acid-Base Management Acid-Base Monitoring Fluid/Electrolyte Monitoring Hemodynamic Regulation Intravenous (IV) Therapy Laboratory Data Interpretation Vital Signs Monitoring	
Impaired Skin Integrity related to thermal injury	Evidence of wound healing	Shave hair to a 2-inch margin from the wound and the area immediately surrounding the burn.	To remove a reservoir for infection
Child's/Family's Defining Characteristics *(Subjective and Objective Data)*	Wounds heal without evidence of damage or inflammation	Thoroughly cleanse the wound and surrounding skin with normal saline and débride devitalized tissue.	To decrease the risk of infection and promote healing
Inflammation at burn site, redness, and swelling	**The Following NOC Concepts Apply to These Outcomes**	Keep child from scratching and picking at the wound. • Keep fingernails clean and clipped short. • Apply socks to hands if necessary and elbow restraints as needed. • Administer antipruritic medications. • Provide distraction appropriate to child's age.	To prevent infection and impaired tissue healing
Lack of granulation of burned tissues, no evidence of epithelialization	Tissue Integrity: Skin & Mucous Membranes	Maintain care in handling the wound.	To avoid damaging epithelializing and granulating tissues
Child scratching or picking at wound, causing redness and irritation at the site	Wound Healing: Secondary Intention	Offer high-calorie, high-protein meals and snacks.	To supplement protein and calorie requirements because of increased metabolism and catabolism
		Prevent infection by maintaining sterile technique with dressing changes.	To prevent infection that can delay wound healing and convert partial-thickness wounds to full-thickness wounds
		Administer supplementary vitamins and minerals—vitamins A, B, and C, iron, and zinc.	To facilitate wound healing and tissue epithelialization
		Pad burned ears.	To prevent tissue necrosis caused by minimal blood flow to cartilage
		Monitor for signs and symptoms of wound infection.	To ensure prompt recognition and treatment
		Wrap fingers and toes separately.	To avoid tissue adherence from prolonged contact
		Place on pressure-sensitive mattress if child is on prolonged bed rest.	To prevent pressure point skin breakdown and further tissue damage
		Monitor skin at pressure points.	
		The Following NIC Concepts Apply to These Interventions Infection Control Medication Administration Skin Care: Topical Treatment Skin Surveillance Wound Care	

		Infection Protection Splinting Wound Irrigation	
Impaired Physical Mobility related to pain, impaired joint movement, scar formation **Child's/Family's Defining Characteristics *(Subjective and Objective Data)*** Limited and/or restricted movement in joint or muscle	Child will achieve optimal physical functioning (mobility) **The Following NOC Concepts Apply to These Outcomes** Mobility Transfer Performance Joint Movement: Wrist Joint Movement: Elbow Joint Movement: Ankle Joint Movement: Hip Joint Movement: Knee Joint Movement: Shoulder	Carry out range-of-motion exercises. Administer pain medication (analgesia) 30-45 minutes before physical therapy. Encourage mobility if child is able to move extremities. Ambulate as soon as feasible. Splint involved joints in extension at night and during rest periods. Encourage and promote self-help activities. Encourage participation in activities of daily living and play activities. **The Following NIC Concepts Apply to These Interventions** Body Mechanics Promotion Energy Management Exercise Therapy: Joint Mobility	To maintain optimal joint and muscle function To minimize or obviate pain from mobilization of tight skin at joints To promote mobility To maintain optimal joint and muscle function and decrease the adverse effects of prolonged immobilization on body systems To minimize contracture formation To increase mobility and positive self-esteem To incorporate exercise into enjoyable events
Pain (Acute) related to skin trauma, therapies **Child's/Family's Defining Characteristics *(Subjective and Objective Data)*** Pain on movement, pain associated with treatment, irritation at burn site, pain on extension of joint	Child will experience reduction of pain to a level acceptable to the child **The Following NOC Concepts Apply to These Outcomes** Comfort Level Pain: Disruptive Effects Pain Control	Assess needs for medication. Recognize that burn pain is often overwhelming, engulfing, and irrepressible. Position in extension position. Implement passive and active exercise. Reduce skin irritation from bed linens and other items as applicable. Administer medication for pruritus after therapy and treatments. Touch or stroke unburned areas. Employ appropriate nonpharmacologic pain reduction techniques. Promote control and predictability during painful procedures Anticipate need for pain medication and administer before onset of severe pain at regular intervals. **The Following NIC Concepts Apply to These Interventions** Analgesic Administration Positioning Presence Pain Management Sleep Enhancement Coping Enhancement	To minimize pain To assess pain To minimize pain resulting from exercising to regain extension To minimize contracture formation To prevent increased pain To provide comfort To provide physical contact and comfort To provide comfort and reduce pain To minimize pain and anxiety To prevent pain recurrence

Nursing Care of the Child with Psychophysiologic Dysfunction

NURSING CARE PLAN

The Child Who Is Maltreated

Nursing Diagnosis	Expected Patient Outcomes	Nursing Interventions	Rationale
Risk for Trauma related to the child, caregiver(s) environment	Child will not experience any maltreatment	Observe child for physical and behavioral evidence of abuse.	To assess for child maltreatment, a significant social problem in the United States
	Child will be protected from further abuse	Report suspicions to appropriate authorities.	To prevent further injury or neglect
Child's/Family's Defining Characteristics ***(Subjective and Objective Data)*** ***Physical Neglect*** Failure to thrive Malnutrition Poor hygiene Poor health care Frequent injuries ***Emotional Neglect*** Failure to thrive Enuresis Sleep disorders ***Physical Abuse*** Bruises Burns Fractures or dislocation Lacerations Intracranial hemorrhage ***Sexual Abuse*** Torn or bloody underclothing Bruises, bleeding, lacerations of external genitalia, anus, mouth or throat Genital discharge or odor Recurrent urinary tract infection (UTI)		Assist in removing child from unsafe environment.	
	Child and family will receive adequate support	Refer family to social agencies.	To provide assistance for physical needs that may help prevent neglect and abuse
	Child is able to express feelings about returning to the home or foster home		To provide counseling and education so that parents learn appropriate parenting skills
		Collaborate with multidisciplinary team.	To allow several disciplines to provide expertise in prevention of future neglect or abuse
	Child and family, including foster parents if appropriate, will be prepared for discharge	Keep factual, objective records of child and parental behaviors.	To facilitate documentation and action planning by authorities
		Be aware of signs for continued abuse or neglect.	To prevent further injury or neglect
		Help families identify circumstances that precipitate an abusive act.	To promote more effective parenting skills
		Assist families with realizing abuse has occurred.	To promote awareness of what has happened
	The Following NOC Concepts Apply to These Outcomes Abuse Support Abuse Recovery: Physical Abuse Recovery: Sexual Anxiety Self-Control Fear Self-Control Coping Personal Safety Behavior Safe Home Environment	**The Following NIC Concepts Apply to These Interventions** Abuse Protection Support: Child Coping Enhancement: Environment Management: Violence Prevention	

Fear/Anxiety related to negative interpersonal interaction, repeated maltreatment, powerlessness, potential loss of parents	Child exhibits minimal fear and anxiety	Provide consistent caregiver during hospitalization.	To promote trust
	Child engages in positive relationships with caregivers	Demonstrate acceptance of the child.	To minimize feelings of shame and guilt
	Child grieves loss of parent	Praise child's abilities.	To promote self-esteem
Child's/Family's Defining Characteristics *(Subjective and Objective Data)*	**The Following NOC Concepts Apply to These Outcomes**	Treat child as one with a specific physical problem, not as "abused" victim.	To promote self-esteem and minimizes feelings of guilt
Withdrawn and depressed	Anxiety Self-Control	Avoid asking too many questions.	To prevent upsetting the child by probing investigation; may interfere with interrogation
Change in behavior	Fear Self-Control	Use play to communicate.	To allow child to communicate the relationship perceived by the child
Inappropriate responses	Coping	Encourage child to talk about feelings.	To facilitate coping
Fear of strangers		Provide a private time and place to talk.	To foster trust
Lack of engagement with others		Help child grieve for loss of parents if parental rights are terminated.	To support child who will likely be attached to parents despite the abuse
No response to painful interventions		Encourage introduction of foster parents before placement if possible.	To give child time to adjust
May not cry or ask for food when hungry		Offer and encourage food intake at usual times.	To promote adequate nutrition
		The Following NIC Concepts Apply to These Interventions	
		Active Listening	
		Calming Technique	
		Counseling	
		Presence	
		Therapeutic Play	
		Provide Distraction	

NURSING CARE PLAN

The Adolescent with an Eating Disorder

Nursing Diagnosis	Expected Patient Outcomes	Interventions	Rationale
Imbalanced Nutrition: Less Than Body Requirements related to altered self-image, inadequate nutrient intake, and chronic vomiting **Child's/Family's Defining Characteristics** ***(Subjective and Objective Data)*** Body weight 20% or more under ideal Reported food intake less than RDA Perceived inability to ingest food Aversion to eating Poor muscle tone Excessive hair loss Misconceptions	Nutrient intake is sufficient to maintain optimal cellular and metabolic function **The Following NOC Concepts Apply to These Outcomes** Weight Control Nutritional Status: Food & Fluid Intake	If adolescent's life is in immediate danger as a result of malnutrition, implement plan for restoring physiologic homeostasis: electrolyte and fluid replacement, enteral feedings as required, monitoring of vital signs, and restoration of fluid and electrolyte balance.	To prevent death or multiorgan failure To restore fluid and electrolyte imbalance
		Develop a mutually agreeable targeted daily caloric intake goal.	To give adolescent sense of control over nutrient intake and establish realistic plan for weight gain
		Observe eating behaviors.	To detect detrimental habits such as purging or bingeing
		Monitor nutritional intake and behavior thereafter for 1 hour.	To detect physiologic changes that may be life-threatening
		Monitor vital signs as warranted by patient status.	To detect life-threatening conditions such as dehydration or hyponatremia
		Monitor fluid and electrolyte status.	To prevent dehydration
		Set mutually agreeable target intake of fluids per day.	To prevent further weight loss
		Establish mutually agreeable targeted goal for daily exercise that is congruent with nutrient intake and weight gain.	To prevent self-harm
		Monitor activities for detrimental behaviors such as administering enemas, purging, bingeing (bulimic), and excessive exercise.	To clarify expectations and provide limits for control of behaviors that are not acceptable
		Set limits and clearly define expectations in relation to therapeutic plan to increase nutrient intake.	To establish a mutually agreed-on plan for nutrient intake and weight gain
		Develop a behavioral contract for nutrient intake and cessation of behaviors related to eating that are detrimental.	To promote verbalization of concerns and fears
		The Following NIC Concepts Apply to These Interventions Vital Signs Monitoring Weight Management Nutrition Therapy Behavior Modification Nutritional Counseling Nutritional Monitoring	

Disturbed Body Image related to altered self perception **Child's/Family's Defining Characteristics** ***(Subjective and Objective Data)*** Negative feelings about body Verbalization of feelings that reflect an altered perception of one's body appearance	Adolescent displays evidence of developing and maintaining a positive self-image **The Following NOC Concepts Apply to These Outcomes** Child Development: Adolescence Self-Esteem	Encourage adolescent to verbalize feelings and concerns regarding view of self in relation to peers and family members.	To enhance self esteem and alter misconception of self in relation to others
		Provide opportunity for adolescent to engage in activities that have potential to build self-esteem.	To promote self-esteem
		Encourage self-care in relation to dietary management and weight control.	To set limits for behavior
		Encourage discussion of maladaptive behaviors surrounding food and fluid intake: bingeing, purging, laxative use, excess exercise.	To provide consistency in therapy and allow mutual discussion
		Provide a therapeutic discussion (over time) of personal attributes perceived as positive.	To enhance reality-based self-perception
		Involve adolescent in activities designed to promote positive image of self-worth and accomplishment.	To promote sense of accomplishment and enhance self image
		Involve family members and adolescent in group family counseling to discuss expectations and members' roles within the family.	To promote expression of perceptions about self within family and identify any distorted patterns of interaction that require clarification or modification
		The Following NIC Concepts Apply to These Interventions Emotional Support Socialization Enhancement Body Image Enhancement Self-Esteem Enhancement Mutual Goal Setting Values Clarification	

NURSING CARE PLAN

The Child with Attention Deficit Hyperactivity Disorder (ADHD)

Nursing Diagnosis	Expected Patient Outcome	Nursing Interventions	Rational
Delayed Growth and Development related to impaired cognitive functioning **Child's/Family's Defining Characteristics *(Subjective and Objective Data)*** Obtain a developmental history for evidence of: • Aggressive behavior in early childhood • Excessive fussiness and irritability • Destructive behavior as small child • Disciplinary problems in early childhood	Achieve optimal growth and development potential **The Following NOC Concepts Apply to These Outcomes** Growth Personal Safety Behavior Symptom Severity	Perform a comprehensive age-appropriate physical assessment (neurologic evaluation, hearing and vision screening, developmental assessment).	To promote early detection
		Assist with diagnostic test (e.g., electroencephalogram [EEG]) and obtain blood lead levels and thyroid levels to rule out potential organic causes (e.g., seizures, lead poisoning, and hyperthyroidism).	To assist with diagnosis
		Perform and/or assist with psychometric testing.	To assist with diagnosis
		Identify child with learning and/or behavior problems consistent with ADHD.	To provide early intervention
		Assist in the maintenance of a consistent environment for the child.	To promote the child's organizational skills
		Evaluate effectiveness of behavioral treatment therapies.	To promote appropriate development
		Assist other professionals (teachers, caregivers) in setting up a structured environment that is conducive to learning and has minimal distractions.	To enhance learning
		Administer child's medications on a consistent basis according to the daily routine.	To promote the effects of the medication and avoid disrupting child's daily routine
		Evaluate child's response to medications.	To prevent untoward effects and enhance drug therapy
		Assist parents in providing routine daily schedule for the child, including meals and exercise.	To promote optimal growth and development
		Make parents aware of potential coexisting behavior problems often seen with ADHD.	To promote prompt and effective treatment of coexisting problems, such as depression, substance abuse, and antisocial personality
		Assist in the provision of a structured environment at school and home.	To promote organizational behavior skills
		Evaluate the effectiveness of therapies prescribed (e.g., structured environment at school and home, pharmacotherapy, family and child psychotherapy).	To promote effective management
		The Following NIC Concepts Apply to These Interventions Developmental Enhancement: Child Behavior Modification Behavior Management: Overactivity/Inattention Impulse Control Training Health Education Developmental Enhancement: Child Health Screening Nutrition Management Medication Administration Medication Management Calming Technique	

Interrupted Family Processes related to having child with ADHD	Family will receive adequate information and support	Involve family in seeking professional assistance for child with learning and/or behavior problems.	To promote family interaction in early assessment of child
		Provide family with written information about ADHD and treatments.	To avoid family receiving inappropriate information from other sources
Child's/Family's Defining Characteristics *(Subjective and Objective Data)*	**The Following NOC Concepts Apply to These Outcomes**	Involve family in setting realistic goals for the child's learning activities in the home environment.	To promote child's learning skills
Evidence suggests one parent may have had similar problems as child	Family Coping	Help parents devise appropriate disciplinary strategies for the child.	To prevent further impulsivity and promote child's self-esteem
Note if other children in the family have been diagnosed with ADHD or have behaviors consistent with ADHD	Family Normalization	Assist family with medication administration schedule in the home.	To provide steady-state pharmacologic effects
Any environmental causes of distractions related to learning	Caregiver Emotional Health	Provide family members with information on medication side effects, particularly when changes in dosing occur.	To prevent adverse medication effects
	Parenting Performance	Provide family with information regarding resources and referrals for families with children with ADHD.	To provide support and prevent family isolation
	Family Functioning	Prepare parents by setting long-term goals for the child's treatment in the home to prevent unrealistic expectations surrounding the child's prognosis.	To promote family function
	Psychosocial Adjustment: Life Change	**The Following NIC Concepts Apply to These Interventions**	
	Symptom Severity	Family Support Counseling Family Involvement Promotion Coping Enhancement Family Process Maintenance Caregiver Support Emotional Support Referral Parent Education Attachment Promotion Medication Management	

Nursing Care of the Child with Poisoning

NURSING CARE PLAN

The Child with Toxic Ingestion or Inhalation

Nursing Diagnosis	Expected Patient Outcomes	Nursing Interventions	Rationale
Risk for Injury related to presence of toxic substance Risk for Poisoning related to exposure to toxic substance, developmental ability, and immature judgment of child **Child's/Family's Defining Characteristics** ***(Subjective and Objective Data)*** Assess possible contributing factors in occurrence of injury, such as discipline, parent-child relationship, developmental ability, environmental factors, and behavior problems	Child will not experience bodily harm from exposure to toxin **The Following NOC Concepts Apply to These Outcomes** Safe Home Environment Risk Control Personal Safety Behavior	Discuss with parents how seemingly benign household items may be toxic to the child's system.	To provide education for prevention of exposure
		Advise parents to relocate all toxic or potentially toxic substances including medications in safe storage; lock cabinets where toxins are stored; avoid placing toxins in containers not properly marked as containing toxin.	To make parents aware of dangerous toxins in common household items
		Teach children the hazards of having contact with substances that are unfamiliar to them.	To prevent toxic ingestion or exposure
		Teach parents how to safe-proof the home environment from potentially lethal toxins: plants, lead-based paint, inhaled toxins such as paint fumes, medications, poisons, cleaners.	To prevent toxic ingestion or exposure
		Teach children the dangers of taking medications without adult supervision.	To decrease exposure to poison
		Encourage parents to use a carbon monoxide monitor in the home. Encourage parents to use smoke detectors in the home and discuss escape routes in case of house fire.	To promote primary exposure or ingestion prevention
		If direct contact with toxin or ingestion has occurred, call Poison Control Center immediately for assistance in determining course of action.	To prevent delay in treatment in case of accidental toxin exposure
		Educate other household members and child caretakers regarding family plan for toxin exposure (call Poison Control Center; have fire escape route).	To implement prompt treatment and avoid further complications
		In hospital, interview family regarding type of ingestion, name of toxin.	To implement proper treatment and antidote administration
		Prepare for administration of antidote or for insertion of nasogastric tube for administration of activated charcoal.	To decrease toxic effects of toxic ingestion
		Advise parents against using plants for teas or medicines.	To prevent untoward effects of chemicals on child's system
		Instruct parents in correct administration of drugs for therapeutic purposes, and notify physician of reaction.	To prevent toxic ingestion and subsequent effects on body systems
		Post number of local Poison Control Center with emergency phone list by telephone.	To promote rapid intervention
		Inhalant or toxin exposure: Remove child from inhalant. In hospital: Observe child for signs and symptoms of difficulty breathing, labored respirations, dusky color, decreased oxygen saturation; administer oxygen for respiratory distress; monitor vital signs; have equipment on hand for airway management; have emergency equipment and medications readily available; assist ventilation as needed (humidified air, oxygen); and assist with intubation and/or respiratory support as indicated.	To prevent continued effects of exposure and maximize early intervention and therapy; to decrease toxic effects and implement therapy

		Skin toxin exposure: • Wash skin with soap and water. • Call Poison Control Center with name of toxin to which child has been exposed. **The Following NIC Concepts Apply to These Interventions** Medication Administration Oxygen Therapy Surveillance of Cardiohemodynamics Shock Management Cardiogenic Vasogenic Volume Prevention Fluid Volume Management Safety Health Teaching Home Care Management	To decrease toxic effects and implement therapy
Interrupted Family Processes related to sudden hospitalization and emergency aspects of illness **Child's/Family's Defining Characteristics** ***(Subjective and Objective Data)*** Immature or inappropriate activity level for developmental age or stage Evidence of physical or mental handicap	Child and family will receive adequate emotional support **The Following NOC Concepts Apply to These Outcomes** Family Coping Social Support Family Normalization	Keep parents and child calm. Avoid admonishing or accusing child of wrongdoing. Allow expression of feelings regarding circumstances related to the poisoning. Provide reassurance as appropriate.	To avoid increased stress during an already stressful time. To facilitate coping To decrease fear and anxiety To provide understanding and empathy To provide support and prevent separation
Impaired Parenting related to knowledge deficit **Child's/Family's Defining Characteristics** ***(Subjective and Objective Data)*** Parents verbalize minimal knowledge about care of child Parents verbalize minimal knowledge about caring for a child with a chronic illness	Parents verbalize lack of resources for meeting nutritional and psychosocial needs of child Parents will experience reduction of anxiety Parents demonstrate ability to provide appropriate care for the child Parents will be prepared for home care **The Following NOC Concepts Apply to These Outcomes** Anxiety Self-Control Coping	Explain therapies and tests. Delay prevention education until child's condition stabilizes. Encourage parents to remain with child. Assess home environment and relationships. Continue interventions begun in hospital. **The Following NIC Concepts Apply to These Interventions** Teaching: Infant Safety Caregiver Support Anticipatory Guidance Support System Enhancement	To decrease anxiety and prevent self-blame To avoid decreasing self-esteem To reassure child To avoid additional parental stress To identify need for intervention To ensure adequate care after discharge

Nursing Care of the Terminally Ill or Dying Child

NURSING CARE PLAN

The Child Who Is Terminally Ill or Dying

Nursing Diagnosis	Expected Patient Outcomes	Nursing Interventions	Rationale
Anxiety related to fear or worry about dying **Child's/Family's Defining Characteristics *(Subjective and Objective Data)*** Unstable emotions Aggressive behavior Withdrawn behavior Depression	Child and family will receive appropriate emotional support during the terminal phase of the child's illness Child will express fears and anxiety related to dying Family will support the child's ability to express fears and anxiety Child and family will be informed of symptoms to expect as child nears the end of life Child and family will be informed of procedures and therapies necessary to promote comfort Child and family will be able to cope with the dying process **The Following NOC Concepts Apply to These Outcomes** Anxiety Self-Control Coping Fear Self-Control	Encourage the family to remain near child as much as possible. Encourage child to talk about feelings; help the family as they encourage child to express feelings. Provide safe, acceptable outlets for aggression or for grieving. Answer questions as honestly as possible while maintaining a positive, hopeful approach. Explain progression of physical symptoms as child nears the end of life. Explain all procedures and therapies, especially physical effects child will experience. Help child distinguish between consequences of treatment and manifestations of the disease. Structure hospital or home environment to allow for maximum self-control and independence within the limitations imposed by child's developmental level and physical condition. **The Following NIC Concepts Apply to These Interventions** Active Listening Coping Enhancement Simple Relaxation Touch	To provide support through the presence of a loved one To provide a sense of closeness and understanding among family members To establish that anger and sadness are normal reactions To promote trust as a major strength for therapeutic relationships To promote trust and decreases anxiety To decrease fear of the unknown, which may be more of a concern than the actual procedure or therapy To provide focus on interventions that can minimize discomfort To minimize fear and loss of control
Chronic Pain related to disease process **Child's/Family's Defining Characteristics *(Subjective and Objective Data)*** Crying Withdrawal Aggression Fear of touch Fear of movement	Child exhibits minimal or no evidence of physical discomfort Family is able to participate in the child's care without causing discomfort Family is able to provide comfort measures for child **The Following NOC Concepts Apply to These Outcomes** Comfort Level Fear of touch Pain Control	Assess child's level of comfort. Provide pain management around the clock. Assess child for symptoms associated with pain or its treatment. Provide stool softener, laxative, diphenhydramine as needed. Provide nonpharmacologic interventions child prefers. Administer anticholinergic drugs as needed. Encourage family to provide comfort measures the child prefers.	To ensure child is treated for changes in pain To prevent the recurrence or escalation of pain To ensure child is treated for symptoms accompanying pain or its management To prevent or treat symptoms related to pain or its management To aid pharmacologic management of pain, helping to prevent recurrence or escalation of pain and accompanying symptoms To reduce secretions and lessen "death rattle," which can be distressing to family To provide comfort

		Provide soothing surroundings for child. Avoid excessive noise or light. Pleasant smell, touch, temperature.	To minimize irritation and maximize comfort
		Place all commodities within easy reach for the child.	To minimize discomfort from movement
		Use gentle touch when required to perform physical procedures Avoid pressure on painful areas. Avoid pressure on bony prominences or painful sites.	To minimize pain when possible
		Use pillows or other supports to prop child in a comfortable position.	To make it easier for the child to breathe
		Place absorbent pads under hips if the child is incontinent.	To prevent skin breakdown
		Limit care to essential needs.	To minimize fatigue
		The Following NIC Concepts Apply to These Interventions Analgesic Administration Patient-Controlled Analgesia Positioning Simple Massage Sleep Enhancement Simple Relaxation Therapy	
Anticipatory Grieving related to impending loss of child **Child's/Family's Defining Characteristics *(Subjective and Objective Data)*** Parents' feelings and physical responses of loss and depression Parents' feelings of loss of control and uncertainty Child's or sibling's feelings and physical responses of loss and depression Child's or sibling's feelings of loss of control and uncertainty	Family expresses fears, concerns, and any special desires for terminal care Family demonstrates an understanding of their children's needs Family members are actively involved in their child's care Family members seek resources needed to assist them during the grieving process **The Following NOC Concepts Apply to These Outcomes** Family Coping Grief Resolution	Discuss the grieving process and differences in grieving among men, women, and children with the family and child.	To facilitate understanding of what family members are feeling and experiencing
		Provide opportunities for family members to express emotions independently or together as desired.	To provide an outlet for their emotions
		Facilitate child's or sibling's expression of emotions through art or play activities.	To facilitate expression of their emotions
		Help parents and siblings deal with their feelings about the child's death.	To provide support
		Encourage parents to remain as near the child as possible.	To allow parents to feel they are doing something for their child
		Provide family with information regarding the child's status.	To promote understanding and communication
		Help parents to understand behavioral reactions of their children.	To provide understanding of their children's behaviors
		Encourage family's assistance with child's care.	To assist with coping and minimize loss of control
		Encourage family to maintain own health care needs.	To give families the approval to take care of themselves
		Provide as much privacy as possible without isolating family from nurse's care.	To provide dignity for the grieving process
		Assist family in assessing their needs for referral services.	To facilitate support for families
		Encourage parents to honestly answer children's questions about dying.	To decrease children's fear and anxiety
		Provide resources for family to facilitate discussions with children about dying.	To provide support and facilitates parents' discussion
		Encourage parents to share their moments of sorrow with their children.	To encourage sharing the loss with one another and promote grief expression of children. To facilitate emotions and sharing between family and child

Continued

NURSING CARE PLAN

The Child Who Is Terminally Ill or Dying–cont'd

Nursing Diagnosis	Expected Patient Outcomes	Nursing Interventions	Rationale
Anticipatory Grieving related to impending loss of child—cont'd		Assist family and child with memory-making opportunities.	To facilitate support of child
		Assist child as needed to complete any unfinished business.	To prevent siblings from feeling excluded
		Discuss with parents appropriate involvement of siblings.	To provide support and spiritual care
		Identify family's religious and cultural beliefs related to death.	To provide support and guidance
		Provide preparation for postdeath services.	To provide support and guidance
		Discuss with parents the frequent need of children to be given permission to die.	To allow families to be in control
		Discuss with family their preferences for care if death is imminent.	To provide support
		Facilitate appropriate spiritual care in accordance with family's beliefs or affiliations.	To allow families to choose where the child is to die and provide guidance for this to occur
		Provide support for families who choose home care for their child.	
		The Following NIC Concepts Apply to These Interventions	
		Anticipatory Guidance	
		Anxiety Reduction	
		Caregiver Support	
		Counseling	
		Family Support Family Therapy	

UNIT 5

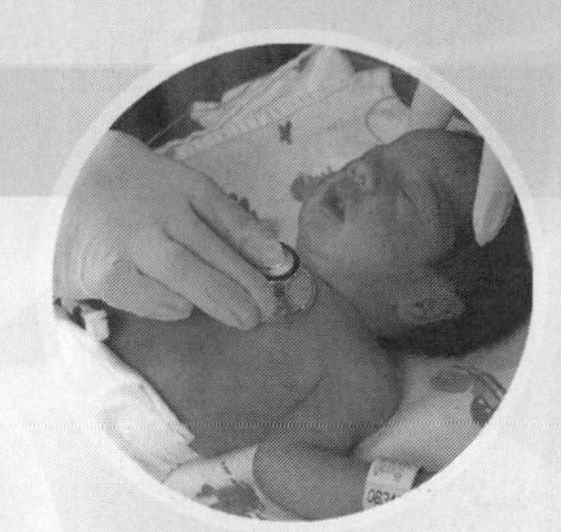

Patient and Family Education: Care in the Home and Community

Symbol ▶ indicates material that may be photocopied and distributed to families.

Preparing the Family for Home Care

The Patient and Family Education (PFE) materials in this unit are provided as a supplement to assist the nurse in preparing the family to manage the child's care at home or in a setting in the community, such as a school or daycare facility. These instructions provide a written reference that the family can use when performing the procedure in the absence of a health professional or when entrusting their child's care to someone else. Each set of instructions can be used as a teaching aid in preparing the patient for discharge from an acute care setting, a long-term care facility, or a clinic, or in the home when increasing the family's participation in the child's care.

The process of patient education involves giving the family information about the child's condition, the regimen that must be followed and why, and other health teaching as indicated. The goal of this education is to enable the family to modify behaviors and adhere to the regimen that has been mutually established.

One common problem with patient education is that the health professional delivers the information and the family listens. This one-way flow of material may not achieve the goal of the education. It is estimated that there is only a 50% compliance rate following patient education. Research has also shown that if family members are provided with written information that they can understand, they are more likely to comply with the regimen. The instructions are written in clear, simple language to accommodate those with about a fifth grade reading level.

To avoid sexist language, but to also retain a personal and casual writing tone, the use of masculine and feminine pronouns is alternated. Unless otherwise indicated, the educational materials apply to both genders.

Every effort has been made to base the instructions on currently available evidence-based practice. For example, the sections on cardiopulmonary resuscitation (CPR), choking, and suctioning reflect the latest research and guidelines. However, most of the content is based on traditional practice because research is not available to define standards of practice for all procedures. Many evidence-based practice guidelines are found in Unit 3. Information on using the dorsogluteal site for intramuscular injections is *not* included, because we believe strongly that unwarranted risks exist with this procedure. The choice has been made to provide instructions for the safest guidelines possible, but health professionals are encouraged to recognize the availability of safer alternatives. The health professional should be aware that new information made available after publication of this book may significantly change the content included in this unit. This is particularly relevant for the instructions on CPR and choking.

How to Use the Patient and Family Education Instructions

To maximize the benefits of patient teaching, these general guidelines should be followed:

1. Establish a rapport with the family.
2. Avoid using *any* specialized terms or jargon. Clarify all terms with the family.
3. When possible, allow family members to decide how they want to be taught (e.g., all at once or over a day or two). This gives the family a chance to incorporate the information at a rate that is comfortable.
4. Provide accurate information to the family about the illness.
5. Assist family members in identifying obstacles to their ability to comply with the regimen and in identifying the means to overcome those obstacles. Then help family members find ways to incorporate the plan into their daily lives.

The PFE materials represent commonly accepted guidelines for performing a procedure, but they may differ from those used in various settings. For this reason, review the instructions carefully and clarify any differences in protocol before giving them to the family. Complete any blanks, such as with names of medication or the frequency of dressing changes. To document discharge teaching, make two copies of the PFE handout, one for the family and one to attach to the patient record or plan of care.

If equipment will be needed at home (e.g., suction machines, syringes), begin making the necessary arrangements in advance so that discharge can proceed smoothly. Whenever possible, make arrangements for the family to use the same equipment in the home that they are using in the hospital. This allows them to become familiar with the items. In addition, the staff can help troubleshoot the equipment in a controlled environment. When the family is being taught at home, individualize the instructions, encourage the family to write notes, and include any adaptations that will be necessary for the family. Plan the teaching sessions well in advance of the time the family will be responsible for performing the care. The more complex the procedure, the more time is needed for training.

Review the instructions with family members. Encourage note taking if they desire. Allow ample practice time under supervision. At least one family member, but preferably two members, should demonstrate the procedure before they are expected to care for the child at home. Provide the family with the telephone numbers of resource individuals who are available to assist them in the event of a problem.

Instructions Related to Hygiene and Care

PATIENT AND FAMILY EDUCATION

Toilet Training Readiness

Signs That Your Child Is Ready to Learn

Physical Readiness

Voluntary control of anal and urethral sphincters, usually by ages 18 to 24 months*
Ability to stay dry for 2 hours; decreased number of wet diapers; waking dry from nap
Regular bowel movements
Gross motor skills of sitting, walking, and squatting
Fine motor skills to remove clothing

Mental Readiness

Recognizes urge to defecate or urinate
Verbal or nonverbal communicative skills to indicate when wet or has urge to defecate or urinate
Cognitive skills to imitate appropriate behavior and follow directions

Psychologic Readiness

Expresses willingness to please parent
Able to sit on toilet for 5 to 10 minutes without fussing or getting off
Curiosity about adults' or older sibling's toilet habits
Impatience with soiled or wet diapers; desire to be changed immediately

Parental Readiness

Recognizes child's level of readiness
Willing to invest the time required for toilet training
Absence of family stress or change, such as a divorce, moving, new sibling, or imminent vacation or travel

Choices

Freestanding potty chair
Allows feeling of security
Planting feet firmly on floor facilitates defecation.
Portable potty seat attached to toilet
May ease transition from potty chair to toilet
Placing a small bench under the feet helps to stabilize the position.
If potty chair or potty seat is not available, have the child sit *facing* the toilet tank for additional support.

Helpful Suggestions

Limit practice sessions to 5 to 10 minutes.
Dress child in clothing that can be easily removed. Avoid clothing with zippers, buttons, snaps, or belt.
Use training pants, panties, or pull-up diapers.
Encourage imitation by watching others. (For boys, imitating older brother or father is a powerful force.)
Use the same words each time to describe the action (e.g., pee-pee or poo-poo).
Avoid words such as "yucky" and "dirty" when referring to stool.
Give clear instructions to explain the steps for "going potty" by demonstration, by using a doll, or by using a potty-training video.
Remind children that when they feel the urge to eliminate, they have time to get to the toilet.
Frequent reminders and trips to the toilet will help avoid accidents.
A parent should stay with the child during the entire session.
Set a good example by washing hands after every session.
Let the child observe the excreta being flushed down the toilet, so he can associate these activities with usual practices.
Always praise the child for cooperative behavior and/or successful evacuation.

Remember

- Bowel training is usually learned before bladder training because of its greater predictability, but this varies among children.
- Daytime accidents are common, especially when the child is busy playing; if not reminded, young children will often wait until it is too late to reach the bathroom.
- Forcing children to sit on the toilet for long periods, verbally scolding them, or spanking them for having accidents should be avoided.

*Although readiness may be demonstrated at these ages, this does not mean the child will achieve toilet training at this time. Some children may not achieve toilet training until 36 to 40 months, depending on the circumstances and the child's development.

Community Resources for Parents

American Academy of Pediatrics, Wolraich ML: *Guide to toilet training,* 2004, Elk Grove Village, Ill, The Academy; (847) 434-4000; *http://www.aap.org.*

American Academy of Pediatrics, Bennett HJ: *Waking up dry,* 2005, Elk Grove Village, Ill, The Academy; (847) 434-4000; *http://www.aap.org.*

Community Resource for Professionals

Schmitt BD: Toilet training: getting it right the first time, *Contemp Pediatr* 21(3):105-122, 2004.

PATIENT AND FAMILY EDUCATION

Caring for Your Child's Teeth

Begin regular visits to the dentist soon after the first teeth erupt, usually around 1 year of age and no later than 15 months.*

Plan the first examination to be a "friendly visit"—meeting the dentist, seeing the room and equipment, and sitting in the chair.

Brushing and Flossing

Begin cleaning the teeth as soon as the first tooth erupts. This is done by wiping it with a cloth.

Begin regular brushing and flossing (twice daily) soon after several baby teeth have erupted. Make mouth care pleasant by talking or singing to child.

Use a small toothbrush with soft, rounded, multitufted nylon bristles that are short and even. Change the toothbrush *often,* as soon as the bristles are bent or frayed.

For young children, place the tips of the bristles firmly at a 45-degree angle against the teeth and gums and move them back and forth in a vibratory motion. Do not move the ends of the bristles forcefully back and forth because this can damage the gums and enamel.

For children whose permanent teeth have erupted, place the sides of the bristles firmly against the gums and brush the gums and teeth in the direction the teeth grow, using a rolling action.

Clean all surfaces of the teeth in this manner, except the inner surfaces of the front teeth. To clean these areas, place the toothbrush vertical to the teeth and move it up and down.

Brush only a few teeth at one time, using six to eight strokes for each section.

Use a battery-powered child-size brush if the child is not afraid of the vibrating motion.

Use a systematic approach so that all surfaces are thoroughly cleaned.

In brushing young children's teeth, use any of the following positions:

- Stand with the child's back toward you.
- Sit on a couch or bed with the child's head in your lap.
- Sit on a floor or stool with the child's head resting between your thighs.

Use one hand to cup the chin and the other hand to brush the teeth.

When child wants to begin brushing his own teeth, let him or her help by brushing before or after.

Floss the teeth after brushing. Wrap a piece of dental floss (about 18 inches long) around the middle finger and grasp it between the index finger and thumb of both hands. With about 1 inch of floss held firmly between the thumbs, insert the floss between two teeth and wrap it around the base of the tooth and below the gum in a C shape. Move the floss toward the top of the tooth in a sweeping motion. Repeat this a few times on every tooth, using a clean piece of floss. Children may find it easier to tie the floss in a circle, rather than wrapping it around the middle finger.

Check the thoroughness of the cleaning by having the child chew a special dental disclosing tablet (available commercially or from dentists) that stains any remaining plaque red. Rebrush any colored areas.

Form the habit of cleaning the teeth after each meal and especially before bedtime. Give the child nothing to eat or drink (except water) after the night brushing.

Use the swish and swallow method of cleaning the mouth at times when brushing is impractical. Have child rinse mouth with water and swallow, repeating this three or four times.

Fluoride

Use a fluoridated toothpaste, but supervise the amount used by the child. Use only a pea-sized amount on the brush, and teach child not to eat toothpaste.

Use a fluoridated mouthrinse if the child is older than 6 years and can safely rinse and spit out the rinse without swallowing. Use only the recommended amount; time the 1-minute rinse with a clock. Give the child nothing to eat or drink for 30 minutes afterward.

If the local water supply is fluoridated, make sure that the child is drinking the water—plain, in juices, in soups, or in other foods prepared with tap water.

If the local water supply is not fluoridated or if the infant after 6 months of age is exclusively breast-fed or given commercial ready-to-feed formula, make sure fluoride supplements are prescribed by a health professional.

When supplemental fluoride is prescribed:

- Give supplements when child has an empty stomach.
- Place the drops directly on the tongue to allow them to mix with saliva and come in contact with the teeth.
- Encourage older children to chew the tablet and swish it around the teeth for 30 seconds before swallowing.
- Give the child nothing to eat or drink for 30 minutes afterward.
- Store fluoride supplements and fluoridated toothpaste and mouthrinse in a safe place away from small children.

*The American Academy of Pediatric Dentistry recommends an oral risk health assessment by the primary health care provider by the age of 6 months; the infant's dental home should be established by 12 months of age. (American Academy of Pediatric Dentistry: *Reference manual 2005-2006: clinical guidelines: guideline on infant oral health care,* Chicago, 2006, The Academy, available online at *http://www.aapd.org.*)

Continued

PATIENT AND FAMILY EDUCATION

Caring for Your Child's Teeth—cont'd

Diet

Keep sweet foods to a minimum, especially sticky or chewy candy and dried fruits (raisins, fruit rolls), chewing gum, and hard candy (lollipops, Life Savers). Read labels on packaged foods (e.g., dry cereals) for hidden sources of sugar, including honey, molasses, and corn syrup.

Remember: *It is how often children eat sweets, rather than the amount of sweets eaten at one time,* that is most important. Plan sweets to follow a meal when the child is likely to brush immediately afterward. Discourage frequent snacking with sweets.

Encourage snacks that are less likely to cause cavities (caries), such as cheese, fresh fruit, raw vegetables, crackers, pretzels, popcorn, peanuts, and artificially sweetened candy, gum, and soda. When choosing snacks for young children, avoid those foods (e.g., grapes, popcorn, nuts) that can cause choking.

If the child takes a bottle to bed, fill it only with water, *never* formula, breast milk, cow's milk, or juice. Avoid frequent or prolonged breast-feeding during sleep times.

Have child drink fruit juice from a cup at meal time or snack time only; avoid child carrying around a cup of juice all day to 'graze' on because this promotes bacterial growth.

Avoid carbonated drinks in the first 30 months of life.

If the child routinely takes any medicine in sweetened liquid or chewable tablet form, clean the teeth immediately afterward or at least have the child drink water to rinse the mouth.

PATIENT AND FAMILY EDUCATION

Measuring Your Child's Temperature

Body temperature changes during the day; it is usually higher in the afternoon than in the early morning. If you are very active, your temperature may be higher than normal. Fever helps protect the body. A rise in body temperature above normal (usually 98.6° F) may mean an infection somewhere. The body temperature may also rise when the child has not consumed enough liquid. Fever helps the body fight the infection. Someone has a fever if the body temperature is higher than 100° F (oral or axillary temperature) or 100.4° F (rectal temperature). If you use the Celsius (°C) system, the conversions from Fahrenheit (°F) are shown in Table 5-1.

You should measure a child's temperature:

1. When the skin feels warm to your touch
2. When the child is not acting like his usual self
3. Before calling your health professional to say that the child is sick

Types of Thermometers

There are many ways to measure your child's temperature. When you buy a thermometer, you should choose one that is easy to use. Because some are more accurate than others, tell your health professional how you measured your child's temperature. Glass mercury thermometers are no longer recommended to take a child's temperature.

Digital Thermometers

Digital thermometers are used just like glass mercury thermometers, but they are safer and much easier to read. They have a button battery-powered heat sensor that measures temperature in less than 1 minute. The temperature is displayed in numbers on a small screen (Figure 1). Digital thermometers are also available within a pacifier. As your child sucks on the pacifier, the temperature is shown on a screen. Read the manufacturer's directions for the length of time to keep the pacifier in the mouth.

Ear Thermometers

Ear thermometers use a probe that is placed in the opening of the ear to measure the temperature of the eardrum (Figure 2). Although this device is expensive, it is easy to use, rapidly measures temperature (in about 1 second), it causes no discomfort to your child, and its use does not require your child's cooperation. However, an ear thermometer must be used correctly for accurate results. The current models are not considered to be accurate for detecting fever in infants and toddlers. Read the manufacturer's instructions for how to place the probe in the ear canal and how to tug the earlobe. Tugging the earlobe straightens the ear canal so the

TABLE 5-1 Conversion of Degrees Fahrenheit (F) to Degrees Celsius (C)

°F	°C	°F	°C	°F	°C
96.8	36.0	100.4	38.0	104.0	40.0
97.7	36.5	101.3	38.5	104.9	40.5
98.6	37.0	102.2	39.0	105.8	41.1
99.5	37.5	103.1	39.5	107.6	42.0

PATIENT AND FAMILY EDUCATION

Measuring Your Child's Temperature—cont'd

probe can measure the temperature of the eardrum. As a general rule, for children younger than 3 years, pull the bottom of the earlobe down and back. For children older than 3 years, pull the top of the earlobe up and back.

Chemical Dot Thermometers

Several types of thermometers have a series of dots that change color as the body temperature goes up or down. Each dot has a specific degree of temperature marked under it; the dot that gets brighter is your child's temperature. Plastic strip thermometers are placed on the child's skin (usually the forehead) and can be kept there to measure temperature continuously without disturbing your child. Another type, Tempa-Dot, is a plastic strip with dots at one end; this end is placed in the child's mouth or under the arm to measure temperature. Read the directions for the length of time to keep the thermometer in the mouth or armpit.

Temporal Artery Thermometers

The temporal artery thermometer measures the heat transmitted from the temporal artery (forehead artery) to a sensitive infrared sensor; the reading is transformed into a body temperature reading by a computer microprocessor, and the thermometer displays the temperature in digital numbers. The temporal artery thermometer is rapid and noninvasive, which makes it ideal for children. However, a number of controlled studies indicate that the temporal artery thermometer is suited for screening children for a fever but not for the actual medical treatment of a fever.

How to Measure Axillary Temperature

Measuring temperature in the axilla (armpit) is the safest way to check if your child has a fever.

1. Tell the child that you are going to measure his temperature.
2. Wash your hands.
3. Look at the thermometer to make sure it is reading below 96° F.
4. Place the thermometer under the child's arm. The thermometer's tip should rest in the center of your child's armpit (Figure 3).
5. Hold the child's arm firmly against his body.
6. Look at the time.
7. The thermometer must remain in place until the alarm or beep sounds. Make sure you hold the thermometer securely.
8. Remove the thermometer and read.
9. PRAISE THE CHILD FOR HELPING.
10. Write down the thermometer reading and the time of day.
11. Clean the thermometer with cool water and soap.

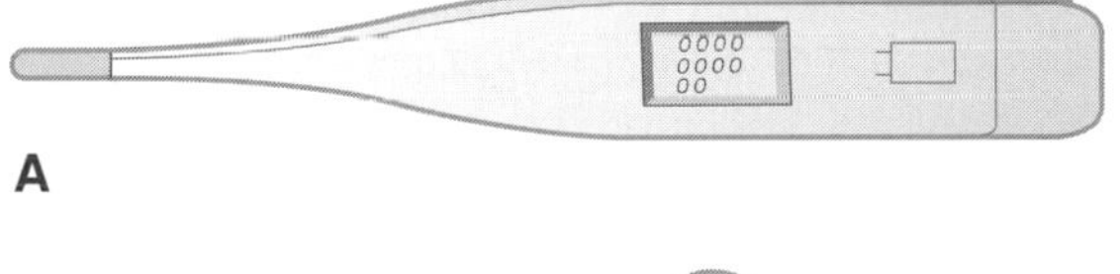

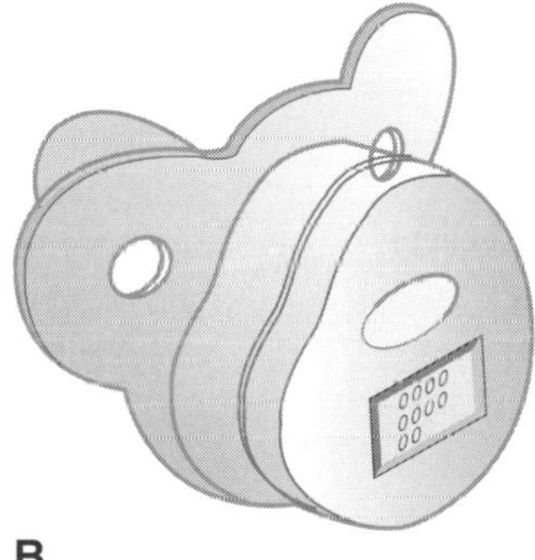

FIGURE 1 Oral digital thermometers. **A,** Oral thermometer. **B,** Digital pacifier thermometer.

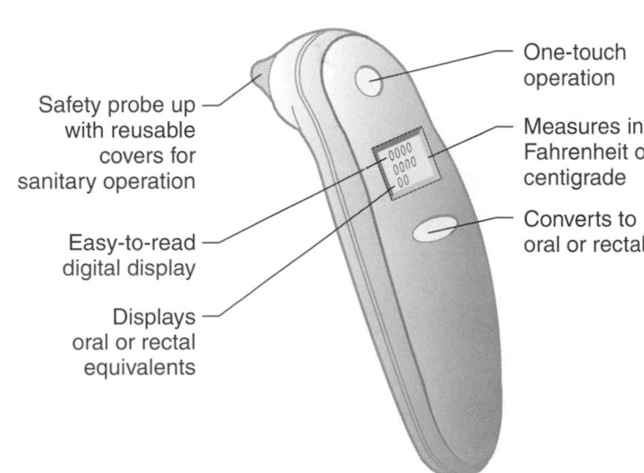

FIGURE 2 Digital ear thermometer.

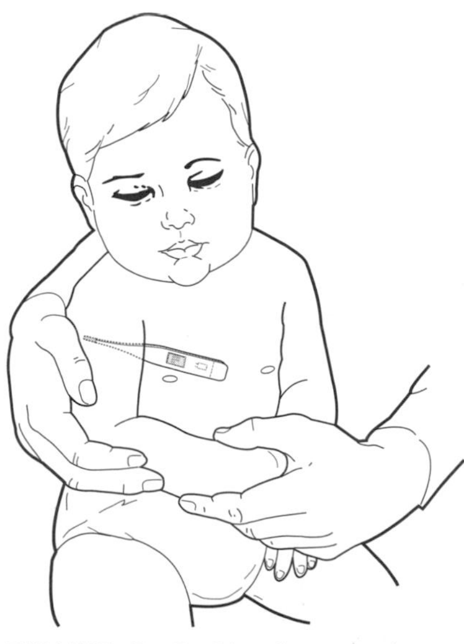

FIGURE 3 Position for measuring axillary temperature.

Continued

5 - PATIENT AND FAMILY EDUCATION

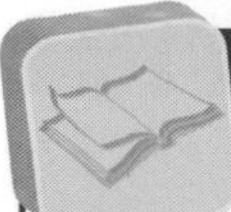

PATIENT AND FAMILY EDUCATION

Measuring Your Child's Temperature—cont'd

How to Measure Oral Temperatures

By 5 or 6 years of age, a child can understand how to safely hold the thermometer in his mouth. If the child has had something to eat or drink, wait 15 minutes before you measure an oral temperature.

1. Tell the child why you want to measure his temperature.
2. Wash your hands.
3. Place the thermometer in the mouth, far back under the tongue (Figure 4). Tell the child to keep the mouth closed, breathe though the nose, and not talk.
4. Make sure the child does not bite the thermometer.
5. Look at the time.
6. Tell the child that the thermometer must stay in place until the alarm or beep sounds.
7. Remove the thermometer and read it.
8. PRAISE THE CHILD FOR HELPING.
9. Write down the thermometer reading and the time of day.
10. Clean the thermometer with cool water and soap.

How to Measure Rectal Temperatures

Rectal temperature measurement is sometimes recommended but is uncomfortable for the child and other methods are considered just as effective. Consult your health professional before taking rectal temperatures on a routine basis. Note that rectal temperatures should not be taken if the child has diarrhea, has had recent rectal surgery, has a rectal defect, or is undergoing cancer chemotherapy. In infants special care must be taken to prevent inserting the thermometer too deeply and puncturing the lower bowel. In taking a child's temperature, use the following procedure:

1. Tell the child that you are going to measure his temperature.
2. Wash your hands.
3. Measure 1 inch on the thermometer or of the thermometer's length.
4. Place the child on his stomach (Figure 5), on one side with the upper leg bent, or on his back with both legs up.
5. Dip the thermometer's tip in a water-soluble lubricant such as K-Y Jelly.
6. Place the end of the thermometer into the child's anus. Do not insert the thermometer any farther than 1 inch (2.5 cm) for a child or 0.6 inch (1.5 cm) for an infant younger than 12 months of age.
7. Hold the thermometer in place until it beeps. Always hold the child so that he cannot twist around.
8. Remove the thermometer and read.
9. PRAISE THE CHILD FOR HELPING.
10. Clean the thermometer with cool water and soap.
11. Wash your hands with soap and water. Count to 10 while washing, then rinse with clear water and dry with a clean paper or cloth towel.
12. Write down the thermometer reading and the time of day.

How to Measure Temporal Artery Temperatures

A temporal artery temperature may be used to screen children for fever if they are older than 3 months of age.

1. Tell the child that you are going to measure his temperature.
2. Wash your hands.
3. Locate the "Scan" button on the temporal artery thermometer.
4. Remove any sweat or hair from child's forehead. Avoid use over an abrasion or wound.
5. Remove the sensor probe cover.
6. With a paintbrush stroke, swipe the thermometer gently across the child's forehead from one side to another while depressing the "Scan" button. The thermometer must come in contact with the child's skin for an accurate reading.

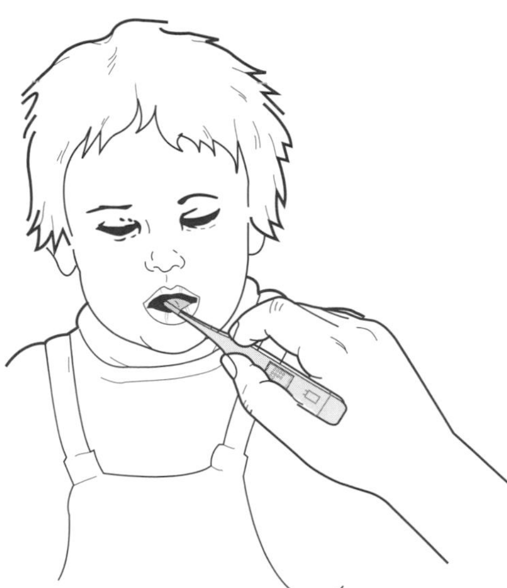

FIGURE 4 Placement of thermometer under tongue, toward back of mouth.

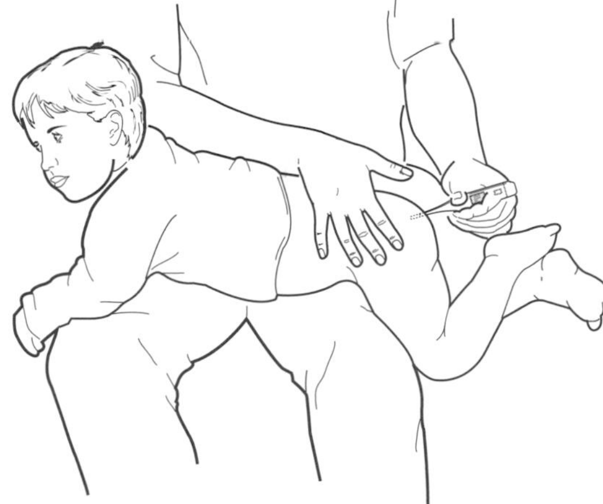

FIGURE 5 Position for measuring rectal temperature. The thermometer is inserted no more than 1 inch into the rectum on a child, and no more than 0.6 inch for an infant younger than 12 months old.

PATIENT AND FAMILY EDUCATION

Measuring Your Child's Temperature—cont'd

7. The digital readout will give a temperature reading.
8. Praise the child for helping.
9. Clean the thermometer scanner with soap and water and a clean cloth or paper towel. Do not submerge in water.

When a Fever Is Present

Call your health professional at _______ *as soon as possible* if (1) the child has a temperature higher than 105° F or (2) a fever (oral or axillary temperature above 100° F or 100.4° F rectally) is present and the child:

- Is less than 2 months of age
- Has a stiff neck, severe headache, stomach pain, persistent vomiting, purplish spots on the skin, or earache along with the temperature
- Has a serious illness in addition to the fever
- Is confused or delirious
- Has trouble breathing after you have cleaned his nose
- Is hard to awaken
- Seems sicker than you would expect
- Cannot be comforted
- Has a temperature that continues to rise after medicine has been given

Call your health professional *during office hours* if:

- The temperature is between 104° F and 105° F, especially if the child is less than 2 years old
- The child has burning or pain with urination
- The fever has been present for more than 72 hours
- The fever has been present for more than 24 hours without a known cause
- The fever went away for more than 24 hours, then returned
- The child has a history of febrile seizures
- You have some questions

The most important thing to remember is not to bundle up the child with extra clothes and blankets, unless the child is shivering. Dress him in light clothing. This will help cool the child by letting air circulate and heat leave the body.

Do not bathe or give the child a sponge bath in cool water. If the temperature is lowered too quickly, the child may shiver, causing the temperature to go up. If shivering occurs, keep the child warm until it stops.

The presence of a fever increases the amount of liquid that is needed by the body. It is important to encourage the sick child to drink fluids. Some things that may help encourage drinking are using straws and small cups instead of a big glass; and giving Popsicles, Jello, and soft drinks with the fizz removed (flat). The carbonation can be removed by leaving the soft drink uncovered, by warming the soda in a microwave or on a stove, or by stirring in ¼ teaspoon sugar.

Medicines should not be used routinely to lower the temperature. If the child is uncomfortable, and the fever needs to be treated with more than light clothes and increased fluids, then drugs can be used. Do not avoid giving fever-reducing medicine before taking the child to the health professional if the child is uncomfortable, has a fever above 100.4° F, and the time period since the last dose given is that recommended on the medicine label.

Be sure to give the right amount (dose) and type of medicine. Use the child's weight as a guide to the right dose. If using infant drops, do not replace with the syrup (elixir) because the amount of medicine in these bottles is different.

See the following tables for recommended dosages of acetaminophen and ibuprofen.

Recommended Dosages of Acetaminophen for Children by Age and Weight*

	Age								
	3 mo	**4-11 mo**	**12-23 mo**	**2-3 yr**	**4-5 yr**	**6-8 yr**	**9-10 yr**	**11 yr**	**12 yr and over**
Weight (lb)	6-11	12-17	18-23	24-35	36-47	48-59	60-71	72-95	96 and over
Dose (mg)	40	80	120	160	240	320	400	480	650
Type of Medicine									
Liquids									
Drops (1 dropper = 80 mg/0.8 ml)	½	1	1-1½	2	—	—	—	—	—
Elixir/suspension 160 mg/5 ml (1 tsp)		½ tsp	¾ tsp	1 tsp	1½ tsp	2 tsp	2½ tsp	3 tsp	
Tablets									
Chewable tablets (80 mg/tablet)	—	—	—	2	3	4	—	—	—
Swallowable or chewable caplets/tablets (160 mg/tablet)	—	—	—	1	1½	2	2½	3	4
Capsules (80 mg)	—	—	—	2	3	4	—	—	—
Capsules (160 mg)	—	—	—	1	—	2	—	3	4
Suppository									
Infant strength (80 mg)	½†	1	—	—	—	—	—	—	—
Child strength (120 mg)	—	½†	1	1	2	—	—	—	—
Junior strength (325 mg)	—	—	—	—	—	1	1	1½†	2

Some Acetaminophen Brand Names

Drops	Tablets	Suppository
Panadol	Chewable Anacin 3	Fever-all
Tylenol	Chewable Tylenol	
Tempra	St. Joseph Aspirin-Free Chewable	
Liquiprin	Junior Strength Tylenol	
	Paracetamol	

*Recommendation: Do not exceed five doses in 24 hours.
†Cut suppository in half.

Caution: Acetaminophen may be found in other medications being taken by the child. Some cold and flu remedies contain acetaminophen. Check with your health professional or pharmacist to make sure the child is not receiving too much of this medication.

Another suggestion to prevent accidental overdosing of this medication is to use a medication record such as the one found on p. 522. Place the paper on the refrigerator door for other family members to see so they will then know not to give additional medication until the right time.

In the event of an accidental administration of an extra dose contact the National Poison Control Center immediately at (800) 222-1222.

Recommended Dosages of Ibuprofen for Children by Age and Weight*

	Age							
	6-11 mo	12-23 mo	2-3 yr	4-5 yr	6-8 yr	9-10 yr	11 yr	12 yr and over
Weight (lb)	12-17	18-23	24-35	36-47	48-59	60-71	72-95	96 and over
Dose (mg)	50	75	100	150	200	250	300	400
Type of Medicine								
Drops (50 mg per dropper)	1 dropper (1.25 ml)	1½ dropper (1.875 ml)	—	—	—	—	—	—
Suspension 100 mg/5 ml (1 tsp)	¼ tsp	½ tsp	1 tsp	1½	2	2½	3	4
Chewable 50-mg tablets	—	—	2	3	4	5	6	8
Swallowable or chewable 100-mg caplets or tablets	—	—	—	1½	2	2½	3	4
Swallowable 200-mg gelcaps or tablets	—	—	—	—	1	1½	1½	2

SOME IBUPROFEN BRAND NAMES

Children's Motrin
Children's Advil

*Recommendation: Administer every 6 to 8 hours.

PATIENT AND FAMILY EDUCATION

Obtaining a Urine Sample

Children who are 8 years of age and older may be able to obtain the sample by themselves. Tell the child how to clean herself and how to obtain the sample. Help the child if needed. Children under 8 years of age will need your help. Young children may not be able to urinate on request. Use the child's words and usual place for urinating to obtain the sample if possible. To help the child urinate, have her blow through a straw or listen to running water while you hold the specimen cup. Do not give the child more than one glass of liquid to drink. Large amounts of liquid can affect the result of the urine test. If you think the child does not understand, have her practice one time, then collect the specimen the next time.

Instructions for the Toilet-Trained Child

Equipment

Urine specimen cup
Potty chair, potty hat, or toilet
Soap and water
Washcloth or paper wipes

Routine Urine Sample (Boys and Girls)

1. Tell the child that you need to get some urine. Use the child's word for urine.
2. If the child is able to obtain the sample of urine, have the child wash her hands.
3. Wash your hands.
4. Gather the equipment needed.
5. Open the urine container, being careful not to touch the inside of the cup or lid.
6. Have the child urinate directly into the cup (or potty hat if more convenient for female).
7. Replace the lid on the cup.
8. Label the cup with the child's first and last name.
9. PRAISE THE CHILD FOR HELPING.
10. Wash your hands with soap and water. Count to 10 while washing, then rinse with clear water and dry with a clean paper or cloth towel.
11. Have the child wash her hands (if she helped).

Urine Sample for Culture (Boys)

If you are told that a clean-catch specimen is needed, follow steps 1 through 5 for routine urine sample, then do the following:

6. If paper wipes are provided, use these instead of a washcloth; rinsing is not necessary with the wipes.
7. Wash the tip of the penis with a wipe or soap and water. Rinse well if soap is used. If the child is uncircumcised, pull back the foreskin only as far as it will easily go, then wash and rinse the tip of the penis with a clean part of the washcloth. Make sure the foreskin is pushed back toward the tip after cleaning.
8. Have the child begin to urinate in the potty chair or toilet.
9. Tell him to stop.
10. Have the child begin to urinate into the cup. If he cannot stop the flow of urine, place the urine cup so that you can catch some of the urine.
11. Replace the lid on the cup.
12. Label the cup with the child's first and last name.
13. PRAISE THE CHILD FOR HELPING.
14. Wash your hands with soap and water. Count to 10 while washing, then rinse with clear water and dry with a clean paper or cloth towel.

Urine Sample for Culture (Girls)

If you are told that a clean-catch specimen is needed, follow steps 1 through 5 for routine urine sample, then do the following:

6. If paper wipes are provided, use them instead of a washcloth; rinsing is not necessary with the wipes.
7. Spread the child's labia (lips) (Figure 1) with your fingers. Wash the area with a paper wipe or soap and water; rinse well if soap is used. Wash from front to back (top to bottom), rinsing well with a clean part of the washcloth.
8. Have the child begin to urinate into the potty chair, potty hat, or toilet.
9. Tell her to stop.
10. Hold the cup in place, and tell her to start to urinate into the cup. If she cannot stop the flow of urine, place the cup so that you can catch some of the urine.
11. Replace the lid on the cup.
12. Label the cup with the child's first and last name.
13. PRAISE THE CHILD FOR HELPING.
14. Wash your hands with soap and water. Count to 10 while washing, then rinse with clear water and dry with a clean paper or cloth towel.

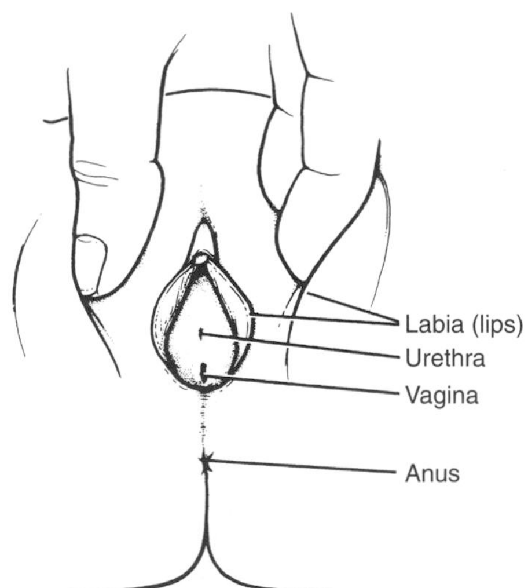

FIGURE 1 Finger position to spread labia for cleaning before obtaining a urine sample for culture.

Spanish translation of this handout available at *http://evolve.elsevier.com/Wong/clinical.*

PATIENT AND FAMILY EDUCATION

Obtaining a Urine Sample—cont'd

Instructions for the Child Who Is Not Toilet Trained

Equipment

Urine specimen cup
Urine collection bag
Soap and water
Washcloths or paper wipes
Clean diaper

Instructions

If the child is very active, you will need help to put on the urine bag.

1. Wash your hands with soap and water. Count to 10 while washing, then rinse with clear water and dry with a clean paper or cloth towel. Your helper should also wash his hands.
2. Tell the child what you are going to do.
3. Gather the needed equipment.
4. Place the child on her back.
5. Remove the child's diaper.
6. If the urine sample is for culture, clean the child's genital area with soap and water as described on the previous page.
7. Rinse thoroughly and pat dry.
8. Have your helper hold the child's legs apart while you apply the bag.
9. Hold the urine collector with the bag portion downward.
10. Remove the bottom half of the adhesive protector.

For Girls

1. Spread the labia and buttocks, keeping the skin tight.
2. Begin with the bottom of the adhesive. Place the sticky portion of the bag as flat as possible against the skin (Figure 2).
3. Smooth the plastic to avoid any wrinkles.
4. Remove the top half of the adhesive protector, and smooth it also on the labia.

For Boys

1. Place the boy's penis and scrotum into the bag if possible. If only the penis fits in the bag, put the sticky part of the bag on the scrotum (Figure 3).
2. Smooth the sticky portion of the bag on the skin, taking care to avoid making any wrinkles.
3. Remove the top half of the adhesive protector and smooth the top part on the skin to remove any wrinkles.

Check the bag often and remove it as soon as the child urinates.

To remove the bag, hold it against the child's skin at the bottom and carefully peel it off by pulling the sticky part parallel to the skin. Cut a corner of the bag to pour the urine into the urine cup or give to health professional as available.

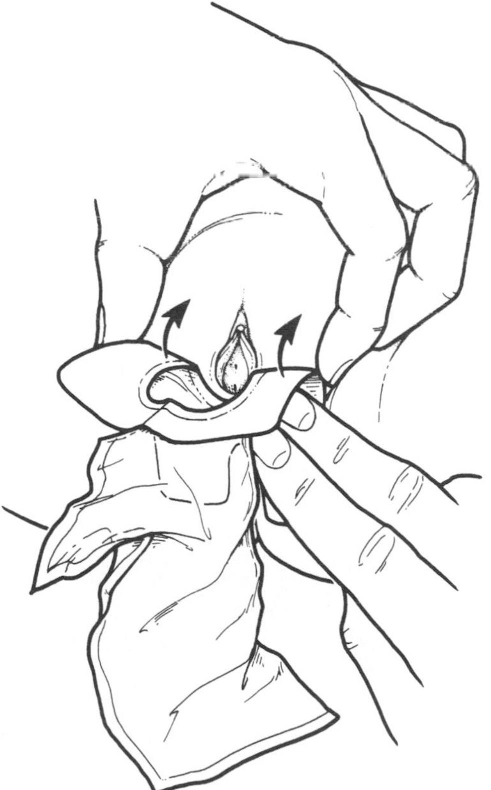

FIGURE **2** Putting the urine bag on a girl, starting from back and proceeding to front.

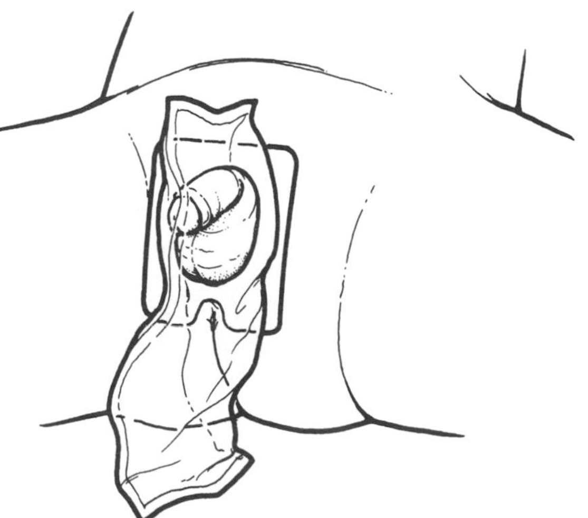

FIGURE **3** Putting the urine bag on a boy, with the penis and scrotum inside the bag.

PATIENT AND FAMILY EDUCATION

Obtaining a Stool Sample

Children who are 8 years of age and older may be able to obtain the sample by themselves. Tell the child how to clean herself and how to obtain the sample. Young children may not be able to defecate on request. Use the child's words and usual place for defecating to obtain the sample, if possible. Have the child tell the parent when they think they are going to have a bowel movement. To help the child defecate have child bear down or hold their breath to facilitate evacuation of the stool. If the child is not potty trained the child's stool can be collected from the diaper.

Equipment

Specimen container
Potty chair or toilet
Clean potty hat
Soap and water
Disposable nonsterile gloves
Washcloth or paper wipes

General Instructions

1. Explain to the child that a stool sample is needed.
2. Instruct the child to let the parent know when she feels the urge to defecate.
3. Have child urinate first if possible. If child is bedridden, empty bedpan or potty chair of urine.
4. After urination, place the clean potty hat in reverse position in the toilet.
5. Retrieve stool from container with a specimen stick (or tongue blade) and place in specimen container.
6. Replace lid on specimen container.
7. Label the container with child's first and last name as well as the date and time.
8. Praise the child for helping.
9. Wash your hands with soap and water. Count to 10 while washing, then rinse with clear water and dry with a clean paper towel
10. Have child wash her hands with soap and water.
11. Store the specimen as indicated by laboratory or by health professional.
12. Children not toilet trained will pass the stool into the diaper.
13. To collect a sample from the diaper, remove the diaper from the child and open.
14. Collect a sample of the stool with a gloved hand, a sample scoop (plastic), or a tongue blade. If the stool is liquid, collect as many small pieces of fecal matter as possible and place into the specimen cup.
15. If liquid stool soaks into diaper, line the inside of a clean diaper with plastic wrap. Place the clean diaper on the child and collect the next stool sample from the plastic liner as directed in step 14.
16. Wash hands with soap and water. Wash child's hands with soap and water. Wash child's diaper area with warm water and soap after each stool to prevent skin irritation.
17. Label the container with child's first and last name as well as the date and time.
18. Store stool sample as directed by health professional.

Cast Care

K—Keep cast exposed to air dry. Do not use a warm blow dryer. Avoid exposure in shower or bath by wrapping fiberglass cast. Plaster cast should not be exposed to water.

E—Elevate casted extremity for 24 hours after application. After that when child is sitting down or resting elevate extremity to avoid swelling.

E—Evaluate condition of toes, fingers or other limb that is distal to the cast. Evaluate for swelling, color, feeling or sensation, movement, and sudden pain not relieved by prescribed analgesic. Notify health professional if any of these occurs.

P—Plaster cast should be handled with palms of hand until completely dry.

D—Do not place any objects such as knitting needles or clothes hangars inside cast.

R—Recreation. Encourage child to limit strenuous activities for the first few days.

Y—Y is for itching. When itching occurs, apply ice pack or cool compress for 15 minutes. May also administer a mild antihistamine to minimize itching. Contact health professional for prolonged itching and discomfort.

PATIENT AND FAMILY EDUCATION

Caring for the Child in a Cast

Casts are made from many different types of material and used on different parts of the body. A cast was put on your child so that the injured area could heal well. The care of the cast will vary slightly, depending on the type of cast that was put on.

Before the cast is applied, a synthetic padding material is used to protect the skin. The cast is then put on over this padding. At first, the cast will feel warm; this will last for about 10 to 15 minutes. A plaster cast will remain damp for many hours, whereas a fiberglass cast will dry within 30 minutes. Do not put anything in the cast while it is drying or afterward. During the drying time, touch the cast as little as possible. If you have to touch the plaster cast, use the palms of your hands, not the fingers (Figure 1). Turning the child in a plaster body cast at least every 2 hours will help the cast dry. Do not use a heated fan or dryer. A regular fan can be used in humid weather to circulate the air.

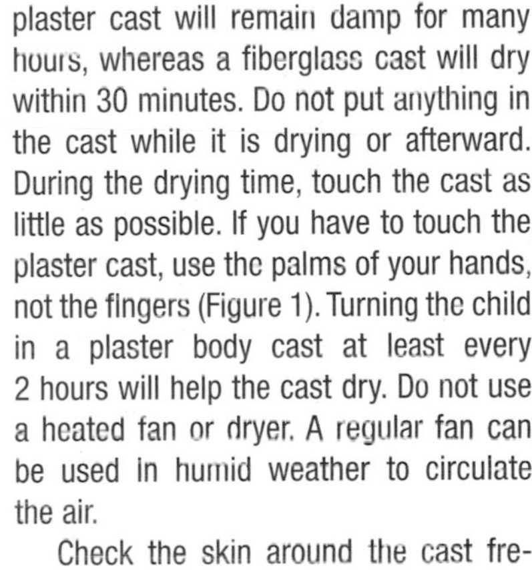

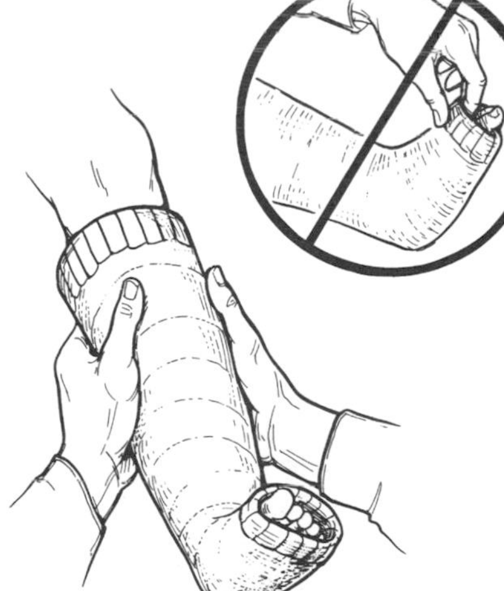

FIGURE **1** When the cast is drying, lift it with the palms of the hands, not the fingers *(inset)*, to avoid making dents in the cast.

Check the skin around the cast frequently. Notify your health professional at ___________ if any of these occur:

- Numbness
- Tingling
- Unrelieved pain
- Burning
- Odor
- Strange feelings
- Temperature change
- Fluid coming through cast
- Cast becomes soft, broken, or cracked
- Toes cannot be seen at edge of cast (for a foot cast)

If it is a leg or arm cast, check the color of the toes or fingers. They should be pink and warm to the touch. When the skin in these areas is lightly pressed and released, the skin color should return quickly. To help prevent swelling, raise the arm or leg in the cast above the level of the child's heart (Figure 2) by resting the cast on several pillows or blankets. If an arm is in a cast, a sling helps support the arm during the day and pillows can be used at night. For leg casts, loosen the covers on the bed at nighttime and place some pillows by the feet to keep the blanket from putting pressure on the toes.

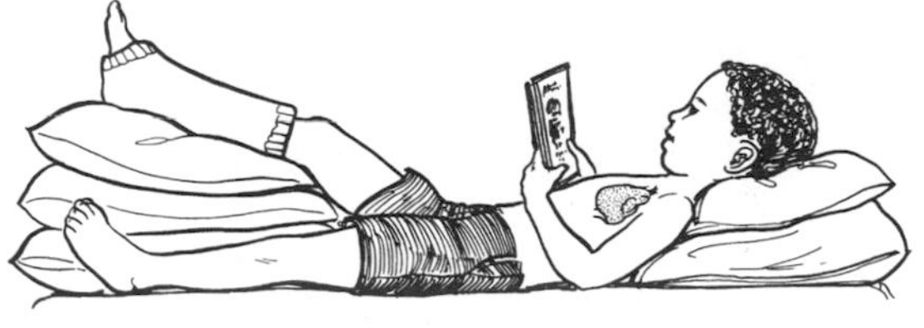

FIGURE **2** Position cast above level of heart to prevent swelling.

Continued

PATIENT AND FAMILY EDUCATION

Caring for the Child in a Cast—cont'd

Some leg casts are made so that the child can walk with the cast. If this type of cast (i.e., weight-bearing) cannot be used, the older child can be taught how to walk with crutches. When crutches are needed, follow your health professional's guidelines for the correct size and padding of the crutches.

The cast will be on for about 4 weeks. During this time, the child should exercise the joints and muscles that are not in the cast. Games such as "Simon says" can make movement fun. Your health professional can suggest some exercises for your child.

Skin Care

During the time the cast is on, special care is needed to keep the skin around the cast healthy. The back of the leg may be irritated when the child is in a short leg cast, and the skin between the thumb and the index finger is often a problem with an arm cast. If the cast rubs against the skin, tape can be used to cover the rough edges of a cast. This is called *petaling* and involves these steps (Figure 3):

1. Use adhesive bandages for strips or cut several 3-inch strips of 1- to 2-inch wide adhesive or duct tape.
2. Tape one end of the strip to the inside of the cast.
3. Tape the other end to the outside of the cast, covering the cast edge.
4. Repeat with the other strips of tape. Overlap the edges to make a smooth surface.

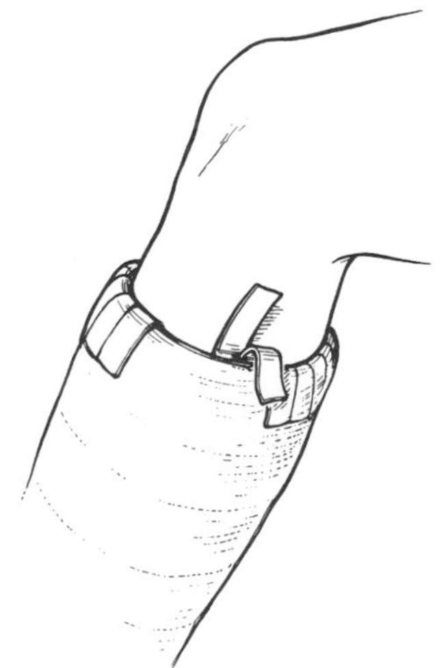

FIGURE 3 "Petaling" the cast to cover rough edges.

Itching

Sometimes the skin under the cast will feel itchy. Do not put anything inside the cast to scratch the skin. Children are often tempted to put forks, knives, food crumbs, combs, and other objects in the cast. Notify your health professional if any object is stuck in the cast. If the skin itches, some things that may make the child more comfortable include the following:

1. Blow *cool* air from a hair dryer into the cast.
2. Rub the opposite arm or leg.
3. Rub the skin around the cast edges.
4. Ask the health professional about a mild antihistamine to help relieve itching.

Baths

Children in body casts and full leg casts should receive sponge baths. A child with a lower leg or arm cast may be bathed or may take a shower if the cast is well covered or kept out of the water. The cast must remain dry. It can be wrapped with a plastic covering or a waterproof cast cover. The plastic cover should be removed and stored safely after the bath or shower. If a plaster cast becomes wet, it will soften and may need to be replaced. When a fiberglass cast becomes wet, it should be thoroughly dried with a fan or hair dryer on the cool setting. If a cast liner is used, the child may get the cast wet. Your health professional will tell you if you need to keep the cast dry.

Cast Care

The surface of fiberglass casts can be easily wiped clean with a damp cloth. However, plaster casts cannot be cleaned. If the cast will be on for a long time, cloth coverings such as a large, stretchy sock or part of an opaque stocking (tights) can be used to protect the cast. These coverings can then be washed and replaced. If a cover is used, it must be fabric and not plastic so that air can circulate through the cast.

Spica Casts (Body Cast)

Body casts are designed to keep the child's hips and thighs from moving. Special care must be taken because the cast covers the child's abdomen (stomach area) and the child is usually unable to move about. A window may be cut in the cast to allow the stomach to expand after meals. The genital area will be left open to allow the child to urinate and have bowel movements without soiling the cast. In the event that a one-way moisture barrier is not applied against the skin when the cast is first placed, certain measures may be taken to prevent skin irritation or breakdown. To protect the cast, duct tape or plastic wrap may be taped to the cast around this opening. This allows urine and stool to be easily wiped off. The other edges of the cast can be petaled to keep rough edges from harming the child's skin. Cotton padding, available from beauty supply stores, can also be used as disposable cushioning inside the edges of the cast. A disposable diaper may also be used to cushion the cast edges and prevent soiling. For the child who is not toilet trained, frequent diaper changes are necessary to prevent skin breakdown.

The child should be lifted with support under the shoulders and hips. Two people may be needed to safely lift the older infant and child (Figure 4). When lifting, avoid twisting the child's body. Never use the bar that keeps the legs separated to lift the child. Placing pressure on this bar can damage the cast. A new cast must be put on if the cast is badly damaged.

Because the child cannot move much, dietary changes may be needed. Three problems that may occur with a body cast include constipation, too much weight gain, and choking. The older infant and child should be given extra liquids and a diet high in fiber, such as fresh fruits, vegetables, beans, and whole grains such as oatmeal and whole wheat bread. If dietary changes do not help, a mild stool softener may be used.

To prevent too much weight gain, avoid sugared drinks such as flavored juices, carbonated soda beverages, and candy because they add empty calories and may

PATIENT AND FAMILY EDUCATION

Caring for the Child in a Cast—cont'd

keep the child from eating foods needed for healing and growth.

Choking is also a concern. Do not feed the child grapes, whole or round pieces of hot dogs, or nuts. These can cause the child to choke. Tell the child to chew carefully.

While in a body cast, the young child cannot move around. You must be responsible for positioning the child and meeting all other needs. Change the child's position frequently. A bean bag chair can be used to place the child upright or to turn the child from side to side. It can also be used to help the child lie on the abdomen with arms over the side to play with toys on the floor.

If the child was able to crawl or walk before being put in a cast, a car mechanic's dolly (a flatbed wagon on wheels) or skateboard can be used to help the child move around. Make sure there are no stairs or loose rugs that can cause injury.

Infants

Feeding the infant in a body cast requires some planning. You can support the child with your arm under the neck and head. Place the infant's hips and legs on a pillow at your side. This position can also be used for bottle- or breast-feeding. You can also hold the child's head and shoulders in front of you with the legs behind your back. If the child is able to sit, a chair or table can be padded to help the child eat and play in a semisitting position.

For infants who are heavy wetters or for nighttime, an extra-absorbent disposable diaper can be used for extra absorbency.

Children in body casts must be safely restrained while riding in cars. Some federally approved car seats can be modified, and a specially designed car restraint is available for purchase. Contact your local SafeKids Coalition chapter or the NHTSA* for more information regarding transporting a child with a body cast.

Older Children

Allow the child to help set the daily schedule. Within reason, the child can decide when meals, activities, schoolwork, and visits from friends take place. Because most clothing will not fit over the cast, some changes must be made. Loose-fitting shorts can be slit on the side seams and self-adhering or other simple fasteners attached so that these can be easily placed on the child.

It is often too difficult for the child to use the standard bathroom commode. A bedpan or urinal should be available for the child to use.

When traveling in a car, the child should lie on the back seat; a special vest should be used with the car seat belts to restrain the child. (The E-Z On vest is available from E-Z On Products, 605 Commerce Way West, Jupiter, FL 33458; [561] 747-6920 or [800] 323-6598 [outside Florida].)

Cast Removal

When the condition has healed, the cast will be removed. A cast is removed by rapid vibrations of the cast cutter. Although the machine makes a loud noise that can be scary, there is little chance that the child can be hurt by it. However, prepare the child for the cast removal. If possible, show the child how the cutter vibrates and give him a chance to get used to the noise. Tell the child there may be a tickling feeling when the cutter is used. Use distraction techniques during the procedure to decrease the child's anxiety.

The skin will appear dry, pale, and scaly when the cast is removed. To soften and remove the dry, dead skin, soak the skin in warm water and use a skin moisturizing lotion. Never scrub the skin to remove the scales. As the old skin comes off, new skin will grow.

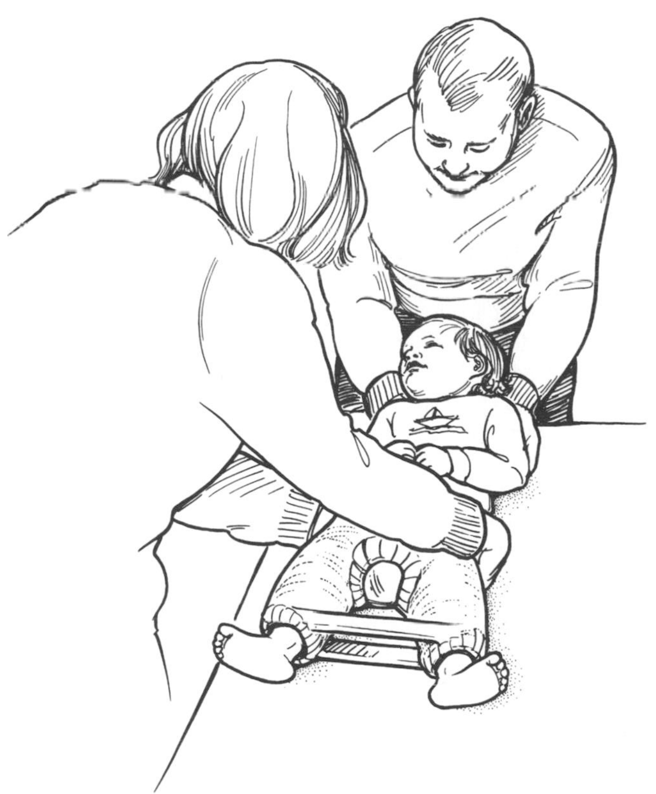

FIGURE **4** Two persons lifting and moving a child in a body cast. The bar between the legs is never used for this purpose.

*National U.S. Department of Transportation, National Highway Traffic Safety Administration, 400 Seventh St SW, Washington, DC 20590; (888) 327-4236; *http://www.nhtsa.dot.gov.*

PATIENT AND FAMILY EDUCATION

Preventing Spread of HIV and Hepatitis B Virus Infections

The child with HIV or hepatitis B virus has an infection that other children and adults can get. To protect all people who come near the child, certain guidelines must be followed. The germs that caused the child's illness can be spread to others by contact with some of the child's body fluids. These may include blood, bloody body fluids, feces, and semen. Needles contaminated with body fluids may also be a source of disease transmission. Instruct your child to avoid contact with any needles or syringes found in the yard, street, or playground. Have the child tell you if such items are seen so they may be disposed of properly to avoid contamination.

Your *best* protection against infection is good hand washing after you have taken care of the child. Always wash your hands with soap and water. Count to 10 while you are washing, then rinse with clear water and dry with a clean paper or cloth towel. If there are any cuts or other open areas on your hands, or if your health professional recommends that you use them, wear gloves when touching any of the child's body fluids. Always follow any contact with the child's body fluids with good hand washing, even if gloves are worn. Always have your child wash his hands after touching body fluids.

Each time you care for the child, you must decide what type of safeguard to use. If the child wears diapers, the disposable, ultra-absorbent kind with leg bands should be used. If the child does not have loose, watery stools and your hands will not come in contact with the urine or stool, then good hand washing after changing the diaper is sufficient. However, if the child has large, loose stools, nonsterile gloves should be worn to provide added protection. You must wash your hands when you are finished, even if gloves were worn. Place all diapers, gloves, wipes, tissues, and used dressings in a plastic bag and throw the bag away.

When feeding an infant, protect your clothes with a waterproof apron or cloth in case the infant has a wet burp or vomits.

Cleaning Body Fluid Spills

If the child vomits, has a nosebleed, or has a loose stool that needs to be cleaned up, you should wear gloves. First, using paper towels, blot the spill to decrease the amount of liquid to be cleaned. Dispose of these towels in a plastic garbage bag. Pour a bleach solution (1 part household bleach mixed in 9 parts water) onto the spill area. Carefully blot with paper towels. Place these towels into a plastic bag. Wash soiled linens and clothes separately in hot water with detergent. Wash your hands with soap and water after removing gloves.

Hepatitis B Vaccine

A vaccine is available to protect people from a type of hepatitis called *hepatitis B.* This vaccine has been added to the list of immunizations that all infants should receive. Three doses must be given. The first dose is given shortly after birth; the child receives the second dose 1 month after the first injection, and the third dose is given 6 months after the first. It can be given at the same time as other immunizations (e.g., DTaP, MMR, Hib) but in different muscles. There are also combination vaccines that contain the hepatitis B vaccine and either one or two to three other vaccines; if your child is eligible to receive a combination vaccine containing hepatitis B vaccine, this will decrease the number of injections your child must have at once. For older children who have not been immunized, especially adolescents, hepatitis B vaccination is now required.

Sexual Activity

At the time of this writing there is no vaccine to prevent HIV infection. This virus may be spread through contact with contaminated needles and mother-to-baby transmission, but most persons who acquire the disease do so through direct sexual contact. Some of the methods previously discussed may help avoid contracting this disease. If persons are engaging in *any* kind of sexual activity involving body fluids, there is a chance of contracting the virus; this includes oral-genital contact. Oral contraceptives and vaccines do not prevent sexually transmitted diseases such as HIV, herpes, papillomavirus, chlamydia, syphilis, or gonorrhea. A condom, when used properly, may prevent the spread of HIV. An excellent resource on sexually transmitted diseases is the Centers for Disease Control and Prevention website; *http://www.cdc.gov/std/default.htm;* or call (800) 232-4636.

Spanish translation of this handout available at *http://evolve.elsevier.com/Wong/clinical.*

Newborn Jaundice

WHAT IS NEWBORN JAUNDICE?

Jaundice commonly occurs in the newborn period. With jaundice the newborn's skin looks yellow, depending on the parents' ethnicity. It is common for Asian, American-Indian, and some Middle Eastern infants to look yellow. The whites of the newborn's eyes will also look yellow when jaundice occurs.

Jaundice occurs when the newborn's liver is not able to get rid of extra bilirubin on its own. Bilirubin is a yellow chemical that accumulates in the blood when red blood cells are naturally broken down as new red blood cells are formed. This is a natural process that occurs in almost all newborns, but sometimes the liver is not able to get rid of the extra bilirubin. In most cases jaundice will appear at about the second or third day of life and disappear by 2 weeks of age. Newborns who do not nurse well may have more jaundice; this is often called *breast-feeding jaundice,* and it commonly occurs in the first 6 to 10 days of life.

A newborn may also become jaundiced after the first week of life when breast-feeding; this is called *breast milk jaundice.*

In newborns with a maternal blood incompatibility such as ABO or Rh, the jaundice may appear sooner than 24 hours of life. This requires medical attention.

Before your newborn is discharged from the hospital a blood test may be done to check for jaundice (this blood test measures the amount of bilirubin in the bloodstream).

WHAT CAN A PARENT DO TO DECREASE THE EFFECTS OF NEWBORN JAUNDICE?

One of the most important things you can do is to make sure your newborn is receiving enough milk. Breast-fed newborns should be fed approximately every 1½ to 2½ hours during the first few weeks of life. If your newborn sleeps more than 4 hours at night, wake him up for a feeding. Formula-fed newborns should be fed about every 3 to 4 hours during the first week.

Call your health professional right away if your newborn:

- Is feeding poorly or is losing weight
- Has a temperature higher than 99.7° F, or 37.6° C (taken under the arm)
- Has skin color that is orange in regular light of day
- Starts to look or act sick, or has any of the following:
  - Vomiting or diarrhea
  - Breathing changes
- Has a low temperature (below 97.5° F, or 36.4° C)
- Demonstrates behavior changes such as being sleepy and not waking up for more than one feeding

Call your health professional during regular office hours if your newborn has any of the following:

- Yellow-colored skin that does not go away by 2 weeks of age
- Fewer than one or two good-sized bowel movements per day (24 hours)
- Fewer than six wet diapers per day (24 hours)

HOME PHOTOTHERAPY

Your baby may need home phototherapy for newborn jaundice. About 50% of all healthy full-term newborns become jaundiced after birth, but this lasts only a few days. Jaundice just means that the baby's skin color is yellow. Phototherapy light waves decrease the baby's jaundiced skin color. Phototherapy helps remove bilirubin—the substance formed when red blood cells break down naturally in the body. Phototherapy has been used to treat newborn jaundice for more than 50 years, and there have been few, minor side effects noted. Some babies get a rash that goes away in a few days; some have loose, gassy stools; and some babies lose body fluid through frequent, loose stools. Should any of these occur during treatment, call your health professional. Most babies need phototherapy for 2 to 3 days.

What You Will Need

Mask to cover newborn's eyes

Phototherapy light—either a bank of lights or a fiberoptic blanket

Newborn diaper

Procedure

If only a bili-blanket is used to treat jaundice, ask your health professional about the use of a mask.

Place the eye shield mask over your newborn's eyes. Most masks fasten with a Velcro attachment or gauze netting. Make sure the mask does not slip over the bridge of your newborn's nose and interfere with breathing. Place your ear next to newborn's nose to hear breathing.

Expose as much of your baby's skin as possible by removing all clothing except a diaper.

Place baby on his back under lights (should be at least 12 to 18 inches from bank light source, not blanket), or lay newborn on bili-blanket. The blanket may be wrapped around the newborn's nude trunk if indicated by the baby's health professional. Make sure the blanket has a see-through cover if recommended by the manufacturer.

Follow the manufacturer's recommendations carefully for use of phototherapy equipment.

Check your baby's temperature under the arm after 1 hour of phototherapy to make sure the infant is not too warm or too cool (see Measuring Your Child's Temperature box).

Follow your health professional's recommendations for time of exposure to lights. In most cases your newborn may be removed from the phototherapy apparatus for brief periods to be fed and cuddled. The bili-blanket does not need to be removed except for bathing.

Remove the mask for feedings, and turn off the phototherapy lights.

Precautions

If your baby is receiving phototherapy he or she will have a simple blood test to make sure the treatment is working. A home health professional will come to the home to do the test, or you may have to take the baby to an outpatient laboratory for this blood test.

Other important care for your baby while under phototherapy include:

- Do not expose your baby's skin to direct sunlight.
- If your baby has loose, gassy stools, cleanse the diaper area skin with soap and water and rinse well.
- Ask your health professional about the use of creams, ointments, or pastes during light treatment. Do not use skin lotion on your baby's exposed skin.

Instructions Related to Administration of Medications

PATIENT AND FAMILY EDUCATION

Giving Medications to Children

It is necessary for you to give the child medicine called________________________________. This medicine will have the following benefits: ____.

You will need to give the drug as follows:

Amount: ____

How often: ____

Special instructions: ____

Your health professional has written on the chart below when the medicine should be given. Give the drug at the same time each day so that it becomes part of the daily routine for you and the child.

For the child to get the most value from this medicine, it must be given until your health professional tells you to stop. Even though the child does not seem ill any longer, the medicine must be given for the prescribed time period.

Some common side effects of the drug are: ____.

If you have any problems that concern you, or if you notice any unexpected reactions from the medicine, notify your health professional at ____.

Drug Schedule

	Sunday	Monday	Tuesday	Wednesday	Thursday	Friday	Saturday
When child wakes up							
Breakfast 1 hour before							
with							
2 hours after							
Lunch 1 hour before							
with							
2 hours after							
Dinner 1 hour before							
with							
2 hours after							
Bed time							
During the night							

Check the box for the correct day and time. If the drug is given at times that differ from the suggested ones, write in the hour where appropriate.

5 - PATIENT AND FAMILY EDUCATION

This section may be photocopied and distributed to families with specific instructions for medication administration route.

PATIENT AND FAMILY EDUCATION

Giving Oral Medications

Your health professional has prescribed special medicine for the child that must be taken by mouth. This is a good time to teach the child about medicines as special things we take to get better. Do not tell her that the drug is candy. If the child thinks that the medicine is candy, and if the bottle is ever left in a place where she can reach it, she may take an overdose. Tell the child to take drugs *only* from you or other special people, such as grandparents or babysitters. Store *all* drugs in a safe place such as a locked cabinet. The storage area should be cool and dry. Bathrooms are usually too warm and moist for storing tablets or capsules. *Always* keep drugs in the original container, with the childproof cap tightly closed. Place drugs that need to be refrigerated on a high shelf toward the back of the refrigerator, not in the door.

To Encourage the Child

Unpleasant-tasting drugs can be mixed with a small amount of a pleasant-tasting food such as applesauce, juice, pudding, jelly, flavored ice, ice cream, or other, more flavorful foods. Allow the child to choose the food; this will encourage her to eat or drink all of the medicine. Tell the child what you have done so that she does not think the food always tastes like the drug-food combination. Do not add drugs to essential foods and liquids (milk, formula, orange juice, cereal) because the child may refuse them later. When mixing a drug with food or liquids, add it to a *small* amount (1 or 2 teaspoons) so that the child will have to eat or drink only that small amount to get all of the medicine. Offer the child a drink of water or other liquid to rinse away the taste of the drug.

If the drug tastes unpleasant, the child can suck on a small ice cube or Popsicle to decrease the taste. Also, you can cut a straw in half and have the child sip the medicine through a straw or have the child pinch her nose while taking the medicine. Not smelling the drug will lessen the unpleasant taste.

Some drugs taste better if served cold rather than at room temperature.

Give the child a gold star or sticker for taking the drug. These can be placed on the drug schedule sheet that you were given. The child can keep track of the number of times she has taken the medicine and how many doses are left. The stars or stickers also provide a record of her help.

Tablets and Capsules

Many tablets are pleasantly flavored, and the child can either swallow the tablet whole or chew the tablet. If a half-tablet is prescribed, only scored tablets (those with a visible groove on the tablet) can be broken in half. An unscored tablet may break into unequal portions. Pill cutters can be used to cut the tablet in half. They are sold in most drug stores. This does not matter if the child is taking the whole tablet. Tablets may also be cut in half if they are too large for the child to swallow whole.

If the child cannot swallow the tablet, you can crush the tablet between two spoons or a spoon and a piece of wax paper. However, before crushing any tablet, check with your health professional or pharmacist to make sure the tablet can be crushed. After the tablet is crushed, you can mix it with a nonessential food such as applesauce, jam, or fruit juice. Make sure all of the crushed tablet is added. If you have added medicine to the food, tell the child.

If the medicine is a capsule, do not open the capsule unless you have been told to do so by the pharmacist or your health professional. If it can be opened, add it to food as described above. Praise the child after she has taken the medicine.

Liquid Medicines

Many medicines are liquid. You can give the liquid in a measuring spoon, dropper, syringe, calibrated spoon, nipple, or medicine cup (Figure 1). *Do not* use household teaspoons or tablespoons. These are not standard sizes and will not measure the correct amount of medicine. Use a measuring spoon or the special measuring device sometimes supplied with the drug.

Measuring Spoon	Metric Equivalent
¼ teaspoon	1.25 ml
½ teaspoon	2.5 ml
¾ teaspoon	3.75 ml
1 teaspoon	5 ml
1 tablespoon	15 ml
1 liquid ounce	30 ml

Instructions

1. Read the label to make certain you have the right drug and to check the right amount of medicine to give the child. Shake the bottle well to mix the medicine if the label says to do this.
2. Pour out the exact amount of the drug into the measuring spoon.
   OR
   Fill the syringe or dropper with the drug to the right amount. Read the amount at the bottom of the semicircular line around the top of the liquid (Figure 2).

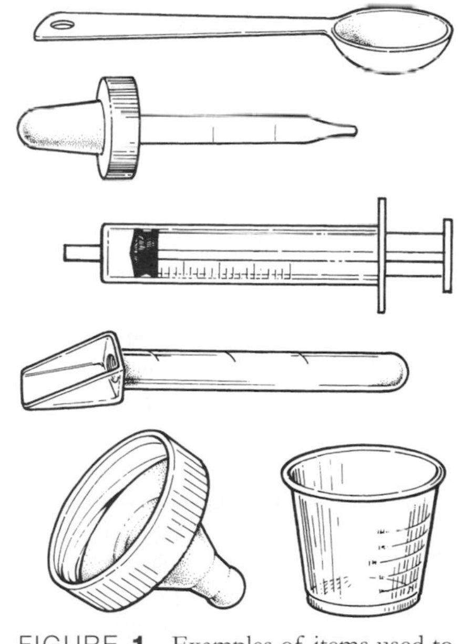

FIGURE 1 Examples of items used to give liquid medications.

Continued

5 - PATIENT AND FAMILY EDUCATION

This section may be photocopied and distributed to families.

Spanish translation of this handout available at *http://evolve.elsevier.com/Wong/clinical.*

PATIENT AND FAMILY EDUCATION

Giving Oral Medications—cont'd

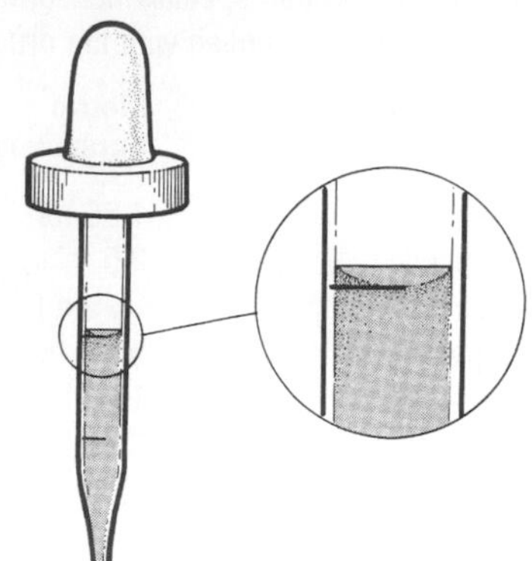

FIGURE 2 Checking correct amount.

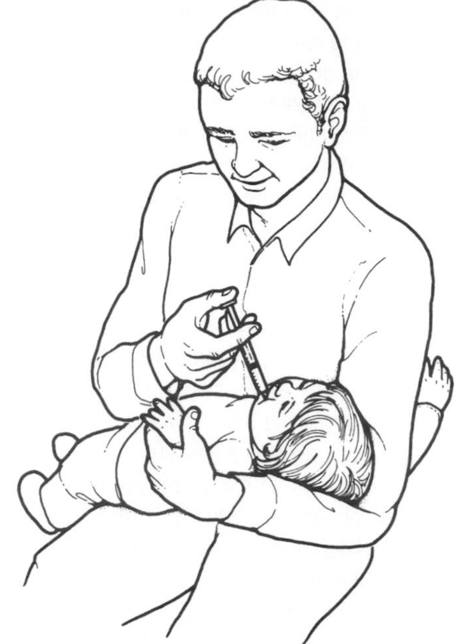

FIGURE 3 Giving oral medication using a syringe. Note how the child's arms are placed.

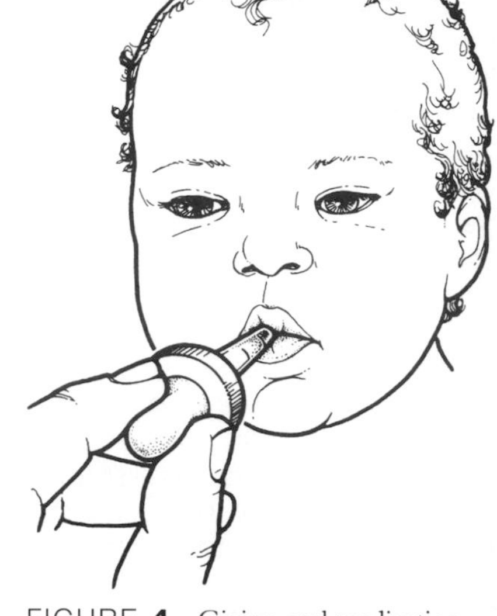

FIGURE 4 Giving oral medication using a dropper.

3. Give the medicine to the child in a quiet place so that you will not be disturbed.
4. Tell the child what you are going to do.
5. If needed, hold the infant or young child in your lap. Place whichever of her arms is closer to you behind your back. Firmly hug her other arm and hand with your arm and hand; snuggle her head between your body and your arm (Figure 3). Sometimes you may also want to grasp her legs between yours. Your other hand remains free to give the child the drug.
6. Allow the child to sip the drug from the spoon. If it is a large amount of medicine and the child can drink from a cup, you can measure the drug into a small cup. Make sure that the child takes all of the drug. You may have to add a small amount of water to rinse the drug from the sides of the cup.
   OR
   Gently place the dropper or syringe in the child's mouth along the inside of the cheek (Figure 4). Allow the child to suck the liquid from the dropper or syringe. If the child does not suck, squeeze a small amount of the drug at a time. This takes longer, but the child will swallow the medicine and be less likely to spit it out or choke on it.
   OR
   Place an empty bottle nipple in the child's mouth, add the drug to the nipple, and allow the child to suck the nipple (Figure 5).
7. Rinse the child's mouth with plain water to remove any of the sweetened drug from the gums and teeth. This can be done by wrapping a paper towel around your finger, soaking it in plain water, then swabbing the gums, cheeks, palate, and tongue.
8. Return the drug to a safe place out of the child's reach. Place it in the refrigerator if the label says to do this.
9. Write down the time you gave the child the medicine, and check for the time you need to give the next dose.
10. PRAISE THE CHILD FOR HELPING.

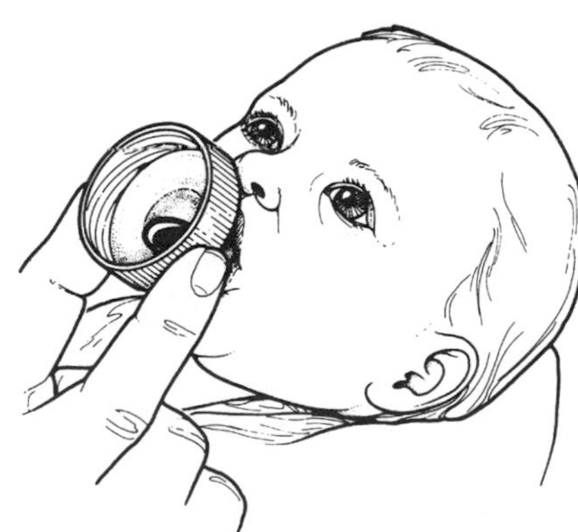

FIGURE 5 Giving oral medication using a bottle nipple.

PATIENT AND FAMILY EDUCATION

Giving Intramuscular (IM) Injections

Your health professional has prescribed special medicine for the child, which must be given by injection. This is a good time to teach the child about medicines as special things that we need to take to get better. Several things can be done to make the injection less painful:

1. Apply a topical anesthetic (see p. 546) to the place you will give the injection 2½ hours before the medicine is due, OR spray the area with the topical anesthetic medicine ordered by your health professional right before you give the injection.
2. Give the child something to do, such as squeezing someone's hand, humming, or counting.
3. Keep the child involved in talking, singing, or watching TV.

Equipment

Alcohol swabs
Syringe and needles
Drug stored at room temperature

Instructions

1. Gather all equipment.
2. Wash your hands with soap and water. Count to 10 while washing, then rinse with clear water and dry with a clean paper or cloth towel.
3. Open the packet containing a new syringe.
4. Clean the top of the drug bottle with alcohol. Do not touch the top after you have cleaned it.
5. Remove the cap from the syringe. Do not touch the needle.
6. Pull back the plunger to fill the syringe with the same amount of air as the drug dose (Figure 1).
7. Put the needle into the drug bottle. Turn the bottle upside down. Push the plunger to inject the air into the drug bottle (Figure 2). Take care not to cause bubbles.
8. With the tip of the needle in the liquid drug, pull back the plunger to fill the syringe with the amount needed (Figure 3).
9. Remove any air bubbles in the syringe. Hold the syringe with the needle pointing upward, and firmly tap the syringe with a finger of the free hand. When all the bubbles are at the top of the syringe, push the plunger gently to remove the bubbles.
10. Make sure the drug dosage is the right amount. The top of the black rubber stopper should be on the desired amount (not bottom of stopper).
11. Turn vial right-side up, then remove the needle from the bottle.
12. Put the cap back on the needle loosely.
13. Use the injection spot circled in the accompanying diagram (Figure 4).
14. Have the child lie or sit down and remove all clothing from the injection area.
15. Have someone hold the child if you think the child will not be able to sit or lie still.
16. Using a circular motion, clean the injection spot with alcohol.
17. Let the skin dry.
18. Place your hand on the landmarks shown in Figure 4 to locate the correct injection spot.
19. Grasp the muscle firmly between your thumb and fingers. This steadies the muscle and allows for the drug to be injected into the deepest part of the muscle.
20. Place the needle cap between the index and middle fingers, and pull out the syringe.
21. With a quick darting motion, insert the needle into the injection spot (Figure 5).

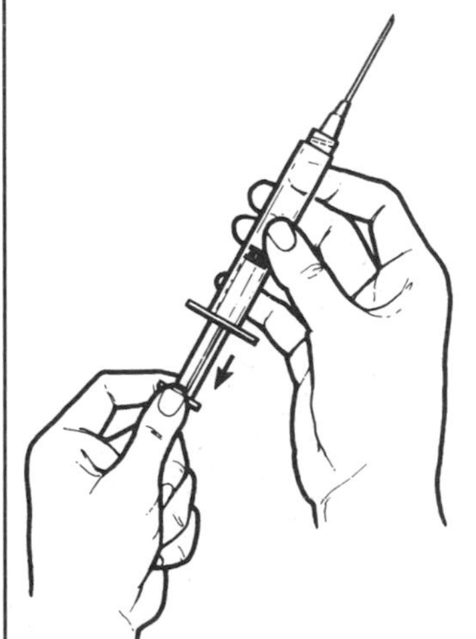

FIGURE **1** Filling the syringe with air.

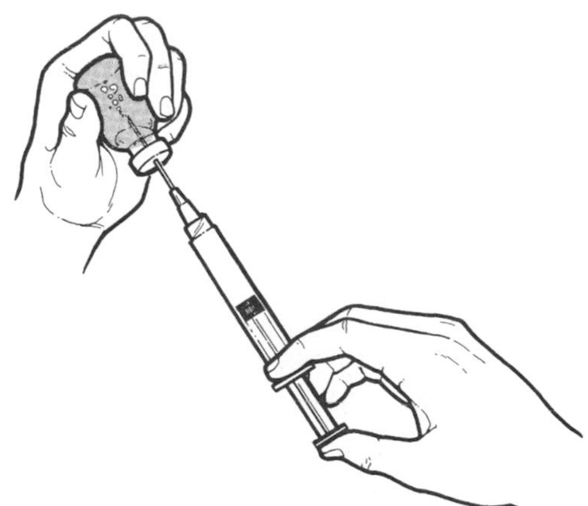

FIGURE **2** Putting air into the drug bottle.

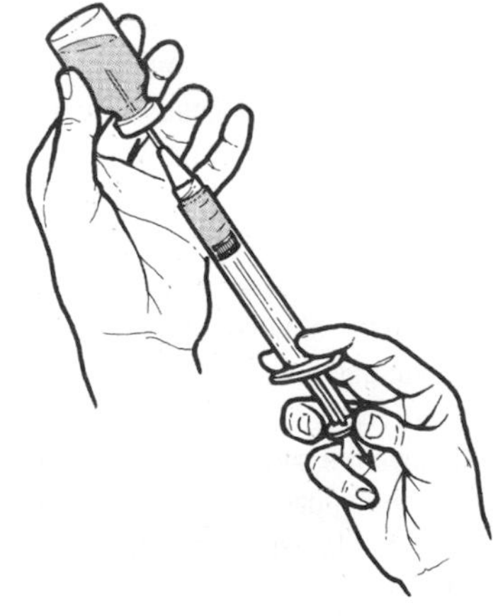

FIGURE **3** Filling the syringe with the drug.

Additional resources for disposal of needles and lancets used in the home are listed in the Community Focus box Safe Disposal of Needles and Lancets.

Continued

5 - PATIENT AND FAMILY EDUCATION

PATIENT AND FAMILY EDUCATION

Giving Intramuscular (IM) Injections—cont'd

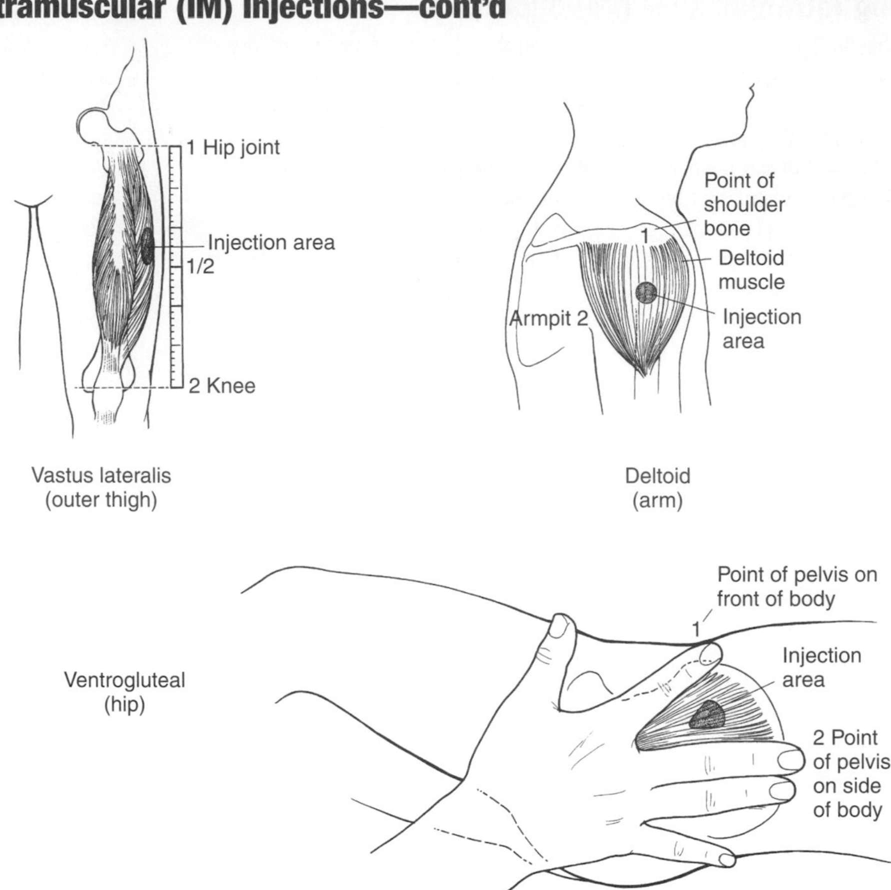

FIGURE **4** Ask your health care professional to mark the area where you need to give the injection.

22. Pull back the plunger slightly and check to see if there is any blood in the syringe.
    a. If there is blood, remove the needle, change needles, and begin again after making sure the medication dose is still right. Place the needle in an area slightly away from the first spot.
    b. If there is no blood, push the plunger slowly until the syringe is empty.
23. Remove the syringe quickly from the site, and apply gentle pressure with a dry sterile pad or a clean tissue.
24. Throw the used needle and syringe into a puncture-resistant container, such as an empty plastic milk carton or aluminum can. Once the injection has been given *do not* attempt to replace the needle cap on the needle. Place the top securely on the container.
25. Place a small bandage on the injection spot.
26. Comfort the child, and make sure that he knows the drug is necessary if he is to get better. It is important that the child does not think that the injections are punishment.
27. PRAISE THE CHILD FOR HELPING.
28. Return the drug to a safe place out of the child's reach.
29. Write down the date and time of the dose and which injection site was used. Check the time that the next dose needs to be given. Use a different area for the next injection.
30. Follow your health professional's instructions for throwing away the used equipment. If you used needles, put them into a rigid container, such as a used bleach bottle, to prevent other people from being stuck. Make sure you do not mix the container with other materials to be recycled. You may want to label the container, "NOT FOR RECYCLING."

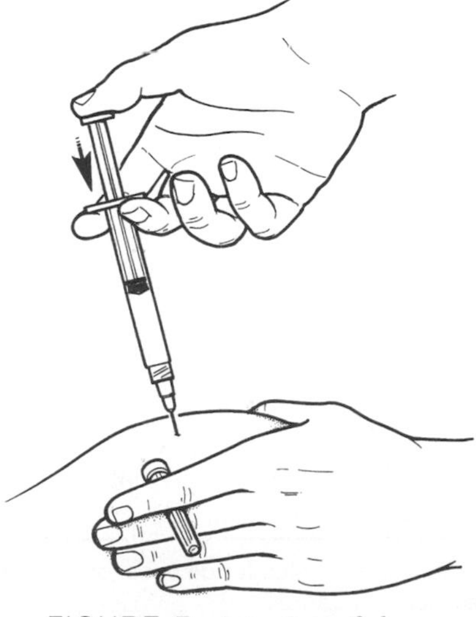

FIGURE **5** Injection of drug.

COMMUNITY FOCUS

Safe Disposal of Needles and Lancets

The growing number of persons being cared for in home settings has increased the amount of medical waste that communities must properly dispose of to prevent accidental needle sticks and the spread of diseases such as hepatitis and HIV. Many states have programs to assist with the disposal of sharps such as needles and lancets to prevent environmental contamination and accidental mishaps involving needle exposures. Contact one of the resources listed below to obtain further information about needle disposal in your state, or discuss the proper disposal of sharp medical equipment with your health professional.

If your state or community does not have programs for safe needle disposal, an option is to place sharps in a rigid container such as a bleach bottle or metal coffee can. Place the lid on the container to prevent accidental needle exposure. Once the container is about ¾ full and ready to be discarded, you may add to it a liquid mixture such as cement or plaster to harden the contents and prevent needle exposure. Special devices that break off the needle into a rigid container are also available in some communities.

Additional information can be found at any one of these resources: Centers for Disease Control and Prevention, *http://www.cdc.gov/needledisposal;* Coalition for Safe Community Needle Disposal, (800) 643-1643; and Environmental Protection Agency, *http://www.epa.gov.*

PATIENT AND FAMILY EDUCATION

Giving Subcutaneous (Sub Q) Injections

Your health professional has prescribed special medicine for the child, which must be given by injection. This is a good time to teach the child about medicines as special things that we need to get better. Several things can be done to make the injection less painful.

1. Apply a topical anesthetic (see p. 546) to the place you will give the injection before the medicine is due OR spray the area with the medicine ordered by your health professional right before you give the medicine.
2. Give the child something to do, such as squeezing someone's hand, humming, or counting.
3. Keep the child involved in talking, singing, or watching TV.

Equipment

Alcohol swabs
Syringe and needles
Medicine stored at room temperature

Instructions

1. Gather all equipment.
2. Wash your hands with soap and water. Count to 10 while washing, then rinse with clear water and dry with a clean paper or cloth towel.
3. Open the packet containing a new syringe.
4. Clean the top of the drug bottle with alcohol. Do not touch top after you have cleaned it.
5. Remove the cap from the syringe. Do not touch the needle.
6. Pull back the plunger and fill syringe with the same amount of air as the drug dose (Figure 1).
7. Put the needle into the drug bottle. Turn the bottle upside down. Push the plunger to inject the air into the medication bottle (Figure 2). Take care not to cause bubbles.
8. With the tip of the needle in the drug, pull back the plunger to fill the syringe with the amount needed (Figure 3).
9. Remove any air bubbles in the syringe. Hold the syringe with the needle pointing up, and firmly tap the syringe with a finger of the free hand. When all the bubbles are at the

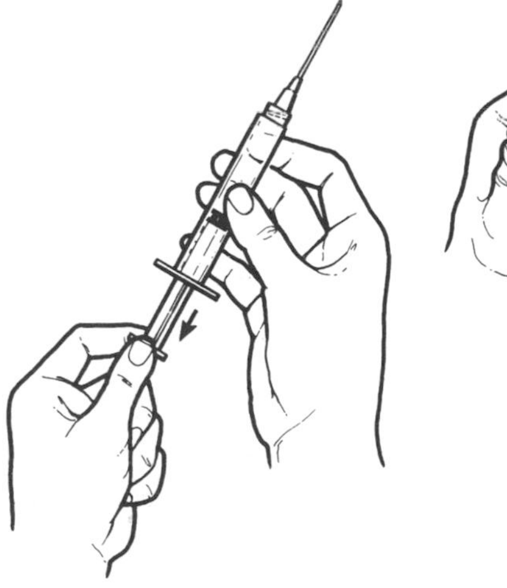

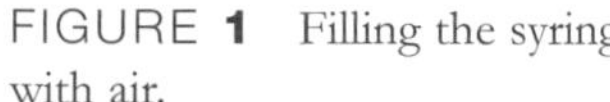

FIGURE **1** Filling the syringe with air.

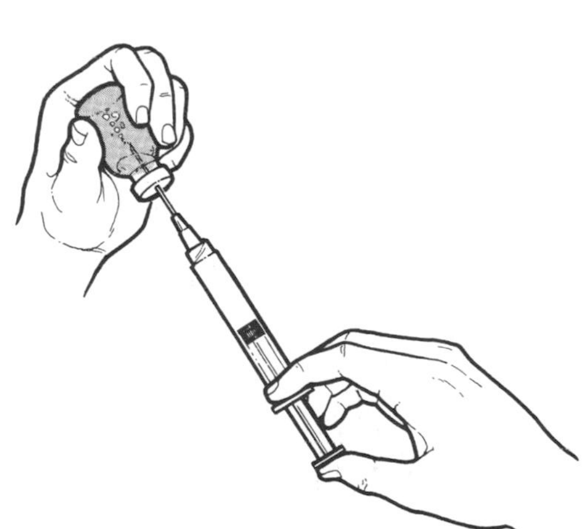

FIGURE **2** Putting air into the drug bottle.

*NOTE: Your health care practitioner may suggest using a 45-degree angle and not pulling back on the syringe (to aspirate for blood). In either case, continue grasping the skin during the injection.

Continued

Spanish translation of this handout available at *http://evolve.elsevier.com/Wong/clinical.*
Source: Wilson D, Hockenberry MJ: *Wong's clinical manual of pediatric nursing*, ed 7. Copyright © 2008, Mosby, St Louis.

PATIENT AND FAMILY EDUCATION

Giving Subcutaneous (Sub Q) Injections—cont'd

top of the syringe, push the plunger gently to remove the bubbles.

10. Make sure the drug dose is the right amount. Top of black rubber stopper should be on the desired amount (not bottom of stopper).
11. Turn the vial right-side up, then remove the needle from the bottle.
12. Put the cap back on the needle loosely.
13. Have the child lie or sit down, and remove all clothing from the injection area.

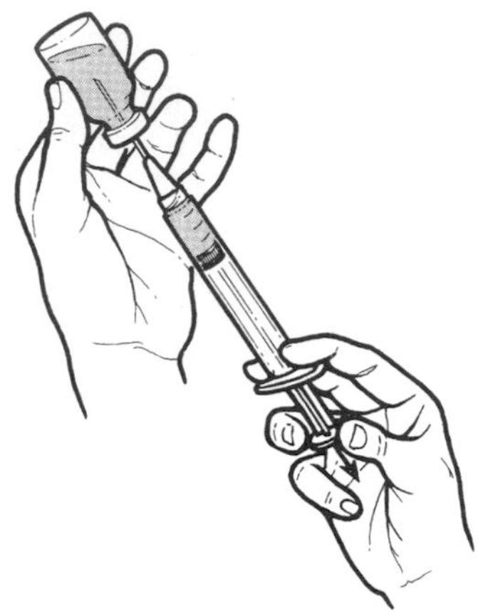

FIGURE 3 Filling the syringe with the drug.

14. Have someone hold the child if you think the child will not be able to lie still.
15. Using a circular motion, clean the injection spot with alcohol.
16. Let the skin dry.
17. Grasp the skin around the injection spot firmly, raising only the skin ½-1 inch (Figure 4).
18. Place the cap between the two fingers (index and middle fingers) that are grasping the skin and pull out the syringe.
19. With a quick darting motion, insert the needle bevel up (see inset in Figure 4) into the injection site at a 90-degree angle.*
20. Release your grasp on the child's skin.
21. Pull back the plunger gently and check to see if there is any blood in the syringe.*
    a. If there is blood, remove the needle, change needles, and begin again after making sure the medication dose is still right. Place the needle in an area slightly away from the first spot.
    b. If there is no blood, push the plunger slowly until the syringe is empty.
22. Remove the syringe and needle quickly from the site, and apply gentle pressure with a dry sterile pad or a clean tissue. Do not massage. Do not attempt to place the cap back on the needle.
23. Throw the used needle and syringe into a puncture-resistant container, such as an empty plastic milk carton.
24. Place a small adhesive bandage on the injection spot.
25. Comfort the child, and make sure that he knows the drug is necessary if he is to get better. It is important that the child does not think that the injections are punishment.
26. PRAISE THE CHILD FOR HELPING.
27. Return the drug to a safe place out of the child's reach.
28. Write down the date and time of the dose and which injection site was used. Check the time that the next dose needs to be given. Use a different area for the next injection.
29. Follow your health professional's instructions for throwing away the used equipment. If you used needles, put them into a rigid container, such as a used bleach bottle, to prevent other people from being stuck. Make sure you do not mix the container with other materials to be recycled. You may want to label the container, "NOT FOR RECYCLING."

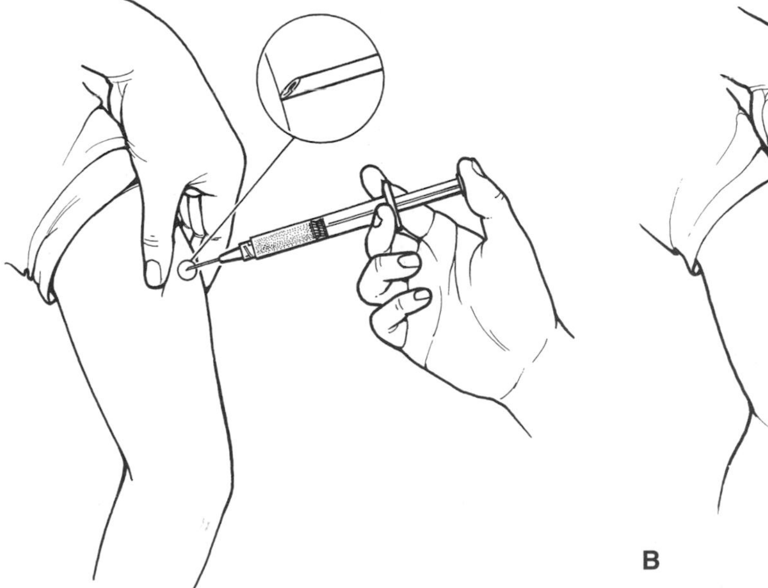

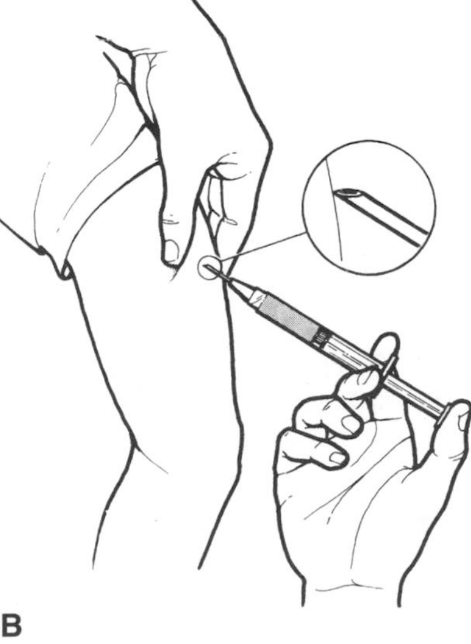

FIGURE 4 Injection of drug with bevel of needle pointing up *(insets)*. **A,** Using 90-degree angle. **B,** Using 45-degree angle.

PATIENT AND FAMILY EDUCATION

Insulin Administration

Insulin is administered as a subcutaneous injection using the same principles as those discussed previously, with some minor variations in the steps.

1. Gather all equipment.
2. Wash hands with soap and water as described previously.
3. Open the packet containing a new insulin syringe. Use *only* an insulin syringe marked in insulin units to draw up and administer insulin.
4. Clean the top of the drug bottles with alcohol. Do not touch tops after you have cleaned them.
5. If you are administering only one type of insulin at a time, follow the directions previously described for subcutaneous administration.
6. If a combination of insulin types is being administered, the clear insulin (usually rapid or short-acting insulin [regular]) is drawn up *first,* then the cloudy (intermediate-acting insulin).
7. Remove the protective cap from the syringe. Do not touch the needle.
8. Pull back the plunge, and fill syringe with the same amount of air as the insulin (cloudy) dose.
9. Put the needle into drug bottle A, but do not allow needle to touch the medication solution in the vial (as in Figure 1, *A*). Inject the air into the bottle. Withdraw needle.
10. Using the same needle and syringe, repeat steps 8 and 9 with vial B (Figure 1, *B*), but do not withdraw needle once air has been injected into vial B.
11. Turn vial B upside down, and fill syringe with proper volume (dose) of *clear* insulin.
12. Calculate the total volume of medication (insulin) by adding the volume of both prescribed doses. For example, if 10 units of regular insulin and 8 units of NPH insulin are prescribed, the total dose will be 18 (10 units + 8 units = 18 units).
13. Insert the needle of syringe into vial A, being careful not to push the plunger and expel the medication into vial. Turn the vial upside down, and carefully withdraw the amount of medication required into syringe (Figure 1, *C*).
14. If there is an air bubble in the syringe, carefully expel the air by holding the syringe with the needle pointed up. Tiny air **bubbles** may be left in the syringe as long as the dosage of insulin is not modified by these bubbles.

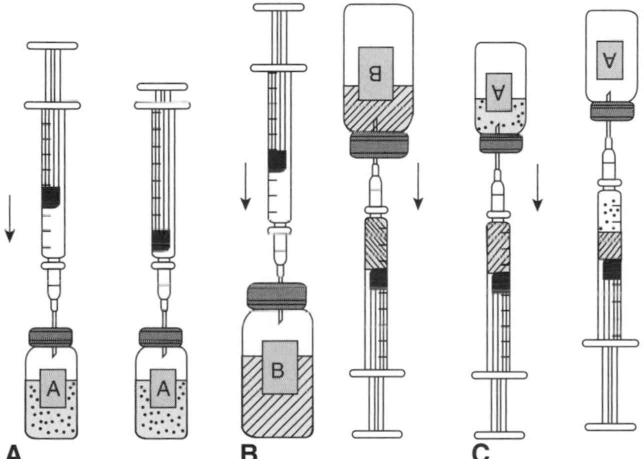

FIGURE **1** The clear insulin is in vial B and the cloudy is in vial A. **A,** Injecting air into vial A. **B,** Injecting air into vial B and withdrawing dose. **C,** Withdrawing medication from vial A; medications are now mixed. (From Potter PA, Perry AG: *Fundamentals of nursing,* ed 6, St Louis, 2005, Mosby.)

NOTE: Insulin may be administered without pulling back on the syringe (aspirating for blood).

PATIENT AND FAMILY EDUCATION

Blood Glucose Monitoring

Depending on the child's age and capability the health care health professional has reviewed steps for testing your child's blood glucose (sugar), or for having the child test his own blood glucose. There are many different types of blood glucose monitors on the market with minor variations in self-testing among the types. Follow the directions given by the health professional for your type monitor. The following instructions are of a general nature and may be exactly as your health professional taught, or there may be minor variations.

1. Gather all equipment.
2. Wash your hands and the child's hands with soap and water.
3. Position the hand below the heart for a few minutes before performing the skin puncture.
4. Turn on the glucose monitor. Some monitors automatically turn on when the strip is inserted.
5. Remove an unused reagent meter strip from the container and insert into the glucose monitor. Make sure the reagent strip is inserted correctly (see manufacturer's directions for meter used if necessary).
6. Choose a finger to puncture (prick)—the side of the finger is best—do not puncture the center of the fingertip.
7. Remove a clean lancet from container and insert in automatic lancing device as indicated by manufacturer.
8. Remove lancet tip cover to expose tip. Take care not to touch lancet tip.
9. Cleanse area of finger to be punctured with an alcohol preparation or warm water. Allow finger to dry completely. It may be helpful to warm the selected finger with a warm moist cloth before performing the puncture.
10. Place automatic lancing device firmly against side of finger selected for lancing and push the release button on the lancing device, causing the lancet to pierce the skin.
    NOTE: Use distraction techniques outlined in Unit 3 with small children who experience pain or fear the pain of the lancet puncture. Letting the child be in control of pushing the release button on the lancet device may also help diminish the effects of the pain. (See also Atraumatic Care.)
    NOTE: Some of these **automatic** lancing devices can be adjusted to decrease the pain associated with lancing.
11. Lightly squeeze finger above the puncture site until a drop of blood appears. (Some meters recommend wiping away the first drop of blood with a cotton ball. Follow the manufacturer's or health professional's directions.)
12. Hold reagent strip pad next to drop of blood so the blood is transferred to the reagent strip. If a sufficient amount of blood is not transferred to the reagent strip, the meter may not read properly and another puncture may be necessary.
13. The meter timer is activated once blood transfer is complete on many meters. Some meters require a timer button to be pressed.
14. Apply gentle pressure to the puncture site for 1 to 2 minutes with a clean cotton ball or clean tissue (follow your health professional's directions).
15. Read the meter once the timer sounds.
16. Dispose of reagent strip, used lancet, and cotton ball in a proper receptacle.
17. Record glucose meter reading in log or diary as requested by health professional.

ATRAUMATIC CARE

Minimizing Pain of Blood Glucose Monitoring

To enhance blood flow to the finger, hold it under warm water for a few seconds before the puncture.

When obtaining blood samples, use the ring finger or thumb (blood flows more easily to these areas), and puncture the finger just to the side of the finger pad (more blood vessels and fewer nerve endings).

To prevent a deep puncture, press the platform of the lancet device lightly against the skin and avoid steadying the finger against a hard surface.

Use lancet devices with adjustable-depth tips. Begin with the most shallow setting.

Use glucose monitors that require small blood samples (e.g., Ascensia Elite) to avoid repeated punctures.

Discuss the use of a topical anesthetic such as EMLA or LMX4.

Discuss Alternate Site Testing (AST) with your health professional; alternate sites for blood glucose monitoring other than the finger include forearm, upper arm, palm, abdomen, thigh, and calf. These sites may not be as painful to prick, but a different glucose monitor may be required (Bui H, Perlman K, Daneman: Self-monitoring of blood glucose in children and teens with diabetes, *Pediatr Diabetes* 6[1]:50, 2005).

PATIENT AND FAMILY EDUCATION

Caring for an Intermittent Infusion Device

A small tube (catheter) was placed in the child for the administration of intravenous (IV) drugs at home. This tube is known as an *intermittent infusion device.* Look at the spot where the tube enters the skin several times each day. Notify your health professional at ________ if you observe any of the following signs around the device:

- Redness
- Swelling or puffiness
- Leaking or drainage
- Red streak along the skin near the device
- Pain around the entry spot

A clear adhesive or tape dressing is usually placed over the device to protect it. The child may wash around the fingers but should not get the dressing or any exposed part of the tube wet. During a bath or shower, cover the tube and dressing with plastic wrap, such as Saran Wrap, or a plastic bag to keep the area dry. The device may need to be changed by your health professional, especially if any problems develop.

These instructions describe the use of needleless devices on the syringe and medicine bottle (also called a *vial*). The type of the needleless devices you use may differ from the type described here, but the same basic methods are used for all of them. Be sure to ask your health professional to show you how your device works. Information for using a needle on the syringe is also given, but be very careful to avoid sticking yourself or someone else with the needle.

Flushing

The inside of the catheter must be rinsed (flushed) with a solution, usually heparin (a special drug called an *anticoagulant*) or saline (a special sterile salt water solution) to prevent any blood clots from forming, which can clog the tube. The small amount of solution that you are using will rinse the entire length of the tube. The tube must be flushed ________ time(s) each day and after any drug or fluid is given through the tube.

Equipment

Needleless cannula and syringe or needle and syringe
Alcohol swabs
Bottle of flush solution at room temperature
Needleless adapter for the bottle

Instructions

1. Gather equipment that you will need on a clean dry surface.
2. Wash your hands with soap and water. Count to 10 while washing, then rinse with clear water and dry with a clean paper or cloth towel.
3. Open the package of alcohol swabs.
4. Wipe the top of the bottle with one of the swabs for about 10 seconds. Let the bottle top dry. Do not touch the bottle top after you have cleaned it.
5. Open the package of the bottle adapter, and push the pointed end straight into the rubber top of the bottle. It may take some force to do this, but do not try to twist the adapter into the bottle top.
6. Open the package containing a new syringe, and remove the cap from the tip of the syringe. Do not touch the exposed part.
7. Open the package of the needle cannula by pulling apart the wrapping at the top of the package. Connect the tip of the syringe to the opening of the cannula by twisting the two pieces together.
8. Remove the cover of the cannula. Do not touch any part of it. If you do touch it, use another new one.
9. If you are using a syringe with a needle, you do not need the bottle adapter. Just follow steps 6 through 8, substituting the needle for the cannula. Sometimes the syringe and needle are already attached.
10. Pull back the plunger and fill syringe with the same amount of air as the dose (Figure 1).
11. Put the cannula into the adapter or the needle into the rubber stopper of the bottle. Turn the bottle upside down. Push the plunger to inject the air into the bottle (Figure 2). Take care not to cause lots of bubbles.

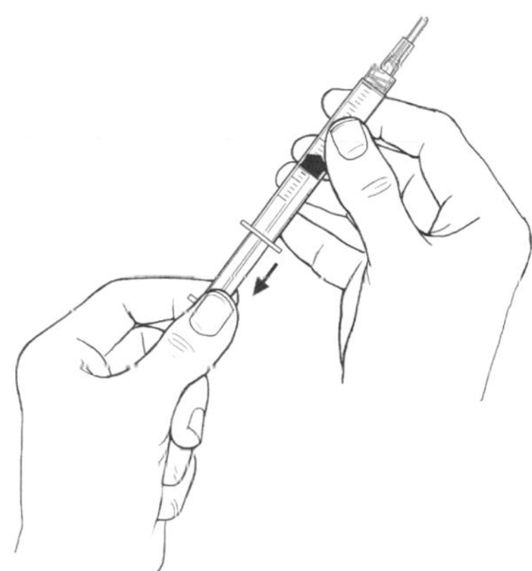

FIGURE 1 Filling the syringe with air by pulling back on plunger.

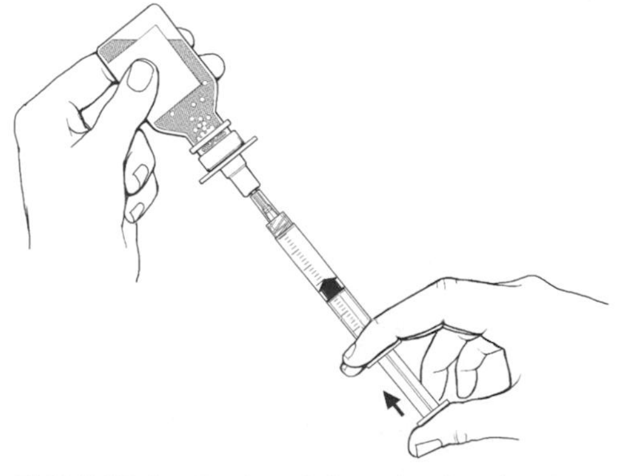

FIGURE 2 Putting air into the drug bottle by pushing forward on the plunger.

Continued

PATIENT AND FAMILY EDUCATION

Caring for an Intermittent Infusion Device—cont'd

12. With the tip of the cannula or needle in the solution, pull back the plunger to fill the syringe with the amount needed (Figure 3).
13. Remove any air bubbles in the syringe. Hold the syringe with the cannula or needle pointing up, and firmly tap the syringe with a finger of the free hand. When all the bubbles are at the top of the syringe, push the plunger gently to remove the bubbles.
14. Make sure you are using the right amount of solution.
15. Turn vial right-side up, then remove the syringe from the bottle and place the cover back on the cannula or needle.
16. With the second alcohol swab, wipe the cap on the catheter or on the end of extra tubing that has been attached to the catheter for about 10 seconds. Let the cap dry. Do not touch it after you have cleaned it.
17. Insert the cannula or needle in the cap. If you are using the cap on the device, hold the plastic just below the rubber cap to make it easier to insert the cannula or needle (Figure 4). If the tubing is clamped, unclamp it now.
18. Slowly push the plunger of the syringe to put the solution into the tubing.
19. *Stop* pushing if there is pressure or pain. Call your health professional, and go to step 21.
20. If there is extra tubing, hold the clamp on the tubing with your free hand. Slide the clamp to close the tubing as you push the last 0.2 ml of solution (Figure 5).
21. Remove the syringe from the cap.
22. PRAISE THE CHILD FOR HELPING.
23. Return the solution to a safe place out of the child's reach.
24. Write down the date and time of the dose and check the time that the next dose needs to be given.
25. Follow your health professional's instructions for throwing away the used equipment. If you used needles, put them into a rigid container, such as a used bleach bottle, to prevent other people from being stuck. Make sure you do not mix the container with other materials to be recycled. You may want to label the container, "NOT FOR RECYCLING."

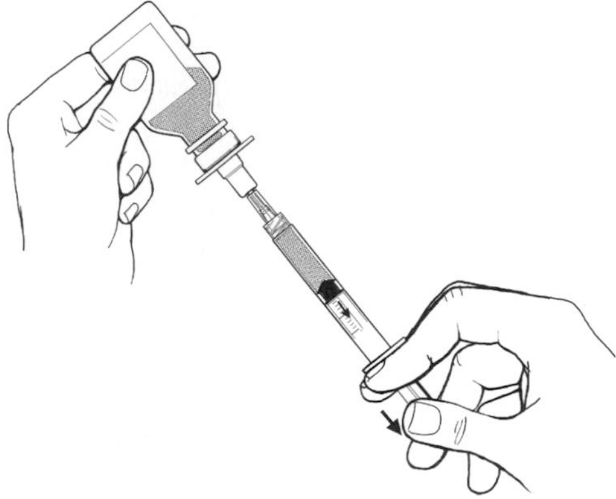

FIGURE **3** Filling the syringe with solution by pulling back on the plunger.

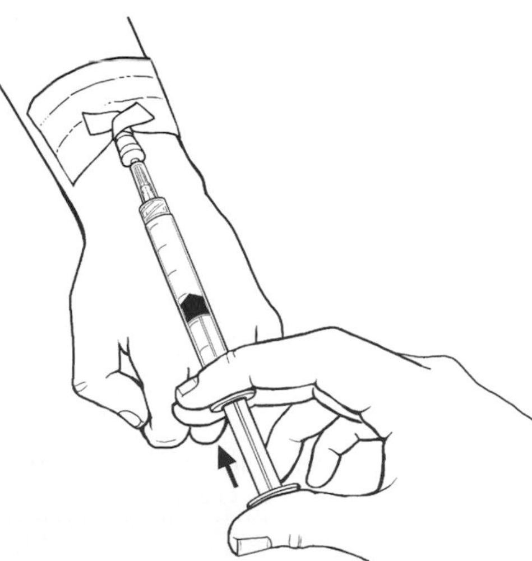

FIGURE **4** Injecting solution into the intermittent infusion device by pushing slowly forward on the plunger.

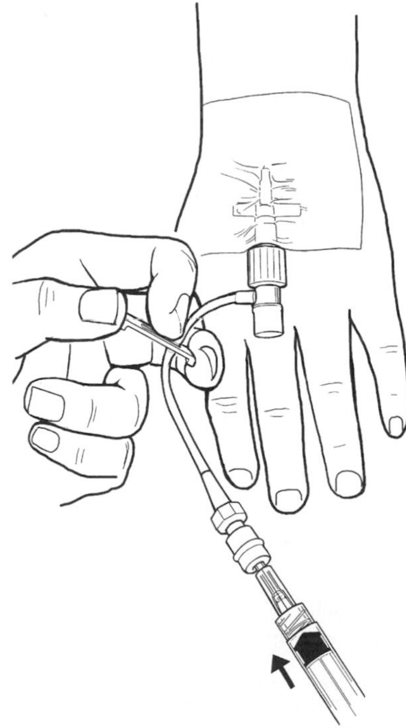

FIGURE **5** Injecting solution into the tubing attached to the infusion device by pushing slowly forward on the plunger and closing the clamp as the last 0.2 ml is given.

PATIENT AND FAMILY EDUCATION

Caring for a Central Venous Catheter

A catheter (tube) was placed in your child so that an intravenous (IV) line will be available for long-term treatment. This tube can be used to give medications, fluids, and nutrients and possibly to obtain blood specimens. Several different types of catheters can be used, such as the Broviac or the Groshong. Both types of catheters are inserted under the skin and into a major blood vessel near the heart (Figure 1).

A peripherally inserted central catheter (PICC) may also be used to give medications over a long-term period. This catheter is placed in a vein in an extremity such as the arm; the catheter will be advanced through the vein to a large vein in the chest. Because the PICC line is not tunneled under the skin as a Broviac or Groshong catheter is, there is greater chance for it to become dislodged, pulled out, or kinked. The PICC line insertion site is covered by a dressing, which is usually changed by the nurse. Unless special teaching is provided by your health care practitioner, it is recommended that the home health nurse or practitioner be called for problems with the PICC line. The PICC line is flushed in the same manner as an intermittent infusion device. Follow the practitioner's guidelines for the number of times the PICC line must be flushed and the type of solution to be used for flushing.

Special Considerations

A young child, either the child with the tube or a playmate, may want to handle the tube and as a result may accidentally pull it out. To prevent the child from playing with the tube, keep a T-shirt on the child, use one-piece outfits such as overalls, or select out-fits that open in the back. Never leave the child alone when she is undressed. Keep all sharp objects, especially scissors, out of the reach of young children in the home.

When the child is bathed, keep the skin dry where the tube enters the body. Plastic wrap can be taped over a gauze dressing, or a transparent dressing can be used to protect the site.

All people who care for the child should be taught about the catheter. At school tell both the child's teacher and the school nurse so that an adult can help the child if needed.

Your health professional should be notified if the tube becomes damaged. The tube should be repaired as soon as possible because of the risk of infection. If the child has a Broviac catheter, clamp the tube at once. The Groshong catheter does not need to be clamped.

Flushing the Tube

The care of each catheter is slightly different. These written instructions will help you to care for the tube at home. Catheter care should always be done in a quiet place where you will not be disturbed. If the child is active, you will need a helper. The helper can keep the child still while you do the catheter care.

The inside of the Broviac must be flushed (rinsed) with a heparin solution (heparin is a special drug called an *anticoagulant*). This will help prevent any blood clots from forming. If blood clots form, the tube may become plugged. The small amount of heparin that you are using will rinse the entire length of the tube. If the child has a Groshong catheter, no heparin flushes are needed, only weekly saline (special sterile salt water) rinses. The Broviac must be flushed ________ time(s) each day, and both types of tube are rinsed (flushed) after giving any drug or fluid through the tube.

These instructions describe the use of needleless devices on the syringe and medicine bottle (also called a *vial*).

The type of needleless device you use may differ from the type described here, but the same basic methods are used for all of them. Be sure to ask your health professional to show you how your device works. Information for using a needle on the syringe is also given, but be very careful to avoid sticking yourself or someone else with the needle.

Equipment

Needleless cannula and syringe or needle and syringe (10-ml size)
2 antiseptic swabs or wipes
Bottle of heparin (concentration will be determined by the practitioner) at room temperature (Broviac) or bottle of sterile injectable saline at room temperature (Groshong)
In some situations a bottle of heparin mixed with saline may be used
Needleless adapter for the bottle

Instructions

1. Gather equipment that you will need, and place on a clean, dry surface.
2. Wash your hands with soap and water. Count to 10 while washing, then rinse with clear water and dry with a clean paper or cloth towel.

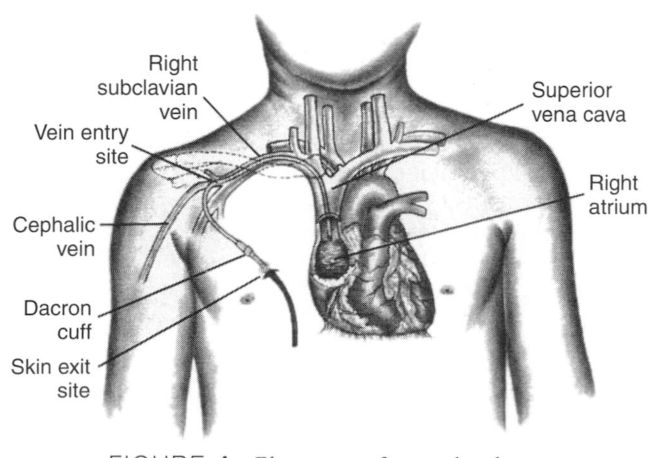

FIGURE 1 Placement of central catheter.

Continued

5 - PATIENT AND FAMILY EDUCATION

PATIENT AND FAMILY EDUCATION

Caring for a Central Venous Catheter—cont'd

3. Open the package of antiseptic swabs.
4. With one of the swabs, scrub the top of the solution bottle for about 10 seconds. Let the bottle top dry. Do not touch the bottle top after you have cleaned it.
5. Open the package of the bottle adapter, and push the pointed end straight into the rubber top of the bottle. It may take some force to do this, but do not try to twist the adapter into the bottle top.
6. Open the package containing a new syringe, and remove the cap from the tip of the syringe. Do not touch the exposed part.
7. Open the package of the needle cannula by pulling apart the wrapping at the top of the package. Connect the tip of the syringe to the opening of the cannula by twisting the two pieces together.
8. Remove the cover of the cannula. Do not touch any part of it. If you do touch it, use a new one.
9. If you are using a syringe with a needle, you do not need the bottle adapter. Just follow steps 6 through 8, substituting the needle for the cannula. Sometimes the syringe and needle are already attached.
10. Pull back the plunger, and fill the syringe with the same amount of air as needed (Figure 2).
11. Insert the cannula into the adapter or the needle into the rubber stopper of the bottle. Turn the bottle upside down. Push the plunger to inject the air into the bottle (Figure 3). Take care not to cause lots of bubbles.
12. With the tip of the cannula or needle in the solution, pull back the plunger to fill the syringe with the amount needed (Figure 4).
13. Remove any air bubbles in the syringe. Hold the syringe with the cannula or needle pointing up, and firmly tap the syringe with a finger of the free hand. When all the bubbles are at the top of the syringe, push the plunger gently to remove the bubbles.
14. Make sure the heparin or saline is the right amount.
15. Remove the syringe from the bottle.
16. Place the cannula or cover over the needle, and set aside.
17. With the second alcohol swab, wipe the cap on the catheter for about 10 seconds. Let the cap dry. Do not touch it after you have cleaned it.
18. Insert the cannula or needle in the cap.
19. If the tubing is clamped, unclamp it now.
20. Slowly push the plunger of the syringe to push the solution into the tubing (Figure 5).
21. *Stop* pushing if there is pressure or pain. Call your health professional and go to step 23.
22. If the tubing has a clamp, hold the clamp on the tubing with your free hand. Slide the clamp to close the tubing as you push the last 0.2 ml of solution.
23. Remove the syringe and needle (or cannula) from the cap.

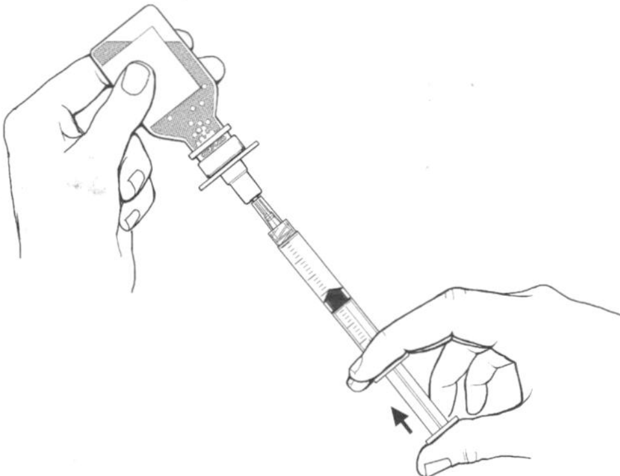

FIGURE 3 Putting air into the drug bottle by pushing forward on the plunger.

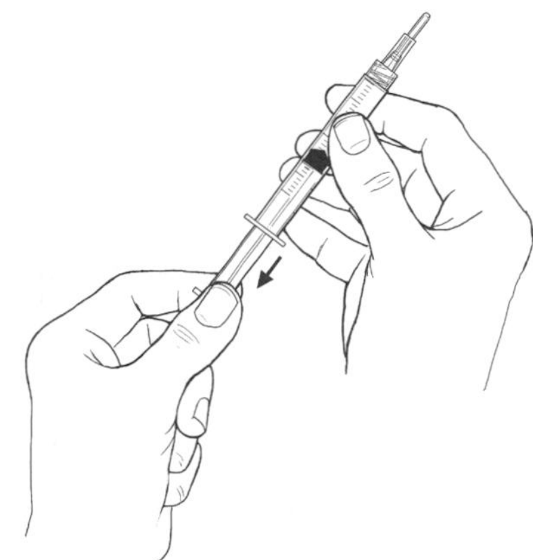

FIGURE 2 Filling the syringe with air by pulling back on the plunger.

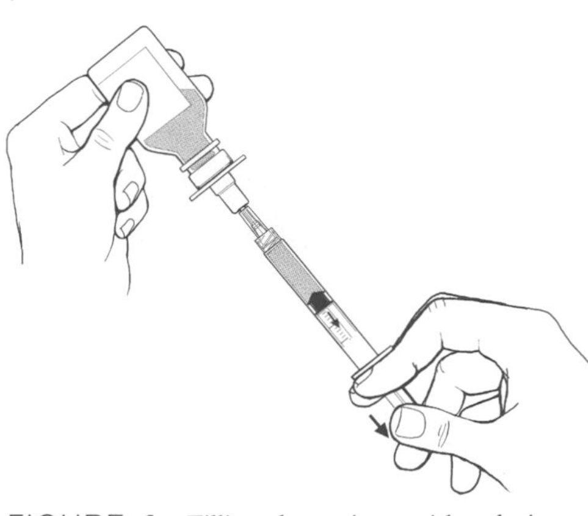

FIGURE 4 Filling the syringe with solution by pulling back on the plunger.

PATIENT AND FAMILY EDUCATION

Caring for a Central Venous Catheter—cont'd

24. PRAISE THE CHILD FOR HELPING.
25. Return the solution to a safe place out of the child's reach.
26. Write down the date and time of the dose, and check the time that the next dose needs to be given.
27. Follow your health professional's instructions for throwing away the used equipment. Do not attempt to place the cap back on the needle. If you used needles, put them into a rigid container, such as a used bleach bottle, to prevent other people from being stuck. Make sure you do not mix the container with other materials to be recycled. You may want to label the container, "NOT FOR RECYCLING."

Changing the Injection Cap

The cap should be changed ________ time(s) per week. If the cap is changed at the time of rinsing, the heparin or saline is given (flushed) through the new injection cap.

Equipment

Antiseptic swab
Injection cap
Sterile gloves (as recommended by health care practitioner)

Procedure

1. Gather the equipment you will need.
2. Wash your hands with soap and water. Count to 10 while washing, then rinse with clear water and dry with a clean paper or cloth towel.
3. Clamp the tube midway between the skin and the end of the tube or on the reinforced clamping sleeve that is on some catheters; do not clamp a Groshong catheter.
4. With the swab, clean around the tip of the tube below the injection cap.
5. Open the new injection cap package but do not remove the cap.
6. Put on sterile gloves.
7. Remove the used injection cap from the tube, handling only the injection cap end, and attach the new injection cap (Figures 6 and 7). Turn the new cap to the right until it is firmly attached.
8. Remove the clamp from the catheter (not needed with Groshong).

Dressing Change

After the catheter has been in your child for a short time, a dressing may or may not be placed over the area where it enters the skin. Your health professional will tell you if a dressing is needed and how often to change it. Usually, a clear, transparent dressing is used. This lets you see the child's skin around the tube. Look at the skin around the tube each day. Call your health professional at once if you see any redness, drainage, or swelling; if the area around the tube is painful; or if the child has a temperature above 100.4° F.

Equipment

Adhesive remover pad
Transparent dressing
Antiseptic swabs
Bag for disposing of used supplies and dressing
Tape

Instructions

1. Gather the equipment on a clean, dry surface.
2. Wash your hands with soap and water. Count to 10 while washing, then rinse with clear water and dry with a clean paper or cloth towel.
3. Gently peel off the edges of the old dressing, using adhesive remover if necessary. Peel off one edge at a time. Another way to remove the dressing is to grasp opposite corners of the plastic film and pull them away from each other to stretch and

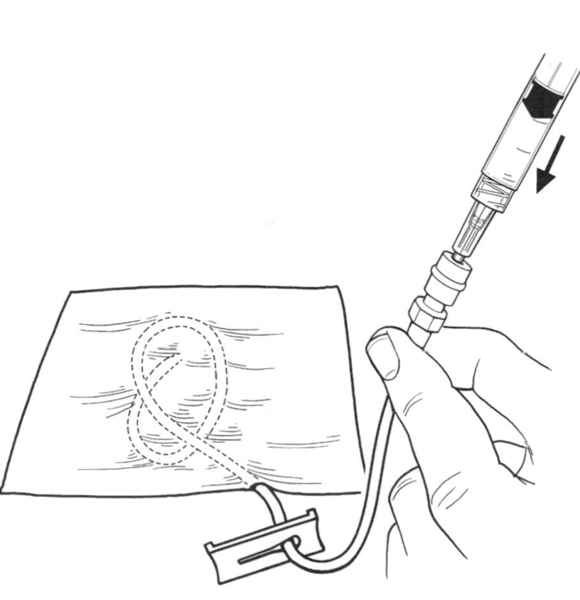

FIGURE 5 Injecting solution into central venous catheter by pushing slowly forward on the plunger.

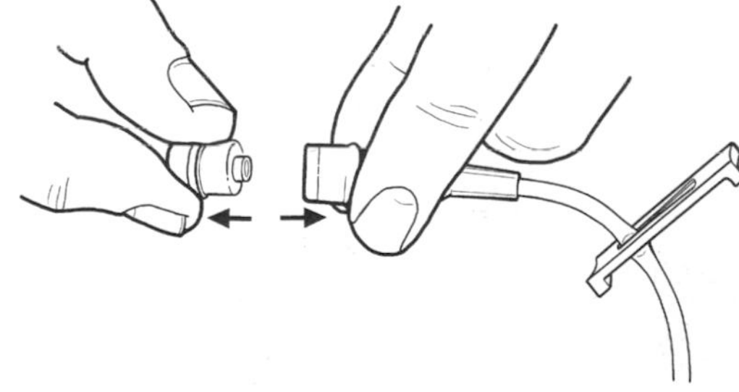

FIGURE 6 Removing used cap.

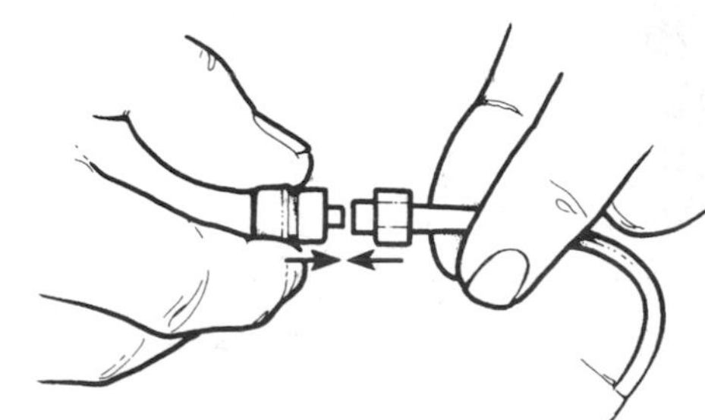

FIGURE 7 Attaching new injection cap.

Continued

PATIENT AND FAMILY EDUCATION

Caring for a Central Venous Catheter—cont'd

loosen the film. After the film begins to loosen, grasp the other two corners of the film and pull. This method is easier and more comfortable than pulling the dressing up and off the skin.

4. Carefully look at the skin around the tube for redness or drainage.
5. Using each antiseptic swab only once, clean the skin where the tube enters the body. Use a circular motion starting at the tube and moving out about 3 inches from the tube (Figure 8).
6. Loop the tube around the entry site, leaving the injection cap below the dressing.
7. Carefully place the dressing on the child's skin. Hold the dressing in both hands. When the top of the dressing is on the skin, slowly bring the dressing toward the bottom of the window frame, making sure that it attaches to the skin (Figure 9).
8. Secure the end of the tube with tape to keep it from dangling.
9. Place all used items in a paper bag. Close the bag and throw it away.
10. PRAISE THE CHILD FOR HELPING.

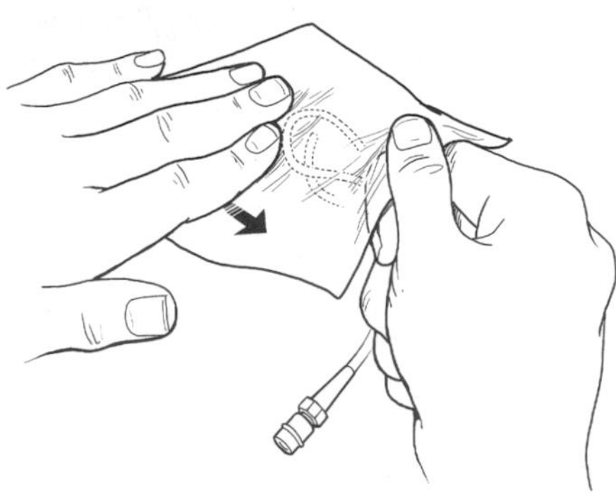

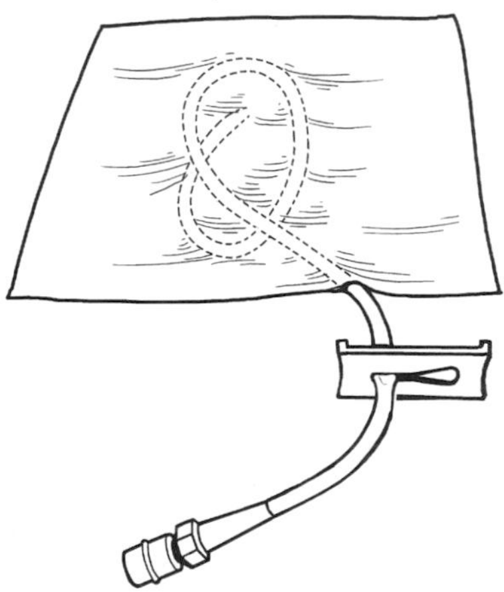

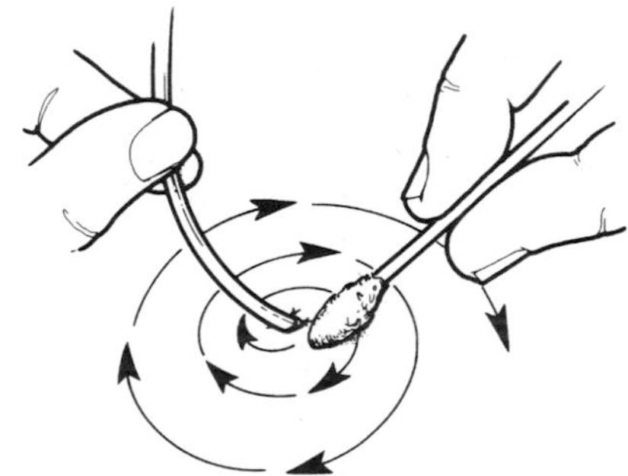

FIGURE **8** Cleaning the skin in a circular motion, beginning at the catheter and moving outward.

FIGURE **9** Applying transparent dressing, beginning at the top and carefully bringing the dressing to the bottom.

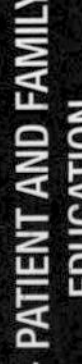

PATIENT AND FAMILY EDUCATION

Caring for an Implanted Port

Use of the Implanted Infusion Port

The implanted port is used much like a regular intravenous (IV) line. The port is usually placed by the surgeon on the chest (Figure 1); the port is implanted under the skin so there is less restriction on the child's activities, and dressing changes are not required once the incision heals. In order to access the port, a special needle is inserted through the skin into the rubber-like top of the port (Figure 2). Insertion of the needle is usually not painful, but if it is uncomfortable for your child, the area may be numbed first with a topical anesthetic such as EMLA or LMX4 (see p. 546 for instructions for applying a topical anesthetic). Because the anesthetic takes a while to work it is best to plan ahead; the anesthetic may need to be placed over the site before leaving home if a scheduled visit to the health care center is planned. The needles are made straight or bent; the bent shape permits delivery of fluids or medications over a period of time. Your child may even receive medicine at home via an ambulatory infusion pump. Blood samples can also be drawn from the port. When the treatment is completed, the needle can be removed. If the child is undergoing a treatment that goes for several days, the same needle can stay in for up to a week before it needs to be changed.

Care for the Implanted Infusion Port

Because no part of the catheter or port is outside the body, the child can carry on normal activities, including showering and swimming, provided he is not receiving treatment. In caring for the implanted port, you will need to:

1. **Watch for infection.** Notify your child's doctor or nurse if any of the following signs or symptoms develops:
   - Fever or chills
   - Pain or redness around the port
   - Drainage at incision site
   - Shortness of breath
   - Chest pain
2. **Prevent blocking off the catheter.** To keep the catheter from becoming blocked between uses, it must be flushed every 4 to 6 weeks. The nurse can do this during your child's regular clinic or doctor's office visits. Heparin is the drug used; it can keep the blood from clotting inside the catheter.
3. **Protect the needle during infusion and maintain the dressing.** Your child may receive treatment over a number of days using an ambulatory infusion pump. During the infusion it will be necessary for you to make certain the needle does not become dislodged. You may need to reinforce the dressing with tape or even change the dressing. If you notice any swelling about the port or if the child is experiencing unusual stinging or pain in the area of the port, call your child's doctor or nurse right away.
4. **Have the needle removed from the port.** When your child's treatment is completed, the nurse will remove the needle after flushing the port with a heparin solution. Once the needle is removed, a dressing is no longer necessary.
5. **Protect the skin over the port.** In order to protect the skin over the port from irritation, avoid bra straps and seat belts that may rub or place pressure on the port area.

Duration of the Implanted Infusion Port

The implanted port can stay in place as long as your child's physician feels it is necessary. It can be surgically removed when no longer needed. With good care and in the absence of infection, the port can remain in place for years if desired.

The implanted infusion port is one way to help make treatments easier. If you have any questions, be sure to ask your child's primary nurse or practitioner, _________.

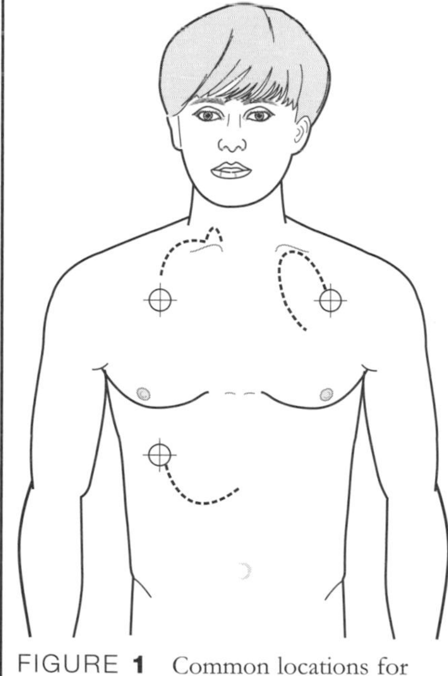

FIGURE **1** Common locations for catheter insertion.

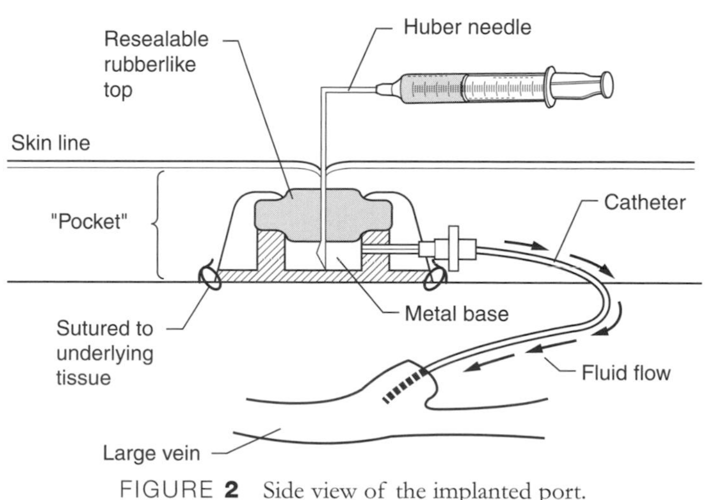

FIGURE **2** Side view of the implanted port.

5 - PATIENT AND FAMILY EDUCATION

PATIENT AND FAMILY EDUCATION

Giving Rectal Medications—Suppositories

Medicines can be given rectally if the child cannot eat or drink. If you have been told to give only half of a suppository, cut the suppository in half *lengthwise.*

Equipment

Suppository
Warm water

Instructions

1. Gather equipment.
2. Wash your hands with soap and water. Count to 10 while washing, then rinse with clear water and dry with a clean paper or cloth towel.
3. Remove the wrapper from the suppository.
4. The index finger or the pinky (fifth finger) should be used to put in the suppository. Use the pinky if the child is small. Make sure the fingernail is short and smooth. As a covering, you can use plastic wrap or a plastic sandwich bag on the finger. Disposable gloves and finger cots can also be bought and used.
5. Remove the child's underpants or diaper.
6. Have child lie on his left side, with right leg slightly bent.
7. With water, wet the finger or covering you will use to insert the suppository.
8. Wet the suppository with warm (not hot) water. Do not use Vaseline or any other kind of grease or lubricant. These may affect how the medicine works.
9. Insert the suppository, with the rounded (not pointed) end first, 1 inch into the child's rectum (Figure 1).
10. If the child is too young to help, hold the buttocks together for at least 5 minutes. This prevents the suppository from being pushed out.
11. Wash your hands as above.
12. PRAISE THE CHILD FOR HELPING.

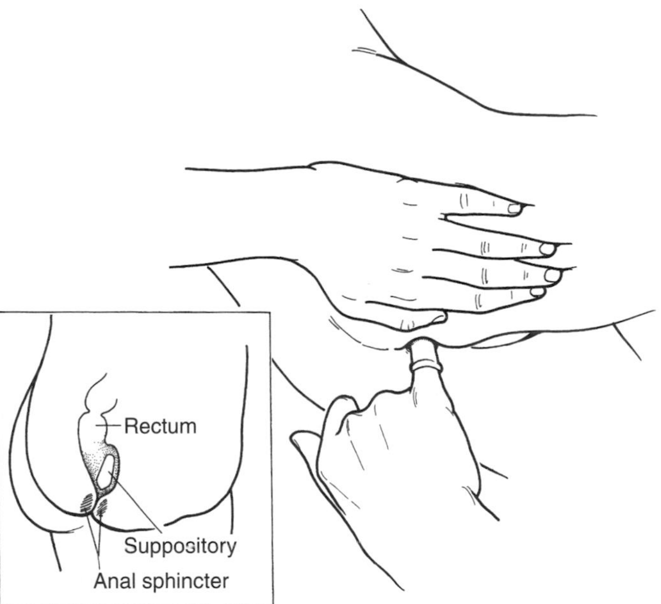

FIGURE **1** Using smallest finger to insert rectal suppository with rounded end first.

5 - PATIENT AND FAMILY EDUCATION

PATIENT AND FAMILY EDUCATION

Giving Eye Medications

Your health professional has prescribed a special drug for the child's eye(s). For this drug to have the most benefit, it is important that you closely follow these procedures.

Equipment

Dropper
Medicine at room temperature
Clean tissue, clean washcloth, warm water

Instructions for Eye Drops

1. Gather equipment.
2. Wash your hands with soap and water. Count to 10 while washing, then rinse with clear water and dry with a clean paper or cloth towel.
3. Remove any discharge from the eye with a clean tissue. Wipe from nose to ear.
4. If the eye has crusted material around it, wet a washcloth with warm water and place this over the eye. Wait about 1 minute. Gently wipe the eye from the nose side outward with the washcloth, place it on the eye, and wait again. If you cannot remove the crusting, rewet the washcloth. Then try to gently remove the crusted drainage. Continue using the warm, moist washcloth and gently wiping until all the crusting is removed. If both eyes need cleaning, use separate cloths for each eye. Launder the washcloth(s) before using again.
5. Have the child lie on his back on a flat surface. If the child will not lie still, you can hold the child by sitting on a flat surface such as the floor or bed. Place the child on his back with his head between your legs and his arms under your legs. If needed, you can cross your lower legs over the child's legs to keep him from moving. Place a pillow under the child's shoulders, or a rolled-up towel under his neck so that his head is tilted back and to the same side as the eye to be treated (right eye, turn head to right; left eye, turn head to left). The eye drops should flow *away* from the child's nose.
6. Open the bottle of eye drops. Do not let the dropper portion touch anything.
7. Tell the child to look up and to the other side (away from the eye into which you are putting the drops). Choose something specific for the child to look at. If the child is young, you can make a game of giving the eye drops. Tell the child to open his eyes on the count of 3. Then count to 3. When you say 3, drop the eye drops into the child's eye. Even if the child will not open the eyes on 3, keep him lying down until he decides to open the eyes. The medicine will flow in the eye.
8. Note that the wrist of the hand you will be using to give the drops is placed on the child's forehead. This will help steady your hand.
9. Gently pull down the child's lower eyelid with the other hand by placing gentle downward pressure below the eyelashes (Figure 1).
10. Position the bottle so that the drug will fall into the lower eyelid, *not* directly onto the eyeball.
11. Squeeze the bottle for the required number of drops.
12. Tell the child to close the eye, then to blink. This helps spread the drug around the eye.
13. Remove any extra drug with a clean tissue, wiping from the nose outward. Putting gentle pressure on the inner corner of the eye for 1 minute prevents any medicine from dripping into the back of the throat and causing an unpleasant taste.
14. If both eyes are to be given the drug, repeat with the other eye.
15. Hold and comfort the child.
16. PRAISE THE CHILD FOR HELPING.
17. Write down the time you gave the child the drug, and check for the time you need to give the next dose.

Instructions for Ointments

When both drops and ointment are needed, give the drops before the ointment. If the ointment is used only once each day, apply the ointment at bedtime because it will blur the child's vision.

1. Follow steps 1 through 9 for eye drops.
2. Position the tube at the inner part of the eye near the nose (Figure 2).
3. Squeeze a ribbon of the ointment onto the inside of lower eyelid. Begin at the side of the eye near the nose, and go toward the outer edge of the eye. Avoid touching the eye with the ointment container.
4. Give the tube a half-turn. This helps "cut" the ribbon of medicine.
5. Finish with steps 12 through 17 for eye drops.

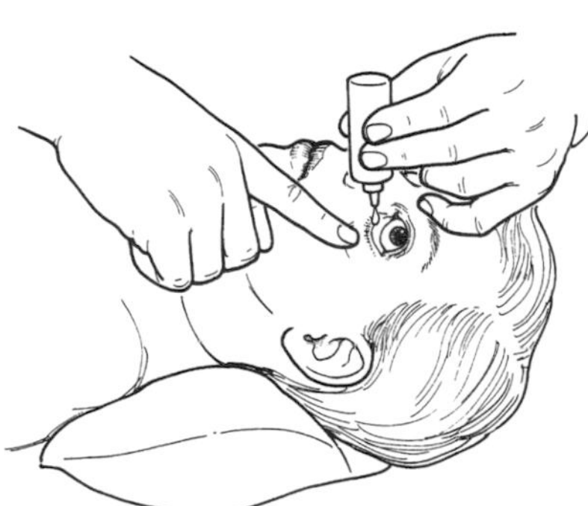

FIGURE 1 Dropper and hand position for giving eye drops.

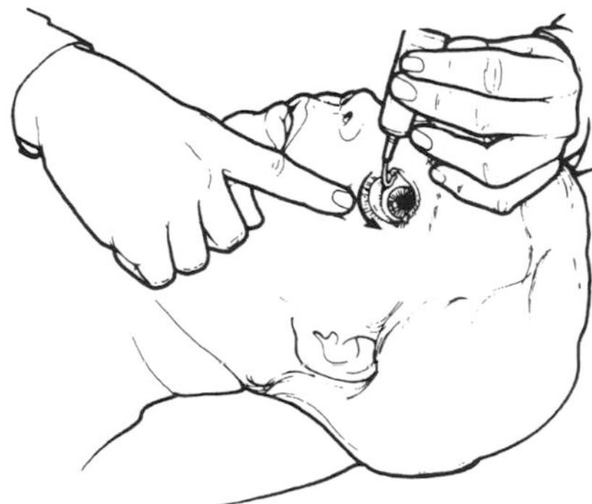

FIGURE 2 Tube and hand position for applying eye ointment.

PATIENT AND FAMILY EDUCATION

Giving Ear Medications

Your health professional has prescribed a special drug for the child's ear(s). For this drug to have the most benefit, it is important that you follow these instructions.

Equipment

Medicine
Container of warm water
Clean tissue or cotton-tipped applicator and cotton ball if desired

Instructions

1. Gather equipment.
2. Wash your hands with soap and water. Count to 10 while washing, then rinse with clear water and dry with a clean paper or cloth towel.
3. Place the drug bottle in warm water. Cold drops in the ear are uncomfortable.
4. Feel a drop to make sure the drug is warm, not too cold or too hot.
5. Have the child lie on the side opposite the ear into which you will be putting the drug (right ear, on left side; left ear, on right side). If the child will not lie still, you can hold the child by sitting on a flat surface, such as the floor or bed. Place the child on her back with her head between your legs and her arms under your legs. If needed, you can cross your lower legs over the child's legs to keep her from moving.
6. Check the ear to see if any drainage is present. If there is drainage, remove it with a clean tissue or cotton-tipped applicator. *Do not* clean any more than the outer ear.
7. Open the bottle of ear drops. Do not let the dropper portion touch anything.
8. The wrist of the hand you will be using is placed on the cheek or head. This will help steady your hand.
9. You will need to straighten the child's ear canal. For children who are 3 years old and younger, pull the outer ear *down* and toward the *back* of the head (Figure 1). For older children, pull the outer ear *up* and toward the *back* (Figure 2).
10. Position the bottle so that the drops will fall against the side of the ear canal.
11. Squeeze the bottle for the right number of drops.
12. Keep the child lying on that side with the medicated ear up for 1 minute. Gently rub the skin in front of the ear (Figure 3). This helps the drug flow to the inside of the ear.
13. If any drug has spilled on the skin, wipe the outer ear. A cotton ball can be loosely placed in the ear, but it must be changed each time drops are given.
14. If both ears need the drug, repeat with the other ear after a 1-minute wait.
15. Hold and comfort the child.
16. PRAISE THE CHILD FOR HELPING.
17. Write down the time you gave the child the drug, and check for the time you need to give the next dose.

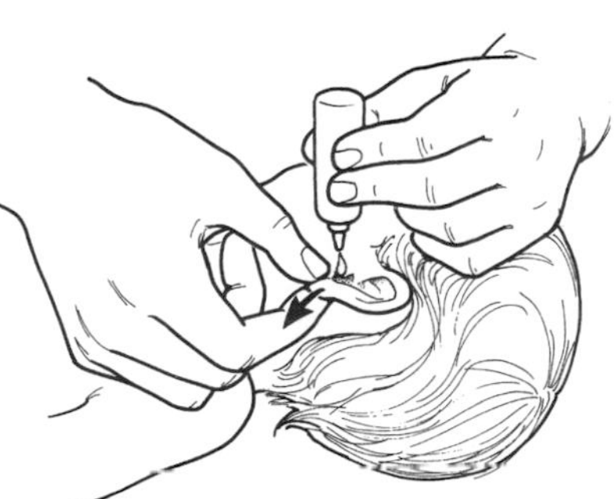

FIGURE **1** Hand and dropper position for children 3 years old and younger, with earlobe pulled down and back.

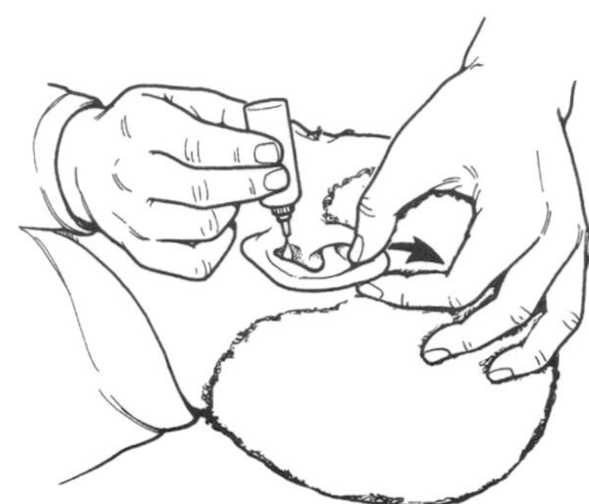

FIGURE **2** Hand and dropper position for older children, with earlobe pulled up and back.

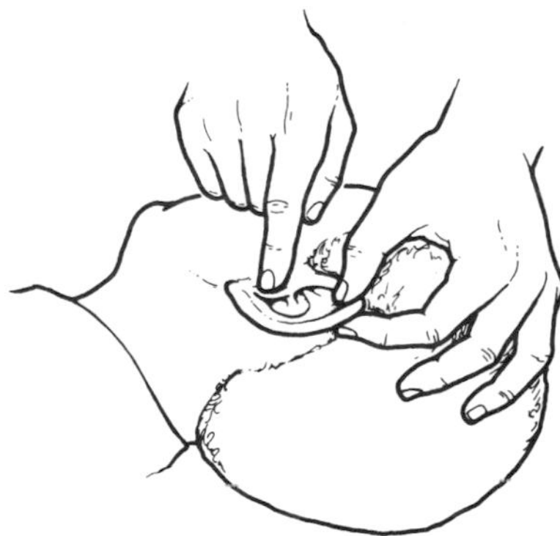

FIGURE **3** Rubbing ear to help drug flow to inside of ear.

PATIENT AND FAMILY EDUCATION

Giving Nose Drops

Your health professional has prescribed a special drug. This drug is placed in the child's nose. If the child is having trouble breathing and eating because of a stuffy nose, these nose drops may help the child. For this drug to have the most benefit, you should follow these instructions.

Equipment

Drug at room temperature

Clean tissues, clean washcloth, warm water

Instructions

1. Gather equipment.
2. Wash your hands with soap and water. Count to 10 while washing, then rinse with clear water and dry with a clean paper or cloth towel.
3. Remove any mucus from the nose with a clean tissue.
4. If the nose has crusted material around it, wet a washcloth with warm water and place this around the nose. Wait about 1 minute. Gently wipe the nose with the washcloth. If you cannot remove the crusting, rewet the washcloth and again place it around the nose. Continue using the warm, moist washcloth and gently wiping until all of the crusting is removed. Launder the washcloth before using it again.
5. Place the child on his back.
6. If the child will not lie still, have a helper hold the child. If you are alone, you can hold the child by sitting on a flat surface such as the floor or a bed. Place the child on his back with his head between your legs and his arms under your legs. If needed, you can cross your lower legs over the child's legs to keep him from moving (Figure 1).
7. Tilt the child's head backward by placing a pillow or rolled-up towel under the child's shoulders or letting the head hang over the side of a bed or your lap (Figure 2).
8. Open the bottle of nose drops.
9. Place the right number of drops in each side of the nose.
10. Keep the child's head tilted back for at least 1 minute (slowly count to 60) to prevent gagging or tasting the drug.
11. Hold and comfort the child.
12. PRAISE THE CHILD FOR HELPING.
13. Return the drug to a safe place out of the child's reach.
14. Write down the time you gave the child the drug, and check for the time you need to give the next dose.

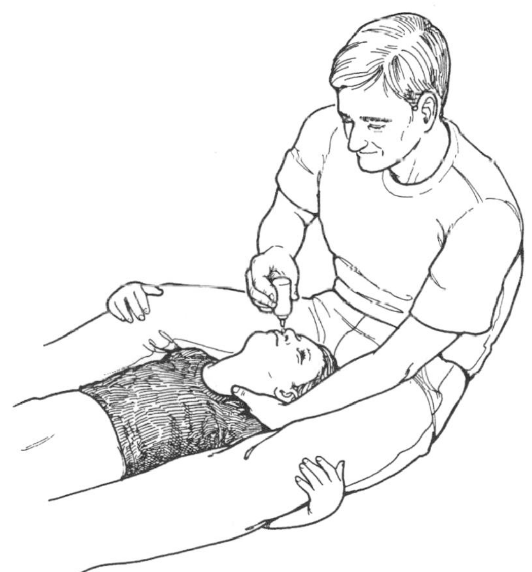

FIGURE 1 Safely holding child while giving nose drops.

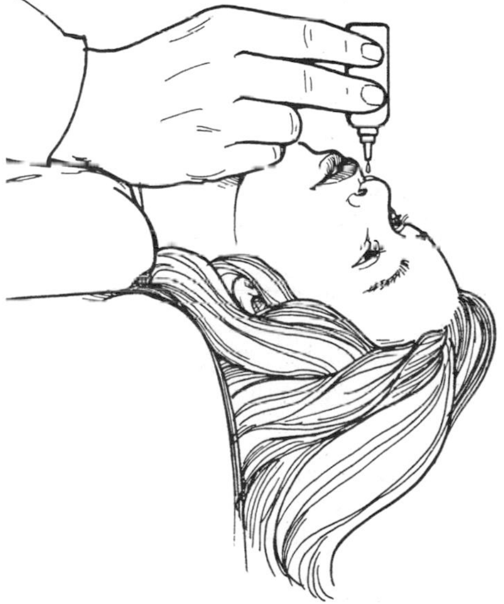

FIGURE 2 Correct position of child's head and neck for giving nose drops.

Spanish translation of this handout available at *http://evolve.elsevier.com/Wong/clinical.*

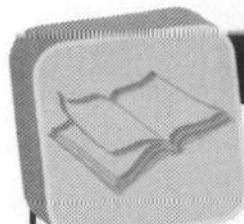

PATIENT AND FAMILY EDUCATION

Giving Inhaled Medications

Instructions

1. Remove the cap and hold inhaler upright.
2. Shake the inhaler.
3. Tilt your head back slightly, take a deep breath, and breathe out slowly.
4. Position the inhaler in one of the ways shown (Figure 1 or 2 is best, but Figure 3 is acceptable for those who have difficulty with 1 or 2. Figure 3 is required for breath-activated inhalers.) Figure 4 demonstrates a dry powder inhaler.
5. Press down on the inhaler to release medication as you start to breathe in slowly.
6. Breathe in slowly (3 to 5 seconds).
7. Hold your breath for 10 seconds to allow the medicine to reach deeply into your lungs.
8. Repeat puff as directed. Waiting 1 minute between puffs may permit second puff to penetrate your lungs better.
9. Spacers or holding chambers are useful for all patients. They are particularly recommended for young children and older adults and for use with inhaled steroids.

Avoid common inhaler mistakes. Follow these inhaler tips:

- Breathe out *before* pressing your inhaler.
- Inhale *slowly, evenly, and deeply.*
- Breathe in through your mouth, not your nose.
- Press down on your inhaler at the *start* of inhalation (or within the first second of inhalation).
- Keep inhaling as you press down on inhaler.
- Press your inhaler only *once* while you are inhaling (one breath for each puff).
- Make sure you breathe in evenly and deeply.

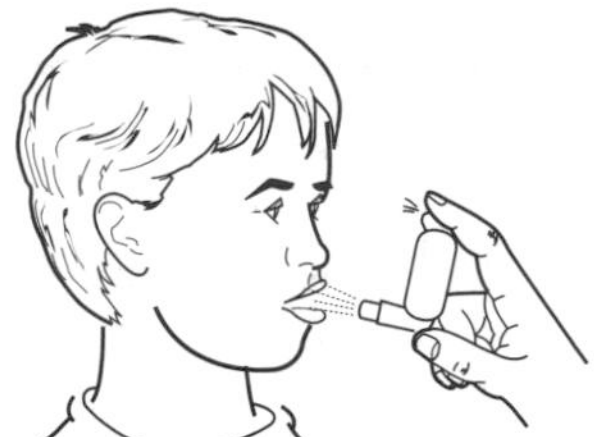

FIGURE **1** Open mouth with inhaler 1 to 2 inches away.

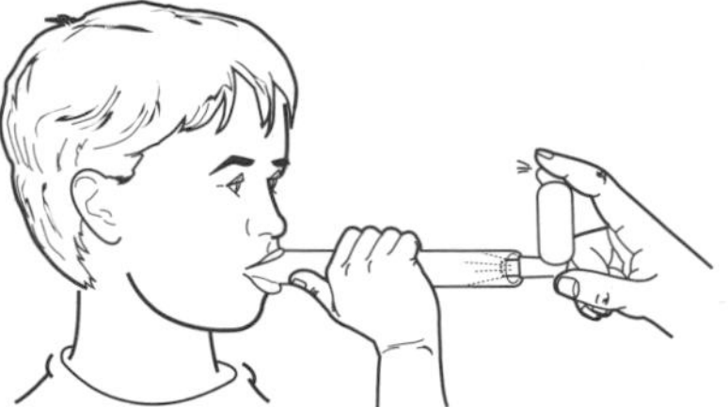

FIGURE **2** Use spacer or holding chamber (recommended especially for young children and for people using corticosteroids).

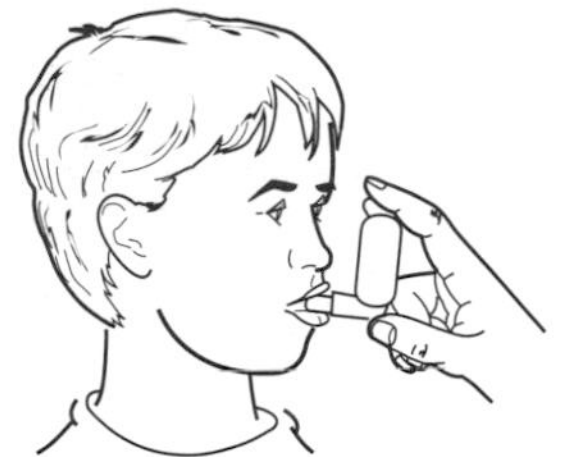

FIGURE **3** In the mouth. Do not use for corticosteroids.

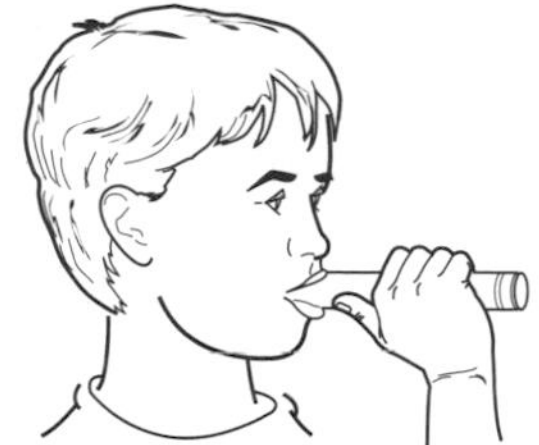

FIGURE **4** NOTE: Inhaled dry powder capsules require a different technique. To use a dry powder inhaler, it is important to close the mouth tightly around the mouthpiece of the inhaler and to inhale rapidly. (Figures 1 to 4 redrawn from the National Asthma Education and Prevention Program.)

Spanish translation of this handout available at *http://evolve.elsevier.com/Wong/clinical.*

PATIENT AND FAMILY EDUCATION

Asthma Medicine Plan

Asthma Medicine Plan

Name: ______________________

Doctor: ______________ **Date:** ________

Phone for doctor or clinic: ______________

Emergency contact phone and name: ______________

You can use the colors of a traffic light to help learn about your asthma medicines.

1. **Green** means **Go.** Use preventive medicine.
2. **Yellow** means **Caution.** Use quick-relief medicine.
3. **Red** means **Stop.** Get help from a doctor.

1. Green — Go

- Breathing is good
- No cough or wheeze
- Can work and play

Peak flow number ______ to ______

Personal best peak flow ________

Use preventive medicine.

Medicine	How much to take	When to take it

5 to 60 minutes before exercise, use this medicine: ______________

2. Yellow — Caution

Cough Wheeze Tight chest

Wake up at night

Peak flow number ______ to ______ (50 to 80% of my best peak flow)

Take quick-relief medicine to keep an asthma attack from getting bad

Medicine	How much to take	When to take it
(short-acting beta$_2$ agonist)		

If symptoms return to Green Zone after 1 hour of taking above quick-relief medication, take ________ (medicine) and ________ (medicine).

If symptoms **do not** return to Green Zone after 1 hour of taking the quick-relief medication, take ________ (medicine) and add ________ (medicine).
(short-acting beta$_2$ agonist) (oral steroid)

Call your doctor if symptoms do not improve within ____ hours after taking the oral steroid or if your symptoms are in the Red Zone.

3. Red — Stop — Danger

- Medicine is not helping
- Breathing is hard and fast
- Nose opens wide
- Can't walk
- Ribs show
- Can't talk well

Peak flow number ______ to ______ (50% or less of personal best)

Get help from a doctor now!
Take these medicines until you talk with the doctor.

Medicine	How much to take	When to take it
(short-acting beta$_2$ agonist)		
(oral steroid)		

Go to the emergency department immediately or call the ambulance if you cannot reach your doctor and you are still in the Red Zone after 15 minutes.

These signs signal **DANGER**:
- Difficulty walking or breathing
- Mental confusion
- Fingernails or lips are blue

Call the ambulance.

FIGURE **1** Example of an asthma action plan. (Redrawn from the National Asthma Education and Prevention Program. National Heart, Lung and Blood Institute: *Asthma management and prevention: global initiative for asthma,* NIH Publication No. 96-3659A, Washington, DC, 1995, National Institutes of Health.)

5 - PATIENT AND FAMILY EDUCATION

PATIENT AND FAMILY EDUCATION

Giving Aerosolized Medications (Nebulizer Treatments)

Nebulization is commonly referred to as a breathing treatment. It combines medications with humidified air to increase the effect of the medication on the child's airways and lungs.

Equipment

Medication ordered
Diluent such as normal saline (if needed)
Nebulizer medication chamber and tubing assembly
Small-volume nebulizer machine or oxygen (as directed by health professional)
Pediatric-sized aerosol mask, face tent, or tracheostomy mask.

Instructions

1. Inform child and family of the procedure.
2. Wash your hands with soap and water. Count to 10 while washing, then rinse with clear water and dry with a clean paper or cloth towel.
3. Assemble the nebulizer medication chamber and tubing according to manufacturer's instructions.
4. Attach aerosol tubing to nebulizer outlet port.
5. Place prescribed amount of medication in the nebulizer medication chamber.
6. Attach child's appliance (mouthpiece or mask).
7. Check to make sure connections are tight.
8. Have child hold the mouthpiece between the lips with gentle pressure.
9. Use a face mask for an infant or small child who is fatigued, who is not able to participate, or who will benefit from a mask (usually a child under 18 months gets better effect from treatment if a mask is used).
10. Use an adaptor or tracheostomy mask for child with a tracheostomy.
11. Turn on the nebulizer. A fine mist should appear in the mouthpiece or mask when the machine is working properly.
12. Have child sit in upright position. Most nebulizers work best when medication chamber is kept upright (if it is not upright, air bypasses the medication chamber and a mist is not formed). Infants can be placed upright in an infant seat or on the parent's lap facing away from the parent or held in a semisitting position cradled in one arm.
13. Tap nebulizer cup frequently to facilitate even distribution of medication.
14. Have child breathe normally during the treatment. There is no need for deep breathing. If the infant or toddler is crying, the medication will still be effective if administered according to these steps.
15. When the liquid medication is gone and mist no longer forms, turn off machine.
16. If steroids were nebulized, have child gargle with warm water after the treatment.
17. Observe the child's response to the treatment with regard to ease of breathing, wheezing, color, and activity.
18. Repeat the treatment as necessary according to child's status and health professional's directions. In some situations, the health professional may recommend repeating the treatments three times back to back (check with health professional before doing this).
19. Clean the medication chamber, mouthpiece, and T-piece with soap and water after each use. Set pieces out on a clean surface to dry. *Do not wash the tubing.*
20. Replace filter and tubing per manufacturer's recommendations.

GUIDELINES

Administering Digoxin at Home

Give digoxin at regular intervals (usually every 12 hours, such as at 8 AM and 8 PM; in some children it may be give every 24 hours).

Plan the times so that the drug is given *1 hour before* or *2 hours after* feedings.

Use a calendar to mark off each dose that is given; or post a reminder, such as a sign on the refrigerator.

Have the prescription refilled *before* the medication is completely used.

Do not mix it with other foods or fluids, because refusal to consume these results in inaccurate intake of the drug.

If the child has teeth, give water after administering the drug; whenever possible, brush the teeth to prevent tooth decay from the sweetened liquid.

If a dose is missed and more than 4 hours have elapsed, withhold the dose and give the next dose at the regular time; if less than 4 hours have elapsed, give the missed dose.

If the child vomits within 1 hour of receiving the dose, do not give a second dose.

If more than two consecutive doses have been missed, notify the physician or other designated health professional.

Do not increase or double the dose for missed doses.

Avoid administration with herbal preparations such as St. John's wort or Siberian ginseng because these may change the medication's intended effect on the heart.

Notify your child's health practitioner if you need to give the child any over-the-counter medications.

If the child becomes ill with any of the following, notify the physician or other designated health professional immediately:

- Diarrhea
- Nausea
- Vision changes
- Lack of appetite
- Vomiting

Keep digoxin in a safe place, preferably a locked cabinet.

In case of accidental overdose of digoxin, call the nearest poison control center immediately or the national number, (800) 222-1222; the number is usually listed in the front of the telephone directory.

See also Giving Oral Medications, p. 523.

PATIENT AND FAMILY EDUCATION

Applying a Topical Anesthetic

Your health professional has prescribed a topical anesthetic medicine for your child to decrease pain associated with a procedure such as an injection or accessing an implanted port. There are several topical anesthetics available; the time it takes the medication to actually "work" and numb the site varies, so it is important to follow the health professional's directions carefully. Some general guidelines are presented for two common topical anesthetics, EMLA and LMX4. EMLA stands for *eutectic mixture of local anesthetics.* A topical anesthetic is a medicine that is placed on normal, healthy skin to make it numb. EMLA contains two anesthetics, lidocaine and prilocaine. Be sure to tell your health professional if your child has an allergy to either of these medicines before using EMLA. Use only the amount of EMLA that has been prescribed.

EMLA comes in a cream; the anesthetic disk is no longer available. The cream must be covered with the dressing that comes with the 5-g tube. There is also a 30-g tube that is useful if you need to apply the cream several times. A transparent dressing, which is a clear plastic film with adhesive (sticky) edges, is placed over the cream. If you do not have this dressing, you can cover the cream with ordinary plastic film, such as Saran Wrap, and seal the edges of the plastic to the skin with tape. You cannot use ordinary Band-Aids because the cream will leak out.

LMX4 is a 4% liposomal lidocaine preparation that is applied just like EMLA; the main difference is that LMX4 is reported to numb the skin within 30 minutes. The site should not have any alcohol-based product before application of this anesthetic. This topical anesthetic is available without a prescription; however, you should consult your health professional regarding the size of the tube to be purchased.

In Canada a 4% amethocaine topical gel (Ametop) may be used. This topical anesthetic is applied in the same manner as EMLA but takes only 30 minutes to be effective. Consult your health professional for use of Ametop gel.

The general directions that follow address EMLA; however, keep in mind that except for the time of application, all three are essentially applied in the same manner.

Equipment

EMLA cream or LMX4 cream
Transparent dressing
Plastic film and tape (if needed)
Ballpoint pen or marker
Tissue or paper towel

General Instructions

1. Make sure that the area to which you apply the topical anesthetic is clean and dry and that the skin has no open areas or sores. Do not apply the medicine near the eye, in the ear, or in the mouth.
2. If you are not sure of where to apply the topical anesthetic, ask your health professional to mark the place on the drawing in Figure 1 (next page).
3. For a blood sample or when an intravenous (IV) line is needed, apply to two or more areas in case more than one try is needed to get into the vein.
4. If your child is young and afraid of needles, you can tell your child that the topical anesthetic is like a "magic cream that takes hurt away." Tap or lightly scratch an area of skin to show your child that "the skin is now awake." After removing the topical anesthetic again tap or lightly scratch the skin to show your child that "the skin is now asleep" so that it cannot feel a needle.
5. To prevent small children from playing with the cream under the clear dressing, cover it with a tissue or paper towel and a little tape.
6. Leave the topical anesthetic EMLA on the skin for at least 60 minutes for a puncture, such as a vein or fingerstick, and at least 2 to 2½ hours for an intramuscular (IM) injection or biopsy. EMLA may need to be kept on longer if your child has dark or thicker skin. LMX4 and Ametop usually require application for only 30 minutes before the procedure. LMX4 should not be left on the skin longer than 2 hours.
7. After removing the cream, see if the skin is pale or reddened. If there is no visible skin change, leave EMLA on longer, but not longer than 4 hours.
8. PRAISE THE CHILD FOR HELPING.
9. Return the drug to a safe place out of the child's reach.

Instructions for EMLA Cream and LMX4 cream

1. Unscrew the cap, and puncture the metal covering of the tube with the point on the top of the cap.
2. EMLA: Apply half of the 5-g tube in a thick layer to about a 2-inch by 2-inch area of skin where the procedure will be done (Figure 2). If the puncture area is very small, such as a finger stick, you can use a third of the tube.

   LMX4: Apply a pea-sized amount to the area of skin to be numbed and rub it in for approximately 30 seconds. Then apply a larger dollop (approximately 2.5 g or ½ of a 5-g tube) over the area and apply the dressing.
3. Remove the center cutout piece of the transparent dressing (Figure 3).
4. Peel the paper liner from the paper-framed dressing (Figure 4).
5. Cover the topical anesthetic cream so that you get a thick layer underneath. Do not spread out the cream. Smooth down the dressing edges carefully, and be sure it is secure to avoid leakage (Figure 5).

5 - PATIENT AND FAMILY EDUCATION

PATIENT AND FAMILY EDUCATION

Applying a Topical Anesthetic—cont'd

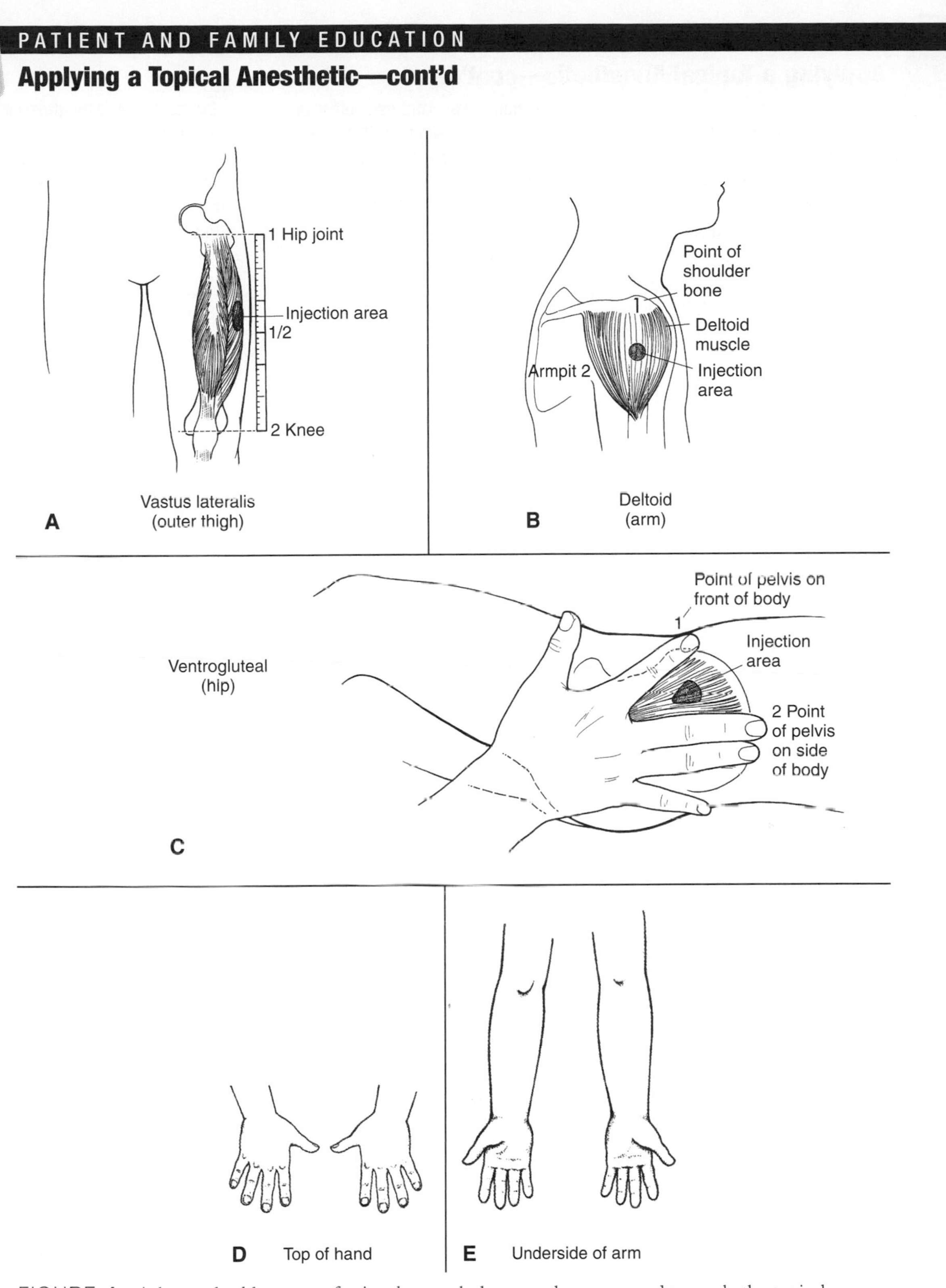

FIGURE **1** Ask your health care professional to mark the area where you need to apply the topical anesthetic. The numbers on **A** to **C** mark the places used to find the injection areas.

Continued

PATIENT AND FAMILY EDUCATION

Applying a Topical Anesthetic—cont'd

6. Remove the paper frame (Figure 6). Mark directly on the occlusive dressing the time you applied the cream.
7. To remove the transparent dressing, grasp opposite sides of the film and pull the sides away from each other to stretch and loosen the film. After the film begins to loosen, grasp the other two sides of the film and pull. This method is easier and more comfortable than pulling the dressing up and off the skin.
8. Wipe off the topical anesthetic cream with a tissue. The numbing effect can last 1 hour or more after removing the dressing.

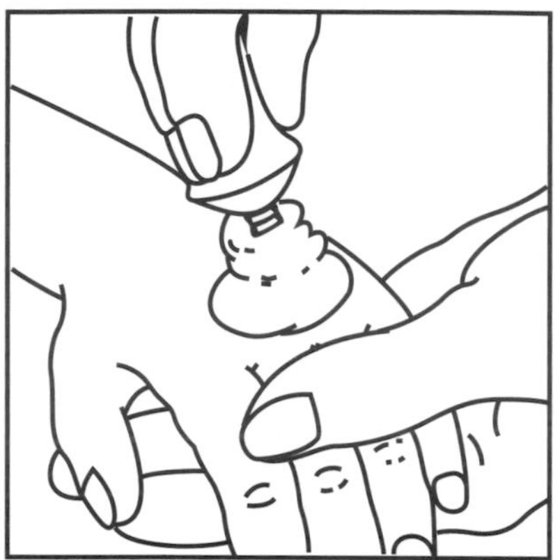

FIGURE **2** Apply 2.5 g of topical anesthetic cream (half the 5-g tube) in a thick layer at the site.

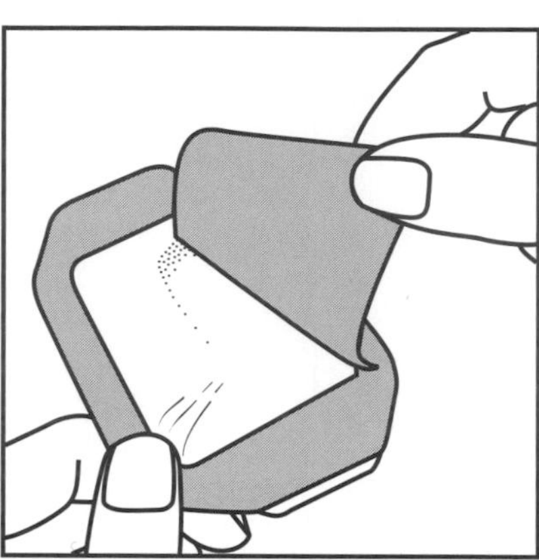

FIGURE **3** Take an occlusive (transparent) dressing and remove the center cutout piece.

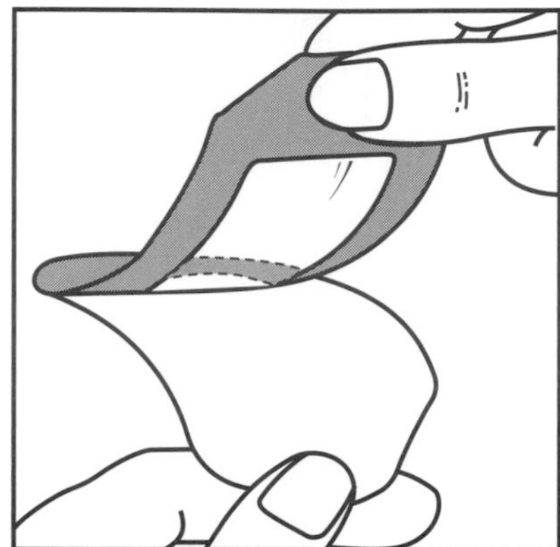

FIGURE **4** Peel the paper liner from the paper-framed dressing.

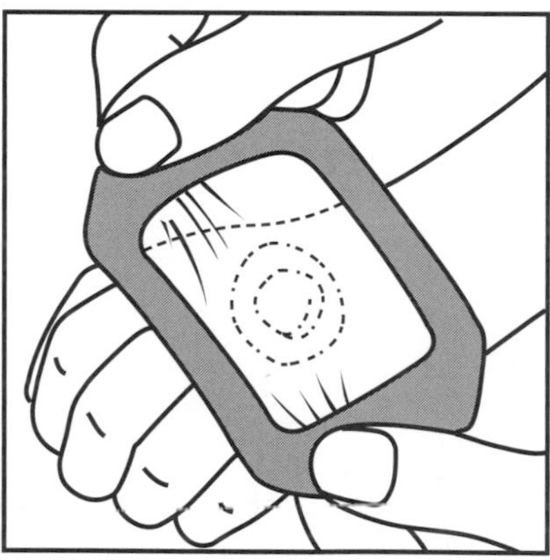

FIGURE **5** Cover the topical anesthetic cream so that you get a thick layer underneath. Smooth the dressing edges carefully to avoid leakage.

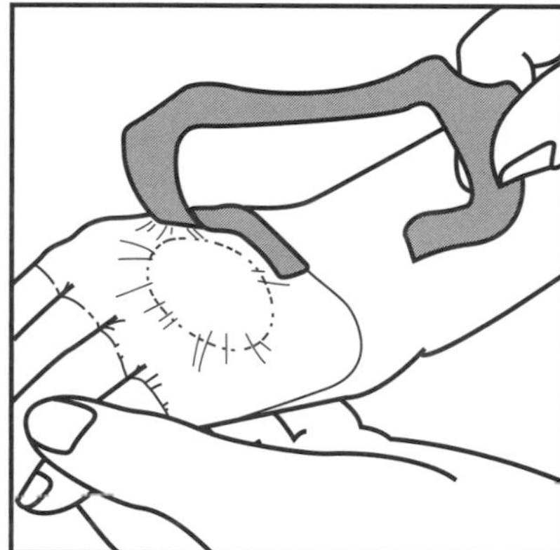

FIGURE **6** Remove the paper frame. Mark the time of application directly on the occlusive dressing. (Figures 2 to 6: EMLA® Cream is a registered trademark of Abraxis BioScience, Inc., and is manufactured by Abraxis BioScience, Inc., for use in the United States only.)

Instructions Related to Alternative Feeding Techniques and Elimination

PATIENT AND FAMILY EDUCATION

Giving Nasogastric Tube Feedings

For the child to obtain enough food to grow, you must feed her by tube. If the child is active, you will need someone to hold the child while you insert the tube. After the tube is securely in place, you should hold and cuddle the child during the feeding.

You should give the child _________ ounces of _________ every _________ hours.

Call your health professional at ____________________ if any of the following occur:

- Vomiting
- Change in color of stomach contents
- Increased amount of stomach contents before feeding
- Increased bowel movements
- You are unable to put in the tube.
- The child becomes very irritable.
- Two meals are missed because of too much food in the stomach.

Equipment

Liquid food at room temperature and water in pour container
Feeding tube
½-inch tape
Water
Syringe
Stethoscope

Instructions

1. Gather equipment.
2. Wash your hands with soap and water. Count to 10 while washing, then rinse with clear water and dry with a clean paper or cloth towel.
3. Cut a piece of tape. You will need this to mark the right distance and to hold the tube in place during the feeding.
4. Tell the child (even if infant) what you will be doing.
5. Place the child on your lap, on her right side, or reclining in an infant seat.
6. Use a pacifier for the infant to enjoy sucking during the feeding.
7. Measure the tube for the exact distance you will have to insert it.
   a. Hold the tip of the tube on the child's stomach (midway between the bellybutton and the highest point of the lower rib cage).
   b. Extend the tube up to the child's earlobe, then out to the nose (Figure 1).
   c. Mark the spot at the nose with the piece of tape.
8. Dip the tip of the tube in clear water to moisten.
9. Insert the tip of the tube into one nostril, guiding it toward the back of the child's throat.
10. If the child is able to help, have her swallow the tube to help it pass.
11. Quickly insert the tube to the tape mark on the tube. If the child begins coughing or has any other problems, remove the tube at once.

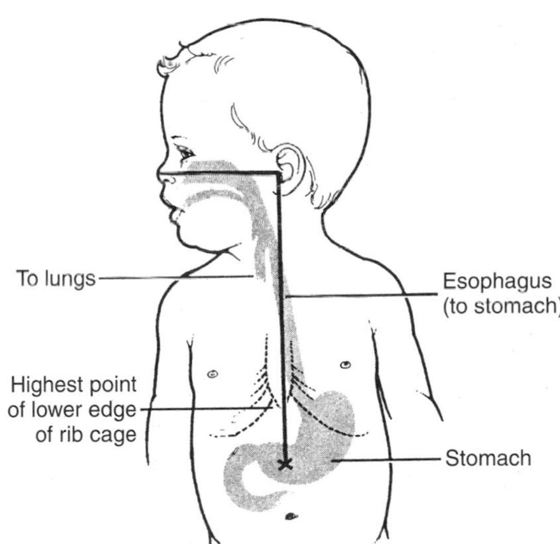

FIGURE 1 Measuring length of tube to insert: from midway between bellybutton and highest point of lower rib cage; to earlobe; to nose.

Continued

5 - PATIENT AND FAMILY EDUCATION

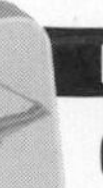

PATIENT AND FAMILY EDUCATION

Giving Nasogastric Tube Feedings—cont'd

12. Tape tube to child's upper lip and cheek (Figure 2). If child wants to pull the tube, tape it down the back to keep it out of reach. Be sure tube is not compressed or kinked.
13. Check the placement of the tube.*
    a. Place 5 ml of air in the syringe. Connect the syringe to the tube.
    b. Place the stethoscope over the child's stomach area.
    c. Inject the air quickly into the tube while listening for the sound of gurgling through the stethoscope.
    d. Remove the air by gently pulling plunger back to the 5-ml mark.
    e. If stomach contents appear in the tube as you pull the plunger back, the tube is in the correct place.
    f. If you are unable to see any stomach contents in the tube, place the child on the left side or advance the tube a short distance. Pull plunger back again to check for stomach contents.
    g. If more than one fourth of the last feeding is still present, return the food to the stomach and wait 30 to 60 minutes. When there is less than one fourth of the amount of food, return the stomach contents and feed the child.
14. Check temperature of food to be given; it should be room temperature.
15. Disconnect the syringe from the tube, and remove the plunger from the syringe.
16. Reconnect the syringe to the tube.
17. Fill the syringe with the right amount of food.
18. If necessary, push gently with the plunger to start the flow of food; then remove the plunger and allow the food to flow by itself. Do not forcefully push on plunger to speed up the feeding. If the feeding is pushed back into the feeding syringe instead of flowing by gravity, leave the plunger in the barrel of the syringe until the feeding is completed.
19. The bottom of the syringe should never be held higher than the child's chin, or 6 inches above the level of the child's stomach (Figure 3).
20. Continue adding food until the right amount has been fed. Do not allow the syringe to become empty.
21. When the food is at the bottom of the syringe, add 1 to 2 teaspoons (5 to 10 ml) (or the amount specified by your health professional) of water to rinse the tube.
22. Place the clamp on the tube if it will be left in place between feedings.
23. Hold, cuddle, and burp the child.
24. PRAISE THE CHILD FOR HELPING.
25. Write down the time and amount of the child's feeding. Use the other nostril for the next insertion.

To Remove the Tube

1. Loosen the tape holding the tube.
2. Fold the tube, and pinch it tightly together.
3. Pull the tube out quickly.
4. Hold, cuddle, and burp the child.

Care of the Nasogastric Tube and Syringe

Wash with soap and water, and rinse the inside well with clear water. Dry the syringe, plunger, and tube. Put plunger in syringe when dry, and store everything in a clean, dry container (e.g., plastic bag, margarine container).

If the tube remains in place between feedings, look at the nose before each feeding for redness. *Always* check to make sure the tube is in the right place before adding formula (step 13). Change the tube every ________ days.

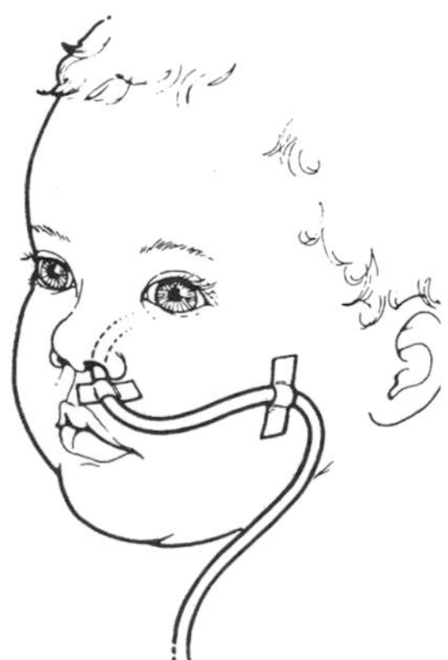

FIGURE 2 Taping tube to keep from injuring child's nose.

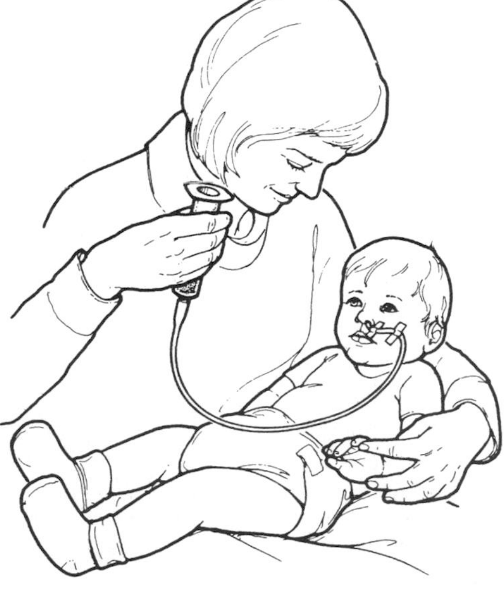

FIGURE 3 Comforting child during feeding.

*If your health professional advises you to test the stomach contents' pH (acidity), as well as to listen with a stethoscope to confirm placement, follow directions for pH testing. At the time of this writing, a pH greater than or equal to 5 obtained on stomach aspirate is confirmation of adequate placement in children (Ellett MLC, Croffie JMB, Cohen MD, Perkins SM: Gastric tube placement in young children, *Clin Nurs Res* 14(3):238-252, 2005).

PATIENT AND FAMILY EDUCATION

Giving Gastrostomy Feedings

To help the child get enough food to grow, an opening was made into the child's stomach for a gastrostomy feeding tube. There are several types of gastrostomy feeding devices. Your health professional chose the one that is best for your child. It is very important that the brand and size of the feeding and/or decompression tube match the device in the child. If a gastrostomy tube has been put into this opening, you can now feed the child through this. If your child has a skin-level device instead of a tube, instructions for feeding are on p. 552. You should hold and cuddle the child during the feeding.

You should give the child ________ ounces of ________ every ________ hours.

Call your health professional at ________ if any of the following occurs:

- Vomiting
- Change in color of stomach contents
- Increased amount of stomach contents before feeding
- Change in color of mucus
- Increased bowel movements
- The child becomes very irritable.
- Increased redness around gastrostomy site
- Two meals are missed because of too much food in the stomach.

Gastrostomy Tube Feeding

Equipment

Liquid food at room temperature in pour container
Water to rinse tube
Syringe

Instructions

1. Gather equipment.
2. Wash your hands with soap and water. Count to 10 while washing, then rinse with clear water and dry with a clean paper or cloth towel.
3. Tell the child (even if infant) what you will be doing.
4. Place the child on your lap or reclining in an infant seat. The older child can sit in a chair or on a bed.
5. Use a pacifier for the infant to enjoy sucking during the feeding.
6. Attach the syringe to the gastrostomy tube.
7. Unclamp the tube.
8. Pull back gently on the plunger to see the amount of food left in the child's stomach.
9. If more than one fourth of the last feeding is still present, return the food to the stomach and wait 30 to 60 minutes. When there is less than one fourth of the amount of food, feed the child.
10. Remove the plunger from the syringe. Hold syringe and tubing below stomach level when filling syringe to prevent excess air getting into stomach.
11. Fill syringe with the right amount of food.
12. A gentle push with the plunger of the syringe may be necessary to start the flow of food; then remove the plunger and allow the food to flow by itself. Do not forcefully push on plunger to speed up the feeding. If the feeding is pushed back into the feeding syringe instead of flowing by gravity, leave the plunger in the barrel of the syringe until the feeding is completed.
13. Never hold the bottom of the syringe higher than the child's chin (Figure 1).
14. Continue adding food to the syringe until you have finished the right amount. Do not let the syringe become empty.
15. When the food is at the bottom of the syringe add water (1 to 2 teaspoons [5 to 10 ml] or the amount specified by your health professional) to rinse the tube and keep it from clogging.
16. Clamp the tube and remove the syringe.
17. Gently pull the tube to allow the balloon to rest against the inside of the stomach at the opening.

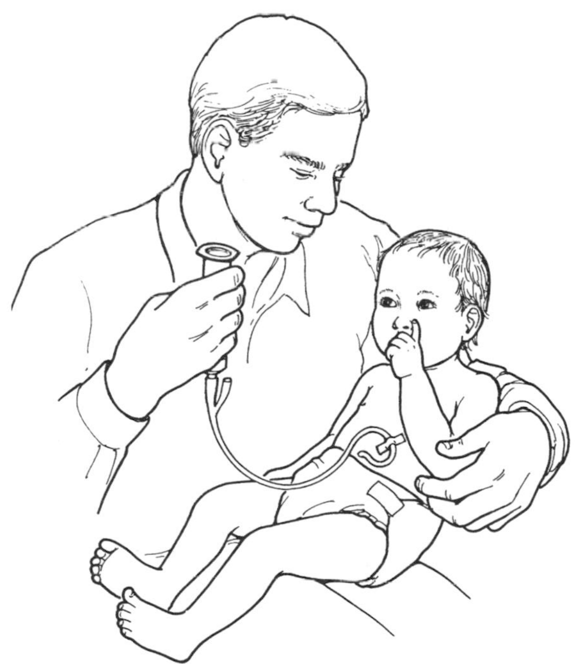

FIGURE 1 Feeding the child with a gastrostomy tube. Note that the bottom of the syringe is at the level of child's shoulder.

Continued

PATIENT AND FAMILY EDUCATION

Giving Gastrostomy Feedings—cont'd

18. Tape the tube to the skin to prevent it from advancing or allowing stomach contents to leak on the skin.
19. Hold and cuddle child after the feeding.
20. PRAISE THE CHILD FOR HELPING.

Wash the syringe in soap and warm water using a bottle brush. Rinse the inside well with clear water. Dry the syringe and plunger. Put plunger in syringe when dry, and store in a clean dry container between feedings (e.g., plastic bag, margarine container).

Care of a Gastrostomy Tube

Some gastrostomy tubes can be removed at home for placement of a new tube. Consult your child's health care practitioner about the type of gastrostomy tube your child has to make sure it can be safely removed by a parent or caretaker. This procedure describes the care of the Foley-type gastrostomy tube.

The gastrostomy tube should be changed ______________________.
If the tube accidentally comes out, it should be put back into the opening in the stomach as quickly as possible with the same tube or a new tube of the same size. Tape the tube to prevent it from coming out. A moist gauze bandage can be placed over the opening until you can get to a quiet place where you can reinsert the tube. When you are away from home and the child will need to be fed, you should carry an extra gastrostomy tube with you in case something happens to the tube that is in place.

Equipment

Gastrostomy tube
Water for lubricant
Small syringe
Water or air if needed for balloon
Tape

Removing the Tube

Remove the tube just before feeding so that there will be only a small amount of liquid in the child's stomach.

1. Gather equipment.
2. Wash your hands with soap and water. Count to 10 while washing, then rinse with clear water and dry with a clean paper or cloth towel.
3. Tell the child what you will be doing.
4. Lay the child flat to ensure a straight tract to insert tube into.
5. Attach the small syringe to the tube at point A (Figure 2).
6. Unclamp the tube and withdraw the air or water from the balloon.
7. Reclamp the tube and quickly remove it, holding the tip up to prevent stomach contents from dripping.
8. Place it out of the child's reach while you replace the new tube.

Inserting the Tube

1. Wet the tip of the clean tube with water.
2. Put the tip of the tube through the opening into the child's stomach.
3. Insert the tube beyond the balloon on the tip (Figure 3).
4. Connect the syringe, containing ________ ml of air or water, to the tube at point A.
5. Inject the air or water into the tube at point A.
6. Gently pull on the tube to make sure the balloon is inflated and the tube is in position.
7. Tape the tube securely to the child's abdomen.
8. Clamp the new tube until you are ready for the next feeding

The gastrostomy tube that you have removed should be cleaned in soap and water. Rinse the inside of the tube well with clear water. Dry the tube and store in a clean, dry container (e.g., plastic bag, margarine container).

Skin-Level Device Feeding

Equipment

Liquid food at room temperature in pour container
Feeding tube with adapter.
Clamp (usually on the feeding tube)
Water to rinse tube
Syringe

Instructions

1. Gather equipment.
2. Wash your hands with soap and water. Count to 10 while washing, then rinse with clear water and dry with a clean paper or cloth towel.
3. Tell the child (even if infant) what you will be doing.
4. Place the child on your lap or reclining in an infant seat. The older child can sit on a chair or a bed.
5. Use a pacifier for the infant to enjoy sucking during the feeding.

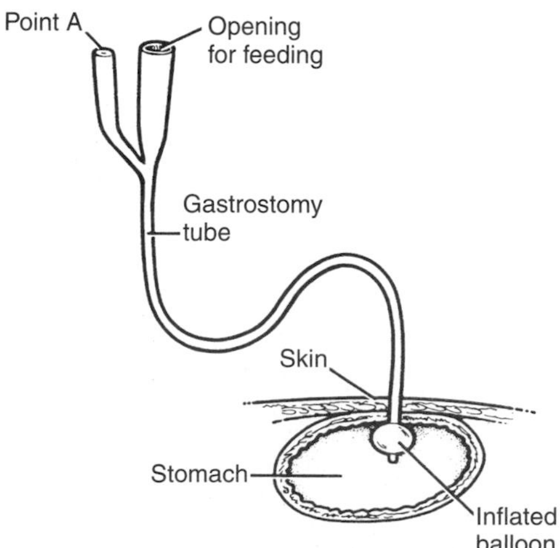

FIGURE 2 Diagram of a gastrostomy tube. Point A is used to inflate the balloon. The other opening is for the feeding syringe.

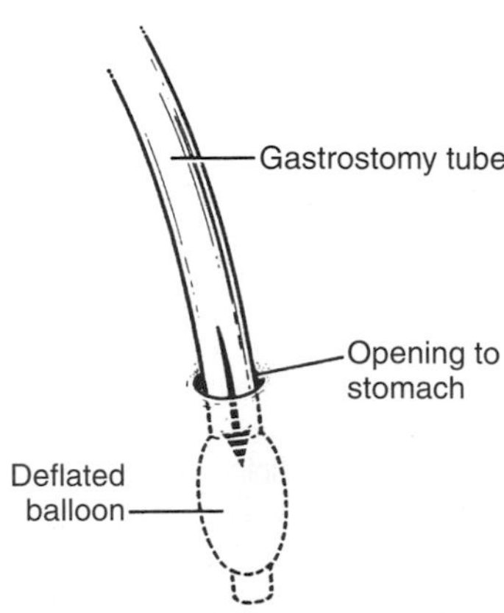

FIGURE 3 Gastrostomy tube in stomach with balloon deflated.

PATIENT AND FAMILY EDUCATION

Giving Gastrostomy Feedings—cont'd

6. If the stomach seems full and gassy, air can be removed by putting the feeding tube adapter into the skin-level device and opening the safety plug on the skin-level device.
7. Align the black line on the feeding tube adapter with the black line on the skin-level device.
8. Turn the feeding tube adapter to the right to lock the feeding tube in place and prevent accidental disconnection and leaking (Figure 4).
9. Attach syringe to the tubing and unclamp the tubing. If more than a fourth of the previous feeding comes out, wait 1 hour before feeding and try again.
10. Place the desired amount of formula or liquid food in the syringe. This keeps too much air from going into the stomach.
11. A gentle push with the syringe plunger may be necessary to start the flow of food; then remove the plunger and allow the food to flow by itself. Do not forcefully push on plunger to speed up the feeding. If the feeding is pushed back into the feeding syringe instead of flowing by gravity, leave the plunger in the barrel of the syringe until the feeding is completed.
12. Avoid holding the bottom of the syringe higher than the child's chin.
13. Continue adding formula or food to the syringe until you have finished the right amount. Do not let the syringe become empty.
14. When the food is at the bottom of the syringe, add 1 to 2 teaspoons (5 to 10 ml) (or the amount specified by your health professional) of water to rinse the tube.
15. Clamp the tubing and remove the tube from the G-button device by unlocking the adapter and feeding tube.
16. Replace the safety plug on the device.
17. Hold and cuddle the child after the feeding.
18. PRAISE THE CHILD FOR HELPING.

Rinse the tubing and syringe with water after each feeding. Each day, wash the syringe and tube in warm, soapy water. Use a bottle brush for the syringe, and pipe cleaners for the tubing. Rinse the inside well with clear water. If a milky coating is on the inside of the syringe or tubing, use a solution of 1 part vinegar to 2 parts water to clean the inside before the soapy wash and rinse.

Care of the Skin-Level Device (G-Button)
Clean around the site each day with mild soap and water. Clean the button with a cotton-tip applicator to remove encrusted formula.

Turn the button around in a complete circle to make sure it is completely cleaned. Dry the area and leave it exposed to air for about 20 minutes so it can dry completely. When your child is allowed tub baths, always close the safety plug of the device before placing your child in the water. If the device is leaking contact your health professional; a small amount of leakage (less than 1 teaspoon) may occur on occasion, but more than that may lead to problems with the skin around the hole.

Check the device at least once a week (or more if leakage is noted) by placing a 6-ml syringe on the side port and withdrawing the water from the balloon to make sure it is properly inflated. Keep your hand on the device to prevent it from coming out while the balloon is deflated—it may be necessary to have a helper keep pressure on the button device while doing this. Most skin-level devices have a balloon that requires 5 ml (1 teaspoon) of water—proper inflation maintains the seal and prevents leaking.

Medications can plug the device. Medicines in tablet form should be crushed well and mixed with water or food before putting them in the feeding syringe. Thick liquids can be mixed with warm water to make them thinner. The medicine should be given before the feeding, to make sure the medicine goes into the stomach. If it is not time for a feeding, rinse the tubing with 1 to 2 teaspoons (5 to 10 ml) of water after giving the medicine.

If your child is on continuous feedings, flush the device and tubing with water (1 to 2 teaspoons [5 to 10 ml] or the amount specified by your health professional) to rinse the tube and keep it from clogging.

Troubleshooting the Skin-Level Device
If the device accidentally comes out, it is not an emergency. Do not throw the device away. Place a clean dressing over the site and call your child's health professional. Once the tube tract has formed (usually 6 to 12 weeks), the surgeon will approve of you changing the tube if it comes out. Follow the directions given by the health professional in charge of the child's gastrostomy tube care, or follow these steps if the device comes out:

- Examine the device carefully; if the balloon has completely deflated or is partially empty, attach a 6-ml syringe to the port on the side of the button device and try to inflate the balloon.

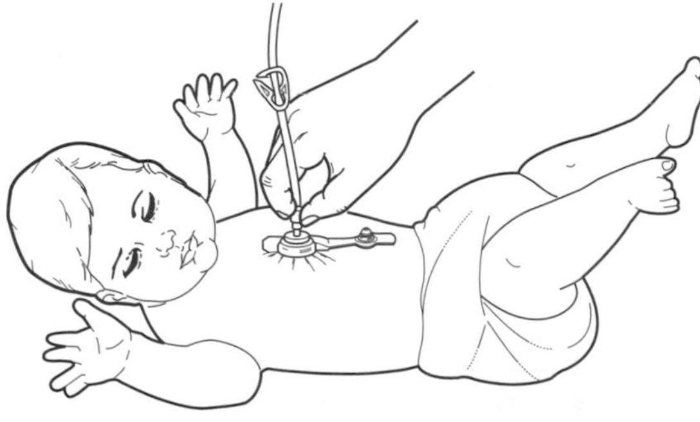

FIGURE 4 Example of skin level device (G-button).

Continued

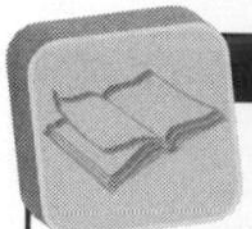

PATIENT AND FAMILY EDUCATION

Giving Gastrostomy Feedings—cont'd

- If the balloon will not inflate and appears to be ruptured, apply a small amount of water-soluble lubricant to the tip of the tube and replace the tube into the stomach hole and tape it in place.
- If the balloon has simply discharged some or all of its water but still inflates, withdraw all the water from the balloon with the 6-ml syringe, apply a small amount of water-soluble lubricant to the tip of the tube, and insert the tube into the stomach hole. Then reinflate the balloon by pushing 5-ml of water into the side port with the 6-ml syringe. The balloon will inflate and hold the tube in place as shown in Figure 2 on p. 552. If the device comes out and you cannot replace the tube into the stomach hole, place a gastrostomy tube into the opening as you were taught, or follow the instructions on p. 552. Use the gastrostomy tube for feedings until you can contact your health professional.*

Skin Care

Keep the skin around the gastrostomy tube or skin-level device clean and dry. A bandage does not have to be put over the area. A cloth diaper or cotton cloth can be wrapped around the child's abdomen and secured with tape. This will keep the child from playing with the tube. Other ways to keep the tube out of reach are to use one-piece outfits, tube tops, the tops of panty hose, or children's tights with the legs cut off.

Zinc oxide ointment, Duoderm-CGF (a thin dressing that can be kept on the skin for 7 days), Pro Shield Plus Skin Protectant, Cavilon No Sting Barrier Film (spray or foam), or any other skin barrier can be used on the skin around the gastrostomy tube or skin-level device. A single-layer 2 × 2 gauze pad may also be placed around the tube or device. (Do not use a large or thick dressing under the skin-level button device unless directed by the health professional because this may stretch the feeding tube and eventually cause more leaking.) It should be changed at least daily or when soiled. These measures will provide protection for the skin in case there is a small leakage of gastric fluid. If the area becomes red or sore or if drainage continues to be a problem after every feeding, call your health professional at ________________ for further directions.

Clothing

Dress the child in loose-fitting clothing that does not press the gastrostomy tube against the skin. Bib-type overalls are preferable to pants. The overalls cover the tube, making it less likely that the child or other children will play with the tube. Also, wearing overalls avoids tight elastic around the child's waist.

*See also Burd A, Burd RS: The who, what, why, and how-to guide to gastrostomy tube placement in infants, *Adv Neonatal Care* 3(4):197-205, 2003.

PATIENT AND FAMILY EDUCATION

Performing Clean Intermittent Bladder Catheterization*

The child is unable to empty the bladder of urine. A catheter (tube) can be put into the bladder to let the urine come out by itself. This will help the child to remain dry and will help prevent bladder infections.

Catheterization should be done when the child wakes up in the morning, before bedtime, and every ________ hours during the day. If the child is unable to do the catheterization alone, someone at school should be taught to help the child. Stopping fluids 2 hours before bedtime may help the child stay dry through the night.

In some situations a record should be kept of all that the child drinks and the amount of urine that was obtained by catheterization. (See sample on p. 556.) A description of the urine is helpful so that you can notice changes that may be caused by an infection. Look at the urine to see if it is cloudy or clear, pale yellow or dark amber. Smell it to tell if a strange odor is present.

Call your health professional at ______________ if any of these occurs:

- Temperature above 101° F
- Trouble inserting the tube
- Change in the amount of urine
- Change in the way the urine looks or smells
- Pain with insertion

Equipment

Catheter and storage container
Soap and water with washcloth or unscented towelettes or baby wipes
Urine container or absorbent diaper
Water-soluble lubricant†

Instructions for Boys

1. Have equipment ready; keep the tube in its container until you are ready to use it.
2. Wash your hands with soap and water. Count to 10 while washing, then rinse with clear water and dry with a clean paper or cloth towel.
3. Tell the child what you will be doing.
4. Catheterization can be done sitting, standing, or lying down.
5. Remove or arrange the child's clothing so that it will not get wet and the urine can flow.
6. Wet the first 2 inches of the tube, either by placing lubricant on your

*You can use these instructions if your child does self-catheterization, but be sure your child washes his hands before and after the procedure.
†Your health professional may recommend the use of a lidocaine lubricant to decrease the discomfort of urinary catheterization.

PATIENT AND FAMILY EDUCATION

Performing Clean Intermittent Bladder Catheterization—cont'd

finger and spreading it on the tube or by dipping the catheter into the lubricant on a clean tissue or paper towel.

7. Hold penis straight; if the child is uncircumcised, pull the foreskin back as far as it will go without forcing it.
8. Wipe the tip of the penis with towelette, baby wipe, or a clean washcloth with soap and water.
9. Hold the penis upright. Push the tube into the urinary opening gently (Figure 1). Just before the bladder you may feel some resistance. Do not push the tube in and out if resistance is met. Hold the tube and continue to move it in slowly, using gentle but firm pressure until the muscle relaxes.
10. Tell the child to take a deep breath and slowly let it out. This helps the child to relax.
11. Continue to insert the catheter until urine begins to flow. Then insert the tube about another ½ inch and hold it there until urine stops flowing. Allow the urine to drain into a container or absorbent diaper, which can then be discarded.
12. Push the foreskin forward if needed. Do not leave it pulled back.
13. Let all of the urine flow out.
14. Tell the child to squeeze his belly as if he were having a bowel movement or to blow bubbles or a pinwheel. This helps empty all the urine out of the bladder.
15. Slowly remove the tube; if urine begins to flow again, stop removing the tube and allow it to empty.
16. Wash your hands and the catheter with soap and water. Rinse the inside of the tube well with clear water.
17. PRAISE THE CHILD FOR HELPING.
18. Dry the catheter with a clean paper or cloth towel, and store in a clean, dry container (e.g., plastic bag or margarine container).
19. Write down the time; whether the underwear or diaper was wet, damp, or dry; and the amount and the way the urine looks.
20. Never reuse a catheter that appears rough, stiff, kinked, worn, discolored, or damaged in any way.
21. Your health professional will tell you how often a new catheter should be used.

Instructions for Girls

1. Gather equipment; keep the tube in its container until you are ready to use it.
2. Wash your hands with soap and water. Count to 10 while washing, then rinse with clear water and dry with a clean paper or cloth towel.
3. Tell the child what you will be doing.
4. Remove or arrange the child's clothing so it will not get wet and urine can flow.
5. Position the girl as comfortably as possible, either lying down with her knees bent in a froglike position, or sitting with legs spread apart for self-catheterization.
6. Separate the labia with the thumb and forefinger and locate the urinary opening (urethra) (Figure 2). A mirror can be used to teach the child self-catheterization.
7. Wash the labia one or two times with the unscented towelette, baby wipe, or a washcloth with warm soap and water. Be sure to wash from front to back and never go back and forth across the opening.
8. Wet the first 2 inches of the tube, either by placing lubricant on your finger and spreading it on the tube or by dipping the catheter into the lubricant on a clean tissue or paper towel.
9. Insert the tube gently into the urethra until urine begins to flow. Then move it slowly about another ½ inch (Figure 3).
10. Allow all the urine to flow out into a container or absorbent diaper.
11. Tell the child to squeeze her belly as if she were having a bowel movement or to blow bubbles or a pinwheel. This helps empty all the urine out of the bladder.
12. Slowly begin to remove the tube when the urine stops. More urine will flow as you remove the tube.

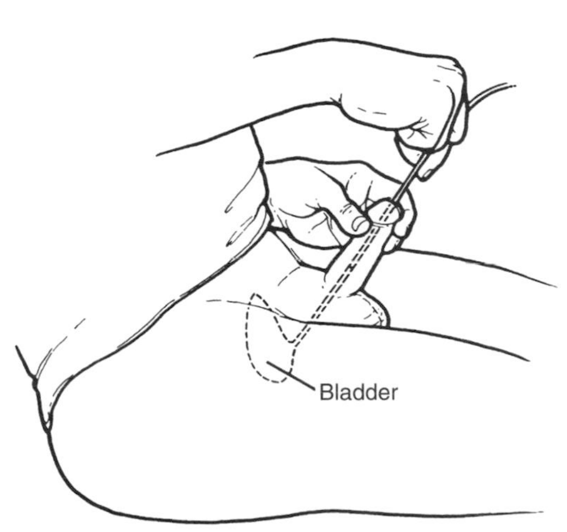

FIGURE 1 A boy doing intermittent self-catheterization.

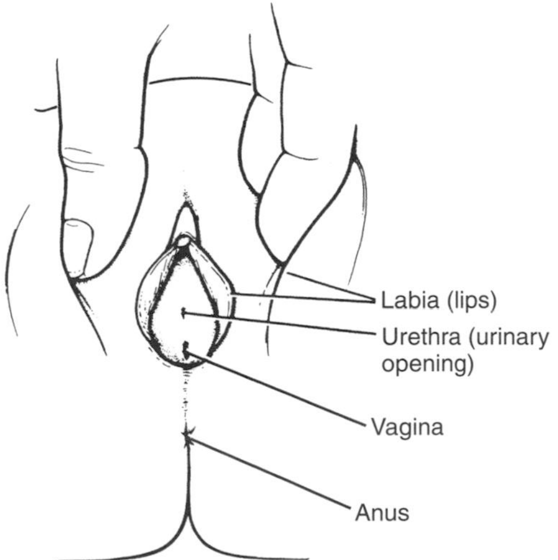

FIGURE 2 Female anatomy showing urinary opening (urethra).

Continued

PATIENT AND FAMILY EDUCATION

Performing Clean Intermittent Bladder Catheterization—cont'd

13. Wash your hands and the catheter with soap and water. Rinse the inside of the tube well with clear water.
14. Dry the tube with a clean paper or cloth towel, and store in a clean, dry container (e.g., plastic bag or margarine container).
15. PRAISE THE CHILD FOR HELPING.
16. Write down the time; whether the underwear or diaper was wet, damp, or dry; the amount of urine; and the way the urine looks.
17. Never reuse a catheter that appears rough, stiff, kinked, worn, discolored, or damaged in any way.
18. Your health professional will tell you how often a new catheter should be used.

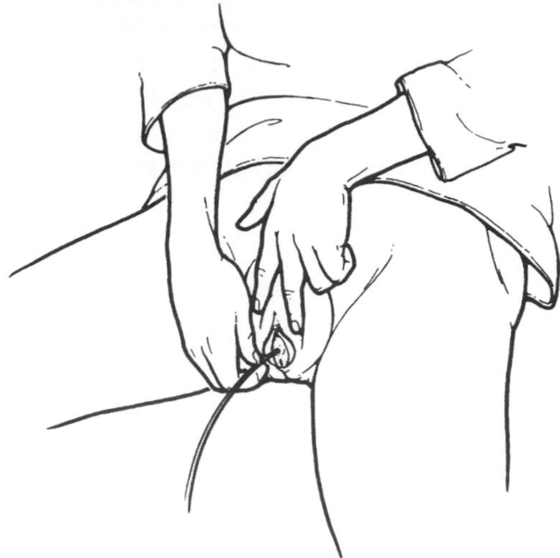

FIGURE 3 A girl doing intermittent self-catheterization.

Sample Record

Day and Time	Amount Fluid In	Amount Fluid Out	Wet/Damp/Dry	Appearance

PATIENT AND FAMILY EDUCATION

Caring for the Child with a Colostomy

The child has had surgery that has changed the way in which he has a bowel movement. An opening was made in the abdomen, and the bowel was attached to the skin. This allows the bowel to empty through the opening (stoma) instead of the rectum. Therefore the area must be kept clean to prevent the skin from becoming irritated. An ostomy appliance (pouch) is placed over the stoma to collect the stool.

You will need to do the ostomy care for the infant and young child. The child can assist according to his developmental level. For example, the child can gather the equipment and hand you supplies. As the child grows, allow him to increase his responsibility for the care of the ostomy. By the age of 8 or 10 years, most children can do the care by themselves.

Ostomy care should be taught to other people who will be caring for the child. At school, tell both the child's teacher and the school nurse so that adult help is available if needed. An extra set of clothing can be kept at the school in case the ostomy appliance leaks. This will help spare the child any embarrassment.

Dress the child in loose-fitting clothing that does not press on the colostomy. Bib-type overalls or dresses are preferable to pants. The overalls or dress will cover the ostomy and avoid the elastic waistband on pants, which may irritate the ostomy.

Call your health professional at ____________ if any of these occurs:

- Bleeding from the stoma more than usual when cleaning stoma
- Bleeding from skin around stoma
- Change in bowel pattern
- Change in the size of stoma
- Change in color of stoma
- Temperature above 100.4° F

Ostomy Care (with a Pouch or Appliance)

The pouch will remain intact for different lengths of time. The pouch should be changed on a routine schedule or sooner if it leaks. Each time the pouch is changed the area needs to be clean and dry and a new barrier must be applied. During the day, the stool can be removed and rinsed from the pouch, then the pouch can be clamped. Two-piece pouches are also available.

Equipment

Washcloth
Skin barrier or wafer
Stoma paste
Pouch or appliance
Rinse bottle

Instructions

1. Gather equipment.
2. Wash your hands with soap and water. Count to 10 while washing, then rinse with clear water and dry with a clean paper or cloth towel.
3. Tell child what you are going to do. (Have him do it if old enough. Be sure he washes his hands before and after the procedure.)
4. Remove old pouch and wafer or skin barrier.
5. Wash the skin, and gently pat dry.
6. Look for any redness or irritation.
7. Cut the new wafer or skin barrier to size if necessary.
8. Apply the wafer or skin barrier. If using the type of wafer that has an adhesive backing, remove the paper seal first.
9. Remove the covering from the adhesive backing on the pouch.
10. Center the pouch over the stoma and press gently, moving from the stoma edge out.
11. Close the end of the pouch with a clamp or rubber band.
12. PRAISE THE CHILD FOR HELPING.
13. Wash your hands as described previously.

Emptying the Pouch

1. When the pouch is one third filled with stool, open the lower end of the pouch over the toilet or another container and let the stool drain out.
2. Rinse the inside of the pouch each day with a squeeze bottle of cool water to remove all the stool. Fill the pouch with a small amount of clear water, and swish it around to thoroughly clean pouch. Then empty pouch over the toilet or a diaper.
3. Make a wick from toilet tissue to dry the inside lower 1 inch of the pouch. Wipe off the outside, and reattach the clamp or rubber band.
4. PRAISE THE CHILD FOR HELPING.
5. Wash your hands as described previously.

Skin Care*

Protection of the skin around the colostomy is a very important part of the child's care. If the skin around the colostomy becomes irritated (moist or red), it is important to help heal the area as fast as possible. A skin barrier should always be used to keep the stool, which may be mainly liquid, off the skin. A barrier can be made by mixing zinc oxide ointment and karaya powder. The paste can be smoothed on the skin around the ostomy. Duoderm-CGF is a readymade wafer-type barrier that is placed on the skin for up to 7 days.

Cavilon No Sting Barrier Film (3M) and AllKare Protective Barrier wipe (ConvaTec) are also available barriers which can be used in children. Consult with your child's discharge nurse, home health nurse, or the enterostomal specialist (a skin care specialist) for the best barrier for your child's skin and the type of appliance to be used.

To help the pouch stay on securely, an adhesive spray must be used before the pouch is applied.

If a pouch is not used, petrolatum (Vaseline) can be applied over the ointment to keep the diaper from sticking to the ointment. When stool is on the skin around the ostomy, clean off the stool and petrolatum, but keep the barrier ointment on to protect the healing skin. Apply more petrolatum before diapering the child.

*See also Skin Care: Neonatal Guidelines, pp. 266-267.

Community Resources for Parents and Professionals

Rogers VE: Managing preemie stomas: More than just the pouch, *J Wound Ostomy Continence Nurs* 30(2):100-110, 2003.
United Ostomy Associates of America; *http://www.uoaa.org;* (800) 826-0826.

PATIENT AND FAMILY EDUCATION

Giving an Enema

An enema is needed when stool must be removed from the bowel or intestine. However, simple constipation in children should not be treated with enemas but with changes in the child's diet. Increasing the amount of liquids to at least 1 quart each day and the amount of fiber in foods (especially whole grains, bran cereals, fresh vegetables, and fruit with the skin on) should increase the size and number of the child's bowel movements.

Large amounts of milk, rice, bananas, and cheese can cause constipation. The child should eat small amounts of these items. If your child is an infant, ask your health professional before changing the feedings.

If the child has persistent constipation, a complete medical evaluation is necessary to determine the cause. If you have been told by a health professional to give an enema (usually only one or two enemas in a day) to the child, use these instructions.

Age	Amount of Lukewarm Water	Approximate Amount of Salt	Distance to Insert Tube
Infant	½-1 cup (120-240 ml, or 4-8 oz)	¼-½ tsp (1.25-2.5 ml)	1 inch (2.5 cm)
2-4 yr	1-1½ cups (240-360 ml, or 8-12 oz)	½-¾ tsp (2.5-3.75 ml)	2 inch (5.0 cm)
4-10 yr	1½-2 cups (360-480 ml, or 12-16 oz)	¾-1 tsp (3.75-5.0 ml)	3 inch (7.5 cm)
11 yr	2-3 cups (480-720 ml, or 16-24 oz)	1-1½ tsp (5.0-7.5 ml)	4 inch (10 cm)

Enema Bag

Equipment

Lukewarm water (water that feels comfortably warm)
Salt
Measuring spoon
Enema bag or kit
Lubricant such as K-Y Jelly
Potty chair or toilet

Instructions

1. Gather equipment.
2. Wash your hands with soap and water. Count to 10 while washing, then rinse with clear water and dry with a clean paper or cloth towel.
3. Refer to the above chart for the right amount of water and salt for the child's age; never use plain tap water.
4. Mix the lukewarm water and salt.
5. Measure the rectal tube for the correct distance.
6. Check to make sure the tube is clamped shut. Then fill the enema container with the solution.
7. Place the child in one of the following positions:
   a. Lying face down on belly with the knees and hips bent toward the chest (Figure 1)
   b. Lying on the left side with the left leg straight and the right leg bent at the hip and knee and placed comfortably on top of the left leg (Figure 2)
   c. Sitting on the potty chair or toilet (Figure 3)
8. Unclamp tube to allow the liquid to flow through and remove air that is present. Clamp the tube.
9. Place a small amount of lubricant on your finger or on a tissue, and spread the lubricant around the tip of the tube, being careful not to plug the holes with lubricant (Figure 4).
10. Gently put the tube into the child's rectum to the marked distance (Figure 5).
11. Holding the bottom of the container no more than 4 inches above the child, open the clamp and allow the liquid to flow, holding the tube in place.

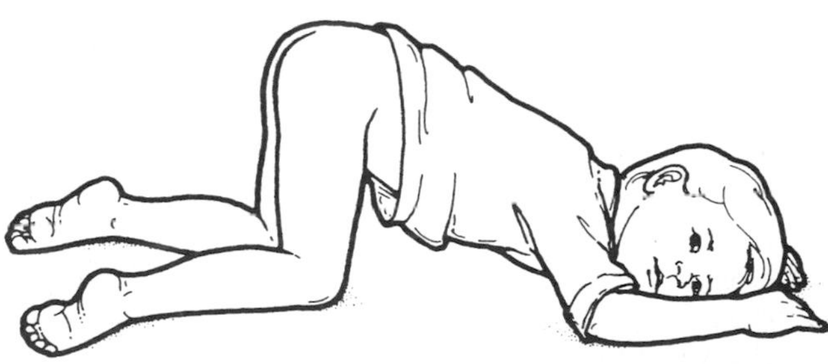

FIGURE 1 Knee-chest position for receiving an enema.

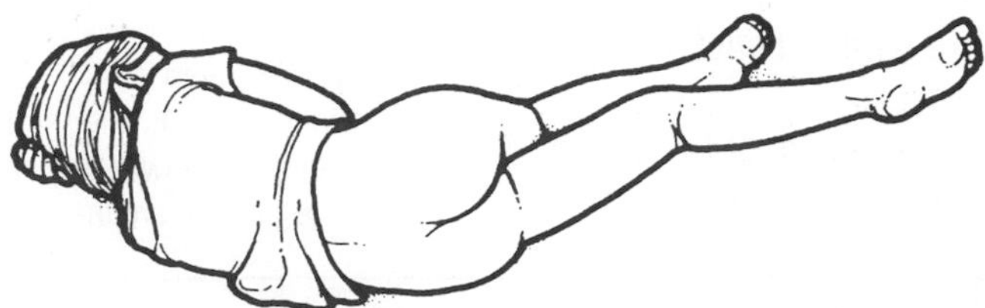

FIGURE 2 Side-lying position for receiving an enema.

PATIENT AND FAMILY EDUCATION

Giving an Enema—cont'd

12. When the container is empty, remove the tube.
13. Have the child keep the liquid inside for 3 to 5 minutes. If the child is too young to follow instructions, then hold the buttocks together to keep the liquid inside. For an older child, encourage slow deep breathing, or read a book to take the child's mind off the time.
14. Help the child to the toilet or potty chair, or allow the child to release the liquid into a diaper.
15. PRAISE THE CHILD FOR HELPING.
16. Write down the appearance of the results of the enema.
17. Wash your hands as above.

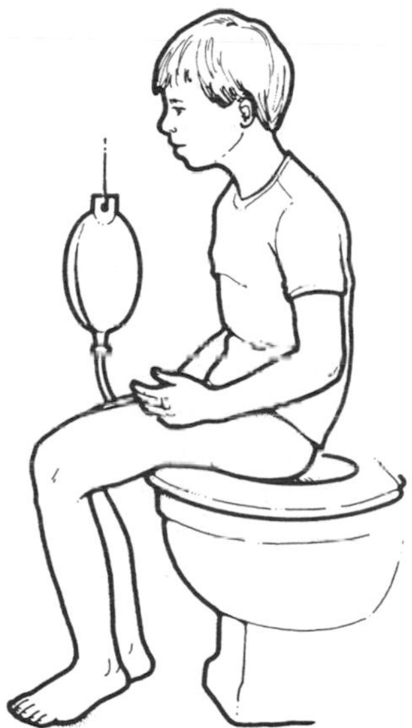

FIGURE **3** Position for receiving an enema on toilet.

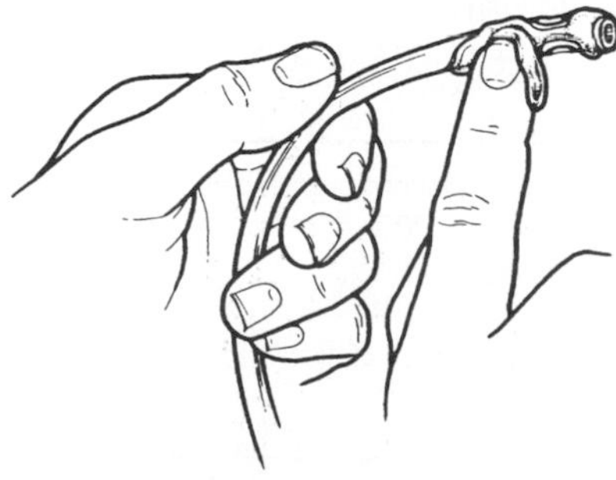

FIGURE **4** Putting lubricant on the tip of the enema tube.

Prepackaged Enema

Ready-to-use enemas are available in varying amounts and solutions for infants, children, and adults. Use the amount and type of solution recommended by your health care professional.

Equipment

Basin of warm water
Prepackaged enema
Potty chair or toilet

Instructions

1. Warm the liquid in a basin of warm water.
2. Wash your hands with soap and water. Count to 10 while washing, then rinse with clear water and dry with a clean paper or cloth towel.
3. Place the child in one of the following positions:
   a. Lying face down on belly with the knees and hips bent toward the chest (see Figure 1)
   b. Lying on the left side with the left leg straight and the right leg bent at the hip and knee and placed comfortably on top of the left leg (see Figure 2)
   c. Sitting on the potty chair or toilet (see Figure 3)
4. Remove the cap (Figure 6). Put the tip, which is already lubricated, into the child's rectum the right distance (Figure 7).
5. Gently squeeze the enema container to empty. A small amount will remain in the container after squeezing.
6. Remove the tip.
7. Have the child keep the liquid inside for 3 to 5 minutes. If the child is too young to follow instructions, then hold the buttocks together to keep the liquid inside.
8. Help the child to the toilet or potty chair, or allow the child to release the solution into a diaper.
9. PRAISE THE CHILD FOR HELPING.
10. Write down the appearance of the results of the enema.
11. Wash your hands as in step 2.

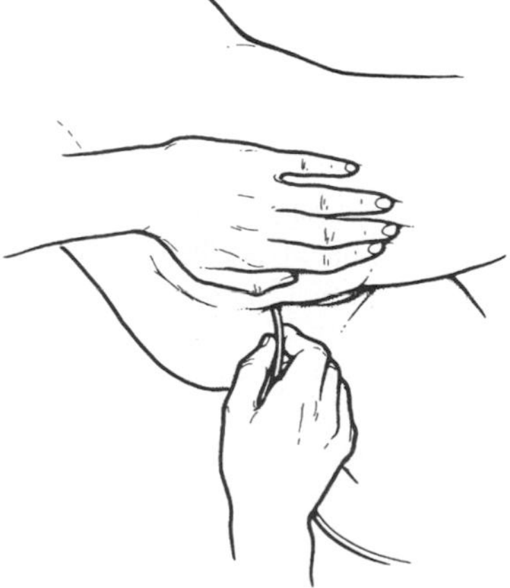

FIGURE **5** Gently placing the tube in the child's rectum. Make sure the tube is not put in farther than the marked distance.

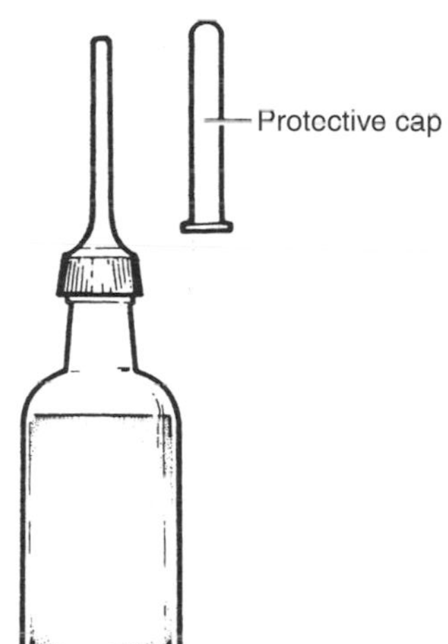

FIGURE **6** Prepackaged enema with the protective cap removed.

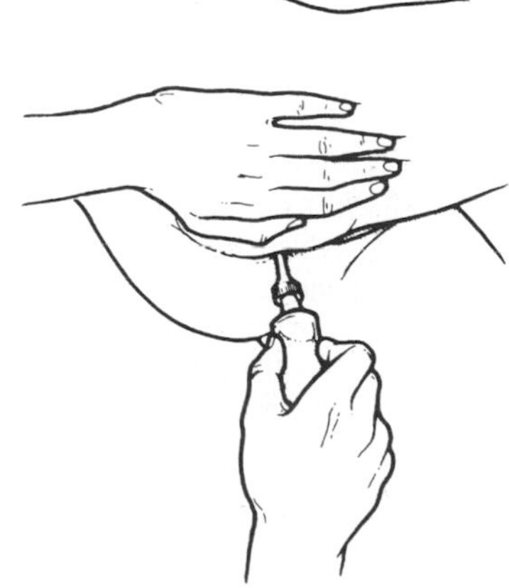

FIGURE **7** Gently placing tip of prepackaged enema in the child's rectum.

PATIENT AND FAMILY EDUCATION

Oral Rehydration Guidelines*

Plan A (to Prevent Dehydration)

Use this plan if your child has:

- Been seen at a health care facility and was found to have no signs of dehydration
- Been treated at a health care facility with treatment plan B until dehydration was corrected
- Recently developed diarrhea but has not yet been seen at a health care facility

Guidelines for Plan A

Give the child more fluids than usual to prevent dehydration.

Give the child plenty of food to prevent undernutrition.

Take the child to a health care facility if the diarrhea does not get better or if signs of dehydration or other serious illness develop.

Fluids to Give

Pedialyte, Gastrolyte, Infalyte (formerly Ricelyte), or other commercial oral rehydration solution

WHO oral rehydration salt packet mixed in 1 liter of water

A homemade sugar-salt solution may be made if none of the above are available; however the above solutions are readily available and preferred to the homemade solution.

- 1 liter (33.8 ounces or 2.1 pints) of clean water
- 8 level teaspoons of sugar
- 1 level teaspoon of salt
- ½ cup orange juice to provide potassium and improve taste

Fluids to Avoid

Carbonated drinks

Tea, coffee, or other caffeinated beverages

High-sugar sports drinks

Commercial juices or flavored juice drinks with a high concentration (>5g) of simple carbohydrate

How Much Fluids to Give by Mouth

Give this much fluid after each loose stool; repeat after every stool until diarrhea stops.

- Age less than 2 years: 50 to 100 ml (approx. 1½ to 3¼ ounces)
- Ages 2 to 10 years: 100 to 200 ml (approximately 3¼ oz to 6½ oz)
- Age over 10 years: as much as child wants

Food to Give

Breast-feeding should be continued without interruption.

Infants taking a cow milk–based formula should continue the full-strength formula.

For children old enough to eat, give soft or semisolid foods and offer small, frequent feedings every 3 to 4 hours.

When to Change the Plan

If the child's diarrhea stops, then return to normal diet.

If the child develops signs of dehydration, take him to a health care facility for evaluation.

Plan B (to Correct Mild to Moderate Dehydration)

Use this plan if your child shows signs of mild or moderate dehydration (see below).

Guidelines for Plan B

Give only rehydration fluids for first 3 to 4 hours.

Continue breast-feeding. Infant may need to be breast-fed more often than usual to achieve adequate intake.

For infants who are fed a cow milk–based formula, continue giving the full-strength formula. If the child vomits, offer small amounts of rehydration solution (Pedialyte, Gastrolyte, Infalyte, or other) and then resume milk once the vomiting ceases.

Resume other foods after 4 hours. (See Plan A for food guidelines.)

Fluids to Give

Pedialyte, Gastrolyte, Infalyte (formerly Ricelyte), or other commercial oral rehydration solution

WHO oral rehydration salt packet mixed in 1 liter of water

Fluids to Avoid

Carbonated drinks

Tea, coffee, or other caffeinated beverages

High-sugar sports drinks

Commercial juices or flavored juice drinks with a high concentration (>5g) of simple carbohydrate

How Much Fluid to Give by Mouth

Children younger than 2 years: 5 ml (1 teaspoon) every 3 to 5 minutes by spoon or medicine syringe (without needle)

Children over 2 years: 5 to 10 ml (1 to 2 teaspoons) every 5 to 10 minutes; increase amount as tolerated.

- If the child vomits, wait 10 minutes and then continue giving oral fluid. A syringe (without a needle) especially designed for giving oral medications may also be used.
- If the child will drink more than the estimated amount of fluid and is not vomiting, give more.
- If the child refuses to drink the determined amount, and the signs of dehydration have disappeared, change to Plan A.
- If the child is breast-fed, continue breast-feeding in addition to administering oral rehydration fluids.

When to Change the Plan

If the dehydration worsens, seek medical attention promptly.

If the signs of dehydration resolve, switch to Plan A.

*Adapted from the World Health Organization, Geneva, Switzerland; and Centers for Disease Control and Prevention: Managing acute gastroenteritis among children: oral rehydration, maintenance, and nutritional therapy, *MMWR* 52(RR-16):1-16, 2003.
For more information on oral rehydration see the Rehydration Project website at *http://www.rehydrate.org/*.

5 - PATIENT AND FAMILY EDUCATION

PATIENT AND FAMILY EDUCATION

Oral Rehydration Guidelines—cont'd

	Degree of Dehydration and Associated Symptoms		
	Minimal or No Dehydration	**Mild to Moderate Dehydration**	**Severe Dehydration**
Loss of body weight	<3%	3%-9%	>9%
Fluid volume loss	<50 ml/kg	50-90 ml/kg	>100 mg/kg
Mental status	Well, alert	Normal, fatigued or restless, irritable	Apathetic, lethargic, unconscious
Skin color	Pale	Gray	Mottled
Extremities	Warm	Cool	Cold, mottled, cyanotic
Thirst	Drinks normally; may refuse liquids	Thirsty; eager to drink	Drinks poorly; unable to drink
Breathing	Normal	Normal to fast	Deep
Tears	Present	Decreased	Absent
Skin elasticity (turgor)	Decreased	Poor	Very poor
Mucous membranes—mouth and tongue	Dry	Very dry	Parched
Urinary output	Normal or decreased	Decreased	Minimal to no urine
Blood pressure	Normal	Normal or lowered	Lowered
Pulse quality	Normal or increased	Increased	Rapid and thready, or not palpable
Capillary filling time	<2 seconds	2-3 seconds	>3 seconds
Eyes	Normal	Slightly sunken	Deeply sunken

Instructions Related to Maintaining Respiratory Function

PATIENT AND FAMILY EDUCATION

Monitoring Peak Expiratory Flow

The peak expiratory flow rate measures the maximum amount of air the child can forcefully exhale. The peak expiratory flow rate helps determine the severity of the child's asthma at the time it is used; this will often determine the type of medications needed to help the child breathe better. Peak flow values vary according to the child's height, weight, gender, and race. In general a peak flow rate is monitored twice a day for 2 to 3 weeks to determine how the child is responding to asthma medications. Once a child's personal best peak flow rate is established, this will serve as a point of reference for future measurements, especially if the child has an illness such as a cold. Follow the directions your health professional provides for using the peak flow meter; the directions below are of a general nature and may serve as a guide.

Equipment

Peak expiratory flow meter
Paper and pencil

Instructions

1. Wash your hands with soap and water. Count to 10 while washing, rinse with clear water, and dry with a clean paper or cloth towel.
2. Have the child wash his hands in the same manner.
3. Lower the sliding marker or arrow on the peak flow meter until it is pointing to the zero or is at the bottom of the numbered scale.
4. Ask the child to remove any gum or food from the mouth.
5. Have the child stand up straight.
6. Instruct the child to take a deep breath and then let it out.
7. Instruct the child to place the flow meter mouthpiece in the mouth and close the lips tightly, keeping the tongue away from the mouthpiece.
8. Have the child take a breath and blow as hard as possible into the mouthpiece over 1 to 2 seconds, keeping the lips around the mouthpiece. If a few practice sessions are needed for the child to get used to the mouthpiece, do not count these in the readings.
9. Check the number where the arrow or marker stopped on the flow meter after the child blew into the meter. Write this number on the piece of paper.
10. Repeat steps 7 and 8 two more times. Before each repetition, lower the marker as you did in step 3 and note the child's top numbers for each time. The top number is the child's personal best when he or she is well.
11. See Guidelines box on Interpreting Peak Expiratory Flow Rates.

GUIDELINES

Interpreting Peak Expiratory Flow Rates*

Green (80% to 100% of personal best) signals all clear. Asthma is under reasonably good control. No symptoms are present, and the routine treatment plan for maintaining control can be followed.

Yellow (50% to 79% of personal best) signals caution. Asthma is not well controlled. An acute exacerbation may be present. Maintenance therapy may need to be increased. Call the practitioner if the child stays in this zone.

Red (below 50% of personal best) signals a medical alert. Severe airway narrowing may be occurring. A short-acting bronchodilator should be administered. Notify the practitioner if the peak expiratory flow rate does not return immediately and stay in yellow or green zone.†

*These zones are guidelines only. Specific zones and management should be individualized for each child.
†See also Asthma Medicine Plan, p. 543.

GUIDELINES

Allergy-Proofing the Home

Keep humidity between 30% and 50%; use dehumidifier and/or air conditioner if available; keep air conditioners clean and free of mold; do not use vaporizers or humidifiers.

Encase pillows in zippered, allergen-impermeable covers, or wash pillows in hot water (at least 54.4° C [130° F]) every week.

Encase mattress and box springs in zippered, allergen-impermeable covers.

Use foam rubber mattress and pillows or Dacron pillows and synthetic blankets.

Wash bed linens every 7 to 10 days in hot water (at least 54.4° C).

Encase polyester comforters in allergen-impermeable covers or wash in hot water (at least 54.4° C) every week; if possible, use cotton blankets instead of comforters.

Do not use a canopy above the bed; children should not sleep on a bottom bunk bed.

Store nothing under the bed; keep clothing in a closet with the door shut.

Use washable window shades; avoid heavy curtains; if curtains are used, launder them frequently.

Remove all carpeting if possible; if not possible, vacuum carpet once or twice a week while the child wears a mask; have child remain out of the room while vacuuming and for 30 minutes after vacuuming.

If possible, use a central vacuum cleaner with a collecting bag outside the home; or use cleaner filters (e.g., high-efficiency particulate air [HEPA] filters).

Have air and heating ducts cleaned annually; change or clean filters monthly; cover heating vents with filter material (e.g., cheesecloth) to prevent circulation of dust, especially when heat is turned on in the fall.

Remove unnecessary furniture, rugs, stuffed or real animals, toys, books, upholstered furniture, plants, aquariums, and wall hangings from child's room.

Use wipeable furniture (wood, plastic, vinyl, leather) in place of upholstered furniture; avoid rattan or wicker furniture.

Cover walls with washable paint or wallpaper.

Limit child's exposure to animals (e.g., rabbits, gerbils, hamsters) at school; keep pets out of the child's bedroom and keep the bedroom door closed if pets are in the house. Keep pets off the sofa.

Change child's clothes after child plays outdoors; wash child's hair nightly if child has been outside and pollen count is high.

Keep child indoors while lawn is being mowed, bushes or trees are being trimmed, or pollen count is high.

Keep windows and doors closed during pollen season; use air conditioner if possible or go to places that are air conditioned, such as libraries and shopping malls, when the weather is hot.

Wet-mop bare floors weekly; wet-dust and clean child's room weekly; child should not be present during cleaning activities.

Wash showers and shower curtains with bleach or all-purpose cleaner containing ammonia at least once a month.

Limit or avoid child's exposure to tobacco and wood smoke.

Do not allow cigarette smoking in the house or car; parents (and others) should not smoke in vehicle when child is in the vehicle; smokers should change clothing after smoking and before coming in close contact with small infants and children

Select daycare centers, play areas, restaurants, and stores that are smoke-free.

Avoid odors, dust, or sprays (e.g., perfumes, talcum powder, room deodorizers, chalk dust at school, fresh paint, cleaning solutions).

Do not use the cellar (basement) as a play area if it is damp; use a dehumidifier in a damp basement.

Cover all food, including pet food, and put food away in cabinets.

Store garbage in closed containers.

Use pesticide sprays, roach bait traps, and boric acid powder to kill cockroaches; if living in an apartment or adjacent housing, encourage neighbors to work together to get rid of cockroaches and mice.

Repair leaking or dripping faucets; seal cracks and crevices in cabinets and pantry areas (to prevent mold).

Community Resources for Parents

Asthma and Allergy Foundation of America; (800) 727-8462; *http://www.aafa.org*
Allergy and Asthma Network/Mothers of Asthmatics; (800) 878-4403; *http://www.aanma.org*
American Academy of Allergy, Asthma, and Immunology; (800) 822-2762; *http://www.aaai.org*
American Lung Association; (800) 548-8252; *http://www.lungusa.org*

PATIENT AND FAMILY EDUCATION

Suctioning the Nose and Mouth

The child needs help to keep the mouth and nose clear of mucus. Suctioning equipment, a humidifier, and other supplies will be needed. While the child is in the hospital, you should practice using the same suction machine that you will be using at home. This allows you a chance to become familiar with the equipment. You will also need a mucus trap or nasal aspirator that can be used to remove mucus when you and the child are away from home. Practice with these items while the child is in the hospital.

Certain guidelines are helpful for the child who has problems clearing mucus from the back of the nose and mouth (pharynx). To keep the mucus liquid so that it is easy to remove by both suctioning and coughing, added moisture is needed. Encourage the child to drink at least 1 quart (four 8-ounce cups) of liquid a day, and place a cool mist humidifier in the room where the child sleeps. Change the water in the humidifier each day and clean the humidifier regularly, according to the manufacturer's instructions.

All the people who provide care for the child must know how to suction the child so that they can assist you. On each telephone in the house, tape emergency phone numbers such as 911 (if available in your area), the numbers for the local hospital and your health professional, and any other numbers that are necessary. Notify your health professional at ____________ if any of the following occurs:

- Temperature is above 100.4° F.
- Yellow or green mucus is present.
- A change in the smell of the mucus occurs.
- The amount of mucus increases.
- The child is very irritable.
- The child is having difficulty breathing.

Suctioning

Suctioning keeps the airway (nose and mouth, Figure 1) clear of mucus to help the child breathe more easily. Suctioning is not done routinely, but only when needed. Suction when the following occur:

- The child is having trouble breathing.
- The child appears very restless.
- The child has difficulty eating or sucking.
- The child's color becomes paler.
- The child's nostrils flare (spread out).
- You hear the sound of air bubbling through the mucus.

When the child has a cold, more mucus is produced, so you will probably need to suction more often. The child may cough or gag when you insert or remove the suction catheter. Gently tell the child when you are almost finished. If the child is old enough, teach him how to help you by holding the supplies.

Preparing the Supplies

Clean Jars and Containers

Wash plastic containers and glass jars with lids in a dishwasher or in hot, soapy water and rinse well. Use a clean towel to dry or allow to air dry. Keep a supply of containers washed and dried.

Salt Solution (Saline)

Boil water for 5 minutes. Add ¾ teaspoon of salt to each 2 cups of water when you are heating the water. Let cool, then pour into a clean glass jar and cover. Store the sterile saline in the refrigerator.

Equipment

Suction machine with tubing
Suction catheters
Saline or water (cool)
White vinegar
Clean container for rinsing catheter

Instructions

1. Gather all the equipment you will need.
2. Wash your hands with soap and water. Count to 10 while washing, then rinse with clear water and dry with a clean paper or cloth towel.
3. Open the suction catheter package, and connect the catheter to the suction machine.
4. Make sure the suction machine is plugged in and working.
5. Measure the tube for the distance you will have to insert it. Place the tip of the catheter at the child's earlobe, and mark the distance to the tip of the child's nose. Hold the catheter at this mark (Figure 2).
6. Place the tip of the catheter in the sterile saline and place your thumb over the opening to obtain suction. The saline wets the catheter (Figure 3).

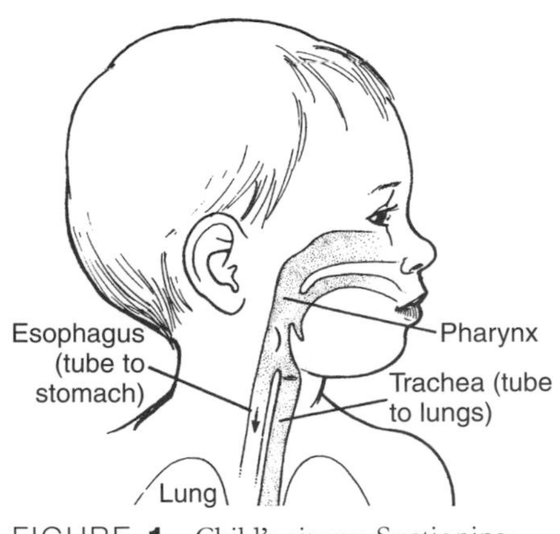

FIGURE 1 Child's airway. Suctioning should clear the pharynx of mucus.

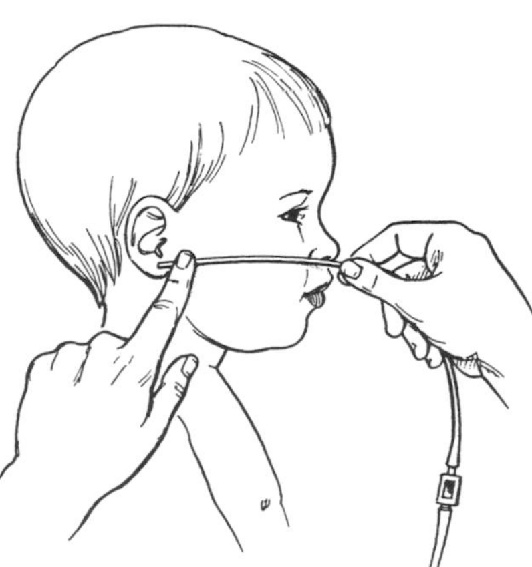
FIGURE 2 Measuring length to insert suction catheter.

PATIENT AND FAMILY EDUCATION

Suctioning the Nose and Mouth—cont'd

7. Tell the child to take a deep breath.
8. With your thumb off the opening (no suction), insert the suction catheter in one nostril up to the measured distance (Figure 4, *A*).
9. Place your thumb on the suction port to obtain suction.
10. Rotate or twist the catheter as you remove it with a slow steady motion (see Figure 4, *B*). Both inserting the catheter and suctioning should take no longer than 5 seconds. Remember, the child may not breathe while you are suctioning.
11. Look at the mucus. Check the color, smell, and consistency for any change.
12. Rinse the suction catheter in the sterile saline or water with your thumb on the suction port.
13. Allow the child to take a few deep breaths.
14. Repeat steps 7 through 13 up to two times if needed (for large amounts of mucus), then repeat for the other nostril.
15. After suctioning the nose, you can use the same catheter to clear the child's mouth.
16. Place the tip of the catheter in the saline, and place your thumb over the opening to obtain suction.
17. Tell the child to take a deep breath.
18. With your thumb off the opening (no suction), insert the suction catheter in the child's mouth along one side of the mouth until it reaches the back of the throat.
19. Place your thumb on the suction port to obtain suction.
20. Rotate or twist the catheter as you remove it with a slow steady motion. Both inserting the catheter and suctioning should take no longer than 5 seconds. Remember, the child may not breathe while you are suctioning.
21. Look at the mucus. Check the color, smell, and consistency for any change.
22. Rinse the suction catheter in the saline or water with your thumb on the suction port.
23. Allow the child a chance to take a few deep breaths.
24. Repeat steps 17 through 23 up to three times.
25. Hold and comfort the child.
26. PRAISE THE CHILD FOR HELPING.
27. After each use, throw away the saline or water and clean the container. The suction machine should be clean and ready for the next time that you will have to use it.
28. Your health professional will instruct you on the care of the suction catheters, or use the method described in the following pages.
29. Wash your hands as in step 2.

Instructions for Cleaning the Suction Catheters

1. Rinse the suction catheters in cool tap water. Do not use hot water because it "cooks" the mucus, which makes it more difficult to remove.
2. Place the catheters in a clean jar filled with hot, soapy water.
3. Rinse both the inside and outside of the tube under hot, running water. Hold the tube with kitchen tongs so that you don't burn yourself.
4. Shake off the excess water.
5. Mix 1 part white vinegar and 3 parts water in a clean container.
6. Place the clean catheters in this solution for 30 minutes.
7. Remove the catheters from the liquid and rinse thoroughly with clean water

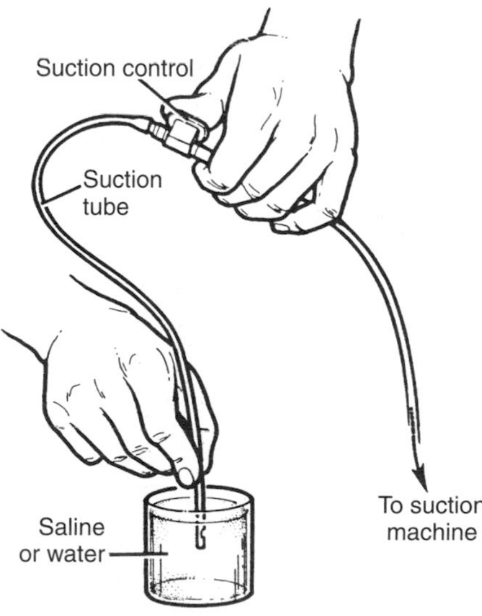

FIGURE 3 Rinsing and lubricating catheter with thumb on suction control.

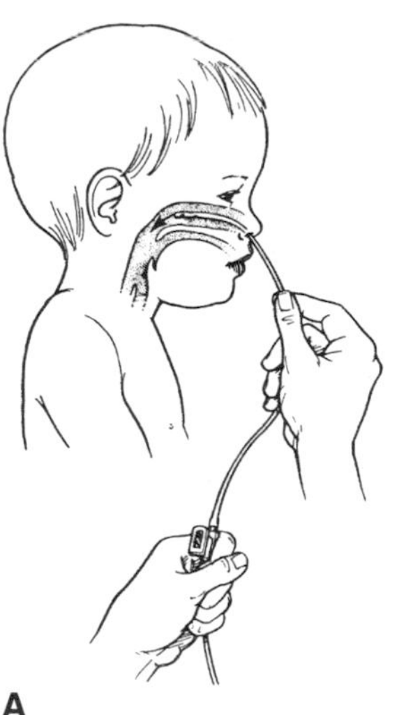

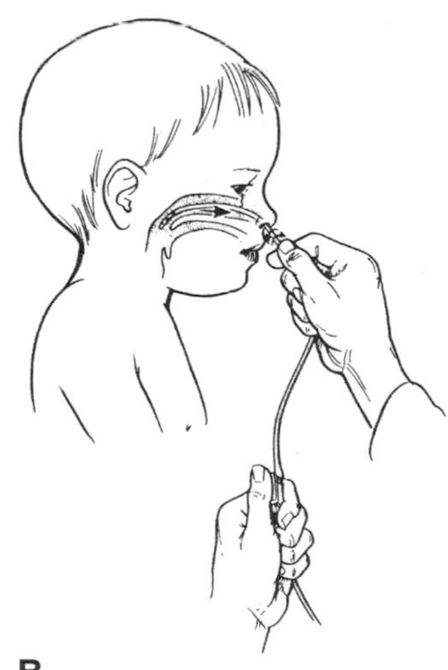

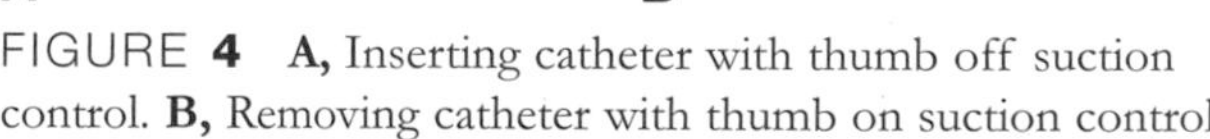

FIGURE 4 **A,** Inserting catheter with thumb off suction control. **B,** Removing catheter with thumb on suction control.

Continued

PATIENT AND FAMILY EDUCATION

Suctioning the Nose and Mouth—cont'd

8. Shake off the excess water.
9. Place on a clean paper towel to dry. When the tube is completely dry, place it in a clean plastic bag.
10. Close the bag and store until the next time you suction the child.
11. If you notice any moisture in the bag, repeat the entire cleaning procedure.

Instructions for Using a Nasal Aspirator

When the child's nose is plugged with loose, runny mucus, the nasal aspirator is very helpful in removing it. The aspirator can also be used when the nose is plugged with dry, crusted mucus. Nose drops must first be used to moisten the mucus before it can be removed. Saline nose drops are the safest product to use. These can be purchased or made at home. To make the nose drops at home, mix ¾ teaspoon (4 ml) salt with 1 pint (2 cups or 500 ml) tap water or the mixture prescribed by your health professional. The solution can be stored in any clean, covered container but should be mixed fresh each day. Use a clean eyedropper to put the solution into the child's nose, or wet a cotton ball and let the saline drip into the nose. Once the dried mucus is softened, then the nasal aspirator can be used.

Instructions

1. Squeeze the rounded end of the bulb to remove air (Figure 5).
2. Place the tip of the bulb snugly into one side of the nose (nostril).
3. Let go of the bulb slowly; the bulb will suck the mucus out of the nose (Figure 6).
4. When the bulb is reinflated, remove it from the nose (Figure 7).
5. Squeeze the bulb into a tissue to get rid of the mucus.
6. Repeat steps 1 through 5 for the other side of the nose.
7. Hold and comfort the child.
8. Repeat this process as often as needed to keep the nose clear.

Cleaning the Nasal Aspirator

Clean the nasal aspirator by filling it with tap water. Then squeeze the bulb to remove the water and the mucus. Refill the bulb with water and boil for 10 minutes. Let the bulb cool, and squeeze out the water before using it again.

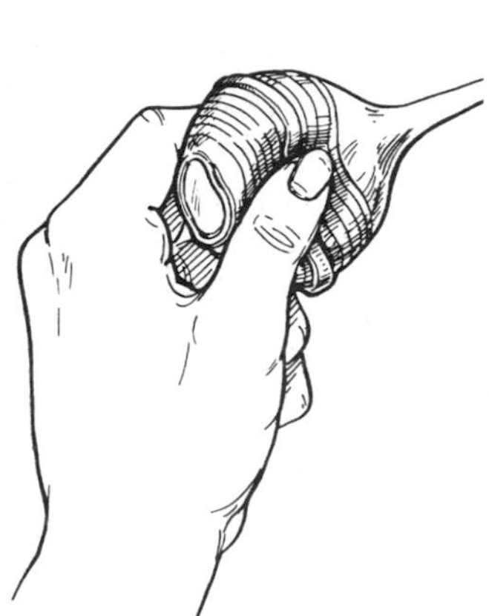

FIGURE 5 Squeezing nasal aspirator to remove air.

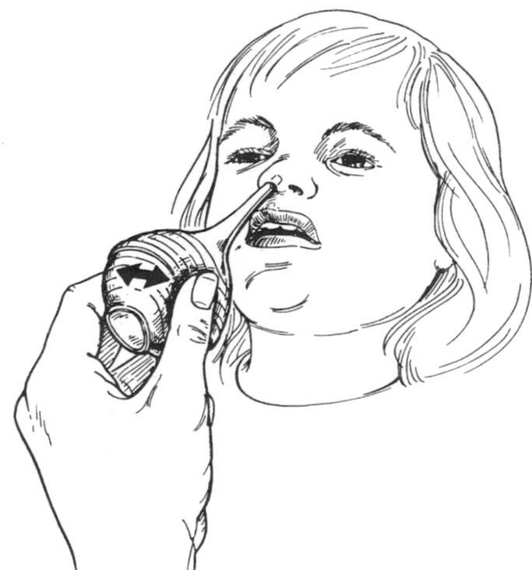

FIGURE 6 Releasing grasp to suck mucus from nose.

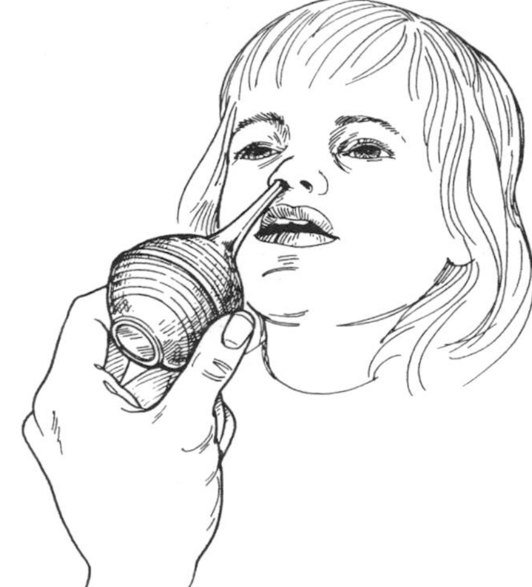

FIGURE 7 Removing aspirator from nose when bulb is reinflated.

PATIENT AND FAMILY EDUCATION

Performing Postural Drainage

Mucus is a protective covering of the inside of the lungs and airways. Mucus traps dust and dirt in the air that we breathe and helps prevent these from irritating the lungs. When an infection or other irritation is present, the body produces more thick mucus to help the lungs get rid of the infection. Some illnesses, such as cystic fibrosis, also cause too much thick mucus. When this thick mucus blocks the airways, breathing becomes more difficult. To help the body get rid of the extra mucus, postural drainage is done. This series of activities helps move thick mucus from the lungs into the trachea (windpipe), where it can be coughed out. The airways can be compared with a freshly opened catsup bottle. Even when the bottle is held upside down, it takes several sharp blows to the bottom of the bottle to make the catsup start flowing.

The postural drainage needs to be carried out ________ times per day. This should be done when the child wakes up; before bedtime; and about 1½ hours before lunch and the evening meal. It should not be done after meals because the exercises and coughing may cause the child to vomit. The exercises should be finished 30 to 45 minutes before the meal so that the child has a chance to rest and feel like eating.

The child must be placed in several different positions for the postural drainage. You must adapt the procedure for the child's age and strength. Each session should usually last 20 to 30 minutes and involve four to six positions. The remaining positions are then used at the other postural drainage times throughout the day.*

Techniques You Will Need

Cupping (Percussion)

Position your hand as if you were holding a liquid or powder, then turn it upside down (Figure 1). When the child is in the drainage position, rapidly strike the child's chest with your hand. The entire oval of your hand should make contact with the child's chest. If your child is very small, you may be given a special device to use instead of your hand. The drawings that follow have a shaded area to show where to place your hand for each position. Cupping is carried out for about 1 minute in each position. Have the child wear a shirt so that your hand does not touch the child's bare skin during cupping. Remember, cupping is not the same as hitting. When done right, cupping does not hurt the child or cause the skin to become red, which occurs when the skin is slapped.

Vibration

Learning to vibrate may take a little practice. First, place one of your hands on top of the other; then rapidly tighten and loosen the muscles of your lower arm (Figure 2). This creates a vibration that, when applied to the skin, is passed through to the lungs to loosen mucus. Now, have the child take a deep breath and while she is breathing out, place your hands over the lung segment to be drained and vibrated. An electric vibrator (massager) or a padded electric toothbrush (for infants) can be used as well as your hands for vibration.

Positioning Aids

Infants and small children can be positioned in your lap. For older children, a padded slant board can be used. If a slant board is not available, a bed or couch at a comfortable height can be used. Pillows are helpful to position the child comfortably.

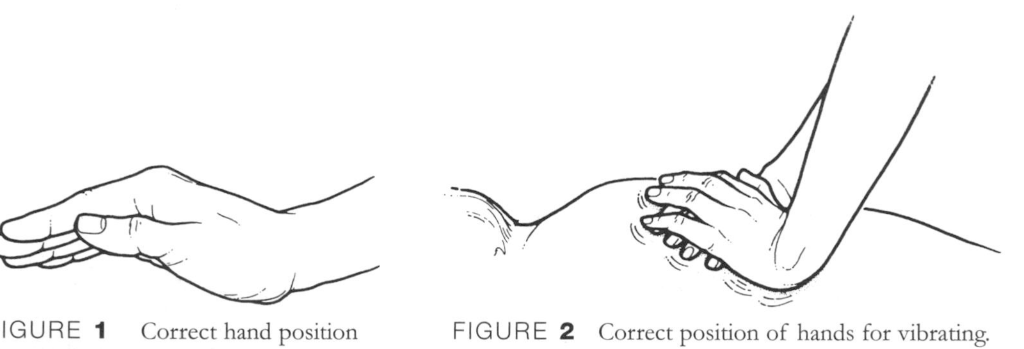

FIGURE 1 Correct hand position for cupping.

FIGURE 2 Correct position of hands for vibrating.

*The postural drainage positions pictured include head-down positions. Some experts caution about the use of the head-down position in infants and small children with gastroesophageal reflux. Ask your health practitioner about using these positions before doing so.

Continued

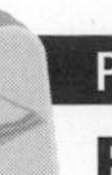

PATIENT AND FAMILY EDUCATION

Performing Postural Drainage—cont'd

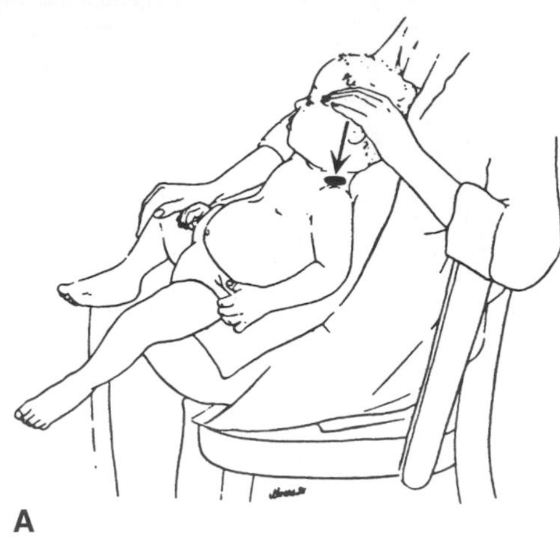

A

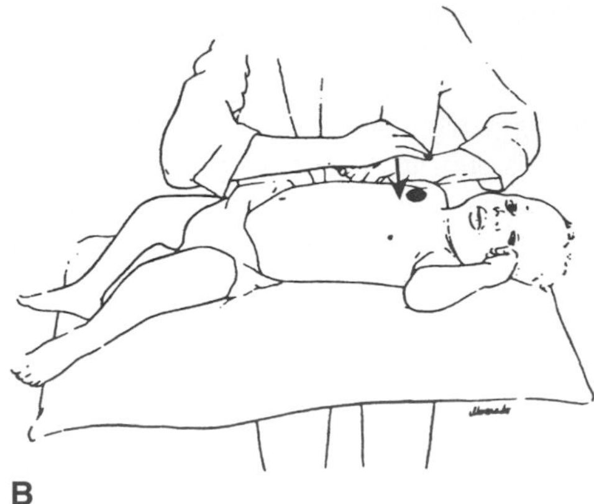

B

Instructions

1. Place the child in the position in Figure 3, *A*.
2. Tell the child to take several deep breaths. The child can also use special blow bottles, try to blow up a balloon, blow a pinwheel, or blow bubbles. These help the child to take deep breaths and may cause the child to cough.
3. Cup the area shaded in the picture for about 1 minute.
4. After cupping, have the child take a deep breath and vibrate the area as she breathes out. Repeat this for three breaths. If the child is too young to understand how to breathe deeply and slowly, just vibrate during a few breaths.
5. Tell the child to cough. Because she may not be able to cough when lying down, help her to a sitting position to produce a good, deep cough.
6. Repeat steps 1 through 5 for each of the other positions (Figure 3, *B* through *I*).
7. Only one side is shown in the figure, but remember that the procedure must be repeated for both left and right sides.

Remember: Spend about 20 to 30 minutes at each session. Watch the child carefully for signs of tiredness. The postural drainage should be stopped before she becomes tired. It can be continued after the child has had an opportunity to rest.

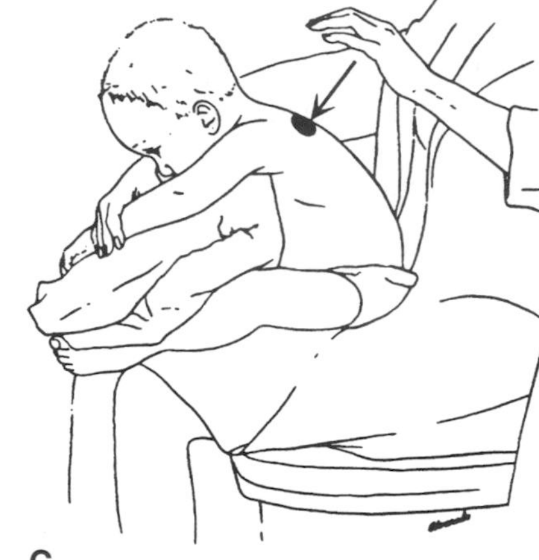

C

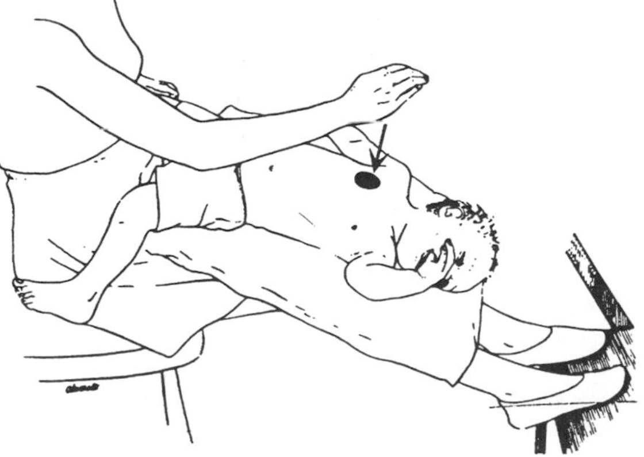

D

FIGURE **3** Positions for postural drainage. (Modified from Cystic Fibrosis Foundation: *Infant segmental bronchial drainage,* Rockville, Md, The Foundation.)

PATIENT AND FAMILY EDUCATION

Performing Postural Drainage—cont'd

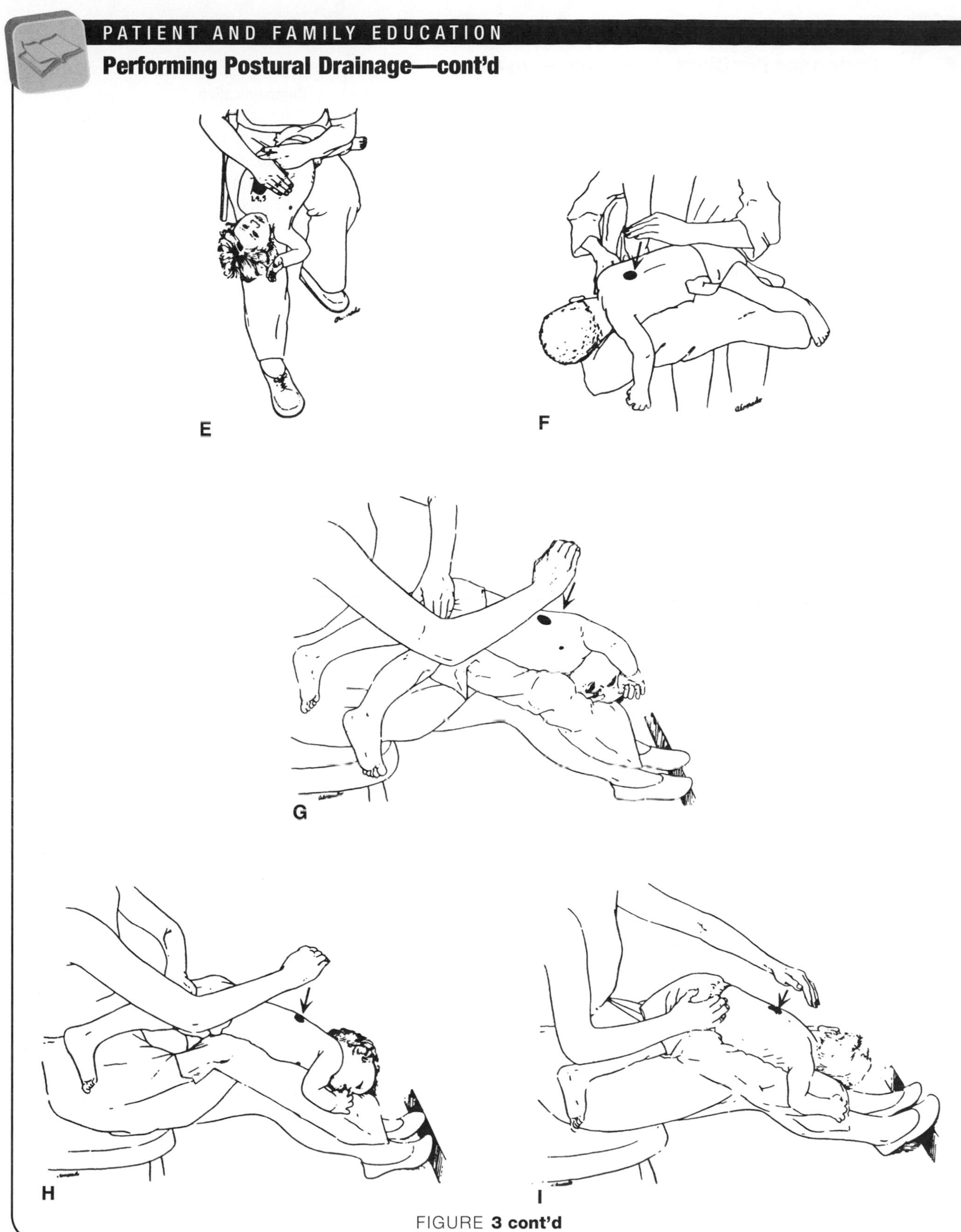

FIGURE **3 cont'd**

PATIENT AND FAMILY EDUCATION

Caring for the Child with a Tracheostomy

A small opening (stoma) was made in the child's windpipe (or trachea, Figure 1) to help her breathe more easily. The tracheostomy ("trach") will require special care while you are at home. Suctioning equipment, a humidifier, and other supplies will be needed. While the child is in the hospital, you should practice using the same suction machine (and monitor) that you will be using at home. This helps you to become familiar with the equipment.

Supplies that you will need when you are outside the house are the following: a mucus trap that can be used when the suction machine is not available, sterile saline, water-soluble lubricant, trach tube with ties attached, scissors, and emergency phone numbers. These items should be kept in a to-go bag that is ready at all times. Practice with these items while the child is in the hospital.

Special Considerations

Certain precautions are needed for the child with a trach. Because the air that the child breathes no longer passes through the nose and mouth, it is no longer warmed, moistened, and filtered before it enters the lungs. To keep the mucus liquid, so that it is easy to remove by both suctioning and coughing, added moisture is needed. Your health professional will advise you on the amount of liquid that should be given to the child to drink throughout the day.

When the child is out in hot, dry, or cold weather or on very windy days, wrap a handkerchief or scarf around the child's neck. This will help warm and filter the air the child breathes. Humidifying or filtering devices can also be bought. Heat and moisture exchange (HME), also called *artificial nose,* provides humidification when you are not using the mist collar and heated humidifier. Children in stable condition who are not requiring supplemental oxygen can wear the HME as tolerated, usually not longer than 4 hours. The tracheostomy mist collar is recommended for sleeping. To keep food and liquids from falling into the trach, use a cloth bib with short ties when the child is eating.

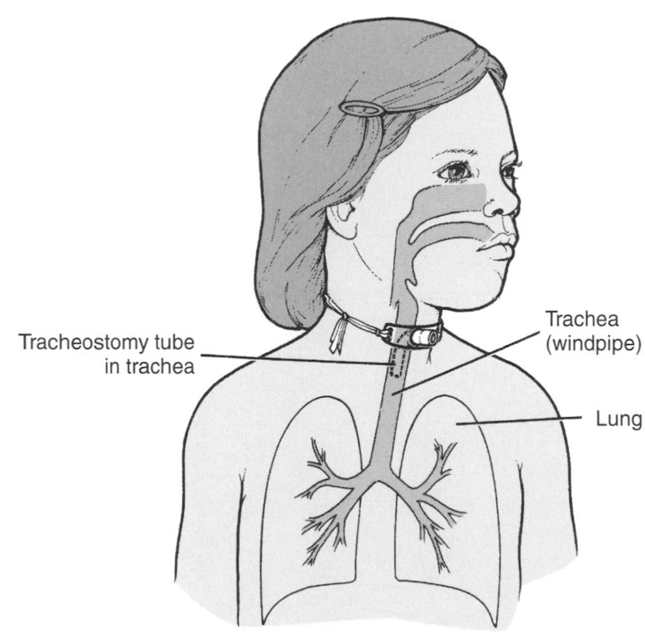

FIGURE 1 Diagram of breathing system with tracheostomy tube in place.

Communication

The trach makes it harder for the child to make her needs known. Nursery monitors or intercoms can be used to listen for changes in the child's breathing while you are in another room. This may signal that the child needs you.

Older children can use bells to call you, or talking boards, where they can point to different words. If the child is old enough to write, the child may choose to communicate in this way. Some children are able to talk by placing their finger over the trach for short periods of time.

A Passy-Muir valve can be attached to the tracheostomy tube, which allows for vocalization and an audible cry. This usually requires a speech therapy consultation but can be of great value to families and may foster parent-infant bonding and allow the parent to better meet the infant's or child's needs.

Skin Care

The moist secretions from the trach can irritate the skin. It is important to keep the area around the tracheostomy clean and dry to prevent skin irritation and infection. Wash the skin with soap and water, and dry well. Change the trach ties each day or if they become wet or dirty. Tie the knot in a new place each time to keep from irritating the skin. Do not apply any ointments or other medications on the skin unless you are told to do so by your health professional.

No dressing is necessary; a dressing may add moisture to the site and encourage a yeast rash.

Barrier creams or ointments (Desitin, Vaseline, ilex, etc.) or barrier wafers, wipes, or dressings (Cavilon No Sting barrier film, AllKare Protective Barrier Wipe, Stomahesive Skin Barrier, Coloplast Skin Barrier) can be used to protect the skin around the tube if leaking occurs.

Safety

Careful adult supervision is needed when the child is near water. Tub baths can be given, but be careful not to allow water into

NOTE: For some children, additional instructions on stoma care and/or use of monitor may be needed. Patient and Family Education instructions are available for CPR and postural drainage.

PATIENT AND FAMILY EDUCATION

Caring for the Child with a Tracheostomy—cont'd

the trach. Swimming and boating must be avoided; however, the child can use a wading pool with supervision.

Any smoke, aerosol sprays, powder, or dust can irritate the lining of the child's trachea. Therefore the child should not be in the same room with anyone who is smoking or where aerosol sprays (e.g., hairspray, antiperspirants) are being used. Strong cleaning liquids such as ammonia are also irritating. Hair from animals that shed can clog the child's trachea. Avoid stuffed animals and toys with small parts that can be removed and put into the trach by a curious child.

All the people who provide care for the child must be aware of how to suction the trach so that they can help you. Anyone caring for the child alone must also know cardiopulmonary resuscitation (CPR). Tape a list of emergency phone numbers to each telephone in the house. Include 911 (if available in your area), numbers for the local hospital and your health professional, and any other numbers that are needed.

Call your health professional at ______________ if any of the following occurs for 12 to 24 hours:

- The child is very irritable.
- The child is having trouble breathing.
- Temperature is above 100.4° F
- Yellow or green mucus from trach or stoma is present.
- Bright red blood from the trach is present.
- The smell of the mucus changes.
- The amount of mucus increases.
- The tracheostomy comes out and you are unable to replace it.

Suctioning

You will need to suction the child's trach to keep the airway clear of mucus. Suctioning helps the child to breathe more easily. Suctioning should be done when the child wakes up and before sleep. Suction the child when any of the following occurs:

- She is having trouble breathing.
- She appears very restless.
- She has trouble eating or sucking.
- Her color becomes paler.
- Her nostrils flare (spread out).
- You hear either the sound of air bubbling through the mucus or stridor (whistling or crowing).

When the child has a cold, more mucus is produced so you will need to suction more often. But suction only when needed; suctioning too often can cause the body to make more mucus.

Preparing the Supplies

Clean Jars and Containers

Wash plastic containers or glass jars with lids in a dishwasher or hot soapy water, and rinse well. Use a clean towel to dry, or allow to air dry. Keep a supply of them washed and dried.

Sterile Saline

Boil water for 5 minutes. Add ¾ teaspoon of noniodized salt (check the ingredients on the box) to each 16 ounces (2 cups) of water when you are heating the water. Let cool, then pour into a clean glass jar and cover. Store the sterile saline in the refrigerator.

Tracheostomy Ties

Use ½-inch seam binding, which is available in the sewing department of many stores. Self-sticking (Velcro) ties are also available but are safe only if the child cannot pull them apart.

Equipment

Suction machine with tubing
Cardiorespiratory monitor (if ordered)
Suction catheters
Clean plastic container for rinsing catheter
Nonsterile gloves.

Instructions

1. Gather all the equipment you will need.
2. Wash your hands with soap and water. Count to 10 while washing, then rinse with clear water and dry with a clean paper or cloth towel. Put on gloves.
3. Open the suction catheter package, and connect the catheter to the suction machine.
4. Make sure the suction machine is plugged in and working. Check that the suction pressure is not above 80 mm Hg for infants or 120 mm Hg for older children.
5. Before suctioning, you must measure the right distance to insert the catheter. Holding the extra trach in one hand, place the suction catheter next to the trach tube. Slowly push the catheter until it is at the tip of the trach tube opening or less than ¼ inch (½ centimeter) longer than the trach tube. Hold this spot with your fingers or mark it with a pen. Now measure the distance from the tip of the catheter to the spot you are holding. Write it down: ____________. This is how far you should insert the catheter each time you suction.
6. Place the tip of the catheter in the sterile saline or water, and place your thumb over the opening to get suction. The sterile saline lubricates the catheter (Figure 2).
7. With your thumb off the opening (no suction), insert the suction catheter to the premeasured distance at the

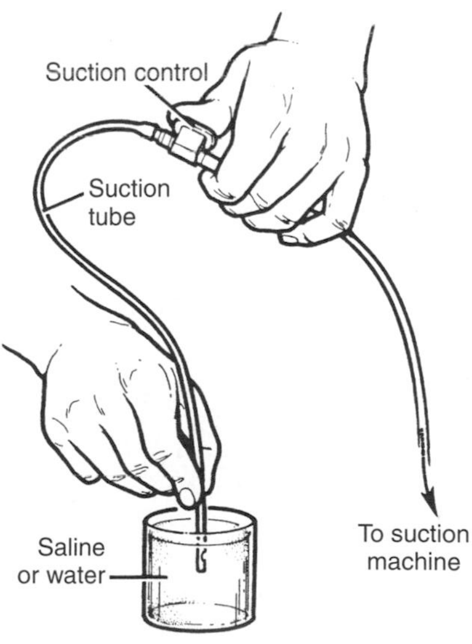

FIGURE 2 Rinsing and lubricating suction catheter with thumb on suction control.

Continued

PATIENT AND FAMILY EDUCATION

Caring for the Child with a Tracheostomy—cont'd

tip of the trach tube opening or less than ¼ inch (½ centimeter) longer than the tube (Figure 3).

8. Place your thumb on the suction port to obtain suction. Rotate or twist the catheter as you remove it with a slow, steady motion (Figure 4). Both inserting the catheter and suctioning should take no longer than 3 or 4 seconds. Remember, the child cannot breathe during suctioning. As a reminder, count 1—one thousand, 2—one thousand, and so on.
9. Look at the mucus. Check the color, smell, and thickness for any change.
10. Rinse the suction catheter in the sterile saline or water with your thumb on the suction port.
11. Allow about 30 seconds before suctioning again.
12. Repeat steps 5 through 11 up to three times.
13. Hold and comfort the child.
14. PRAISE THE CHILD FOR HELPING.
15. After each use, discard the saline and clean the container. Clean the suction machine to have it ready for the next time.
16. Use the following instructions, or ask your health professional to discuss the care of the suction catheters.
17. Wash your hands with soap and water, even if you wore gloves. Count to 10 while washing, then rinse with clear water and dry with a clean paper or cloth towel.

Changing the Tracheostomy Tube

A plastic or metal tracheostomy tube may be used. Your health professional will provide you with any specific instructions needed.

The tracheostomy tube is changed once a month (per manufacturer's recommendation) or any time the parent suspects a plug obstructing airflow to allow for a thorough cleaning of the tube. The change should be done 2 to 3 hours after meals to avoid any chance of the child vomiting. When you change the tube, check the skin around the trach for any redness, swelling, cuts, or bruises.

Equipment

Clean trach tube with trach ties attached (Figure 5) and obturator, if needed
Suction machine with catheters
Sterile saline in clean container
Pipe cleaners
Hot, soapy water
White vinegar

Instructions for Changing the Tube

1. Gather all the equipment you will need.
2. Wash your hands with soap and water. Count to 10 while washing, then rinse with clear water and dry with a clean paper or cloth towel.
3. Place the child in an infant seat or sitting upright.
4. If the child is unable to help, have your helper hold the child's arms while the tube is being changed.
5. Suction the trach until it is clear. (See instructions for suctioning.)
6. Untie or carefully cut the old trach ties. Use scissors with rounded tips.
7. Remove the trach tube (Figure 6).
8. Quickly check the skin.
9. Quickly dip the clean trach tube in the sterile saline, and shake to remove excess water.
10. Insert the clean tracheostomy tube (with or without an obturator) into the opening (stoma).
11. Remove obturator if used.
12. Secure the tracheostomy ties, either at the side or back of the neck. Change the position of the knot each time the tube or ties are changed. Make sure that the ties are snug enough to let you put only one finger under them (Figure 7).
13. If you are unable to put the new tube in, reposition the child's neck, dip the tube into the saline, and try again. If you still cannot get the tube in, check to see if the child is in distress. If the child is not in distress call your health professional. If the child is having trouble breathing, call

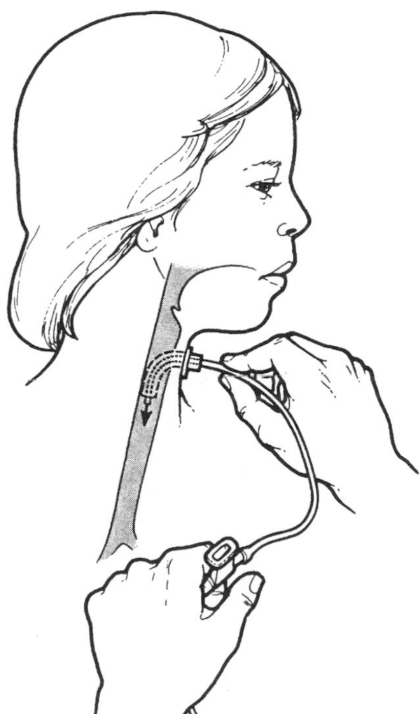

FIGURE **3** Putting the suction catheter in trach tube with thumb off suction control. The premeasured catheter is inserted to the tip of the catheter or no more than ¼ inch (½ centimeter) longer than tube.

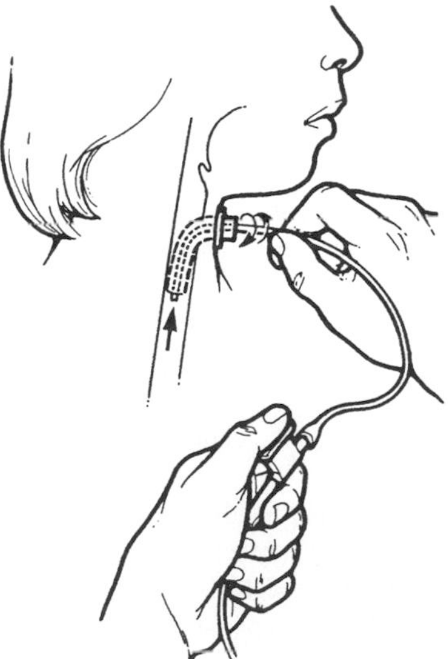

FIGURE **4** Twisting catheter while removing it from tracheostomy tube with thumb on suction control.

PATIENT AND FAMILY EDUCATION

Caring for the Child with a Tracheostomy—cont'd

the emergency numbers and begin rescue breathing if necessary.

14. Hold and comfort the child.
15. PRAISE THE CHILD FOR HELPING.
16. Wash your hands with soap and water. Count to 10 while washing, then rinse with clear water and dry with a clean paper or cloth towel.

NOTE: The child may cough or gag during the insertion or removal of the tracheostomy tube. Gently tell the child when you are almost finished. If the child is old enough, teach her how to help you by handing you the supplies.

Your health professional will instruct you on the care of the suction catheters, or use the following method.

Instructions for Cleaning Suction Catheters

1. Rinse the suction catheters in cool tap water. Do not use hot water because it "cooks" the mucus and makes it more difficult to remove.
2. Place the catheters in a clean jar filled with hot, soapy water.
3. Rinse both the inside and outside of the tube under hot, running water. Hold the tube with kitchen tongs so that you don't burn yourself.
4. Rinse the inside and outside with sterile saline.
5. Shake off the excess water.
6. Mix 1 part white vinegar and 3 parts water in a clean container.
7. Place the clean catheters in this solution for 30 minutes.
8. Remove the catheters from the liquid, and rinse thoroughly with clean water.
9. Shake off the excess water.
10. Place on a clean paper towel to dry. When the tubes are completely dry, place them in a clean plastic bag.
11. Close the bag, and store until the next time you suction the child.
12. If you notice any moisture in the bag, repeat the entire cleaning procedure.

Instructions for Cleaning the Tracheostomy Tube

1. Rinse the trach tube in cool tap water. Hot water "cooks" the mucus, which makes it harder to remove.
2. Place the trach tube in a clean jar filled with hot, soapy water.
3. Scrub the tube with pipe cleaners while it is in the jar.
4. While holding it by the area where the ties are attached, rinse both the inside and outside of the tube under hot, running water. You can hold it with kitchen tongs so that you do not burn yourself.
5. Rinse the inside and outside of the tube with sterile saline.
6. Shake off the excess water.
7. Mix 1 part white vinegar and 3 parts water in a clean container.
8. Place the clean tube in this solution for 30 minutes.
9. Remove the tube from the liquid, and rinse thoroughly with clean water.
10. Shake off the excess water.
11. Place inside a clean paper towel to dry. Keep the trach tube in a safe place so that it can dry undisturbed.
12. When the tube is completely dry, place it in a clean plastic bag.
13. Close the bag, and store until the next tube change.
14. If you notice any moisture in the bag, repeat the entire cleaning procedure.

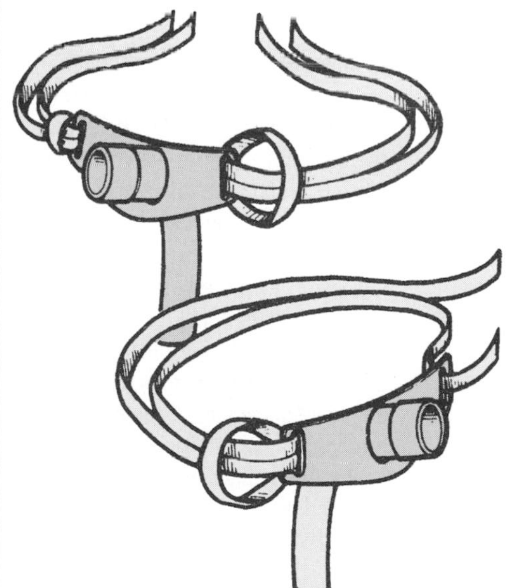

FIGURE **5** Tracheostomy tube with ties. Knot will be tied either in back *(top example)* or on side *(bottom example)*.

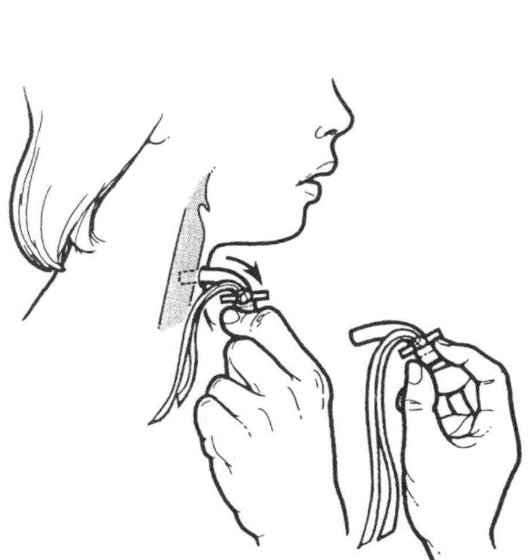

FIGURE **6** Removing tracheostomy tube with left hand. Right hand has clean tube ready to insert.

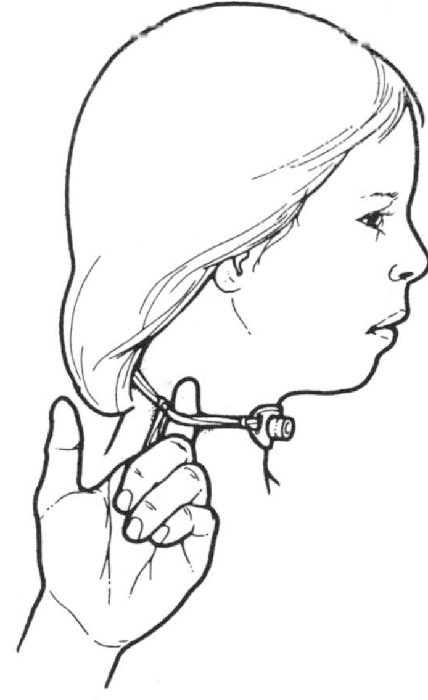

FIGURE **7** Tracheostomy ties are tight enough if only one finger fits under them.

PATIENT AND FAMILY EDUCATION

Home Apnea Monitoring

Prolonged apnea is defined as a lack of breathing for 20 seconds or more or a shorter time period if the child develops a bluish or pale color, the heart rate drops, or both. Many infants will not breathe for approximately 15 seconds. This is considered normal when the child does not have any color change or a significant drop in heart rate and begins breathing without stimulation.

When the child has apnea, it is necessary for his breathing and heart rate to be monitored at home using special equipment called an *apnea monitor.* You also need to keep a record and write down a description of each apneic episode. This description includes the date, time, and the child's condition. This record will help your health professional to evaluate the need for continued home monitoring. The child should be on the apnea monitor at all times, except at bath time.

Equipment

Apnea monitor (respiratory and heart rate)
Electrodes and belt
Clock or watch with second hand in the room where the baby sleeps
Apnea recording sheet and pencil or pen near monitor
Emergency numbers attached to all telephones in the house

Instructions

Follow the manufacturer's instructions for applying the electrodes or belt to the child and setting up the monitor. The monitor requires electricity to operate. Most monitors are equipped with battery packs that allow you to take short trips with the child. Carefully read the manufacturer's instructions for the care of the batteries. All adolescents and adults in the home should be familiar with the monitor, cardiopulmonary resuscitation (CPR), and the following information. You will be taught about the care and use of your specific monitor.

The monitor can be used anywhere in the home and is easily moved. Place the monitor on a sturdy, flat surface in the room, out of the reach of any other children. The monitor will sound an alarm if breathing stops for more than 20 seconds. When an alarm sounds, you must determine if the infant has stopped breathing; if the child is able to begin breathing without stimulation; and if the machine is working properly.

Placement of Electrodes and Belt

Correct placement of the electrodes is important for the monitor to be useful. Place your index and middle fingers just below the child's nipple (use only one finger for small infants). Slide the fingers over to the side edge of the child's chest. Place one electrode here. Do the same for the other side, and place the second electrode (Figure 1). If your monitor has a belt, the electrodes are attached to the belt, then the belt is placed on the child's chest. Put the belt on the child, making sure the electrodes are placed as described previously.

Care of Skin Electrodes

If skin electrodes are used, they should be changed every 2 to 3 days or when they become loose. To change the electrodes, carefully peel them off the child's chest. Wash the skin with soap and water to remove all the adhesive, and dry thoroughly.

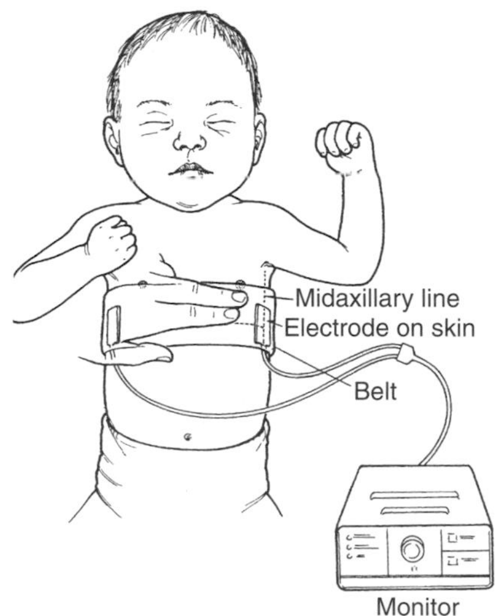

FIGURE 1 Placement of electrodes or belt for apnea monitoring.

Attach the monitor leads to the new electrodes before you apply them to the skin. Peel the backing of one of the electrodes, and apply it to the skin. Attach the other electrode in the same manner. Notify your health professional if there are signs of redness at the site of the electrodes.

Procedure for Alarms Sounding

1. Calmly check the time.
2. Do not touch the child. Observe the child for another 10 seconds. If the child is not awake:
   a. Look at the child's color to see if it is the usual color.
   b. Place your ear by the child's nose and mouth, and listen for air moving.
   c. Look to see if the child's chest is moving.
3. If the child's color is good and the child is breathing without difficulty, wait 10 seconds; then check the monitor to make sure the connections are intact, and reset the alarm. Write down the event on the record sheet.
4. If there is a change in the skin color or the child has not resumed breathing, gently rub the child's back or chest. Wait 10 seconds, then look to see if the infant begins breathing. If he does, observe him for another 10 seconds. If the color and breathing have returned to normal, check the monitor to make sure the connections are intact and reset the alarms. Write down the event on the record sheet.
5. If the child has not resumed breathing, gently slap the bottom of his feet. Never vigorously shake the child. Wait 10 seconds and look to see if he begins breathing. If he does, observe for another 10 seconds. If the color and breathing have returned to normal, check the monitor to make sure the connections are intact and reset the alarms. Write down the event on the record sheet.
6. If the child has not responded to measures such as slapping the feet, begin CPR.

5 - PATIENT AND FAMILY EDUCATION

PATIENT AND FAMILY EDUCATION

Measuring Oxygen Saturation with Pulse Oximetry

Your health professional may request that you periodically measure the child's oxygenation status using a pulse oximeter monitor. This monitor is noninvasive and will provide information about the child's breathing or oxygenation status. The pulse oximeter consists of a cable with a light-emitting diode (LED) that transmits data to a small hand-held machine. The LED measures the child's oxygen saturation in the arteries under the skin where it is placed. The sensor is usually applied to a finger or toe, or in small infants it may attach to the bottom of the foot. There are two types of sensors: one is shaped like an alligator clip and the finger is placed in the bed of the clip; this type is more suitable for older children who can sit still for a few minutes. The other type of sensor is a small adhesive strip that can be wrapped around a finger or toe to obtain a reading. The following steps are of a general nature. Follow the directions give by the health professional or equipment company for the pulse oximeter you have.

Instructions

1. Wash hands with soap and water.
2. Turn the machine on.
3. Make sure the finger or toe to be used is clean and free of any ointment or dressing.
4. For the infant using an adhesive strip sensor, remove the clear strip covering the adhesive strip so that the sticky side is exposed. Avoid touching the sticky side of the adhesive strip.
5. Place the light on the sticky side of the adhesive strip against the side of the finger or toe so that it is in full contact with the skin.
6. Wrap the remainder of the adhesive strip around the finger or toe so the sensor is attached firmly to the digit.
7. The pulse oximeter will begin searching for a pulse at the site where the sensor is placed; this may take 30 to 60 seconds. If the child is moving or squirming, the sensor may not be able to pick up a signal, so it may be necessary to hold the child's foot or finger still.
8. Once a pulse is detected the monitor will read the oxygen saturation. Many models also give a pulse reading. If the pulse reading does not seem appropriate for the child, the sensor will not read an accurate oxygen saturation. In other words, if the child's pulse is 100 beats per minute but the monitor is showing a pulse of only 50 beats per minute, the oxygen saturation reading will be inaccurate.
9. If the pulse oximeter reading is to be left on the child continuously, change the sensor to another finger or toe as recommended by the manufacturer or health professional or at least every 5 to 6 hours. Clean the previously used digit well with soap and water.
10. The alligator clip may be used in an older child; simply make sure the finger is clear of any ointment or nail polish, and have the child place a finger inside the bed of the alligator clip against the sensor light. A reading is usually obtained within 30 to 60 seconds if the child is still. Movement can make the alligator sensor unable to read the oxygen saturation. In such cases the adhesive strip may need to be used.
11. Record the oxygen saturation as requested by the health professional. Note that the oxygen saturation monitor will give a reading only between approximately 21 and 100. Check with the health professional for your child's target oxygen saturation range.

This section may be photocopied and distributed to families.

PATIENT AND FAMILY EDUCATION

Infant Cardiopulmonary Resuscitation for the Layperson*†

Cardiopulmonary resuscitation (CPR) is a way to do some of the work of the heart and lungs for a short time. The heart pumps the blood around the body to provide oxygen and nutrients to the different body systems. The lungs are a transfer spot: as the blood flows through the lungs, oxygen is picked up by the blood and carbon dioxide is released. When the infant breathes, oxygen is brought into the body and carbon dioxide is breathed out.

Before beginning CPR, you must assess the infant to determine if both breathing and the heart have stopped. CPR is done when the infant's heart and breathing have stopped. You can breathe for the infant by blowing air into the lungs. Between breaths, the chest falls and air flows out of the lungs. You can do the work of the heart by doing a chest compression. The heart can be squeezed between the breastbone and the backbone to force blood out of the heart and into the arteries that carry it to the rest of the body. When you remove the pressure, the heart fills with blood so that the next squeeze (compression) will force additional blood out to the body.

All the infant's caregivers must be able to perform CPR so that you can have relief and help if needed. Prepare for an emergency before it happens. Keep emergency information for your local emergency medical services handy so visitors, relatives, or babysitters can call in an emergency. Include 911 (if available in your area), the phone number that you are calling from, the address, and directions to the house. When calling in an emergency, be sure to give all this information in addition to a description of what happened, who is involved, and the condition of the infant. Do not hang up the phone until the emergency operator tells you to do so.

Equipment

Emergency telephone numbers
Bulb syringe

Assessment

1. If trauma is suspected, do not move infant's head or neck. Avoid moving him unless he is in danger of further injury. If you need to turn the infant over, roll the head and torso as a unit, supporting head and neck to prevent movement that could cause further injury.
2. Try to wake the infant. Tap the infant, say his name loudly, clap your hands, or flick the bottom of his feet and look for a response or movement. Do not shake the infant.
3. Shout for help.
4. If infant is still unresponsive, begin CPR at once by opening the infant's airway (see below).
5. If there is someone else with you, have that person call the emergency telephone number (911 or other number) for help. If you are alone, do not stop to call, but begin CPR immediately. Do CPR for approximately 2 minutes, then call the emergency number as quickly as possible.

Airway

1. Place the infant on his back on a *firm surface.*
2. Properly position the head and open the airway by placing your hand on the forehead and placing the fingers (not thumb) of your other hand under the bony part of the lower jaw near the middle of the chin. Be careful not to push the forehead too far back or to put too much pressure on the skin under the jaw. Make sure the infant's lips are open. Then lift and slightly tilt the head backward to a sniffing or nose-pointing-to-the-ceiling position. Proper positioning is essential to allow air to enter the windpipe and the lungs).
3. If vomit is present, you must clear the infant's mouth before you breathe for the infant.
4. Quickly remove any mucus or vomit with your fingers or a bulb syringe after turning the infant's head to the side. If using a bulb syringe, squeeze it before placing it in the mouth, then release the pressure in the bulb to remove the material.
   a. If you see an object, vomit, or mucus, insert a finger of your other hand inside the mouth.
   b. Move your finger toward you across the back of the throat. This sweeping action will help remove foreign objects.

Breathing

5. Once the mouth is clear, reposition the head and observe the chest to determine if the infant has begun breathing normally. Place your ear close to the infant's mouth and *look, listen,* and *feel* for breathing for no longer than 5 to 10 seconds.

Procedures based on *BLS for healthcare providers,* Dallas, 2006, American Heart Association (AHA).

NOTE: The 2005 AHA guidelines for CPR state that rescue breathing will not be taught to laypersons except in a Heartsaver Pediatric First Aid Course and that laypersons should not perform ventilations without compressions to save time and lives. Therefore, rescue breathing is not included.

*These guidelines should not be used as substitutes for basic life support (BLS) training. It is important that you participate in an infant-child CPR class in your community. Courses available to the public include Family and Friends CPR Anytime, a 25-minute course sponsored by the AHA, and the Heartsaver CPR course, also by the AHA.

†In 2005 the AHA made changes for laypersons performing CPR; the guidelines on these pages are for laypersons.

Community Resource for Parents and Professionals

American Heart Association; *http://www.americanheart.org;* (800) 242-8721; may contact regarding local availability of CPR classes and materials for learning CPR.

PATIENT AND FAMILY EDUCATION

Infant Cardiopulmonary Resuscitation for the Layperson—cont'd

6. If breathing has not begun, you must breathe for the infant.
   a. Open your mouth wide. Cover the infant's nose and mouth with your mouth.
   b. Give two slow breaths about 1 second in length, pausing to inhale between them. Each breath should be just enough to make the chest rise.
7. If you do not see the chest rise, reposition the head and try again. After repositioning the head, if you still cannot see the chest rise, then follow the instructions for caring for the choking infant (see p. 581).
8. If the infant vomits, turn his head to the side and clean out the mouth with your finger or the bulb syringe.

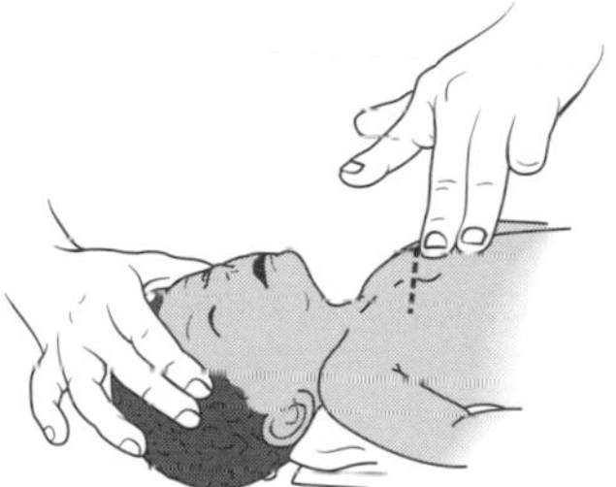

FIGURE 1 Proper location for chest compressions in infant.

Circulation

9. After giving two breaths and seeing the chest rise, if the infant does not start breathing on his own or showing signs of circulation—breathing, coughing, or movement— prepare to do chest compressions.
10. Locate the correct position for chest compressions. Use one hand to hold the infant's head in the correct position. Using the other hand, draw an imaginary line connecting the infant's nipples and place two fingers just below the imaginary line on the breastbone (Figure 1).
11. Using your middle and ring fingers, press straight down on the breastbone for a distance of ½-1 inch. Chest compressions are performed 30 times. After 30 chest compressions, stop and give the infant two breaths of air about 1 second each. The chest should rise gently with each breath. Keep your fingers on the infant's chest while giving the two breaths, and start chest compressions immediately after the two breaths (Figure 2). If the chest does not rise, reposition the infant's head and give another breath. If the breath does not go in, follow the instructions for a choking infant.
12. Compress the chest at a rate of 100 times per minute.
13. After about 2 minutes (five cycles of 30 chest compressions and two breaths), stop and check the infant to see if he has begun breathing or is showing signs of circulation—breathing, coughing, or movement. Call the emergency number (911) if you are alone. If you need to move the infant to get help or to get out of danger, try not to stop CPR for more than 5 seconds.‡
14. CPR may be stopped only if one of the following occurs:
    a. The infant begins breathing.
    b. You are relieved by someone who can do CPR.
    c. You reach medical assistance and other action is begun.
    d. You are exhausted.
15. *Side position*—If the infant begins breathing on his own and there is no suspected injury, place infant on his side with the head resting on his arm and with the top leg slightly bent at the knee and resting on the firm surface (Figure 3). When possible write down a description of what occurred, and immediately call the emergency phone number (911).

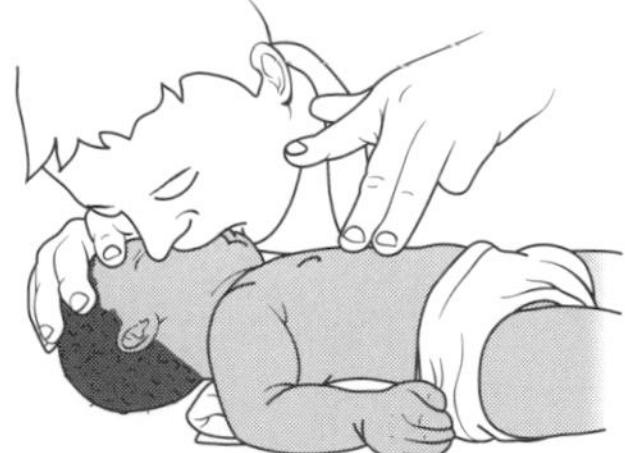

FIGURE 2 Combining breathing with chest compressions.

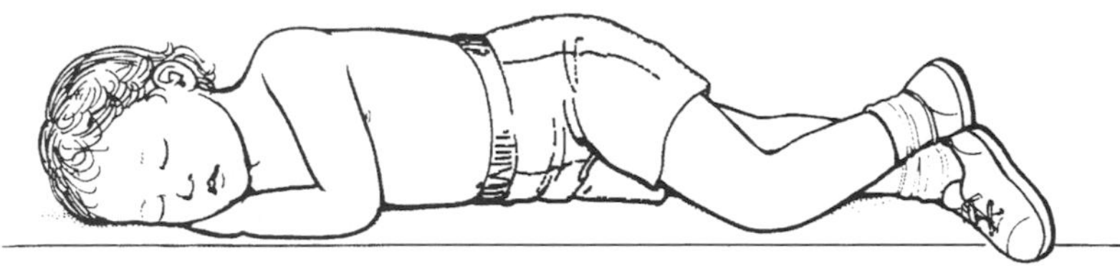

FIGURE 3 Side position.

‡The 2005 AHA guidelines do not include automated external defibrillator (AED) recommendations for infants less than 1 year of age.

PATIENT AND FAMILY EDUCATION

Child Cardiopulmonary Resuscitation for the Layperson*†‡

Cardiopulmonary resuscitation (CPR) is a way to do some of the work of the heart and lungs for a short time. The heart pumps the blood around the body to provide oxygen and nutrients to the different body systems. The lungs are a transfer spot: as the blood flows through the lungs, oxygen is picked up by the blood and carbon dioxide is released. When the child breathes, oxygen is brought into the body and carbon dioxide is breathed out.

Before beginning CPR, you must assess the child to determine if both breathing and the heart have stopped. CPR is done when the child's heart and breathing have stopped. You can breathe for the child by blowing air into the lungs. Between breaths, the chest falls and air flows out of the lungs. You can do the work of the heart by doing a chest compression. The heart can be squeezed between the breastbone and the backbone to force blood out of the heart and into the arteries that carry it to the rest of the body. When you remove the pressure, the heart fills with blood so that the next squeeze (compression) will force additional blood out to the body.

All the child's caregivers must be able to perform CPR so that you can have relief and help if needed. Prepare for an emergency before it happens. Keep emergency information for your local emergency medical services handy so visitors, relatives, or babysitters can call in an emergency. Include 911 (if available in your area), the phone number that you are calling from, the address, and directions to the house. When calling in an emergency, be sure to give all this information in addition to a description of what happened, who is involved, and the condition of the child. Do not hang up the phone until the emergency operator tells you to do so.

Equipment

Emergency telephone numbers

Assessment

1. If trauma is suspected, do not move the child's head or neck. Avoid moving child unless she is in danger of further injury. If you need to turn the child over, roll the head and torso as a unit, supporting head and neck to prevent movement that could cause further injury.
2. Try to wake the child. Tap the child, say her name loudly, clap your hands, or shake shoulders gently to look for a response or movement.
3. Shout for help.
4. If child is still unresponsive, begin CPR at once by opening the child's airway (see Airway section).
5. If there is someone else with you, have him or her call the emergency telephone number (911) for help and obtain an automated external defibrillator (AED). If you are alone, do not stop to call, but begin CPR immediately. Do CPR for 2 minutes, then call the emergency number as quickly as possible. *If the child is 8 years old or older, call the emergency telephone number (911) for help before beginning CPR.**

Airway

1. Place the child on her back on a *firm* surface.
2. Properly position the head and open the airway by placing your hand on the forehead and placing the fingers (not thumb) of your other hand under the bony part of the lower jaw near the middle of the chin. Then lift and slightly tilt the head backward to a sniffing or nose-pointing-to-the-ceiling position. Be careful not to push the forehead too far back or to put too much pressure on the skin under the jaw. Make sure the child's lips are open. Proper positioning is essential to allow air to enter the windpipe and the lungs (Figure 1).
3. If vomit is present, you must clear the child's mouth before you breathe for the child.
4. Quickly remove any mucus or vomit with your fingers after turning the child's head to the side.
   a. If you see an object, vomit, or mucus, insert a finger of your other hand inside the mouth.
   b. Move your finger toward you across the back of the throat. This sweeping action will help remove foreign objects.

Breathing

5. Once the mouth is clear, reposition the child's head and observe the chest to determine if breathing has begun. Place your ear close to the child's mouth and look, listen, and

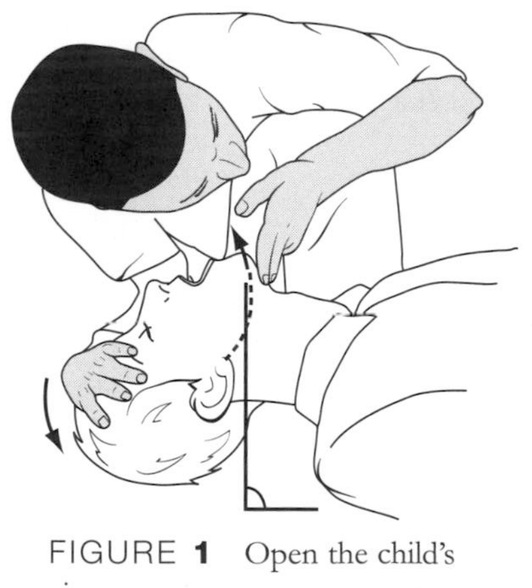

FIGURE 1 Open the child's airway.

Procedures based on *BLS for healthcare providers,* Dallas, 2006, American Heart Association (AHA).
*Instructions are for children between 1 and 8 years old; the sections in italics are for children older than 8 years.
†These guidelines should not be used as substitutes for basic life support (BLS) training. It is important that you participate in an infant-child CPR class in your community.
‡Reflects the AHA 2005 changes for layperson CPR.

5 - PATIENT AND FAMILY EDUCATION

PATIENT AND FAMILY EDUCATION

Child Cardiopulmonary Resuscitation for the Layperson—cont'd

feel for normal breathing for no longer than 5 to 10 seconds. Gasping is not breathing.

6. If breathing has not begun, you must breathe for the child.
   a. Open your mouth and cover the child's mouth with your mouth (Figure 2). For a larger child, pinch the nose closed with the thumb and forefinger of the hand you have on the forehead.
   b. Give two slow breaths about 1 second in length, pausing to inhale between them. Each breath should be just enough to make the chest rise.
7. If you do not see the chest rise, reposition the head and try again. After repositioning the head, if you still cannot see the chest rise, then follow the instructions for caring for the choking child (see p. 582).
8. If the child vomits, turn her head to the side and clean out the mouth with your finger.

Circulation

9. After you have given two breaths and seen the chest rise, if the child does not start breathing on his own or showing signs of circulation—breathing, coughing, or movement—prepare to do chest compressions.[§]

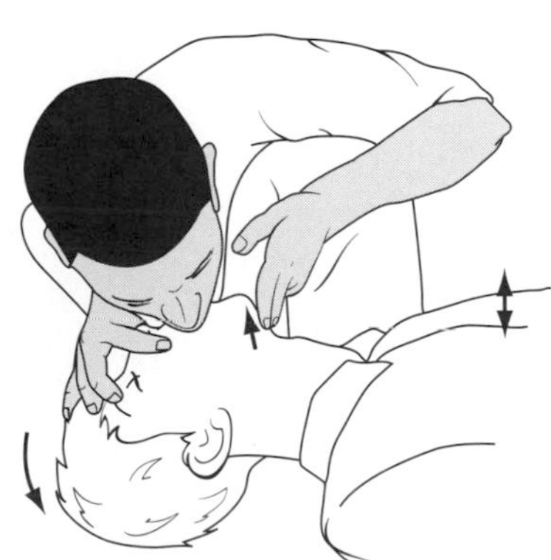

FIGURE 2 Covering the mouth and nose for breathing.

10. Locate the correct position for chest compressions. Use one hand to maintain the child's head position. Place the heel of the other hand in the center of the child's chest (breastbone) at an imaginary line drawn between the nipples. Avoid compressing the child's lower chest where the ribs meet the breastbone. Feel the notch: you must avoid pressing at this spot. The fingers of the hand on the chest should be pointing away from you, across the child's chest (Figure 3).
    For children 8 years old and older, place the heel of the hand on the breastbone between the nipples as described previously. One or two hands may be used to perform chest compressions on the older child. Your fingers can be interlaced or straight; your arms must be straight and your shoulders above your hands.
11. Using one hand, press straight down on the breastbone for a distance of 1 to 1½ inches. Compress the chest 30 times. After each 30 compressions, stop and give the child two breaths of air. If one hand is used for compressions keep your other hand on the head to maintain the head in the right position. If the child resumes breathing, place in the side recovery position (see step 18) (Figure 4).
    a. *For children 8 years old and older, using both hands, press straight down on the breastbone for a distance of 1½ to 2 inches. Compress the chest 30 times. After each 30 compressions, give the child two breaths of air. Remember to correctly reposition the head when you breathe for the child (see step 2).*
    b. *If the child resumes breathing place in the side recovery position* (see step 17).

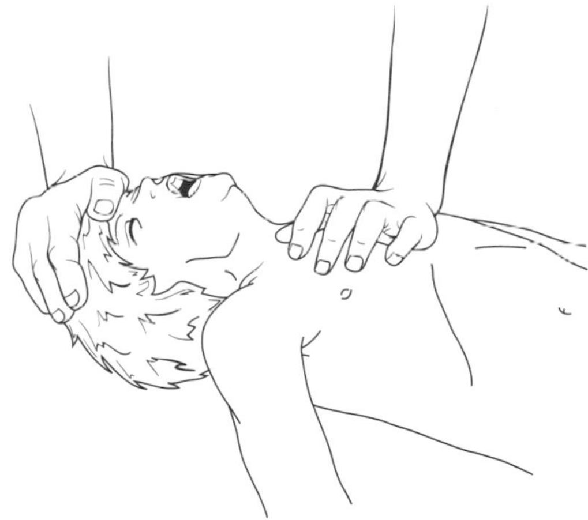

FIGURE 3 Hand position for chest compression in the child.

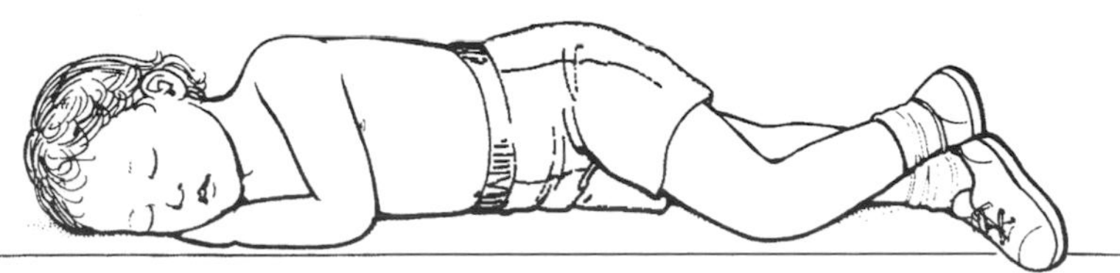

FIGURE 4 Side position.

§NOTE: The 2005 AHA guidelines for CPR state that rescue breathing will not be taught to laypersons except in a Heartsaver Pediatric First Aid Course and that laypersons should not perform ventilations without compressions to save time and lives. Therefore rescue breathing is not included.

Continued

PATIENT AND FAMILY EDUCATION

Child Cardiopulmonary Resuscitation for the Layperson—cont'd

12. Compress the chest at a rate of 100 times per minute.
13. After about five cycles of 30 compressions and two breaths (about 2 minutes), stop and check the child to see if he has begun breathing or is showing signs of circulation—movement or coughing. *For children 8 years old and older, the chest compression rate is also 30, followed by two breaths.*
    Call the emergency number (911) as quickly as possible if you are alone. If an automated external defibrillator (AED) is available, take it to the child's side. If you need to move the child to get help or to get out of danger, try not to stop CPR for more than 5 seconds.
14. If the arrest is *witnessed* the AED should be used to analyze the rhythm *before* CPR is begun. If the arrest is *unwitnessed,* after approximately 2 minutes of CPR have been performed and the child remains unresponsive (not breathing, coughing, or moving), open the AED and place the child pads on the chest at the location indicated on the diagram of the AED (Figure 5). The AED should be able to read a shockable rhythm and have pediatric pads. *Use adult pads for a child 8 years old or older.* In the event that the AED has only adult pads, use these on children 1 to 8 years of age.
15. Administer one shock according to the instructions on the AED, then resume CPR immediately afterward, beginning with chest compressions.
16. CPR may be stopped only if one of the following occurs:
    a. The child begins breathing, and the heart rate returns to normal.
    b. You are relieved by someone who can do CPR.
    c. You reach medical assistance, and other action is begun.
    d. You are exhausted.
17. *Side position*—If normal breathing resumes and there is no suspected injury, roll the child onto his side, moving the head, shoulders, and trunk at the same time without twisting. Place the child's head resting on his hand and slightly bend the top leg at the knee, resting it on the floor or surface (Figure 4). If the child begins breathing on his own, write down a description of what occurred and immediately call the emergency phone number (911)

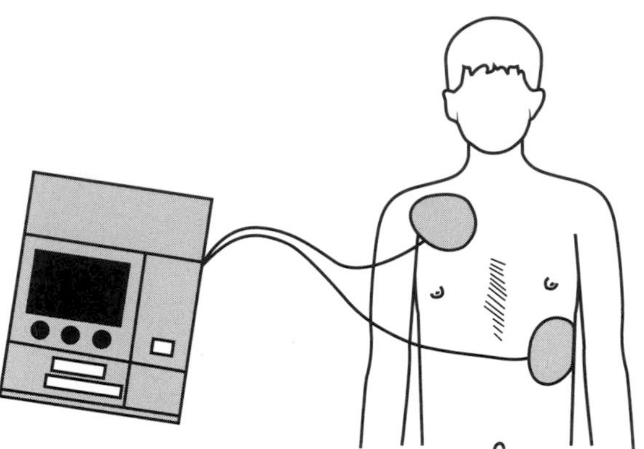

FIGURE 5 Placement of the AED on a child.

PATIENT AND FAMILY EDUCATION

Caring for the Choking Infant*

Choking is a life-threatening event. If the infant begins to choke or is *suddenly* having difficulty breathing, immediate action is needed. When the airway is blocked, the infant cannot cry or make sounds. If the infant is coughing, his color is pink, and he can make sounds, no action may be needed.

Awake and Alert (Conscious) Infant

1. Look at the infant to see if he is having difficulty breathing.
2. If the infant is not making sounds, appears to be choking, has a dusky color, and has difficulty breathing, take action immediately.
   a. Position the infant face down on your forearm. Hold the head and neck firmly with one hand. If the infant is large, it may be necessary to support his weight on your thigh.
   b. Give up to five quick blows between the shoulder blades with the heel of your hand (Figure 1).
3. If this does not remove the object, turn infant over and give up to five chest thrusts. *Do not perform abdominal thrusts in an infant.*
   a. Draw an imaginary line connecting the child's nipples.
   b. Place your middle and ring fingers on the breastbone at the imaginary line.
   c. Thrust straight down on the breastbone at a distance of ½-1 inch (Figure 2).
4. Repeat steps 2 and 3 until the airway is clear and the infant begins breathing or until the infant stops responding.

Infant Stops Responding

1. If the infant stops responding, place him on a *firm,* flat surface and call 911 or call out for help.
2. Start the steps of cardiopulmonary resuscitation (CPR).
3. Each time you open the infant's airway, check the inside of the infant's mouth to see if there is a foreign object.
4. Open the infant's mouth, using your thumb and fingers to grasp both the tongue and lower jaw and lift up gently.
5. If you see an object, insert a finger of your other hand inside the infant's mouth and move your finger toward you across the back of the infant's throat. This sweeping action will help remove the foreign object. Be careful not to push it farther into the throat. If no object is seen, *do not sweep* out the mouth.
6. Perform 5 cycles of 30 compressions and two breaths (about 2 minutes) (Figure 3). If you are alone call 911.
7. Continue with CPR until the infant revives or starts breathing on his own. If the infant does not begin breathing, properly position the head and open the airway by placing your hand on the forehead and place the fingers (not thumb) of your other hand under the bony part of the lower jaw near the middle of the chin. Then lift and slightly tilt the head backward to a sniffing or nose-pointing-to-ceiling position. Proper positioning is essential to allow the air to enter the windpipe and the lungs.

Infant Found Unconscious (Choking Is Suspected)

1. Try to wake the infant. Tap the infant, say his name loudly, clap your hands, or flick the bottom of his feet to look for a response or movement. Do not shake the infant.
2. Shout for help.
3. Begin CPR steps described previously at once if infant is still not breathing, coughing, or moving.
4. If there is someone else with you, have that person call the emergency telephone number (911) for help. If you are alone, do not stop to call, but begin CPR immediately. Do CPR for approximately 2 minutes (five cycles of 30 compressions and two breaths), then call the emergency number as quickly as possible.
5. Perform steps 3 to 5, described previously. Continue with CPR until the infant revives, the infant starts breathing on his own, or medical help arrives.

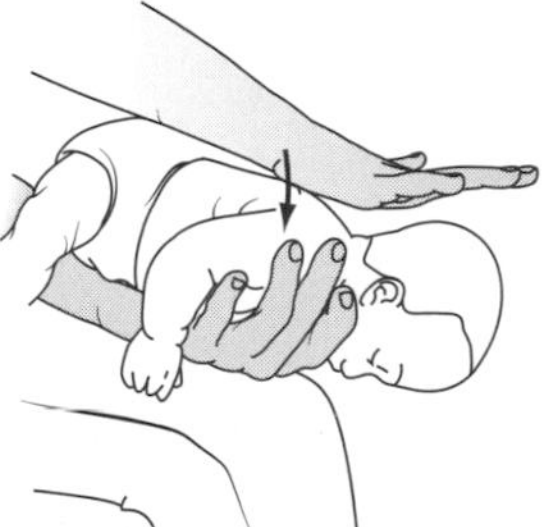

FIGURE **1** Back blows in the infant.

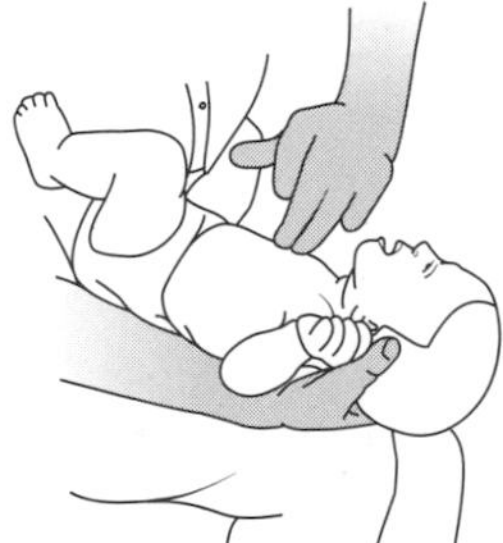

FIGURE **2** Performing chest thrusts in the infant.

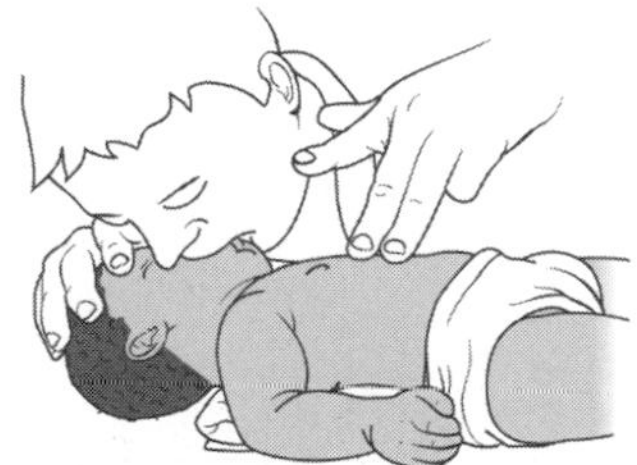

FIGURE **3** Performing chest compressions and breathing for the infant.

5 - PATIENT AND FAMILY EDUCATION

Procedures based on *BLS for healthcare providers,* Dallas, 2006, American Heart Association.
*These guidelines should not be used as substitutes for basic life support (BLS) training. It is important that you participate in an infant-child CPR class in your community.

PATIENT AND FAMILY EDUCATION

Caring for the Choking Child*†

Choking is a life-threatening event. If a child begins to choke or is having difficulty breathing, immediate action is needed. When the airway is blocked, the child cannot talk or make noises. If the child is coughing forcefully and can make sounds, no action is needed; stand by and let the child cough.

Awake and Alert (Conscious) Child—Sitting or Standing

1. Ask the child if he is choking. Check if he can talk or make noise. If the child cannot make any sounds, cannot cry (younger child), has bluish lips or skin, makes the choking sign of clutching neck with both hands, or has high-pitched noisy breathing, then begin emergency treatment.
2. Stand or kneel behind the child (Figure 1).
3. Wrap your arms around the child's waist. Make one hand into a fist.
4. Put your fist, with the thumb side against the child's skin, on the abdomen just above the bellybutton. Make sure you are well below the breastbone.
5. Grab the fist with your other hand. Press into the child's abdomen with upward thrusts until the object comes out or until the child loses consciousness.
6. Each thrust should be a separate movement. This allows enough force to help the child expel the object.
7. If the child still cannot breathe, continue the thrusting while calling for help.
8. Continue your actions until the object is removed, help arrives, or the child becomes unconscious. If the child becomes unconscious, call the emergency telephone number (911) at once.

Awake and Alert (Conscious) Child—Lying Down

1. If the child is on the floor, ask if the child is OK. If she cannot breathe or talk, place the child flat on her back.
2. Kneel on the floor at the child's feet. For a larger child you can straddle the legs.
3. Put the heel of one hand on the child's abdomen just above the bellybutton. Make sure you are well below the breastbone.
4. Put your other hand on top of the first hand and press into the child's abdomen with a quick upward thrust (Figure 2).
5. Repeat the thrusts until the object comes out or until the child becomes unconscious. Each thrust should be a separate movement. This allows enough force to help the child expel the object.
6. Repeat steps 3, 4, and 5 until the object is removed, help arrives, or the child stops responding or becomes unconscious. If the child becomes unconscious, call the emergency number (911) at once.

Child Becomes Unconscious

1. If the child is not already on the floor, place the child on a *firm,* flat surface, such as the floor.
2. Yell for help.

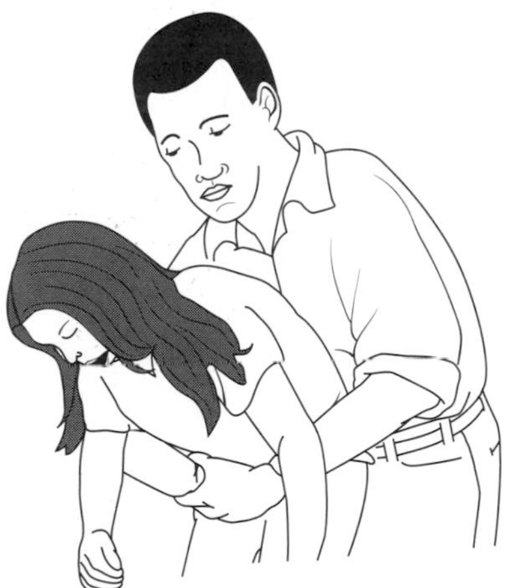

FIGURE **1** Proper hand placement for abdominal thrusts.

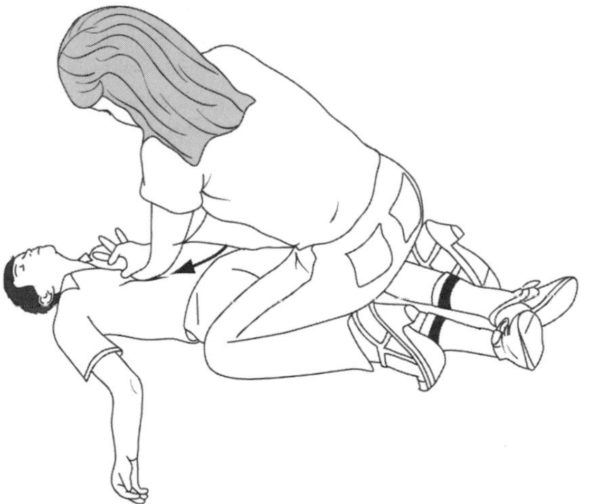

FIGURE **2** Hand placement for abdominal thrusts with the child lying down.

Procedures based on *BLS for healthcare providers,* Dallas, 2006, American Heart Association.

*These guidelines should not be used as substitutes for basic life support (BLS) training. It is important that you participate in an infant-child CPR class in your community.

†These guidelines are for a child 1 year of age and older.

PATIENT AND FAMILY EDUCATION

Caring for the Choking Child—cont'd

3. Kneel on the floor next to the child.
4. Open the child's mouth. Use your thumb and fingers to grasp both the tongue and lower jaw and lift.
5. If you can see an object, insert a finger of your other hand inside the child's mouth. Move your finger toward you across the back of the throat and remove the object. This sweeping action will help remove the foreign object. Be careful not to push it further into the throat. If no object is seen, do not sweep out the mouth.
6. If the child does not begin breathing, open the airway and try to breathe for the child.
   a. To open the airway, gently lift the chin with the fingers of one hand on the lower jaw near the middle of the chin while pushing down on the forehead with your other hand. Tilt the child's head into a sniffing or nose-pointing-to-the-ceiling position.
   b. Lift the chin so that the teeth are almost together while listening for breathing.
   c. If the child does not begin breathing at once, pinch the child's nostrils with your thumb and forefinger while keeping the child's head in the right position.
   d. Open your mouth wide, take a regular breath, make a tight seal over the child's mouth, and try to breathe for child.
   e. Watch to see if the child's chest rises with your breath.
7. If you are alone, begin the steps of CPR.
8. After about five cycles of 30 compressions and two breaths, call 911 then resume CPR. Continue CPR until emergency help arrives or the child revives or starts breathing normally.

Child Found Unconscious (Choking Is Suspected)

1. Try to wake the child. Tap the child, say his name loudly, clap your hands, or shake gently to look for a response or movement.
2. Call for help. If someone comes to help, tell them to call the emergency telephone number (911).
3. If the child is not already on the floor, place the child on a *firm,* flat surface, such as the floor.
4. Kneel on the floor next to the child.
5. If the child is not breathing, open the airway and try to breathe for the child.
   a. To open the airway, gently lift the chin with one hand while pushing down on the forehead with your other hand. Tilt the child's head into a sniffing or nose-to-the-ceiling position.
   b. Lift the chin so the teeth are almost together while you listen for breathing.
   c. If the child does not breathe after 5 seconds, pinch the child's nostrils with your thumb and forefinger while keeping the child's head in the right position.
   d. Open your mouth wide, take a regular breath, make a tight seal over the child's mouth, and attempt to breathe for the child.
   e. Watch to see if the child's chest rises with your breath.
6. If you are alone, perform five cycles of 30 compressions and two breaths, then call the emergency telephone number (911).

Instructions Related to Injury Prevention and First Aid

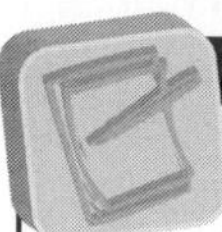

GUIDELINES

Preventing Eye Injuries

Infants and Toddlers

Avoid any toys with long, pointed handles, such as a pinwheel on a stick.

Keep pointed instruments and tools (e.g., scissors, knives, screwdrivers, rulers, pencils, sticks) out of reach.

Do not allow child to *walk* or *run* with any pointed object (e.g., spoon, lollipop, toothbrush) in the hand.

Keep child away from play of older children and adults that involves projectile activities (e.g., throwing a ball, golf, target shooting, swings).

Stress importance of fire safety and poison protection in preventing thermal and chemical burns to the eye.

Shield child's eyes when in direct sunlight.

Preschoolers

Supervise the use of sharp or pointed objects, especially scissors.

Teach proper use of pointed objects, such as toy guns or scissors (namely, to always point them *away* from the face and from anyone else at close range).

Teach child to walk carefully (never run) while carrying any sharp or pointed object.

Keep child away from projectile activities.

Begin teaching respect for firearms.

Avoid play with mirrors, especially where they can reflect sunlight.

School-Age Children and Adolescents

Teach proper use and respect for potentially dangerous equipment such as power tools (objects fly from them), firearms, firecrackers (where legally permitted), and racquet sports.

Stress use of eye protection when riding motorcycles or when using equipment such as power saws or chemistry sets.

Teach child to open soda bottles by pointing screw cap away from face.

Encourage safe use of curling iron.

Advise child of danger of excessive sunlight (ultraviolet burns).

Warn child to never look directly at the sun, even with sunglasses, and to avoid using mirror in sunlight.

Monitor duration of wear of contact lens to prevent corneal scratching and possible scarring.

Emergency Care of Eye Injuries

Foreign Object

Examine eye for presence of a foreign body. (Turn upper lid outward to examine upper eye.)

Remove a freely movable object with pointed corner of gauze pad lightly moistened with water.

Do not irrigate eye or attempt to remove a penetrating object. (See below.)

Caution child against rubbing eye.

Chemical Burns

Irrigate eye copiously with tap water for 20 minutes.

Turn upper lid outward to flush thoroughly.

Hold child's head with eye under tap of running lukewarm water.

Take to emergency room.

Have child rest with eyes closed.

Keep room darkened.

Ultraviolet Burns

If skin is burned, patch both eyes (make sure lids are completely closed); secure dressing with a gauze bandage wrapped around head rather than tape.

Have child rest with eyes closed.

Refer to an ophthalmologist.

Hematoma (Black Eye)

Use a flashlight to check for gross hyphema (hemorrhage into anterior chamber; visible fluid meniscus across iris; more easily seen in light-colored than in brown eyes).

Apply ice for first 24 hours to reduce swelling if no hyphema is present.

Refer to an ophthalmologist immediately if hyphema is present.

Have child rest with eyes closed.

Penetrating Injuries

Take child to emergency room.

Never remove an object that has penetrated eye.

Follow strict aseptic technique in examining eye.

Observe for the following:

- Aqueous or vitreous leaks (fluid leaking from point of penetration)
- Hyphema
- Shape and equality of pupils, reaction to light
- Prolapsed iris (not perfectly circular)

Apply a Fox shield if available (not a regular eye patch), and apply patch over unaffected eye to prevent bilateral movement.

Maintain bed rest with child in 30-degree Fowler position.

Caution child against rubbing eye.

Selected Substances Causing Poisoning in Children

Corrosives (strong acids or alkali)
Drain, toilet, or oven cleaners
Electric dishwasher detergent (liquid, because of higher pH, is more hazardous than granular)
Mildew remover
Batteries
Clinitest tablets
Denture cleaners
Bleach

Signs of Poisoning

- Severe burning pain in mouth, throat, and stomach
- White, swollen mucous membranes; swelling of lips, tongue, and pharynx (respiratory obstruction); oral ulcerations
- Violent vomiting (hemoptysis)
- Drooling and inability to clear secretions from throat
- Signs of shock
- Anxiety and agitation

Comments

- Household bleach is a commonly ingested corrosive but rarely causes serious damage.
- Liquid corrosives cause more damage than granular preparations.
- DO NOT INDUCE VOMITING.
- Call National Poison Control Center—(800) 222-1222

Hydrocarbons
Gasoline
Kerosene
Lamp oil
Mineral seal oil (found in furniture polish)
Lighter fluid
Turpentine
Paint thinner and remover

Signs of Poisoning

- Gagging, choking, and coughing
- Nausea
- Vomiting
- Changes in level of consciousness or awareness, such as lethargy
- Weakness

Respiratory Symptoms of Pulmonary Involvement

- Tachypnea
- Cyanosis
- Retractions
- Grunting

Comments

- Immediate danger is aspiration into lungs (even small amounts can cause bronchitis and chemical pneumonia).
- Gasoline, kerosene, lighter fluid, mineral seal oil, and turpentine cause severe pneumonia.
- DO NOT INDUCE VOMITING.
- Call National Poison Control Center—(800) 222-1222.

Acetaminophen

Signs of Toxic Ingestion

Occurs in four stages:

1. Initial period (2 to 4 hours after ingestion): nausea, vomiting, sweating, pallor
2. Latent period (24 to 36 hours): Patient improves.
3. Hepatic (liver) involvement (may last up to 7 days and be permanent): pain in right upper quadrant, jaundice, confusion, stupor, coagulation abnormalities.
4. Patients who do not die during hepatic stage gradually recover.

Comments

- Most common drug poisoning in children.
- Occurs primarily from acute ingestion.
- Toxic dose is 150 mg/kg or greater in children.
- Call National Poison Control Center—(800) 222-1222.
- Toxicity from chronic therapeutic use is rare but may occur with ingestion of approximately 150 mg/kg/day, or about double the recommended maximum therapeutic dose (90 mg/kg/day) of acetaminophen, for several days (Douidar SM, Al-Khalil I, Habersang RW: Severe hepatotoxicity, acute renal failure and pancytopenia in a young child after repeated acetaminophen overdosing, *Clin Pediatr* 33[1]:42-45, 1994); toxicity is more likely in children with hepatic dysfunction (McDonough J: Acetaminophen overdose, *Am J Nurs* 98[3]:52, 1998).

Aspirin (ASA)

Signs of Toxic Ingestion

- Acute poisoning
  - Nausea
  - Disorientation
  - Vomiting
  - Dehydration
  - Diaphoresis (profuse sweating)
  - Hyperpnea (hyperventilation)
  - Hyperpyrexia (fever)
  - Oliguria (decreased urine output)
  - Tinnitus (ringing in ears)
  - Coma
  - Convulsions (seizures)

Chronic Poisoning

- Same as for acute poisoning, but subtle onset (often mistaken for viral illness)
- Dehydration, coma, and seizures possibly more severe
- Bleeding tendencies

Comments

- May be caused by acute ingestion (severe toxicity occurs with 300 to 500 mg/kg).
- May be caused by chronic ingestion (i.e., more than 100 mg/kg/day for 2 or more days); can be more serious than acute ingestion.

- Time to peak serum salicylate can vary with enteric aspirin or the presence of concretions (bezoars).
- Activated charcoal is important early in ASA toxicity.
- Sodium bicarbonate transfusions to correct metabolic acidosis and urinary alkalinization may be effective in enhancing elimination. Urinary alkalinization is very difficult to achieve. Be aware of the risk for fluid overload and pulmonary edema.
- Use external cooling for hyperpyrexia.
- Administer anticonvulsants.
- Use oxygen and ventilation for respiratory depression.
- Give vitamin K for bleeding.
- In severe cases, hemodialysis (not peritoneal dialysis) may be used.
- Call Poison Control Center—(800) 222-1222.

Iron

Mineral supplement or vitamin containing iron

Signs of Toxic Ingestion

Occurs in five stages:

1. Initial period (½-6 hours after ingestion) (if child does not develop gastrointestinal symptoms in 6 hours, toxicity is unlikely): vomiting, hematemesis (bloody vomiting), diarrhea, hematochezia (bloody stools), stomach pain
2. Latency (2 to 12 hours): Patient's condition improves
3. Systemic toxicity (4 to 24 hours after ingestion): metabolic acidosis, fever, hyperglycemia, bleeding, shock, death (may occur)
4. Hepatic injury (48 to 96 hours): seizures, coma
5. Rarely, pyloric stenosis develops at 2 to 5 weeks.

Comments

- Factors related to frequency of iron poisoning include:
  - Widespread availability
  - Packaging of large quantities in individual containers
  - Lack of parental awareness of iron toxicity
  - Resemblance of iron tablets to candy (e.g., M&Ms)
- Toxic dose is based on the amount of elemental iron in various salts (sulfate, gluconate, fumarate), which ranges from 20% to 33%; ingestions of 60 mg/kg are considered dangerous.
- Call National Poison Control Center—(800) 222-1222.

Plants

- See Box 5-1.

Signs of Toxic Ingestion

- Depend on type of plant ingested
- May cause local irritation of mouth and throat and entire gastrointestinal tract
- May cause respiratory, renal, and neurologic symptoms
- Topical contact with plants can cause dermatitis (rash, itching)

Comments

- Some of the most commonly ingested substances are plants
- Rarely cause serious problems, although some plant ingestions can be fatal
- Can also cause choking and allergic reactions
- DO NOT INDUCE VOMITING.
- Treatment
  - Wash from skin or eyes.
  - Call National Poison Control Center—(800) 222-1222

BOX 5-1 | POISONOUS AND NONPOISONOUS PLANTS

Poisonous Plants*

Apple (leaves, seeds)
Apricot (leaves, stem, seed pits)
Azalea (foliage and flowers)
Buttercup (all parts)
Cherry—wild or cultivated (twigs, seeds, foliage)
Daffodil (bulbs)
Dumb cane, dieffenbachia (all parts)
Elephant ear (all parts)
English ivy (all parts)
Foxglove (leaves, seeds, flowers)
Holly (berries, leaves)
Hyacinth (bulbs)
Ivy (leaves)
Mistletoe (berries, leaves)†
Oak tree (acorn, foliage)
Philodendron (all parts)
Plum (pit)
Pokeweed, pokeberry (roots, berries, leaves [when eaten raw])
Poinsettia (leaves)‡
Poison ivy, poison oak (leaves, fruit, stems, smoke from burning plants)
Pothos [devil's ivy, golden pothos] (all parts)
Rhubarb (leaves)
Tulip (bulbs)
Water hemlock (all parts)
Wisteria (seeds, pods)
Yew (all parts)

Nonpoisonous Plants

African violet
Aluminum plant
Asparagus fern
Begonia
Boston fern
Christmas cactus
Coleus
Gardenia
Grape ivy
Jade plant
Piggyback begonia
Piggyback plant
Prayer plant
Rubber tree
Snake plant
Spider plant
Swedish ivy
Wax plant
Weeping fig
Zebra plant

*Toxic parts in parentheses.
†Eating one or two berries or leaves is probably nontoxic.
‡Mildly toxic if ingested in massive quantities. May cause gastrointestinal upset.

Parental Guidelines for Reducing Blood Lead Levels*

Make sure child does not have access to peeling paint or chewable surfaces painted with lead-based paint, especially windowsills and window wells.

If a house was built before 1960 (and possibly before 1980) and has hard-surface floors, wet mop them at least once a week. Wipe other hard surfaces (e.g., windowsills, baseboards). If there are loose paint chips in an area, such as a window well, use a disposable cloth to pick up and discard them. Do not vacuum hard-surfaced floors or windowsills or window wells, because this spreads dust. Use vacuum cleaners with agitators to remove dust from rugs rather than vacuum cleaners with suction only. If a rug is known to contain lead dust and cannot be washed, it should be discarded.

Wash and dry child's hands and face frequently, especially before eating.

Wash toys and pacifiers frequently.

If soil around home is or is likely to be contaminated with lead (e.g., if home was built before 1960 or is near a major highway), plant grass or other ground cover; plant bushes around outside of house so that child cannot play there.

During remodeling of older homes, be sure to follow correct procedures. Be certain children and pregnant women are not in the home, day or night, until process is completed. Following deleading, thoroughly clean house using cleaning solution to damp mop and dust before inhabitants return.

In areas where lead content of water exceeds the drinking water standard and a particular faucet has not been used for 6 hours or more, "flush" the cold-water pipes by running the water until it becomes as cold as it will get (30 seconds to longer than 2 minutes). The more time water has been sitting in pipes, the more lead it may contain.

Use only cold water for consumption (drinking, cooking, and especially for making infant formula). Hot water dissolves lead more quickly than cold water and thus contains higher levels of lead. May use first-flush water for nonconsumption uses.

Have water tested by a competent laboratory. This action is especially important for apartment dwellers; flushing may not be effective in high-rise buildings or in other buildings with lead-soldered central piping.

Do not store food in open cans, particularly if cans are imported.

Do not store food in pottery or ceramic ware that was inadequately fired or that is meant for decorative use.

Do not store drinks or food in lead crystal.

Avoid folk remedies or cosmetics that contain lead.

Make sure that home exposure is not occurring from parental occupations or hobbies. Household members employed in occupations such as lead smelting should shower and change into clean clothing before leaving work. Construction and abatement workers may also bring home lead contaminants.

Make sure child eats regular meals, because more lead is absorbed on an empty stomach.

Make sure child's diet contains plenty of iron and calcium and not excessive fat.

Basic First Aid

ABRASION OR SCRAPE

The skin may be scraped when the child falls on a rough surface such as cement or asphalt. A scrape only removes the first layer of skin. Cleanse with soap and water; an antibiotic ointment may be applied. The child may find relief from a benzocaine-based spray that temporarily anesthetizes (deadens) the area. A bandage may be used to cover the scrape if clothing comes in contact with the scrape; otherwise, no covering is necessary.

If the scrape tears off larger portions of tissue (first layer of skin or more), bleeding may be stopped by applying a clean cloth on the scrape and applying firm pressure. Clean with soap and water.

Puncture wounds may require suturing (sewing together) or stapling. Apply a clean cloth to the wound and apply firm pressure. It may help to apply an ice pack over the cloth to decrease tissue trauma. Consult a health professional or emergency services if bleeding does not stop within 20 minutes. If an object is embedded in the skin it is best to consult a health professional.

BLOODY NOSE

Blunt trauma may cause the highly vascular nose to bleed, causing concern. Dry environmental air may also cause the child to have a nosebleed during sleep.

Apply pressure to the sides of the bridge of the nose (by pinching) until the bleeding stops. Keep the child seated upright. Keep a terry cloth or towel under the nose to absorb any blood.

If the nosebleed does not stop within 15 minutes, consult a health professional. Additional packing with gauze may be required.

In most cases a simple nosebleed does not require medical attention (unless child has a blood disorder such as hemophilia)—the amount of blood lost is usually not significant, but

*For more information, contact the county or state department of health or environment for information on local water quality. For general information on lead, call the Environmental Protection Agency Safe Drinking Water Hotline, (800) 426-4791; *http://www.epa.gov.*

it looks worse because blood spreads on cloth and the amount looks more threatening than it really is. Consult a health professional if concerns exist or if nosebleeds recur.

BRUISE

Most bruises occur from a fall or sudden moving contact of the body part with a solid object (wood bat, cement, asphalt, play equipment). The immediate care is to stop any bleeding by placing a clean cloth on the area and applying pressure. Swelling may happen, and this can be treated with an ice pack for 15 minutes. The bruise will typically turn red immediately, then blue as dying red cells enter the traumatized tissues. Consult a health professional if trauma involves vital organ or tissue such as the eye or abdomen or occurs around the nose or mouth. If the child shows signs of breathing difficulty, call emergency medical services *immediately*.

A head bruise may cause a bump or knot. Ice may be applied to minimize swelling. If the child loses consciousness or starts vomiting, consult the health professional for further assistance. If there is a laceration or cut, suturing (stitches) may be necessary.

A *concussion* (manifested by dizziness, disorientation, loss of consciousness, unaware of surroundings, blurred vision) requires prompt medical evaluation and intervention.

BROKEN BONE (FRACTURE)

Children frequently fall from trees, playground equipment, and toys such as bicycles or are involved in contact sports activities that may cause a bone to fracture. In some cases the bone may simply bend instead of actually breaking.

The child will usually cry in pain or refuse to use the affected (suspected) limb or joint. It is not necessary to manipulate or handle a suspected fracture except to immobilize or splint. If the bone is obviously broken—compare with opposite limb—apply an immobilizing support or splint loosely. If there is a lot of bleeding or the bone is sticking out of the skin, take child to the nearest health professional or emergency facility immediately.

If the suspected break is minor, apply an immobilizing splint until the health professional is consulted; a rolled towel may be used for the wrist, arm, or finger (toes), and a folded blanket for larger limb such as the leg. Apply an ice pack to the affected area for no more than 15 minutes.

When possible raise the affected limb above the level of the heart.

For pain the child may take Tylenol or ibuprofen. There is no need to wait until you see the health professional for evaluation to administer either of these, provided the child can tolerate either one.

CUT OR LACERATION

Children often experience cuts from sharp or dull objects in the environment. All cuts do not require suturing provided the bleeding stops and the skin edges can be closed effectively. Deeper cuts involving deeper tissue layers may require extensive surgery for proper healing. Most cuts should be evaluated within 8 to 10 hours if suturing is to be performed successfully. Some superficial cuts not involving joints or hair can be "glued" successfully. Staples may be used to join skin lacerations on the scalp (where hair growth hides the scar).

The first priority is to stop the bleeding by placing a clean cloth such as a towel on the cut. Apply firm pressure without cutting off circulation to the extremity distal (on the other side) to the cut (laceration). Tourniquets are not recommended except when used by experienced health care workers.

Deep cuts (more than ⅛ inch) should be evaluated by a health professional.

SPRAIN

Muscle sprains usually involve a sudden shifting of weight or energy in the opposite direction, causing muscle pain, swelling, and possibly some bruising in the area affected.

Ankle sprains are the most common types of muscle sprain seen, especially in children involved in running and jumping or contact and noncontact sports activities.

Treat an ankle sprain by first immobilizing with a loose-fitting wrap such as an Ace bandage. Second, elevate the ankle above the level of the waist or heart and apply an ice pack to the painful area for no more than 15 minutes at a time. Remember the RICE acronym:

R—rest
I—ice
C—containment
E—elevate

Elbow sprains may involve more serious damage and should be evaluated by a health professional. You may use the RICE acronym for immediate treatment initially.

Administer acetaminophen (Tylenol) or ibuprofen per package instructions. These may be administered according to the child's previous ability to take these medications, but with a sprained muscle it is not necessary to avoid pain medication until the health professional is consulted.

Ankle rehabilitation involves exercising the involved muscles in a non–weight-bearing fashion. Point the toes outward and make a circle-8 going in a clockwise fashion; repeat this exercise 10 times several times daily. Another exercise for ankle rehabilitation involves a rubber stretch band. Place the band, which looks like a large rubber band, on the bottom of the affected foot and hold the other end of the rubber band. Push the foot against the rubber band, keeping the knees straight, then return the ankle to its neutral position and stretch the band "out" several times with the ankle. These exercises are aimed at keeping the muscle strengthened and preventing tightness while keeping weight off the affected joint.

Consult a health professional if the pain is severe (weight bearing is impossible) and swelling does not go away in 4 to 5 days.

TOOTH AVULSION (CHIPPED, BROKEN, OR KNOCKED OUT)

A child may fall and break a tooth or chip a portion off the primary tooth. In some cases the pediatric dentist can glue a chipped tooth for cosmetic purposes. At the regular dental visit ask for an information sheet on tooth care.

An avulsed tooth—one that is knocked completely out of the gum—may be replaced, but this often depends on the type of tooth, the tooth location, the dentist's previous experience, and the child's age. Place the avulsed tooth in a liquid solution such as milk, and seek dental care as required.

A tooth that is knocked loose but remains in the socket may be glued in place. Consult the child's dental care health professional for instructions.

TICK REMOVAL

Avoid tick infestation when in an area heavily populated by ticks by using an insect repellant containing dicthyltoluamide (DEET) on the clothing. Use as directed on the container. When feasible wear a long-sleeved shirt and long-legged pants tucked into boots or long socks to prevent ticks from getting on the skin.

Inspect the child daily at bedtime for ticks if you live in an area that has ticks or have been around animals that may carry ticks into the house. Ticks may be found in the hair on the head, behind the ears, or on the neck, groin, or beltline (waist).

Remove the tick with tweezers close to the skin and pull straight out. If tweezers are not available, use a tissue or paper towel to avoid contact with the insect. Wash hands well with soap and water if contact with tick occurs.

UNIT 6

Reference Data

Abbreviations Used in Laboratory Tests

Abbreviation	Term
cap	capillary
CHF	congestive heart failure
conc	concentration
CSF	cerebrospinal fluid
d	day; diem
EDTA	ethylenediaminetetraacetate
g	gram
H^+	hydrogen ion
Hb	hemoglobin
hr	hour
IU	international unit
L	liter
m	meter
mEq	milliequivalent
min	minute
mm	millimeter
mm Hg	millimeters of mercury
mm H_2O	millimeters of water
mm_3	cubic millimeter
mo	month
mol	mole
mOsm	milliosmole
Na	sodium
RBC	red blood cell
s	second
temp	temperature
therap	therapeutic
U	international unit of enzyme activity
uU	picogram unit
vol	volume
WBC	white blood cell
wk	week
yr	year
$>$	greater than
$\geq$	greater than or equal to
$<$	less than
$\leq$	less than or equal to
$\pm$	plus or minus
$\cong$	approximately equal to

The Joint Commission Official "Do Not Use" List*

Do Not Use	Potential Problem	Use Instead
U (unit)	Mistaken for "0" (zero), the number "4" (four), or "cc"	Write "unit"
IU (International Unit)	Mistaken for "IV" (intravenous) or the number "10" (ten)	Write "International unit"
Q.D., QD, q.d., qd (daily)	Mistaken for each other	Write "daily"
Q.O.D., QOD, q.o.d., qod (every other day)	Period after the "Q" mistaken for "I" and the "O" mistaken for "I"	Write "every other day"
Trailing zero (X.0 mg)†	Decimal point is missed	Write "X mg"
Lack of leading zero (.X mg)		Write "0.X mg"
MS	Can mean "morphine sulfate" or "magnesium sulfate	Write "morphine sulfate"
MSO_4 and $MgSO_4$	Confused for one another	Write "magnesium sulfate"

*Applies to all orders and all medication-related documentation that is handwritten (including free-text computer entry) or on preprinted forms.
†**Exception:** A "trailing zero" may be used only where required to demonstrate the level of precision of the value being reported, such as for laboratory results, imaging studies that report size of lesions, or catheter/tube sizes. It may not be used in medication orders or other medication-related documentation.

Prefixes Denoting Decimal Factors

Prefix	Symbol	Amount
kilo	k	one thousand (10^3)
deci	d	one tenth (10^{-1})
centi	c	one hundredth (10^{-2})
milli	m	one thousandth (10^{-3})
micro	mc, μ	one millionth (10^{-6})
nano	n	one billionth (10^{-9})
pico	p	one trillionth (10^{-12})
femto	f	one quadrillionth (10^{-15})

Common Laboratory Tests*

		Normal Ranges	
Test, Specimen	**Age, Gender, Reference**	**Conventional Units**	**International Units (SI)**
Acetaminophen			
Serum or plasma	Therap conc	10-30 mcg/ml	66-200 μmol/L
	Toxic conc	>200 mcg/ml	>1300 μmol/L
Ammonia nitrogen			
Plasma or serum	Newborn	90-150 mcg/dl	64-107 μmol/L
	0-2 wk	79-129 mcg/dl	56-92 μmol/L
	>1 mo	29-70 mcg/dl	21-50 μmol/L
	Thereafter	0-50 mcg/dl	0-35.7 μmol/L
Amylase (serum)	1-19 yr	30-100 U/L	30-100 U/L
Anion gap (sodium-chloride + bicarbonate)		7-16 mEq/L	7-16 mEq/L
Antistreptolysin O titer (ASO)			
Serum	2-4 yr	<160 Todd units	
	School-age children	170-330 Todd units	
Base excess			
Whole blood	Newborn	(−10)-(−2) mEq/L	(−10)-(−2) mmol/L
	Infant	(−7)-(−1) mEq/L	(−7)-(−1) mmol/L
	Child	(−4)-(+2) mEq/L	(−4)-(+2) mmol/L
	Thereafter	(−3)-(+3) mEq/L	(−3)-+3) mmol/L
Bicarbonate (HCO_3)			
Serum	Arterial	21-28 mEq/L	21-28 mmol/L
	Venous	22-29 mEq/L	22-29 mmol/L

Modified from Behrman RE, Kliegman RM, Jenson HB, editors: *Nelson textbook of pediatrics,* ed 17, Philadelphia, 2004, Saunders; McMillan JA, Deangelis CD, Feigin RD, and others, editors: *Oski's pediatrics: principles and practice,* ed 3, Philadelphia, 1999, Lippincott Williams & Wilkins; and Fischbach F: *A manual of laboratory and diagnostic tests,* ed 6, Philadelphia, 2000, Lippincott Williams & Wilkins.

*For a description of abbreviations, see p. 592.

Continued

Test, Specimen	Age, Gender, Reference	Normal Ranges: Conventional Units		Normal Ranges: International Units (SI)	
		Premature (mg/dl)	Full term (mg/dl)	Premature (μmol/L)	Full term (μmol/L)
Bilirubin, total					
Serum	Cord	<2	<2	<34	<34
	0-1 d	<8	<6	<137	<103
	1-2 d	<12	<8	<205	<137
	2-5 d	<16	<12	<274	<205
	Thereafter	<20	<10	<340	<171
Bilirubin, direct (conjugated)					
Serum		0.0-0.2 mg/dl		0-3.4 μmol/L	
Bleeding time					
Blood from skin puncture					
Ivy	Normal	2-7 min		2-7 min	
	Borderline	7-11 min		7-11 min	
Simplate (G-D)		2.75-8 min		2.75-8 min	
Blood volume					
Whole blood	Male	52-83 ml/kg		0.052-0.083 L/kg	
	Female	50-75 ml/kg		0.050-0.075 L/kg	
C-reactive protein (CRP)					
Serum	Cord	52-1330 ng/ml		52-1330 mcg/L	
	2-12 yr	67-1800 ng/ml		67-1800 mcg/L	
Calcium, ionized					
Serum, plasma, or whole blood	Cord	5.0-6.0 mg/dl		1.25-1.50 mmol/L	
	Newborn, 3-24 hr	4.3-5.1 mg/dl		1.07-1.27 mmol/L	
	24-48 hr	4.0-4.7 mg/dl		1.00-1.17 mmol/L	
	Thereafter	4.8-4.92 mg/dl or 2.24-2.46 mEq/L		1.12-1.23 mmol/L	
Calcium, total					
Serum	Cord	9.0-11.5 mg/dl		2.25-2.88 mmol/L	
	Newborn, 3-24 hr	9.0-10.6 mg/dl		2.3-2.65 mmol/L	
	24-48 hr	7.0-12.0 mg/dl		1.75-3.0 mmol/L	
	4-7 d	9.0-10.9 mg/dl		2.25-2.73 mmol/L	
	Child	8.8-10.8 mg/dl		2.2-2.70 mmol/L	
	Thereafter	8.4-10.2 mg/dl		2.1-2.55 mmol/L	
Carbon dioxide, partial pressure (PCO_2)					
Whole blood, arterial	Newborn	27-40 mm Hg		3.6-5.3 kPa	
	Infant	27-41 mm Hg		3.6-5.5 kPa	
	Thereafter: Male	35-48 mm Hg		4.7-6.4 kPa	
	Female	32-45 mm Hg		4.3-6.0 kPa	
Carbon dioxide, total (tCO_2)					
Serum or plasma	Cord	14-22 mEq/L		14-22 mmol/L	
	Premature (1 wk)	14-27 mEq/L		14-27 mmol/L	
	Newborn	13-22 mEq/L		13-22 mmol/L	
	Infant, child	20-28 mEq/L		20-28 mmol/L	
	Thereafter	23-30 mEq/L		23-30 mmol/L	
Cerebrospinal fluid (CSF)					
Pressure		70-180 mm H_2O		70-180 mm H_2O	
Volume	Child	60-100 ml		0.06-0.10 L	
	Adult	100-160 ml		0.10-0.16 L	

		Normal Ranges	
Test, Specimen	**Age, Gender, Reference**	**Conventional Units**	**International Units (SI)**
Chloride			
Serum or plasma	Cord	96-104 mEq/L	96-104 mmol/L
	Newborn	97-110 mEq/L	97-110 mmol/L
	Thereafter	98-106 mEq/L	98-106 mmol/L
Sweat	Normal (homozygote)	<40 mEq/L	<40 mmol/L
	Marginal (e.g., asthma, Addison disease, malnutrition)	45-60 mEq/L	45-60 mmol/L
	Cystic fibrosis	>60 mEq/L	>60 mmol/L
Cholesterol, total			
Serum or plasma†	Acceptable	<170 mg/dl (LDL <110 mg/dl)	<4.4 mmol/L (LDL <2.85 mmol/L)
	Borderline	170-199 mg/dl (LDL 110-129 mg/dl)	4.4-5.1 mmol/L (LDL 2.85-3.35 mmol/L)
	High	≥200 mg/dl (LDL ≥130 mg/dl)	≥5.2 mmol/L (LDL ≥3.35 mmol/L)
Clotting time (Lee-White)			
Whole blood		5-8 min (glass tubes)	5-8 min
		5-15 min (room temp)	5-15 min
		30 min (silicone tube)	30 min
Creatine kinase (CK, CPK)			
Serum	Cord	70-380 U/L	70-380 U/L
	5-8 hr	214-1175 U/L	214-1175 U/L
	24-33 hr	130-1200 U/L	130-1200 U/L
	72-100 hr	87-725 U/L	87-725 U/L
	Adult	5-130 U/L	5-130 U/L
Creatinine			
Serum	Cord	0.6-1.2 mg/dl	53-106 μmol/L
	Newborn	0.3-1.0 mg/dl	27-88 μmol/L
	Infant	0.2-0.4 mg/d	18-35 μmol/L
	Child	0.3-0.7 mg/dl	27-62 μmol/L
	Adolescent	0.5-1.0 mg/dl	44-88 μmol/L
	Adult: Male	0.6-1.2 mg/dl	53-106 μmol/L
	Female	0.5-1.1 mg/dl	44-97 μmol/L
Urine, 24 hr	Premature	8.1-15.0 mg/kg/24 hr	72-133 μmol/kg/24 hr
	Full term	10.4-19.7 mg/kg/24 hr	92-174 μmol/kg/24 hr
	1.5-7 yr	10-15 mg/kg/24 hr	88-133 μmol/kg/24 hr
	7-15 yr	5.2-41 mg/kg/24 hr	46-362 μmol/kg/24 hr
Creatinine clearance (endogenous)			
Serum or plasma and urine	Newborn	40-65 ml/min/1.73 m^2	
	<40 yr: Male	97-137 ml/min/1.73 m^2	
	Female	88-128 ml/min/1.73 m^2	
Digoxin			
Serum, plasma; collect at least 12 hr after dose	Therap conc		
	CHF	0.8-1.5 ng/ml	1.0-1.9 nmol/L
	Arrhythmias	1.5-2.0 ng/ml	1.9-2.6 nmol/L
	Toxic conc		
	Child	>2.5 ng/ml	>3.2 nmol/L
	Adult	>3.0 ng/ml	>3.8 nmol/L

†From National Cholesterol Education Program: Report of the expert panel on blood cholesterol levels in children and adolescents, *Pediatrics* 89(3 pt 2):527, 1992.

Continued

Test, Specimen	Age, Gender, Reference	Normal Ranges: Conventional Units	Normal Ranges: International Units (SI)
Eosinophil count			
Whole blood, capillary blood	50-250 cells/mm³ (µl)	50-250 × 10^6 cells/L	
Erythrocyte (RBC) count			
Whole blood	Cord	3.9-5.5 million/mm³	3.9-5.5 × 10^{12} cells/L
	1-3 d	4.0-6.6 million/mm³	4.0-6.6 × 10^{12} cells/L
	1 wk	3.9-6.3 million/mm³	3.9-6.3 × 10^{12} cells/L
	2 wk	3.6-6.2 million/mm³	3.6-6.2 × 10^{12} cells/L
	1 mo	3.0-5.4 million/mm³	3.0-5.4 × 10^{12} cells/L
	2 mo	2.7-4.9 million/mm³	2.7-4.9 × 10^{12} cells/L
	3-6 mo	3.1-4.5 million/mm³	3.1-4.5 × 10^{12} cells/L
	0.5-2 yr	3.7-5.3 million/mm³	3.7-5.3 × 10^{12} cells/L
	2-6 yr	3.9-5.3 million/mm³	3.9-5.3 × 10^{12} cells/L
	6-12 yr	4.0-5.2 million/mm³	4.0-5.2 × 10^{12} cells/L
	12-18 yr: Male	4.5-5.3 million/mm³	4.5-5.3 × 10^{12} cells/L
	Female	4.1-5.1 million/mm³	4.1-5.1 × 10^{12} cells/L
Erythrocyte sedimentation rate (ESR)			
Whole blood			
Westergren (modified)	Child	0-10 mm/hr	0-10 mm/hr
	<50 yr: Male	0-15 mm/hr	0-15 mm/hr
	Female	0-20 mm/hr	0-20 mm/hr
Wintrobe	Child	0-13 mm/hr	0-13 mm/hr
	Adult: Male	0-9 mm/hr	0-9 mm/hr
	Female	0-20 mm/hr	0-20 mm/hr
Fibrin degradation products (D-dimer), plasma	Adults	68-494 µg/L (mean 207 µg/L)	68-494 µg/L (mean 207 µg/L)
Fibrinogen			
Plasma	Newborn	125-300 mg/d	1.25-3.00 g/L
	Thereafter	200-400 mg/dl	2.00-4.00 g/L
Galactose			
Serum	Newborn	0-20 mg/dl	0-1.11 mmol/L
	Thereafter	<5 mg/dl	<0.28 mmol/L
Urine	Newborn	≤60 mg/dl	≤3.33 mmol/L
	Thereafter	<14 mg/24 hr	<0.08 mmol/d
Glucose			
Serum	Cord	45-96 mg/dl	2.5-5.3 mmol/L
	Newborn, 1 d	40-60 mg/dl	2.2-3.3 mmol/L
	Newborn, >1 d	50-90 mg/dl	2.8-5.0 mmol/L
	Child	60-100 mg/dl	3.3-5.5 mmol/L
	Thereafter	70-105 mg/dl	3.9-5.8 mmol/L
Whole blood	Adult	65-95 mg/dl	3.6-5.3 mmol/L
CSF	Adult	40-70 mg/dl	2.2-3.9 mmol/L
Urine (quantitative)		<0.5 g/d	<2.8 mmol/d
Urine (qualitative)		Negative	Negative

Test, Specimen	Age, Gender, Reference	Normal Ranges: Conventional Units		Normal Ranges: International Units (SI)	
Glucose tolerance test (GTT), oral					
Serum					
Dosages		Normal	Diabetic	Normal	Diabetic
Adult: 75 g	Fasting	70-105 mg/dl	≥126 mg/dl	3.9-5.8 mmol/L	≥7 mmol/L
Child: 1.75 g/kg of ideal weight up to maximum of 75 g	60 min	120-170 mg/dl	≥200 mg/dl	6.7-9.4 mmol/L	≥11 mmol/L
	90 min	100-140 mg/dl	≥200 mg/dl	5.6-7.8 mmol/L	≥11 mmol/L
	120 min	70-120 mg/dl	≥200 mg/dl	3.9-6.7 mmol/L	≥11 mmol/L
Glycohemoglobin hemoglobin (Hb) A1c	1-5 yr	2.1%-7.7% of total Hb		0.021-0.077 fraction of total Hb	
	5-16 yr	3.0%-6.2% of total Hb		0.030-0.062 fraction of total Hb	
Growth hormone (GH, somatotropin)					
Plasma	1 d	5-53 ng/ml		5-53 mcg/L	
	1 wk	5-27 ng/ml		5-27 mcg/L	
	1-12 mo	2-10 ng/ml		2-10 mcg/L	
	Fasting child/adult	<0.7-6.0 ng/ml		<0.7-6.0 mcg/L	
Hematocrit (HCT, Hct)					
Whole blood	1 d (cap)	48%-69%		0.48-0.69 vol fraction	
	2 d	48%-75%		0.48-0.75 vol fraction	
	3 d	44%-72%		0.44-0.72 vol fraction	
	2 mo	28%-42%		0.28-0.42 vol fraction	
	6-12 yr	35%-45%		0.35-0.45 vol fraction	
	12-18 yr: Male	37%-49%		0.37-0.49 vol fraction	
	Female	36%-46%		0.36-0.46 vol fraction	
Hemoglobin (Hb)					
Whole blood	1-3 d (cap)	14.5-22.5 g/dl		2.25-3.49 mmol/L	
	2 mo	9.0-14.0 g/dl		1.40-2.17 mmol/L	
	6-12 yr	11.5-15.5 g/dl		1.78-2.40 mmol/L	
	12-18 yr: Male	13.0-16.0 g/dl		2.02-2.48 mmol/L	
	Female	12.0-16.0 g/dl		1.86-2.48 mmol/L	
Hemoglobin A					
Whole blood		>95% of total		>0.95 fraction of Hb	
Hemoglobin F					
Whole blood	1 d	63%-92% HbF		0.63-0.92 mass fraction HbF	
	5 d	65%-88% HbF		0.65-0.88 mass fraction HbF	
	3 wk	55%-85% HbF		0.55-0.85 mass fraction HbF	
	6-9 wk	31%-75% HbF		0.31-0.75 mass fraction HbF	
	3-4 mo	<2%-59% HbF		<0.02-0.59 mass fraction HbF	
	6 mo	<2%-9% HbF		<0.02-0.09 mass fraction HbF	
	Adult	<2% HbF		<0.02 mass fraction HbF	
Immunoglobulin A (IgA)					
Serum	Cord	1.4-3.6 mg/dl		14-36 mg/L	
	1-3 mo	1.3-53 mg/dl		13-530 mg/L	
	4-6 mo	4.4-84 mg/dl		44-840 mg/L	
	7-12 mo	11-106 mg/dl		110-1060 mg/L	
	2-5 yr	14-159 mg/dl		140-1590 mg/L	
	6-10 yr	33-236 mg/dl		330-2360 mg/L	
	Adult	70-312 mg/dl		700-3120 mg/L	
Immunoglobulin D (IgD)					
Serum	Newborn	None detected		None detected	
	Thereafter	0-8 mg/dl		0-80 mg/L	

Continued

		Normal Ranges	
Test, Specimen	**Age, Gender, Reference**	**Conventional Units**	**International Units (SI)**
Immunoglobulin E (IgE)			
Serum	Male	0-230 IU/ml	0-230 kIU/L
	Female	0-170 IU/ml	0-170 kIU/L
Immunoglobulin G (IgG)			
Serum	Cord	636-1606 mg/dl	6.36-16.06 g/L
	1 mo	251-906 mg/dl	2.51-9.06 g/L
	2-4 mo	176-601 mg/dl	1.76-6.01 g/L
	5-12 mo	172-1069 mg/dl	1.72-10.69 g/L
	1-5 yr	345-1236 mg/dl	3.45-12.36 g/L
	6-10 yr	608-1572 mg/dl	6.08-15.72 g/L
	Adult	639-1349 mg/dl	6.39-13.49 g/L
Immunoglobulin M (IgM)			
Serum	Cord	6.3-25 mg/dl	63-250 mg/L
	1-4 mo	17-105 mg/dl	170-1050 mg/L
	5-9 mo	33-126 mg/dl	330-1260 mg/L
	10-12 mo	41-173 mg/dl	410-1730 mg/L
	2-8 yr	43-207 mg/dl	430-2070 mg/L
	9-10 yr	52-242 mg/dl	520-2420 mg/L
	Adult	56-352 mg/dl	560-3520 mg/L
Insulin (12 hour fasting)	Newborn	3-20 uU/mL	3-20 mU/mL
	Thereafter	7-24 uU/mL	7-24 mU/mL
International Normalized Ratio (INR)—only for patients on coumarin	DVT target INR	2-3 s	2-3 s
	Prosthetic heart valve	2.5-3 s	2.5-3 s
Iron			
Serum	Newborn	100-250 mcg/dl	18-45 μmol/L
	Infant	40-100 mcg/dl	7-18 μmol/L
	Child	50-120 mcg/dl	9-22 μmol/L
	Thereafter: Male	65-170 mcg/dl	12-30 μmol/L
	Female	50-170 mcg/dl	9-30 μmol/L
	Intoxicated child	280-2550 mcg/dl	50.12-456.5 μmol/L
	Fatally poisoned child	>1800 mcg/dl	>322.2 μmol/L
Iron-binding capacity, total (TIBC)			
Serum	Infant	100-400 mcg/dl	17.90-71.60 μmol/L
	Thereafter	250-400 mcg/dl	44.75-71.60 μmol/L
Lead			
Whole blood	Child	<10 mcg/dl	<0.48 μmol/L
	Toxic	≥100 μg/dl	≥4.83 μmol/L
Urine, 24 hr		<80 mcg/L	<0.39 μmol/L
Leukocyte count (WBC count)		×1000 cells/mm^3 (μl)	×10^9 cells/L
Whole blood	Birth	9.0-30.0	9.0-30.0
	24 hr	9.4-34.0	9.4-34.0
	1 mo	5.0-19.5	5.0-19.5
	1-3 yr	6.0-17.5	6.0-17.5
	4-7 yr	5.5-15.5	5.5-15.5
	8-13 yr	4.5-13.5	4.5-13.5
	Adult	4.5-11.0	4.5-11.0

Test, Specimen	Age, Gender, Reference	Normal Ranges		
		Conventional Units		International Units (SI)
Leukocyte count (WBC count)—cont'd		×1000 cells/mm³ (µl)		$\times 10^6$ cells/L
CSF (cell count)	Premature	0-25 mononuclear		0-25
		0-10 polymorphonuclear		0-10
		0-1000 RBCs		0-1000
	Newborn	0-20 mononuclear		0-20
		0-10 polymorphonuclear		0-10
		0-800 RBCs		0-800
	Neonate	0-5 mononuclear		0-5
		0-10 polymorphonuclear		0-10
		0-50 RBCs		0-50
	Thereafter	0-5 mononuclear		0-5
Leukocyte differential count				
Whole blood	Myelocytes	0%	0 cells/mm³ (µl)	Number fraction 0
	Neutrophils—"bands"	3%-5%	150-400 cells/mm³ (µl)	Number fraction 0.03 0.05
	Neutrophils—"segs"	54%-62%	3000-5800 cells/mm³ (µl)	Number fraction 0.54-0.62
	Lymphocytes	25%-33%	1500-3000 cells/mm³ (µl)	Number fraction 0.25-0.33
	Monocytes	3%-7%	285-500 cells/mm³ (µl)	Number fraction 0.03-0.07
	Eosinophils	1%-3%	50-250 cells/mm³ (µl)	Number fraction 0.01-0.03
	Basophils	0%-0.75%	15-50 cells/mm³ (µl)	Number fraction 0-0.0075
Lipase (serum)	1-18 yr old	3-32 U/L		3-32 U/L
Mean corpuscular hemoglobin (MCH)				
Whole blood	Birth	31-37 pg/cell		0.48-0.57 fmol/cell
	1-3 d (cap)	31-37 pg/cell		0.48-0.57 fmol/cell
	1 wk–1 mo	28-40 pg/cell		0.43-0.62 fmol/cell
	2 mo	26-34 pg/cell		0.40-0.53 fmol/cell
	3-6 mo	25-35 pg/cell		0.39-0.54 fmol/cell
	0.5-2 yr	23-31 pg/cell		0.36-0.48 fmol/cell
	2-6 yr	24-30 pg/cell		0.37-0.47 fmol/cell
	6-12 yr	25-33 pg/cell		0.39-0.51 fmol/cell
	12-18 yr	25-35 pg/cell		0.39-0.54 fmol/cell
	18-49 yr	26-34 pg/cell		0.40-0.53 fmol/cell
Mean corpuscular hemoglobin concentration (MCHC)				
Whole blood	Birth	30%-36% Hb/cell or g Hb/dl RBCs		4.65-5.58 mmol Hb/L RBCs
	1-3 d (cap)	29%-37% Hb/cell or g Hb/dl RBCs		4.50-5.74 mmol Hb/L RBCs
	1-2 wk	28%-38% Hb/cell or g Hb/dl RBCs		4.34-5.89 mmol Hb/L RBCs
	1-2 mo	29%-37% Hb/cell or g Hb/dl RBCs		4.50-5.74 mmol Hb/L RBCs
	3 mo–2 yr	30%-36% Hb/cell or g Hb/dl RBCs		4.65-5.58 mmol Hb/L RBCs

Continued

Test, Specimen	Age, Gender, Reference	Normal Ranges: Conventional Units	Normal Ranges: International Units (SI)
Mean corpuscular hemoglobin concentration (MCHC)—cont'd, Whole blood—cont'd	2-18 yr	31%-37% Hb/cell or g Hb/dl RBCs	4.81-5.74 mmol Hb/L RBCs
	>18 yr	31%-37% Hb/cell or g Hb/dl RBCs	4.81-5.74 mmol Hb/L RBCs
Mean corpuscular volume (MCV)			
Whole blood	1-3 d (cap)	95-121 μm^3	95-121 fl
	0.5-2 yr	70-86 μm^3	70-86 fl
	6-12 yr	77-95 μm^3	77-95 fl
	12-18 yr: Male	78-98 μm^3	78-98 fl
	Female	78-102 μm^3	78-102 fl
Osmolality			
Serum	Child, adult	275-295 mOsm/kg H_2O	
Urine, random		50-1400 mOsm/kg H_2O, depending on fluid intake; after 12-hr fluid restriction: >850 mOsm/kg H_2O	
Urine, 24 hr		≅300-900 mOsm/kg H_2O	
Oxygen, partial pressure (Po_2)			
Whole blood, arterial	Birth	8-24 mm Hg	1.1-3.2 kPa
	5-10 min	33-75 mm Hg	4.4-10.0 kPa
	30 min	31-85 mm Hg	4.1-11.3 kPa
	>1 hr	55-80 mm Hg	7.3-10.6 kPa
	1 d	54-95 mm Hg	7.2-12.6 kPa
	Thereafter (decreases with age)	83-108 mm Hg	11-14.4 kPa
Oxygen saturation (Sao_2)			
Whole blood, arterial	Newborn	85%-90%	Fraction saturated 0.85-0.90
	Thereafter	95%-99%	Fraction saturated 0.95-0.99
Partial thromboplastin time (PTT)			
Whole blood (Na citrate)			
Nonactivated		60-85 s (Platelin)	60-85 s
Activated		25-35 s (differs with method)	25-35 s
pH			H^+ concentration
Whole blood, arterial	Premature (48 hr)	7.35-7.50	31-44 nmol/L
	Birth, full term	7.11-7.36	43-77 nmol/L
	5-10 min	7.09-7.30	50-81 nmol/L
	30 min	7.21-7.38	41-61 nmol/L
	>1 hr	7.26-7.49	32-54 nmol/L
	1 d	7.29-7.45	35-51 nmol/L
	Thereafter must be corrected for body temperature	7.35-7.45	35-44 nmol/L
Urine, random	Newborn or neonate	5-7	0.1-10 µmol/L
	Thereafter	4.5-8 (average ≅6)	0.01-32 µmol/L (average ≅1.0 µmol/L)
Stool		7.0-7.5	31-100 nmol/L

Test, Specimen	Age, Gender, Reference	Normal Ranges: Conventional Units	Normal Ranges: International Units (SI)
Phenylalanine			
Serum	Premature	2.0-7.5 mg/dl	120-450 μmol/L
	Newborn	1.2-3.4 mg/dl	70-210 μmol/L
	Thereafter	0.8-1.8 mg/dl	50-110 μmol/L
Urine, 24 hr	10 d–2 wk	1-2 mg/d	6-12 μmol/d
	3-12 yr	4-18 mg/d	24-110 μmol/d
	Thereafter	Trace—17 mg/d	Trace—103 μmol/d
Plasma volume			
Plasma	Male	25-43 ml/kg	0.025-0.043 L/kg
	Female	28-45 ml/kg	0.028-0.045 L/kg
Platelet count (thrombocyte count)			
Whole blood (EDTA)	Newborn (after 1 wk, same as adult)	84-478 × 10^3/mm^3 (μl)	84-478 × 10^9/L
	Adult	150-400 × 10^3/mm^3 (μl)	150-400 × 10^9/L
Potassium			
Serum	Newborn	3.0-6.0 mEq/L	3.0-6.0 mmol/L
	Thereafter	3.5-5.0 mEq/L	3.5-5.0 mmol/L
Plasma (heparin)		3.4-4.5 mEq/L	3.4-4.5 mmol/L
Urine, 24 hr		2.5-125 mEq/d (varies with diet)	2.5-125 mmol/L
Protein			
Serum, total	Premature	4.3-7.6 g/dl	43-76 g/L
	Newborn	4.6-7.4 g/dl	46-74 g/L
	1-7 yr	6.1-7.9 g/dl	61-79 g/L
	8-12 yr	6.4-8.1 g/dl	64-81 g/L
	13 19 yr	6.6-8.2 g/dl	66-82 g/L
Total			
Urine, 24 hr		1-14 mg/dl	10-140 mg/L
		50-80 mg/d (at rest)	50-80 mg/d
		<250 mg/d (after intense exercise)	<250 mg/d (after intense exercise)
CSF		Lumbar: 8-32 mg/dl	80-320 mg/L
Prothrombin time (PT)			
One-stage (Quick)			
Whole blood (Na citrate)	In general	11-15 s (varies with type of thromboplastin)	11-15 s
	Newborn	Prolonged by 2-3 s	Prolonged by 2-3 s
Two-stage modified (Ware and Seegers)			
Whole blood (Na citrate)		18-22 s	18-22 s
RBC count: see Erythrocyte (RBC) count			
Red blood cell volume			
Whole blood	Male	20-36 ml/kg	0.020-0.036 L/kg
	Female	19-31 ml/kg	0.019-0.031 L/kg

Continued

Test, Specimen	Age, Gender, Reference	Normal Ranges: Conventional Units	Normal Ranges: International Units (SI)
Reticulocyte count			
Whole blood	Adults	0.5%-1.5% of erythrocytes or 25,000-75,000/mm^3 (μl)	0.005-0.015 (number fraction) or 25,000-75,000 × 10^6/L
Capillary	1 d	0.4%-6.0%	0.004-0.060 (number fraction)
	7 d	<0.1%-1.3%	<0.001-0.013 (number fraction)
	1-4 wk	<0.1%-1.2%	<0.001-0.012 (number fraction)
	5-6 wk	<0.1%-2.4%	<0.001-0.024 (number fraction)
	7-8 wk	0.1%-2.9%	0.001-0.029 (number fraction)
	9-10 wk	<0.1%-2.6%	<0.001-0.026 (number fraction)
	11-12 wk	0.1%-1.3%	0.001-0.013 (number fraction)
Salicylates			
Serum, plasma	Therap conc	15-30 mg/dl	1.1-2.2 mmol/L
	Toxic conc	>30 mg/dl	>18.5 mmol/L
Sedimentation rate: see Erythrocyte sedimentation rate (ESR)			
Sodium			
Serum or plasma	Newborn	134-146 mEq/L	134-146 mmol/L
	Infant	139-146 mEq/L	139-146 mmol/L
	Child	138-145 mEq/L	138-145 mmol/L
	Thereafter	136-146 mEq/L	136-146 mmol/L
Urine, 24 hr		40-220 mEq/L (diet dependent)	40-220 mmol/L
Sweat	Normal	<40 mEq/L	<40 mmol/L
	Indeterminate	45-60 mEq/L	45-60 mmol/L
	Cystic fibrosis	>60 mEq/L	>60 mmol/L
Specific gravity			
Urine, random	Adult	1.002-1.030	1.002-1.030
	After 12-hr fluid restriction	>1.025	>1.025
Urine, 24 hr		1.015-1.025	
Theophylline			
Serum, plasma	Therap conc		
	Bronchodilator	10-20 mcg/ml	56-110 μmol/L
	Premature apnea	5-10 mcg/ml	28-56 μmol/L
	Toxic conc	>20 mcg/ml	>110 μmol/L
Thrombin time			
Whole blood (Na citrate)		Control time ±2 s when control is 9-13 s	Control time ±2 s when control is 9-13 s
Thyroxine, total (T_4)			
Serum	Cord	8-13 mcg/dl	103-168 nmol/L
	Newborn	11.5-24 mcg/dl (lower in low-birth-weight infants)	148-310 nmol/L
	Neonate	9-18 mcg/dl	116-232 nmol/L
	Infant	7-15 mcg/dl	90-194 nmol/L
	1-5 yr	7.3-15 mcg/dl	94-194 nmol/L
	5-10 yr	6.4-13.3 mcg/dl	83-172 nmol/L
	Thereafter	5-12 mcg/dl	65-155 nmol/L
	Newborn screen (filter paper)	6.2-22 mcg/dl	80-284 nmol/L

Test, Specimen	Age, Gender, Reference	Normal Ranges			
		Conventional Units		International Units (SI)	
Triglycerides (TG)		**Male** (mg/dl)	**Female** (mg/dl)	**Male** (g/L)	**Female** (g/L)
Serum, after ≥12-hr fast (recommended levels)	Cord	10-98	10-98	0.10-0.98	0.10-0.98
	0-5 yr	30-86	32-99	0.30-0.86	0.32-0.99
	6-11 yr	31-108	35-114	0.31-1.08	0.35-1.14
	12-15 yr	36-138	41-138	0.36-1.38	0.41-1.38
	16-19 yr	40-163	40-128	0.40-1.63	0.40-1.28
Triiodothyronine (T_3), free					
Serum	Cord	20-240 pg/dl		0.3-3.7 pmol/L	
	1-3 d	200-610 pg/dl		3.1-9.4 pmol/L	
	6 wk	240-560 pg/dl		3.7-8.6 pmol/L	
	Adults (20-50 yr)	230-660 pg/dl		3.5-10.0 pmol/L	
Triiodothyronine, total (T_3-RIA)					
Serum	Cord	30-70 ng/dl		0.46-1.08 nmol/L	
	Newborn	72-260 ng/dl		1.16-4 nmol/L	
	1-5 yr	100-260 ng/dl		1.54-4 nmol/L	
	5-10 yr	90-240 ng/dl		1.39-3.70 nmol/L	
	10-15 yr	80-210 ng/dl		1.23-3.23 nmol/L	
	Thereafter	115-190 ng/dl		1.77-2.93 nmol/L	
Urea nitrogen					
Serum or plasma	Cord	21-40 mg/dl		7.5-14.3 mmol/L	
	Premature (1 wk)	3-25 mg/dl		1.1-9 mmol/L	
	Newborn	3-12 mg/dl		1.1-4.3 mmol/L	
	Infant or child	5-18 mg/dl		1.8-6.4 mmol/L	
	Thereafter	7-18 mg/dl		2.5-6.4 mmol/L	
Urine volume					
Urine, 24 hr	Newborn	50-300 ml/d		0.05-0.3 L/d	
	Infant	350-550 ml/d		0.35-0.5 L/d	
	Child	500-1000 ml/d		0.5-1 L/d	
	Adolescent	700-1400 ml/d		0.7-1.4 L/d	
	Thereafter: Male	800-1800 ml/d		0.8-1.8 L/d	
	Female	600-1600 ml/d (varies with intake and other factors)		0.6-1.6 L/d	
WBC: see Leukocyte count (WBC count)					

Abbreviations and Acronyms

A substantial number of words and phrases are abbreviated in nursing practice for convenience in communication. Although most of the abbreviations are familiar to health professionals, many are not. In addition, students unfamiliar with the vocabulary used by health professionals are at a particular disadvantage when interpreting communications. This extensive list is compiled to facilitate this process. Because many of the abbreviations can represent several different words or phrases, the user is advised to use caution in their interpretation. For example, *per os* can be interpreted as *by mouth* or *in left eye; D/C* can mean *discharge* or *discontinue.* The meaning of unfamiliar abbreviations should be confirmed with the people who wrote them. If the author of a particular abbreviation is unavailable, check the abbreviation in a dictionary of medical abbreviations, or use a list of hospital-approved abbreviations to verify its meaning.

Abbreviation	Term
AA	Automobile accident; Alcoholics Anonymous
AAMD	American Association on Mental Deficiency
Ab	Antibody
ABG	Arterial blood gases
ABR	Auditory brainstem response
ac	*Ante cibum* (before meals)
ACLS	Advanced cardiac life support
ACT	Activated clotting time
ACTH	Adrenocorticotropic hormone
AD	Autosomal dominant; atopic dermatitis; *auris dextra* (right ear)
ad lib	*Ad libitum* (as desired)
ADA	Adenosine deaminase (deficiency disease)
ADC	Aid to Dependent Children
ADD	Attention deficit disorder
ADDH	Attention deficit disorder, hyperactivity
ADH	Antidiuretic hormone
ADHD	Attention deficit hyperactivity disorder
ADI	Acceptable daily intake
ADL	Activities of daily living
ADP	Adenosine diphosphate
ADR	Adverse drug reaction
ADS	Attention deficit syndrome; antidiuretic substance
AEP	Auditory evoked potential
AF	Atrial fibrillation
AFB	Acid-fast bacillus
AFDC	Aid to Families with Dependent Children
AFP	Alpha-fetoprotein
Ag	Antigen, *argentum* (silver)
AGA	Appropriate for gestational age
AGC	Absolute granulocyte count
AGN	Acute glomerulonephritis
AHC	Acute hemorrhagic conjunctivitis
AHD	Autoimmune hemolytic disease
AHF	Antihemophilic factor; antihemolytic factor
AHG	Antihemophilic globulin; antihuman globulin
AI	Aortic insufficiency
AID	Artificial insemination by donor
AIDS	Acquired immunodeficiency syndrome
AIH	Artificial insemination by husband
AJ	Ankle jerk
ALG	Antilymphocytic globulin
ALL	Acute lymphoid leukemia
ALS	Advanced life support
ALT	Alanine aminotransferase
ALTE	Apparent life-threatening event
AMA	Against medical advice; American Medical Association
AMEND	Aiding Mothers Experiencing Neonatal Death
AMI	Acute myocardial infarction
AML	Acute myelogenous leukemia
amp	Ampule
AMP	Adenosine monophosphate
ANA	Antinuclear antibody; American Nurses Association
ANLL	Acute nonlymphocytic leukemia
ANS	Autonomic nervous system; anterior nasal spine
AODM	Adult-onset diabetes mellitus
AOM	Acute otitis media
AP	Anteroposterior; antepartum; atrioperitoneal
APON	Association of Pediatric Oncology Nurses
aq	*Aqua* (water)
AR	Autosomal recessive
ARC	AIDS-related complex
ARD	Acute respiratory disease
ARDS	Adult respiratory distress syndrome
ARF	Acute renal failure; acute respiratory failure
ARV	AIDS-associated retrovirus
AS	Aortic stenosis; aortic sound; aqueous solution; aqueous suspension; astigmatism; ankylosing spondylitis; *auris sinistra* (left ear)
ASAP	As soon as possible
ASD	Atrial septal defect
ASDH	Acute subdural hematoma

Abbreviation	Term
ASH	Asymmetric septal hypertrophy
ASK	Antistreptokinase
ASO	Antistreptolysin O
ATC	Certified athletic trainer; around the clock
ATG	Antithymocyte globulin
ATN	Acute tubular necrosis
ATO	Alimentary tract obstruction
ATP	Autoimmune thrombocytopenia (purpura); adenosine triphosphate
ATPS	Ambient temperature and pressure, saturated (with water)
ATV	All-terrain vehicle
AU	*Auris uterque* (each ear)
Av	Average; avoirdupois
AV (A-V)	Atrioventricular
AVM	Arteriovenous malformation
AWD	Abdominal wall defect
BA	Bronchial asthma; bone age
BAEP	Brainstem auditory-evoked potential
BAER	Brainstem auditory-evoked response
BAT	Brown adipose tissue
BBB	Blood-brain barrier
BBT	Basal body temperature
BC	Blood culture
BCG	Bacille Calmette-Guérin (tuberculin vaccine)
BCS	Battered child syndrome
BD	Bronchial drainage; birthday; birth defect
BE	Barium enema
BEAM	Brain electrical activity map
BEI	Butanol extractable iodine
BFP	Biologic false positive
BG	Blood glucose
BHI	Biosynthetic human insulin
bid	*Bis in die* (twice a day)
BiPAP	Bilevel positive airway pressure
BJ	Biceps jerk
BM	Bowel movement; bone marrow
BMD	Bone marrow depression
BMR	Basal metabolic rate
BNBAS	Brazelton Neonatal Behavioral Assessment Scale
BOA	Behavioral observation audiometry; born out of asepsis
BP	Blood pressure
BPD	Bronchopulmonary dysplasia
BRAT	Bananas, rice cereal, applesauce, toast
BRP	Bathroom privileges
BS	Blood sugar; bowel sounds; breath sounds
BSA	Body surface area; bovine serum albumin
BSE	Breast self-examination
BSER	Brainstem-evoked response
BSI	Biologic substance(s) isolation; body substance isolation
BSID	Bayley Scales of Infant Development
BT	Bleeding time
BTPS	Body temperature and pressure, saturated (with water)
BUN	Blood urea nitrogen
BW	Birth weight
BWF	Basic waking frequency
BWS	Battered woman syndrome
Bx	Biopsy
$\bar{c}$	*cum* (with)
CA (Ca)	Cancer; chronologic age; calcium
CAH	Congenital adrenal hyperplasia; chronic active hepatitis
CAL	Chronic airflow limitation
cAMP	Cyclic adenosine monophosphate
cap	Capsule
CAPD	Continuous ambulatory peritoneal dialysis
CAT	Computed axial tomography
CAV	Congenital absence of vagina; croup-associated virus
CAVH	Continuous arteriovenous hemofiltration
CB	Chronic bronchitis
CBA	Congenital biliary atresia
CBC	Complete blood count
CBD	Closed bladder drainage
CBF	Cerebral blood flow
CBPU	Care by parental unit
CBV	Cerebral blood volume; cerebral blood (flow) velocity
CC	Chief complaint; Caucasian child; common cold; critical condition; color and circulation; creatinine clearance
CCMS	Clean catch midstream specimen
Ccr	Creatinine clearance
CCS	Crippled Children's Services
CD	Communicable disease; celiac disease; cutdown
CDC	Centers for Disease Control and Prevention
CDGA	Constitutional delay of growth and adolescence
CDH	Congenital diaphragmatic hernia
CDP	Continuous distending pressure
C-E	Croup-epiglottitis syndrome
CF	Cystic fibrosis; cardiac failure; complement fixation
CFF	Cystic Fibrosis Foundation
CFU	Colony-forming units
CHAP	Child Health Assessment Program
CHB	Complete heart block
CHC	Child health conference; community health center
CHD	Congenital heart disease; childhood disease; coronary heart disease
CHF	Congestive heart failure
CHL	Crown-heel length

Abbreviation	Term
CI	Cardiac index; cardiac insufficiency; cerebral infarction
CIC	Clean intermittent catheterization
CID	Cytomegalic inclusion disease; combined immune deficiency
CIE	Countercurrent immunoelectrophoresis
CINAHL	Cumulative Index to Nursing and Allied Health Literature
CK	Creatine kinase
CL	Cleft lip
CLBBB	Complete left bundle branch block
CLD	Chronic lung disease; chronic liver disease
CL (P)	Cleft lip with or without cleft palate
CLP	Cleft lip and cleft palate
cm	Centimeter
CMA	Cow's milk allergy
CMI	Cell-mediated immunity
CML	Chronic myelocytic leukemia
CMPI	Cow's milk protein intolerance
CMR	Cerebral metabolic rate
CMV	Cytomegalovirus
CN	Clinical Nurse
CNA	Canadian Nurses Association
CNM	Certified Nurse Midwife
CNS	Central nervous system; Clinical Nurse Specialist
CNSD	Chronic nonspecific diarrhea
CO	Cardiac output; carbon monoxide
COA	Children of alcoholics; coarctation of aorta
Cocci	Coccidioidomycosis
COHb	Carboxyhemoglobin
COLD	Chronic obstructive lung disease
COPD	Chronic obstructive pulmonary disease
COR	Conditioned orientation reflex
CP	Cleft palate; cerebral palsy; capillary pressure; cor pulmonale; Certified Prosthetist; constant pressure; child psychiatrist; closing pressure (spinal tap); chronic pyelonephritis
CPAP	Continuous positive airway pressure
CPAV	Continuous positive airway ventilation
CPD	Cephalopelvic disproportion; childhood polycystic disease
CPK	Creatine phosphokinase
CPM	Continuous passive motion
CPN	Certified Pediatric Nurse
CPP	Cerebral perfusion pressure
CPPV	Continuous positive pressure ventilation
CPR	Cardiopulmonary resuscitation
CPS	Cycles per second; Child Protective Services
CPSC	Consumer Product Safety Commission
CPT	Chest physiotherapy
CRBBB	Complete right bundle branch block
CRD	Child restraint devices
CRF	Corticotropin-releasing factor
CRP	C-reactive protein
CRS	Congenital rubella syndrome
CS	Clinical Specialist; cesarean section
C&S	Culture and sensitivity
CSA	Colony-stimulating activity
CSD	Cat scratch disease
CSF	Cerebral spinal fluid (cerebrospinal fluid)
CSII	Continuous subcutaneous insulin infusion
CSN	Certified School Nurse
CSOM	Chronic serous otitis media
CT	Computed tomography; circulation time; clotting time; coated tablet; compressed tablet; corneal transplant; Coombs test
CTT	Computerized transaxial tomography
CUG	Cystourethrogram
CV	Closing volume
CVA	Cerebrovascular accident; costal vertebral angle
CVI	Common variable immunodeficiency
CVo_2	Mixed venous oxygen content
CVP	Central venous pressure
CVR	Cerebral vascular resistance
CVS	Clean voided specimen; chorionic villi sampling
CW	Crutch walking
C/W	Consistent with
CXR	Chest x-ray
DA	Developmental age
DASE	Denver Articulation Screening Examination
DAW	Dispense as written
db	Decibel
DC, D/C	Discontinue; dichorionic; discharge
D&C	Dilatation and curettage
DCT	Direct Coombs test
DD	Dry dressing; differential diagnosis; discharge diagnosis; discharge by death; diaper dermatitis
DDH	Developmental dysplasia of the hip
DDST	Denver Developmental Screening Test
DDST-R	Denver Developmental Screening Test, revised
DFA	Diet for age; direct fluorescent antibody
DH	Diaphragmatic hernia
DHHS	Department of Health and Human Services
DI	Diabetes insipidus
D/I	Direct/indirect ratio (bilirubin)
DIC	Disseminated intravascular coagulation
DIP	Desquamated interstitial pneumonitis
DKA	Diabetic ketoacidosis
dl	Deciliter
DLIS	Digoxin-like immunoreactive substance

Abbreviation	Term
DM	Diabetes mellitus; diastolic murmur
DMD	Duchenne muscular dystrophy
DNHW	Department of National Health and Welfare (Canada)
DNR	Do not resuscitate
DOA	Date of admission; dead on arrival
DOB	Date of birth
DOD	Date of discharge; date of death
DOE	Dyspnea on exertion
DP	Dorsalis pedis (artery)
DPNB	Dorsal penile nerve block
DPT	Diphtheria-pertussis-tetanus (vaccine)
DQ	Developmental quotient
DRG	Diagnosis-related group(s)
DS	Down syndrome
DSA	Digital subtraction angiography
DSD	Dry sterile dressing
DSDB	Direct self-destructive behavior
DSM	Diagnostic and Statistical Manual of Mental Disorders
DT	Delirium tremens
DTR	Deep tendon reflex
DU	Diagnosis undetermined
DV	Dilute volume
D&V	Diarrhea and vomiting
DW	Distilled water
D5W	Dextrose 5% in water
Dx	Diagnosis
DZ	Dizygotic
EA	Esophageal atresia
EAM	External acoustic meatus
EBL	Estimated blood loss
EBM	Expressed breast milk
EBV	Epstein-Barr virus
ECC	Emergency cardiac care; extracorporeal circulation
ECD	Endocardial cushion defect
ECF	Extracellular fluid; extended care facility
ECG	Electrocardiogram
ECM	Erythema chronicum migrans
ECMO	Extracorporeal membrane oxygenation
ED	Emergency department
EDC	Estimated date of confinement
EDD	Estimated date of delivery
EEE	Eastern equine encephalitis
EEG	Electroencephalogram
EENT	Eye, ear, nose, throat
EF	Extended field (irradiation)
EFA	Essential fatty acid
EFAD	Essential fatty acid deficiency
EFE	Endocardial fibroelastosis
EFM	Electronic fetal monitoring
EGS	Electric galvanic stimulator
EHBA	Extrahepatic biliary atresia
E-IPV	Enhanced (potency) IPV

Abbreviation	Term
ELBW	Extremely low birth weight
ELISA	Enzyme-linked immunosorbent assay
elix	Elixir
EMG	Electromyogram
EMI	Electromagnetic interference
EMM	Expressed mother's milk
EMS	Emergency medical services
EMT	Emergency medical technician
ENA	Extractable nuclear antigens
EOA	Examination, opinion, and advice
EOM	Extraocular movement; extraocular muscle
EP	Extraperitoneal; evoked potential; erythrocyte protoporphyrin
EPA	Erect posteroanterior
EPCA	Epidural patient-controlled analgesia
EPI	Echo-planar imaging
EPSDT	Early and periodic screening, diagnosis, and treatment
ER	Emergency room; external rotation; expiratory reserve; equivalent roentgen (unit)
ERA	Electric response audiometry
ERG	Electroretinography
ERPF	Effective renal plasma flow
ERV	Expiratory reserve volume
ESI	Early Screening Inventory
ESR	Erythrocyte sedimentation rate
ESRD	End-stage renal disease
ET	Endotracheal; esotropia; eustachian tube
ETA	Estimated time of arrival
E_TCO_2	End-tidal carbon dioxide concentration
ETOH	Ethyl alcohol
ETT	Endotracheal tube
EV	Enterovirus
FAAN	Fellow in American Academy of Nursing
FAB	French-American-British
FAE	Fetal alcohol effect
FAS	Fetal alcohol syndrome
FB	Foreign body
FBA	Foreign body aspiration
FBS	Fasting blood sugar
FDA	Food and Drug Administration
FEP	Free erythrocyte porphyrins
FET	Forced expiratory technique
FEV_1	Forced expiratory volume, 1 second
FEV_5	Forced expiratory volume, 5 seconds
FEVC	Forced expiratory volume capacity
FFA	Free fatty acids
FFP	Fresh-frozen plasma
FH, FHx	Family history
FHS	Fetal hydantoin syndrome
Fio_2, FIO_2	Forced inspiratory oxygen; fraction of inspired oxygen
FISH	Fluorescent in-situ hybridization

Abbreviation	Term
FLM	Fetal lung maturity
FMD	Fibromuscular dysplasia
FMH	Family medical history
FMS	Fat-mobilizing substance
FNP	Family Nurse Practitioner
FRC	Functional residual capacity
FS	Full strength
FSH	Follicle-stimulating hormone
FSP	Fibrin split products
FSS	Family short stature
FTA-ABS	Fluorescent treponemal antibody absorption (test)
FTSG	Full-thickness skin graft
FTT	Failure to thrive
F/U	Follow-up
FUE	Fever of unknown etiology
FUO	Fever of unknown origin
FVC	Forced vital capacity
FWB	Full weight bearing
Fx	Fracture
FYI	For your information
GA	General anesthesia; gestational age
GABHS	Group A β-hemolytic streptococci
GAS	Group A streptococci
GBBS	Group B β-streptococci
GBM	Glomerular basement membrane
GC	Gonococci (gonorrhea); general condition; general circulation
GCS	Glasgow Coma Scale
G&D	Growth and development
GDM	Gestational diabetes mellitus
GER	Gastroesophageal reflux
GFR	Glomerular filtration rate
GGT, GGTP	Gamma-glutamyl transpeptidase
GH	Growth hormone
GHB, GHb	Glycosylated hemoglobin
GHD	Growth hormone deficiency
GHRF	Growth hormone-releasing factor
GH-RH	Growth hormone-releasing hormone
GI	Gastrointestinal
GOT	Glutamic-oxaloacetic transaminase
G6PD	Glucose-6-phosphate dehydrogenase
GSE	Gluten-sensitive enteropathy
GSW	Gunshot wound
gtt	*Guttae* (drops)
GTT	Glucose tolerance test
GU	Genitourinary
GVH	Graft-vs-host
GVHD	Graft-vs-host disease
GVHR	Graft-vs-host reaction
h	*Hora* (hour)
HA	Headache
H-A	*Hartmannella-Acanthamoeba*
HAV	Hepatitis A virus
Hb	Hemoglobin

Abbreviation	Term
HB	Heart block
HBGM	Home blood glucose monitoring
HBIG	Hepatitis B immune globulin
HBO	Hyperbaric oxygen
HbOC	*Haemophilus* b conjugate vaccine (diphtheria CRM_{19}—protein conjugate)
HBsAg	Hepatitis B surface antigen
HBV	Hepatitis B virus; honey bee venom
HC	Hyperosmolar coma
hCG	Human chorionic gonadotropin
HCI	Home care instructions
HCM	Health care management
Hct	Hematocrit
HD	Heart disease
HDCV	Human diploid cell virus
HDL	High-density lipoprotein
HDN	Hemorrhagic disease of the newborn
HEENT	Head, eye, ear, nose, and throat
HELLP	Hemolysis, elevated liver, low platelets
HFJV	High-frequency jet ventilation
HFO	High-frequency oscillation
HFOV	High-frequency oscillatory ventilation
HFPPV	High-frequency positive pressure ventilation
HFV	High-frequency ventilation
Hgb	Hemoglobin
HGH, hGH	Human growth hormone
HHHO	Hypothyroidism, hypoxia, hypogonadism, obesity
HHNC	Hyperosmolar, hyperglycemic, nonketogenic coma
HHNKD	Hyperosmolar, hyperglycemic, nonketotic dehydration
H/I	Hypoxia-ischemia
Hib	*Haemophilus influenzae* type B
HIE	Hypoxic-ischemic encephalopathy
HISG	Human immune serum globulin
HIV	Human immunodeficiency virus
HL	Hearing level
HLA	Human leukocytic antigen; histocompatibility locus antigen
HMD	Hyaline membrane disease
HMO	Health maintenance organization
HO	House officer
HOB	Head of bed
HOME	Home Observation for Measurement of the Environment
HOPI	History of previous (prior) illness
HPA	Hypothalamic-pituitary-adrenal (axis)
HPB	Health Protection Branch (of Canada)
HPC	Healed primary complex
HPLC	High-power liquid chromatography
HPN	Hypertension
HPV	Human parvovirus; human papillomavirus
HR	Heart rate

Abbreviation	Term
HRA	Health risk appraisal
HRF	Health-related facility
HRIG	Human rabies immune globulin
hs	*Hora somni* (hour of sleep; bedtime)
HS	Heart sounds; herpes simplex; house surgeon
HSA	Health systems agency; human serum albumin
HSBG	Heel stick blood gases
HSE	Herpes simplex encephalitis
HSN	Herpes simplex neonatorum
HSP	Henoch-Schönlein purpura
HSV	Herpes simplex virus
HTLV-III	Human T-lymphotropic virus type III
HTN	Hypertensive; hypertension
HTPN	Home total parenteral nutrition
HTSI	Human thyroid stimulator immunoglobulin
HUS	Hemolytic uremic syndrome
Hx	History
IA	Imperforate anus; internal auditory; intra-arterial; intraarticular; infantile apnea
IAA	Insulin autoantibodies
IABP	Intraaortic balloon pump
IAFI	Infantile amaurotic familial idiocy
IAR	Interagency referral
IBC	Iron-binding capacity
IBD	Inflammatory bowel disease
IBO	In behalf of
IBS	Irritable bowel syndrome
IBW	Ideal body weight
IC	Intracutaneous
ICA	Islet cell antibodies
ICC	Intermittent clean catheterization
ICD	International Classification of Diseases
ICF	Intracellular fluid
ICN	Intensive care nursery
ICP	Intermittent catheterization program; intracranial pressure
ICS	Intercostal space
ICSH	Interstitial cell-stimulating hormone
ICU	Intensive care unit
ID	Identification; intradermal; initial dose; infective dose; ineffective dose; inside diameter
IDM	Infant of diabetic mother
IDP	Infant development program
I/E ratio	Inspiratory/expiratory ratio
IEP	Individualized education program; immunoelectrophoresis
IF	Involved field (irradiation); immunofluorescence
IFA	Indirect fluorescent antibody
IFSP	Individualized family service plan
Ig, IG	Immune globulin
IGIV	Immune globulin intravenous

Abbreviation	Term
IgS	Immunoglobulin system
IGT	Impaired glucose tolerance
IH	Infectious hepatitis
IHA	Indirect hemagglutination
IHSS	Idiopathic hypertrophic subaortic stenosis
IIA	Interrupted infantile apnea
IM	Intramuscular; internal medicine; infectious mononucleosis; intramedullary
IMV	Intermittent mandatory ventilation
IND	Investigational new drug
IOL	Intraocular lens
IPH	Intraparenchymal hemorrhage
IPPB	Intermittent positive pressure breathing
IPV	Inactivated polio virus (vaccine)
IQ	Intelligence quotient
IRB	Institutional Review Board
IRV	Inspiratory reserve volume
ISADH	Inappropriate secretion of ADH
ISC	Intermittent self-catheterization; intermittent servocontrol
ISDB	Indirect self-destructive behavior
ISF	Interstitial fluid
ISG	Immune serum globulin
ISP	Infant stimulation program
IT	Intrathecal
ITP	Idiopathic thrombocytopenia; idiopathic thrombocytopenic purpura
ITQ	Infant Temperament Questionnaire
IU	Immunizing unit, international unit
IUCD	Intrauterine contraceptive device
IUD	Intrauterine device
IUFD	Intrauterine fetal death
IUGR	Intrauterine growth restriction
IV	Intravenous
IVC	Inferior vena cava
IVCD	Intraventricular conduction defect
IVDU	Intravenous drug use
IVGG	Intravenous gamma globulin
IVH	Intraventricular hemorrhage
IVP	Intravenous pyelogram
IVT	Intravenous transfusion
IWL	Insensible water loss
JA	Juvenile arthritis
JAS	Juvenile ankylosing spondylitis
JCAHO	Joint Commission on Accreditation of Healthcare Organizations
JCP	Juvenile chronic polyarthritis
JND	Just noticeable difference
JRA	Juvenile rheumatoid arthritis
KD	Kawasaki disease
17-KGS	17-ketogenic steroid
KIDS	Kansas Infant Development Screen
17-KS	17-ketosteroids
KUB	Kidney, ureter, and bladder
KVO	Keep vein open

Abbreviation	Term
LA	Left atrium
LAE	Left atrial enlargement
LAP	Left arterial pressure
LATS	Long-acting thyroid stimulator
LAV	Lymphadenopathy-associated virus
LBCD	Left border of cardiac dullness (sternal border)
LBM	Lean body mass
LBW	Low birth weight; lean body weight
LCM	Left costal margin
LD	Lethal dose; light difference (perception); left deltoid
L&D	Labor and delivery
LDH	Lactic dehydrogenase
LDL	Low-density lipoprotein
LE	Lupus erythematosus; left eye; LE prep; lower extremity
LES	Lower esophageal sphincter; Life Expectancy Survey
LFD	Light for dates
LG	Left gluteal
LGA	Large for gestational age
LH	Luteinizing hormone
LH-RH	Luteinizing hormone releasing hormone
LIP	Lymphoid interstitial pneumonitis
LJM	Limited joint movement
LKS	Liver, kidneys, spleen
LLBCD	Left lower border of cardiac dullness
LLE	Left lower extremity
LLL	Left lower lobe
LLQ	Left lower quadrant
LLT	Left lateral thigh
LMC	Left midclavicular line
LMD	Local medical doctor
LMN	Lower motor neuron
LMP	Last menstrual period
LNMP	Last normal menstrual period
LOC	Level of consciousness; loss of consciousness; locus of control; laxative of choice
LOM	Left otitis media; loss of movement; limitation of motion
LOS	Length of stay
LP	Lumbar puncture
LPN	Licensed Practical Nurse
LQ	Lower quadrant
LRE	Least restrictive environment
LRI	Lower respiratory infection
LS	Lecithin, sphingomyelin
LSB	Left sternal border; left scapular border
LTB	Laryngotracheobronchitis
LTH	Luteotropic hormone
LUE	Left upper extremity
LUL	Left upper lobe
LUOQ	Left upper outer quadrant
LUQ	Left upper quadrant

Abbreviation	Term
LV	Left ventricle
LVG	Left ventrogluteal
LVH	Left ventricular hypertrophy
LVN	Licensed Vocational Nurse
LVO	Left ventricular output
M	Molar; mean; muscle; male
m^2	Meters squared (square meters)
MA	Mental age; menstrual age
MABP	Mean arterial blood pressure
MAC	Maximum allowable concentration
MAMC	Midarm muscle circumference
MAP	Mean arterial pressure; mean airway pressure; most appropriate placement
MAS	Meconium aspiration syndrome
MAWP	Mean arterial wedge pressure
MBC	Minimum bactericidal concentration
MBP	Mean blood pressure
MC	Mucocutaneous lymph node syndrome; maternal child; monochorionic
MCDI	Minnesota Child Development Inventory
mcg	Microgram
MCH	Mean corpuscular (cell) hemoglobin; maternal and child health
MCHC	Mean corpuscular (cell) hemoglobin concentration
MCL	Midclavicular line
MCNS	Minimal change nephrotic syndrome
MCT	Medium-chain triglyceride; mean circulatory time
MCV	Mean corpuscular (cell) volume; mean clinical value
MD	Muscular dystrophy; medical doctor; manic depression; myocardial disease
MDA	Minimal daily allowance
MDI	Medium dose inhalants; metered dose inhaler
MDR	Minimal daily requirement
MDRP	Multidrug-resistant pathogens
MEBM	Maternally expressed breast milk
MED	Minimal effective dose; minimal erythema dose
mEq	Milliequivalents
MFD	Minimal fatal dose
mg	Milligram
MGN	Membranous glomerulonephritis
MH	Melanocytic hormone
MHC	Major histocompatibility complex
MI	Mitral insufficiency; myocardial infarction; myocardial ischemia; mental illness
MIC	Minimum inhibitory concentration
MID	Minimum infective dose
MIF	Migration-inhibiting factor
MLC	Mixed lymphocyte culture
MLD	Minimum lethal dose; median lethal dose
MLNS	Minimal lesion nephrotic syndrome

Abbreviation	Term
MM	Mucous membrane; multiple melanoma
MMEF	Maximal midexpiratory flow
MMPI	Minnesota Multiphasic Personality Inventory
MMR	Morbidity and Mortality Report
MNP	Mononuclear phagocyte
MO	Medical officer
MOD	March of Dimes
MODM	Mature-onset diabetes mellitus
MOF	Multiple organ failure
MOSF	Multiple organ system failure
MPAP	Mean pulmonary artery pressure
MPD	Maximum permissible dose
MPI	Minnesota Preschool Inventory
MPS	Mucopolysaccharidosis
MR	May repeat; measles, rubella; mitral regurgitation; magnetic resonance
MRD	Minimum reacting dose
MRI	Magnetic resonance imaging
MRSA	Methicillin-resistant *Staphylococcus aureus*
MS	Mitral stenosis; multiple sclerosis; mitral sounds; musculoskeletal
MS-1	Hepatitis A
MS-2	Hepatitis B
MSAF	Meconium-stained amniotic fluid
MSAFP	Maternal serum alpha fetoprotein
MSCA	McCarthy Scales of Children's Abilities
MSL	Midsternal line
MSP	Munchausen syndrome by proxy
MST	McCarthy Screening Tests
MTT	Mean transit time
MVA	Motor vehicle accident
MVC	Motor vehicle crash
MVP	Moisture vapor permeable (dressing)
MVV	Maximum voluntary ventilation
MZ	Monozygotic
N	Normal
n	Number
NA	Nutritional assessment; not applicable
NAD	No abnormalities noted; no appreciable disease
NAI	Nonaccidental injury
NANB	Non-A, non-B (hepatitis)
NAPNAP	National Association of Pediatric Nurse Associates and Practitioners
NASN	National Association of School Nurses
NB	Newborn
NBAS	Newborn Behavioral Assessment Scale
NBN	Newborn nursery
NCDB	National Center for Drugs and Biologics
NCDC	National Center for Disease Control
NCHS	National Center for Health Statistics
NCVS	Nerve conduction velocity studies
ND	Not done
NEC	Necrotizing enterocolitis

Abbreviation	Term
NFT	Nonorganic failure to thrive
NG	Nasogastric
NGU	Nongonorrheal urethritis
NH	Neonatal hepatitis
NHL	Non-Hodgkin's lymphoma
NICU	Neonatal intensive care unit
NIH	National Institutes of Health
NIMH	National Institute of Mental Health
NKA	No known allergies
NKDA	No known drug allergies
nl	Normal (value)
NLN	National League for Nursing
NLTR	Non-life-threatening reaction
NM	Neonatal mortality
NMR	Nuclear magnetic resonance; neonatal mortality rates
NND	New and nonofficial drugs
NNS	Nonnutritive sucking
NO	Nitric oxide
NOFT	Nonorganic failure to thrive
NOP	Not otherwise provided for
NOS	Not otherwise specified
NP	Nasopharynx; new patient; not palpable; nerve palsy; Nurse Practitioner
NPN	Nonprotein nitrogen
NR	Normal range; nonreactive; no report; no respirations; not remarkable; no resuscitation; not refillable; normal reaction
NREM	Nonrapid eye movement
NS	Normal saline; not significant
NSAID	Nonsteroidal antiinflammatory drug
NSFTD	Normal spontaneous full-term delivery
NSR	Normal sinus rhythm
NSU	Nonspecific urethritis
NT	Nasotracheal
NTB	Necrotizing tracheobronchitis
NTD	Neural tube defect
NTM	Nontuberculous mycobacterium
NTP	Normal temperature and pressure
NUG	Necrotizing ulcerative gingivitis
NVSS	Normal variant short stature
NWB	Non–weight-bearing
NYD	Not yet diagnosed
OASDL	Ordinary activities and skills of daily living
OBS	Organic brain syndrome
OC	Oral contraceptive; oculocephalic (doll's eye reflex)
OCD	Over-the-counter drug; obsessive-compulsive disorder
OCP	Ova, cysts, and parasites
OD	*Oculus dexter* (right eye); once daily; overdose; outside diameter; optical density
OFC	Occipitofrontal circumference
OG	Orogastric
OHS	Orally administered hydration solution(s)

Abbreviation	Term
OI	Opportunistic infection; osteogenesis imperfecta
OJ	Orange juice
OM	Otitis media; opportunistic mycoses
OME	Otitis media with effusion
OOB	Out of bed
O&P	Ova and parasites
OPC	Outpatient clinic
OPD	Outpatient department
OR	Operating room
ORIF	Open reduction internal fixation
OS	*Oculus sinister* (left eye)
OSA	Obstructive sleep apnea
OSB	Open spina bifida
OT	Occupational therapy; orotracheal; old tuberculin; old term
OTC	Over the counter
OU	*Oculi unitas* (both eyes)
OV	Oculovestibular (cold water caloric test)
P	Probability
PA	Posteroanterior; pernicious anemia; primary amenorrhea; pulmonary artery; prolonged action; Physician's Assistant
PAC	Premature atrial contraction
$Paco_2$	Carbon dioxide pressure (tension), arterial
PACU	Postanesthesia care unit
PAIDS	Pediatric AIDS
PALS	Pediatric advanced life support
PANESS	Physical and neurologic examination for soft signs
Pao_2	Oxygen pressure (tension), arterial
PAP	Primary atypical pneumonia; Papanicolaou smear; passive-aggressive personality; pulmonary artery pressure
PAPVR	Partial anomalous pulmonary venous return
PAR	Postanesthesia room
PAT	Paroxysmal atrial tachycardia
PAWP	Pulmonary artery wedge pressure
PB	Peripheral blood
PBA	Percutaneous bladder aspiration
PBB	Polybrominated biphenyls
PBGT	Personal blood glucose testing
PBI	Protein-bound iodine
PBS	Phosphate-buffered saline
pc	*Post cibos* (after meals)
PC	Purulent conjunctivitis; present complaint
PCA	Patient-controlled analgesia
PCB	Polychlorinated biphenyls
PCC	Poison Control Center
PCM	Protein-calorie malnutrition
Pco_2	Partial pressure (tension), carbon dioxide
PCP	Patient care plan, *Pneumocystis carinii* pneumonia; primary care practitioner; primary care physician

Abbreviation	Term
PCR	Polymerase chain reaction
PCT	Prothrombin consumption test
PCV	Packed cell volume
PCWP	Pulmonary capillary wedge pressure
PD	Pupillary distance
PDA	Patent ductus arteriosus
PDC	Private diagnostic clinic
PDI	Preschool Development Inventory
PDNB	Penile dorsal nerve block
PDQ	Prescreening Developmental Questionnaire
PDR	*Physicians' Desk Reference*
PE	Physical examination; pressure equalizing; probable error; pulmonary embolism; port of entry; point of entry; physical education; pelvic examination
PEEP	Positive end-expiratory pressure
PEEX	Pediatric Early Elementary Examination
PEFR	Peak expiratory flow rate
PEG	Percutaneous endoscopic gastrostomy; pneumoencephalogram
PEN	Parenteral-enteral nutrition
PERL	Pupils equal and react to light
per os	By mouth
PERRLA	Pupils equal, round, react to light and accommodation
PET	Positron emission tomography
PETT	Positron emission transaxial tomography
PF	Pulmonary flow
PFC	Persistent fetal circulation
PFNB	Percutaneous fine needle biopsy
PFT	Pulmonary function test
PG	Prostaglandin; phosphatidylglycerol
pH	Power of hydrogen
PH	Past history; previous history; public health
PHA	Phytohemagglutinin
PHN	Public Health Nurse
PHV	Peak height velocity
PI	Pulmonary insufficiency; present illness
PICC	Percutaneously inserted central catheter
PICU	Pediatric intensive care unit
PID	Pelvic inflammatory disease
PIE	Pulmonary interstitial emphysema
PIH	Pregnancy-induced hypertension
PIP	Peak inspiratory pressure; proximal interphalangeal
PIPP	Peak inspiratory plateau pressure
PKD	Polycystic kidney disease
PKU	Phenylketonuria
PLH	Pulmonary lymphoid hyperplasia
PM	Postmortem
PMC	Pseudomembranous colitis
PMD	Private medical doctor; past (previous) medical doctor
PMH	Past medical history

Abbreviation	Term
PMI	Point of maximum impulse (intensity)
PMN	Polymorphonuclear neutrophil
PMR	Psychomotor retardation; perinatal mortality rate; physical medicine and rehabilitation
PNA	Pediatric Nurse Associate
PND	Paroxysmal nocturnal dyspnea; postnasal drip
PNM	Postnatal mortality
PNP	Pediatric Nurse Practitioner
PNPR	Positive-negative pressure respiration
PO	*Per os* (by mouth); postoperative; phone order; in left eye
Po_2	Partial pressure (tension), oxygen
POA	Primary optic atrophy
POD	Postoperative day
POMR	Problem-oriented medical record
POR	Problem-oriented record
PP	Partial pressure; patient profile; peripheral pulses; postpartum; postprandial; presenting problem
PPC	Progressive patient care
PPD	Purified protein derivative
PPHN	Persistent pulmonary hypertension of the newborn
PPLO	Pleuropneumonia-like organism
PPPA	Poison Prevention Packaging Act
PPS	Peripheral pulmonic stenosis
PPT	Partial prothrombin time
PPV	Positive pressure ventilation
PR	Perfusion rate; peripheral resistance; progress report; pulse rate; public relations
PRA	Plasma renin activity
PRBC	Packed red blood cells
PRESS	Preschool Readiness Experimental Screening Scale
PRN, prn	*Pro re nata* (as necessary); as circumstance may require
PROM	Passive range of motion; premature rupture of membranes
PRP	Persistent recurrent pneumonia
PRP-D	Polysaccharide of *Haemophilus influenzae* type b conjugated to diphtheria toxoid
PS	Pulmonic stenosis; pyloric stenosis
P/SH	Personal social history
PSMA	Progressive spinal muscular atrophy
PSP	Phenolsulfonphthalein test
PSR	Psychological Stimulus Response
PSRO	Professional Standards Review Organization
PSSD	Psychosocial dwarfism
PT	Physical therapy (therapist); prothrombin time

Abbreviation	Term
PTA	Prior to admission; plasma thromboplastin antecedent; percutaneous transluminal angioplasty
PTC	Plasma thromboplastin component; phenylthiocarbamide
PTH	Parathyroid hormone; pseudohyperparathyroidism
PTT	Partial thromboplastin time
PUD	Peptic ulcer disease
PUO	Pyrexia of undetermined (unknown) origin
PV	Parainfluenza virus
PVC	Premature ventricular contraction; polyvinyl chloride
PVD	Percussion, vibration, and drainage
PVH	Periventricular hemorrhage
PVP	Pulmonary venous pressure
PVR	Peripheral vascular resistance; pulmonary vascular resistance
PVS	Percussion, vibration, and suction
PWB	Partial weight-bearing
PWM	Pokeweed mitogen
PWP	Pulmonary wedge pressure
PWS	Port-wine stain; Prader-Willi syndrome
Px	Pneumothorax; prognosis
q	*Quaque* (every)
Qd*	*Quaque die* (every day)
qh	*Quaque hora* (every hour)
q2h	Every 2 hours
qid	*Quater in die* (four times a day)
qn	*Quaque nocte* (every night)
qns	Quantity not sufficient
Qod*	Every other day
QPIT	Quantitative pilocarpine iontophoresis test
qs	Quantity sufficient
RA	Rheumatoid arthritis; return appointment; renal artery; right arm; right atrium; rectal atresia; repeat action; room air
RAE	Right atrial enlargement
RAST	Radioallergosorbent test
RATG	Rabbit antithymocytic globulin
RBC	Red blood cell
RBD	Right border dullness
RBE	Relative biologic effectiveness
RBF	Renal blood flow
RBS	Random blood sugar
RC	Rice cereal; red cell
RCC	Red cell concentrate
RCM	Right costal margin
RD	Retinal detachment; respiratory disease; right deltoid; registered dietitian; respiratory distress

*See The Joint Commission Official "Do Not Use" list.

Abbreviation	Term
RDA	Recommended dietary allowance
RDS	Respiratory distress syndrome
RDSI	Revised Developmental Screening Inventory
RE	Regional enteritis; rear end (accident); right eye; rectal examination
REE	Resting energy expenditure
REM	Rapid eye movement
RF	Rheumatic fever; rheumatoid factor
RG	Right gluteal
RHD	Rheumatic heart disease; relative hepatic dullness
RIA	Radioimmunoassay; radioactive immunoassay
RICE	Rest, ice, compression, elevation
RICM	Right intercostal margin
RLE	Right lower extremity
RLQ	Right lower quadrant
RLT	Right lateral thigh
RMA	Rhythmic motor activities
RML	Right mediolateral; right middle lobe
RMR	Resting metabolic rate
RMSF	Rocky Mountain spotted fever
RN	Registered Nurse
RN, C	Registered Nurse, Certified
RN, CS	Registered Nurse, Certified Specialist
RO	Rule out; routine order
ROM	Range of motion; right otitis media
ROP	Retinopathy of prematurity
ROS	Review of systems
R-PDQ	Revised Prescreening Developmental Questionnaire
RPF	Renal plasma flow
RPR	Rapid plasma reagin
RR	Respiratory rate; recovery room; radiation response; rust ring
RS	Review of symptoms; Reye syndrome; Reiter syndrome
RSB	Right sternal border
RSV	Respiratory syncytial virus
RT	Respiratory therapy (therapist); room temperature
RTA	Renal tubular acidosis
RTI	Respiratory tract infection
RTUS	Real-time ultrasound
RUE	Right upper extremity
RUL	Right upper lobe
RUOQ	Right upper outer quadrant
RUQ	Right upper quadrant
RV	Residual volume; right ventricle
RVG	Right ventrogluteal
RVH	Right ventricular hypertrophy
RVV	Rubella vaccine virus
Rx	Prescription; *recipe* (take)
$\bar{s}$	*Sine* (without)

Abbreviation	Term
SAC	Short arm cast
SAD	Sugar and acetone determination
SAH	Subarachnoid hemorrhage
SAM	Surface active material; Society for Adolescent Medicine
Sao_2	Saturated arterial oxygen
sb	Strabismus
SBE	Subacute bacterial endocarditis
SC	Subcutaneous; servo control
SCB	Strictly confined to bed
SCD	Sudden cardiac death; sickle cell disease
SCFE	Slipped capital femoral epiphysis
SCID	Severe combined immune deficiency disease
SCM	Sternocleidomastoid muscle
SCU	Special care unit
SCV	Smooth, capsulated, virulent
SD	Standard deviation; septal defect; spontaneous delivery; sudden death; shoulder disarticulation
SEA	Seronegative enthesopathy and arthropathy (syndrome)
SES	Socioeconomic status
SFD	Small for dates
SG	Specific gravity; Swan-Ganz
SGA	Small for gestational age
SGOT	Serum glutamic-oxaloacetic transaminase
SGPT	Serum glutamic-pyruvic transaminase
SH	Social history; self help; serum hepatitis; shoulder
SI	*Système International d'Unités*
SIADH	Syndrome of inappropriate ADH
SIDS	Sudden infant death syndrome
SIG	Serum immune globulin
SIMV	Synchronized intermittent mandatory ventilation
SKL	Serum killing levels
SKSD	Streptokinase/streptodornase (control test)
SLC	Short leg cast
SLD	Specific learning disability
SLE	Systemic lupus erythematosus; St Louis encephalitis
SLUD	Salivation, lacrimation, urination, defecation
SLWC	Short leg walking cast
SMA	Smooth muscle antibodies; sequential multiple analyzer
SMBG	Self-monitoring blood glucose
SM-C	Somatomedin-C
SNF	Skilled nursing facility
SNP	School Nurse Practitioner
SNS	Sympathetic nervous system
SOB	Short of breath; see order book
SOM	Serous otitis media
S/P	Status post

Abbreviation	Term
SPA	Suprapubic aspiration; salt-poor albumin
SPF	Sun protection factor
SPL	Sound pressure levels
SPT	Sweat patch test
SQ	Subcutaneous
SR	System review; sinus rhythm; sedimentation rate; stretch reflex; schizophrenic reaction; stimulus response
S-R	Stimulus-response
SRI	Systemic reaction index
SRSA	Slow-reacting substance of anaphylaxis
ss	*Semis* (one half)
S/S	Signs and symptoms
SSE	Soapsuds enema; soap solution enema
SSEP	Somatosensory evoked potential
SSI	Segmental spinal instrumentation
SSSS	Staphylococcal scalded skin syndrome
stat	*Statim* (immediately)
STC	Serum theophylline concentration
STD	Sexually transmitted disease; skin test dose; standard test dose
STS	Serologic test for syphilis
STSG	Split-thickness skin graft
STU	Skin test unit
SubQ	Subcutaneous
supp	Suppository
susp	Suspension
SV	Stroke volume
SVC	Superior vena cava
SVD	Spontaneous vaginal delivery
SVR	Systemic vascular resistance
SVT	Sinus ventricular tachycardia; supraventricular tachycardia
Sx	Symptoms
SxH	Sexual history
T_3	Triiodothyronine
T_4	Thyroxine
TA	Toxin-antitoxin; tricuspid atresia; truncus arteriosus
T&A	Tonsillectomy and adenoidectomy
tab	Tablet
TAPVR	Total anomalous pulmonary venous return
TB	Tuberculosis
TBG	Thyroxine-binding globulin
TBI	Traumatic brain injury; total body irradiation
TBLC	Term birth, living child
TBM	Total body mass
Tbn	Tuberculin
TBSA	Total body surface area
TBT	Tracheobronchial tree
TBW	Total body water
TcB	Transcutaneous bilirubinometer
TCDB	Turn, cough, deep breathe

Abbreviation	Term
$tcPaco_2$	Transcutaneous carbon dioxide pressure (tension)
$tcPao_2$	Transcutaneous oxygen pressure (tension)
TCU	Transitional care unit
Td	Adult tetanus and diphtheria
TD	Typhoid dysentery
Tdap	Tetanus toxoid, diphtheria (reduced), acellular pertussis (adolescent formulation)
TDM	Therapeutic drug monitoring
TE	Expiratory time
TEF	Tracheoesophageal fistula
TEN	Toxic epidermal necrolysis
TENS	Transcutaneous electrical nerve stimulation
TEV	Talipes equinovarus
TEWL	Transevaporative water loss
Tg	Thyroglobulin
TG	Triglyceride(s)
TGA	Transposition of great arteries
TGE	Theoretic growth evaluation
TGV	Transposition of great vessels
TI	Tricuspid insufficiency
TIA	Transient ischemic attack
tid	*Ter in die* (three times a day)
TIPP	The Injury Prevention Program
TKO	To keep open
TLC	Tender loving care; total lung capacity; total lymphocyte count; thin layer chromatography
TM	Tympanic membrane; temperature by mouth; tender midline; transmetatarsal; temporomandibular
TMR	Trainable mentally retarded
TNA	Total nutrient admixture
TNI	Total nodal irradiation
TNR	Tonic neck reflex
TO	Target organ; telephone order
TOF	Tetralogy of Fallot
TORCH	Toxoplasmosis, (other), rubella, cytomegalovirus, herpes simplex
TORCHES	Toxoplasmosis, rubella, cytomegalovirus, herpes simplex, syphilis
Torr	Millimeters of mercury
TPN	Total parenteral nutrition
TPR	Temperature, pulse, respiration; total perfusion resistance
TRH	Thyrotropin-releasing hormone
TS	Terminal sensation; test solution; tricuspid stenosis; Tourette syndrome
TSF	Triceps skinfold
TSB	Total serum bilirubin
TSE	Testicular self-examination
TSH	Thyroid stimulating hormone
TSS	Toxic shock syndrome
TST	Tuberculin skin test
TT	Transit time; tuberculin tested

Abbreviation	Term
TU	Tuberculin units; toxic unit; transmission unit
TV	Total volume; tidal volume
Tx	Treatment; therapy
UA	Urinalysis
UAC	Umbilical artery catheters
UCHD	Usual childhood diseases
UD	Urethral discharge
UDT	Undescended testicle
UGI	Upper gastrointestinal
U/L	Upper/lower body ratio
ULC	Unique-looking child
UMN	Upper motor neuron
UNO	United Network for Organ Sharing
UP	Universal Precautions
UPC	Unplanned pregnancy counseling
UQ	Upper quadrant
UrA	Uric acid
URI	Upper respiratory infection
US	Ultrasound
USA	Ultrasonic aerosol (nebulization)
USPHS	United States Public Health Service
UTI	Urinary tract infection
UV	Ultraviolet
UVA	Ultraviolet A
UVB	Ultraviolet B
VA	Visual acuity
VAD	Venous access devices
VAR	Visual-aural range
VC	Vital capacity
VCA	Viral capsid antigen
VCG	Vectorcardiography
VCT	Venous clotting time
VCUG	Voiding cystourethrogram
VD	Venereal disease
VDG	Venereal disease, gonorrhea
VDRL	Venereal Disease Research Laboratory
VDRR	Vitamin D–resistant rickets
VDS	Venereal disease, syphilis
VDT	Video display terminal

Abbreviation	Term
VE	Vesicular exanthema
VEP	Visual evoked potential
VF	Visual fields
VG	Ventricular gallop
VIG	Vaccinia immune globulin
VLBW	Very low birth weight
VLDL	Very low-density lipoprotein
VM	Vasomotor; vestibular membrane
VNA	Visiting Nurses Association
VO	Verbal order
VP	Venous pressure
VPC	Ventricular premature complex
VRA	Visual reinforced audiometry
VS	Vital signs
VSD	Ventricular septal defect
VSGA	Very small for gestational age
VSS	Vital signs stable
V_T	Tidal volume
VUR	Vesicoureteral reflux
VZIG	Varicella zoster immune globulin
VZV	Varicella zoster virus
WAIS	Wechsler Adult Intelligence Scale
WB	Whole blood
WBC	White blood cell count
WEE	Western equine encephalitis
WHM	Women's health movement
WHO	World Health Organization
WIPI	Word intelligibility by picture identification
WISC-R	Wechsler Intelligence Scale for Children—Revised
WNL	Within normal limits
WPPSI	Wechsler Preschool and Primary Scale of Intelligence
WPW	Wolff-Parkinson-White syndrome
WRAT	Wide Range Achievement Test
XLMR	X-linked mental retardation
XLR	X-linked recessive
XTB	X-ray treated blood
ZIG	Zoster immune globulin
ZIP	Zoster immune plasma

Index

Page numbers followed by *f* indicate figures; those followed by *t* indicate tables; those followed by *b* indicate boxed material.

D

E

F

Conversion of Pounds to Kilograms for Pediatric Weights

Pounds	KILOGRAMS 0	1	2	3	4	5	6	7	8	9
0	0.00	0.45	0.90	1.36	1.81	2.26	2.72	3.17	3.62	4.08
10	4.53	4.98	5.44	5.89	6.35	6.80	7.35	7.71	8.16	8.61
20	9.07	9.52	9.97	10.43	10.88	11.34	11.79	12.24	12.70	13.15
30	13.60	14.06	14.51	14.96	15.42	15.87	16.32	16.78	17.23	17.69
40	18.14	18.59	19.05	19.50	19.95	20.41	20.86	21.31	21.77	22.22
50	22.68	23.13	23.58	24.04	24.49	24.94	25.40	25.85	26.30	26.76
60	27.21	27.66	28.22	28.57	29.03	29.48	29.93	30.39	30.84	31.29
70	31.75	32.20	32.65	33.11	33.56	34.02	34.47	34.92	35.38	35.83
80	36.28	36.74	37.19	37.64	38.10	38.55	39.00	39.46	39.93	40.37
90	40.82	41.27	41.73	42.18	42.63	43.09	43.54	43.99	44.45	44.90
100	45.36	45.81	46.26	46.72	47.17	47.62	48.08	48.53	48.98	49.44
110	49.89	50.34	50.80	51.25	51.71	52.16	52.61	53.07	53.52	53.97
120	54.43	54.88	55.33	55.79	56.24	56.70	57.15	57.60	58.06	58.51
130	58.96	59.42	59.87	60.32	60.78	61.23	61.68	62.14	62.59	63.05
140	63.50	63.95	64.41	64.86	65.31	65.77	66.22	66.67	67.13	67.58
150	68.04	68.49	68.94	69.40	69.85	70.30	70.76	71.21	71.66	72.12
160	72.57	73.02	73.48	73.93	74.39	74.84	75.29	75.75	76.20	76.65
170	77.11	77.56	78.01	78.47	78.92	79.38	79.83	80.28	80.74	81.19
180	81.64	82.10	81.55	83.00	83.46	83.91	84.36	84.82	85.27	85.73
190	86.18	86.68	87.09	87.54	87.99	88.45	88.90	89.35	89.81	90.26
200	90.72	91.17	91.62	92.08	92.53	92.98	93.44	93.89	94.34	94.80

Conversion of Pounds and Ounces to Kilograms for Pediatric Weights

Pounds	Kilograms	Ounces	Kilograms
1	0.454	1	0.028
2	0.907	2	0.057
3	1.361	3	0.085
4	1.814	4	0.113
5	2.268	5	0.142
6	2.722	6	0.170
7	3.175	7	0.198
8	3.629	8	0.227
9	4.082	9	0.255
10	4.536	10	0.283
11	4.990	11	0.312
12	5.443	12	0.340
13	5.897	13	0.369
		14	0.397
		15	0.425

Powers of Ten

Prefix	Power	Decimal	Name
tera	10^{12}	1,000,000,000,000	trillion
giga	10^{9}	1,000,000,000	billion
mega	10^{6}	1,000,000	million
kilo	10^{3}	1000	thousand
milli	10^{-3}	0.001	one-thousandth
micro	10^{-6}	0.000001	one-millionth
nano	10^{-9}	0.000000001	one-billionth
pico	10^{-12}	0.000000000001	one-trillionth
femto	10^{-15}	0.000000000000001	one-quadrillionth